D1736540

Principles and Practice of
PEDIATRIC SLEEP MEDICINE

Stephen H. Sheldon, DO, FAAP
Associate Professor of Pediatrics
Northwestern University
Feinberg School of Medicine
Director, Sleep Medicine Center
Children's Memorial Hospital
Chicago, Illinois

Richard Ferber, MD
Associate Professor of Neurology
Harvard Medical School
Director, Center for Pediatric Sleep Disorders
Children's Hospital Boston
Boston, Massachusetts

Meir H. Kryger, MD, FRCPC
Professor of Medicine
University of Manitoba Faculty of Medicine
Director, Sleep Disorders Center
St. Boniface General Hospital
Winnipeg, Manitoba, Canada

EVIER
SAUNDERS

ELSEVIER
SAUNDERS

PRINCIPLES AND PRACTICE OF PEDIATRIC SLEEP MEDICINE   ISBN 0–7216–9458–6
Copyright © 2005 by Elsevier Inc.

Notice

Medicine is an ever-changing field. Standard safety precautions must be followed, but as new research and clinical experience broaden our knowledge, changes in treatment and drug therapy may become necessary or appropriate. Readers are advised to check the most current product information provided by the manufacturer of each drug to be administered to verify the recommended dose, the method and duration of administration, and contraindications. It is the responsibility of the treating physician, relying on experience and knowledge of the patient, to determine dosages and the best treatment for each individual patient. Neither the Publisher nor the editor assumes any liability for any injury and/or damage to persons or property arising from this publication.

The Publisher

Library of Congress Cataloging-in-Publication Data

Principles and practice of pediatric sleep medicine/Stephen H. Sheldon . . . [et al.].– 1st ed.
   p. cm.
  Includes bibliographical references.
  ISBN 0-7216-9458-6
   1. Sleep disorders in children. 2. Children–Sleep. I. Sheldon, Stephen H.

RJ506.S55P746 2005
618.92'8498–dc22   2004066249

Acquisitions Editor: Dolores Meloni
Project Manager: Joan Nikelsky
Design Coordinator: Ellen Zanolle

Printed in the United States of America.

Last digit is the print number: 9 8 7 6 5 4 3 2 1

We dedicate this book, first to our families and, second, to all of the children and their families who have had the courage to work with us and help us achieve a better understanding of how to recognize and treat sleep problems in the child.

Contributors

Roberto L. Barretto, MD
Clinical Assistant Professor, Department of Otolaryngology—Head and Neck Surgery, University of California, Irvine, School of Medicine, Irvine; Attending Pediatric Otolaryngologist, Children's Hospital of Orange County, Orange, California
Otolaryngologic Management of Sleep-Related Breathing Disorders

Lee J. Brooks, MD
Clinical Associate Professor of Pediatrics, University of Pennsylvania School of Medicine; Attending Physician, Pulmonary Division, The Children's Hospital of Philadelphia, Philadelphia, Pennsylvania
Obstructive Sleep Apnea Syndrome in Infants and Children: Clinical Features and Pathophysiology; Enuresis in Children with Sleep Apnea

Ronald D. Chervin, MD, MS
Associate Professor of Neurology, University of Michigan Medical School; Director, Sleep Disorders Center/Michael S. Aldrich Sleep Disorders Laboratory, Department of Neurology, University Hospital, Ann Arbor, Michigan
Attention Deficit, Hyperactivity, and Sleep Disorders

Richard Ferber, MD
Associate Professor of Neurology, Harvard Medical School; Director, Center for Pediatric Sleep Disorders, Children's Hospital Boston, Boston, Massachusetts

Mark E. Gerber, MD, FACS, FAAP
Assistant Professor, Department of Otolaryngology—Head and Neck Surgery, Northwestern University Feinberg School of Medicine, Chicago; Attending, Children's Memorial Hospital, Chicago, and Evanston Northwestern Healthcare (Evanston, Glenbrook, and Highland Park Hospitals), Evanston, Illinois
Otolaryngologic Management of Sleep-Related Breathing Disorders

Daniel G. Glaze, MD
Associate Professor of Pediatrics and Neurology, Baylor College of Medicine; Medical Director, The Texas Children's Hospital, the Children's Sleep

Center; Medical Director, The Methodist Hospital Sleep Disorders Center, Houston, Texas
Sleep in Neurologic Disorders

David Gozal, MD
Children's Foundation Chair of Pediatric Research and Professor of Pediatrics, Pharmacology and Toxicology, and Psychology and Brain Science, University of Louisville School of Medicine; Director, Comprehensive Sleep Medicine and Apnea Center, Kosair Children's Hospital; Vice Chairman for Research and Director, Kosair Children's Hospital Research Institute, Louisville, Kentucky
Consequences of Obstructive Sleep Apnea Syndrome

John H. Herman, PhD, FCCP, Dipl ABSM
Professor of Psychiatry and Director, Sleep Medicine Fellowship Program, UT Southwestern Medical Center School of Medicine; Director, Sleep Disorders Center for Children, Children's Medical Center of Dallas, Dallas, Texas
Chronobiology of Sleep in Children; Circadian Rhythm Disorders: Diagnosis and Treatment; Pharmacology of Sleep Disorders in Children

Eliot S. Katz, MD
Instructor, Harvard Medical School; Attending, Division of Respiratory Diseases, Children's Hospital Boston, Boston, Massachusetts
Diagnosis of Obstructive Sleep Apnea Syndrome in Infants and Children

Michael Kohrman, MD
Associate Professor of Pediatrics and Neurology, University of Chicago Pritzker School of Medicine; Director, Pediatric Clinical Neurophysiology, University of Chicago Children's Hospital, Chicago, Illinois
Idiopathic Hypersomnia

Suresh Kotagal, MD
Professor and Chair, Division of Child and Adolescent Neurology, Department of Neurology, Mayo Medical School; Consultant, Sleep Disorders Center, Mayo Clinic, Rochester, Minnesota
Narcolepsy in Childhood

Meir H. Kryger, MD, FRCPC

Professor of Medicine, University of Manitoba Faculty of Medicine; Director, Sleep Disorders Centre, St. Boniface Hospital Research Center, St. Boniface General Hospital, Winnipeg, Manitoba, Canada

Differential Diagnosis of Pediatric Sleep Disorders

Mark W. Mahowald, MD

Professor of Neurology, University of Minnesota School of Medicine; Director, Minnesota Regional Sleep Disorders Center, Department of Neurology, Hennepin County Medical Center, Minneapolis, Minnesota

Disorders of Arousal in Children

Carole L. Marcus, MBBCh

Professor of Pediatrics, University of Pennsylvania School of Medicine; Director, Pediatric Sleep Center, The Children's Hospital of Philadelphia, Philadelphia, Pennsylvania

Diagnosis of Obstructive Sleep Apnea Syndrome in Infants and Children; Treatment of Obstructive Sleep Apnea Syndrome in Children

Susanna A. McColley, MD

Associate Professor of Pediatrics, Department of Pediatrics, Northwestern University Feinberg School of Medicine; Division Head, Pulmonary Medicine, Children's Memorial Hospital, Chicago, Illinois

Primary Snoring in Children

Louise Margaret O'Brien, PhD

Research Fellow, Department of Pediatrics, University of Louisville School of Medicine, Louisville, Kentucky

Consequences of Obstructive Sleep Apnea Syndrome

Judith Owens, MD, MPH

Associate Professor of Pediatrics, Division of Ambulatory Pediatrics, Brown Medical School; Director, Pediatric Sleep Disorders Clinic, Hasbro Children's Hospital, Providence, Rhode Island

Epidemiology of Sleep Disorders during Childhood

Gerald M. Rosen, MD, MPH

Associate Professor, Department of Pediatrics, University of Minnesota School of Medicine; Medical Director, Pediatric Sleep Center, Children's Hospitals and Clinics, St. Paul, Minnesota; Pediatric Sleep Specialist, Minnesota Regional Sleep Disorders Center, Hennepin County Medical Center, Minneapolis, Minnesota

Case-Based Analysis of Sleep Problems in Children; Disorders of Arousal in Children

Stephen H. Sheldon, DO, FAAP

Associate Professor of Pediatrics, Northwestern University, Feinberg School of Medicine; Director, Sleep Medicine Center, Children's Memorial Hospital, Chicago, Illinois

Introduction to Pediatric Sleep Medicine; Anatomy of Sleep; Polysomnography in Infants and Children; Physiologic Variations during Sleep in Children; Disorders of Initiating and Maintaining Sleep; Post-Traumatic Hypersomnia; Kleine-Levin Syndrome and Recurrent Hypersomnias; Sleep in Neurologic Disorders; The Parasomnias; Sleep-Related Enuresis; Pharmacology of Sleep Disorders in Children

Julie L. Wei, MD

Assistant Professor, Department of Otolaryngology—Head and Neck Surgery, University of Kansas School of Medicine, Kansas City, Kansas; Attending Physician, Pediatric Otolaryngology, Children's Mercy Hospital, Kansas City, Missouri

Otolaryngologic Management of Sleep-Related Breathing Disorders

Marc Weissbluth, MD

Professor of Clinical Pediatrics, Northwestern University Feinberg School of Medicine; Active Attending, Children's Memorial Hospital, Chicago, Illinois

Sleep and Colic

Preface

Sleep medicine is a unique medical discipline, the one area of specialization that focuses on patients' health and disease during the hours of sleep. Pediatric sleep medicine holds special significance in that it is concerned with about half of the child's life during the important early years of development. Because sleep constitutes such a large proportion of the child's day, and because the development of the neurologic structures responsible for sleep, in patterns of increasing complexity and predictability, occurs so rapidly during the early months and years of life, the maturation of these systems is clearly among the most important of neurodevelopmental milestones to be met. Early disruption of these vital processes has major cognitive and possibly emotional consequences that are only recently becoming clear. Studies have repeatedly confirmed the importance of sleep for the acquisition of new knowledge and for processing and maintaining information previously gained. Knowledge of primary and secondary sleep-related disorders also has been shown to be essential to the understanding of many other childhood disorders and in the development of proper treatment.

Principles and Practice of Sleep Medicine in the Child, first published as a separate volume from *Principles and Practice of Sleep Medicine* (2nd edition) in 1995, helped move the practice of pediatric sleep medicine from the sphere of adult medicine to one that is overseen by professionals who have dedicated their careers to the health and well-being of the pediatric patient. As stated in the Preface to that volume, "In recent years, a robust scientifically based body of knowledge has emerged, and the tools to diagnose and effectively treat children with sleep disorders are now available." *Principles and Practice of Pediatric Sleep Medicine* represents another step in the development of pediatric sleep medicine as a distinct discipline.

Diagnosis and management of sleep disorders in children may hold unique significance in at least three very important ways:

1. Primary sleep-related pathology may directly cause daytime symptoms, and only through treatment of the sleep disorder is resolution possible.
2. Sleep-related pathology may be a co-morbid condition contributing to daytime symptomatology, and through treatment of the sleep-related pathology, the patient becomes more responsive to treatment of the co-existing disorders.
3. A child's sleep difficulties may have greater impact on other family members than on the affected child, causing a caretaker, for example, to be sleep deprived, with medical and emotional compromises (including impaired ability to care for the child). Treating these problems can improve the lives of child and family members alike.

As we continue to gain better understanding of the effect of sleep disorders on children, major advances will be made, with great significance for all three of these scenarios, including insight into the often unclear area of cause and effect—namely, whether disordered sleep is a cause or a result of a specific disease or disorder.

Sleep disorders in infants and children reflect an interplay among many factors, including central nervous system function, parental-child interaction, social stress, patient needs, and other medical conditions. Comprehensive knowledge of these interactions is essential for all child-care professionals who want to deliver optimal management. This book provides resources for sleep medicine specialists as well as primary care practitioners to use to deliver the best possible care to their pediatric patients throughout the 24-hour day.

Stephen H. Sheldon, Chicago

Richard Ferber, Boston

Meir Kryger, Winnipeg

Acknowledgments

The editors wish to thank the entire editorial staff at Saunders/Elsevier for their outstanding efforts in the creation of this book. Specifically, we wish to single out Joan Nikelsky and Delores Meloni for their patience and persistence, without which this project could have never been completed.

We also would like to thank all of the courageous health care professionals who care for children during sleep—for their dedication and foresight to understand the importance of sleep in health and disease in the pediatric patient. Beginning with the scientific foundation laid by pioneers Nathaniel Kleitman, Arthur Parmelee, Jr., and Heinz F.R. Prechtl, many other child health care practitioners have begun to follow in their footsteps, delving into the life of children at night. These researchers and practitioners of pediatric sleep medicine truly are leading the way.

Contents

Introduction to Pediatric Sleep Medicine

Stephen H. Sheldon

FUNCTION OF SLEEP

Although sleep has been studied subjectively and objectively for more than 100 years, the exact function of sleep and its components remains elusive. Historically, physicians have recommended sleep for the treatment of many disorders. This prescription has been based on the assumption that sleep provides a unique restorative purpose. Although the relationship between the immune system and sleep may be important with many clinical implications, no study has documented that sleep cures anything.[1] Circadian rhythms of various biologic processes, for example the immune system, appear to be modulated by sleep, and lymphocyte functions are dramatically altered at sleep onset and during sleep.[2] Specific pokeweed mitogen response and natural killer cell activity are altered by sleep in healthy young men. Interleukin-1–like activities are followed by interleukin 2–like activities during sleep, and interleukins-1 and -2 are disrupted by sleep deprivation.[3] Insomnia has been shown to be associated with nocturnal sympathetic arousal and declines in natural immunity, including a decrease in natural killer cell response.[3a] Narcoleptic patients present disordered diurnal patterns of immune function;[4] however, the clinical effects that these changes produce or how they may be therapeutically modified are unknown.

Theories of sleep function fall into several major categories, with many overlaps. An understanding of these hypotheses provides a basis for comprehension of the varied effects that disordered sleep may have on health and disease.

Restoration Theory

In 1946 Sherington suggested that sleep was a state required for enhanced tissue growth and repair.[5] This hypothesis proposes that certain somatic and/or cerebral deficits occur as a result of wakefulness, and sleep allows or promotes physiologic processes to repair or restore these deficits thereby assuring normal daytime functioning.[6-8] Special focus has been placed on both restoration of somatic function and the central nervous system (CNS) function. Non–rapid eye movement (NREM) sleep is thought to function in reparation of body tissue and REM sleep in restoration of brain tissue. Supporting evidence, however, is indirect. Napping, when its timing and duration are designed properly, has the potential to improve waking function. Even brief napping of less than 30 minutes in duration counteracts decreased alertness and performance under conditions of sleep deprivation.[8a] The role of NREM sleep in repair of somatic tissue comes from investigations that have shown the following:

1. Slow-wave sleep (SWS) increases following sleep deprivation.[9]
2. The percentage of SWS is increased during the developmental years.[10]
3. Total sleep duration increases with body mass.[11]
4. Release of growth hormone occurs at sleep onset and peak levels occur during SWS in prepubertal children.[12]
5. The release of many endogenous anabolic steroids (prolactin, testosterone, and luteinizing hormone) occurs in relation to a sleep-dependent cycle.[13,14]
6. The nadir of catabolic steroid release, such as corticosteroids, occurs during the first hours of sleep, coincident with the largest percentage of SWS.[15]
7. Increased mitosis of lymphocytes and increased rate of bone growth occur during sleep.[16]

1

8. There is a gradual increase in SWS percentage of total sleep time in response to a graded increase in physical exercise.[17]

However, other observations might suggest an influence of sleep on a physiologic process rather than a direct effect. For example, while peak rates of cell division occur during sleep, they do not appear to be due to sleep itself. Increased mitosis is demonstrable after a night without sleep and is positively influenced by oral glucose load and negatively influenced by cortisol secretion.[18] Similarly, in adolescents and adults, somatomedin levels are the highest during wakefulness, not during sleep as it is in prepubertal children.[19]

On the other hand, REM sleep—characterized by intense CNS activation—has been thought to function in the restoration of CNS function. It may have evolved in order to "reprogram" innate behaviors and to incorporate learned behaviors and knowledge acquired during wakefulness.[20] The synthesis of CNS proteins is increased during REM sleep.[21] This sleep state also appears in significantly higher proportions in the fetus and newborn, gradually decreasing over the first few years of life. Increased protein synthesis during REM sleep may be critical in the development of the CNS.

Evolutionary and Adaptive Theories

Development of many physiologic functions follows an orderly progression that mirrors phylogenetic development. It has been suggested that the development of sleep in the human organism also follows this same phylogenetic pattern. Evidence for this theory is scant. Animals sleep in many different ways, often influenced more by the environment and lifestyle than by evolution of the species.[22] SWS and REM sleep rebound are characteristic features seen after sleep deprivation in the dog, cat, rabbit, and human.[23] Definitive REM sleep, however, has never been documented in the dolphin. Dolphins do not have a pulmonary reflex to hypoxemia; therefore, they have complete, voluntary control of breathing, and sleep would presumably be associated with impaired neurorespiratory control. Actually, dolphins appear to exhibit hemispheric sleep. That is to say, when

dolphins appear to sleep, slow-wave patterns are seen over a single hemisphere at a time, while the other hemisphere shows waking rhythm.[24] If the evolutionary theory of sleep is true, animals with highly complex CNS function, such as the dolphin, should follow this pattern. It stands to reason that if the dolphin slept in the same manner as the dog, cat, and human, survival in its aquatic environment would be impossible. Skeletal muscle atonia during REM sleep (as currently understood) would result in drowning. Therefore, the lifestyle and environment of the dolphin play a much more significant role in the pattern of sleep development in these species than phylogeny.

In some species, sleep may function to enhance survival. Animals that graze for food tend to sleep in bursts over a short period of time, a behavior that may provide the time needed for sufficient food-seeking while protecting the animal from predators.[25] Carnivorous animals who do not require large amounts of time for foraging and who are relatively safe from predation tend to sleep for long periods of time.

Sleep may also be an instinctive behavior, a patterned response to stimuli that conserves energy, prevents maladaptive behaviors, and promotes survival.[26] According to the evolutionary theory of sleep, cortical activation in REM sleep may perform additional survival functions.[27]

Energy Conservation Theory

Sleep may function to conserve energy. In fact, mammalian species exhibit a high correlation between metabolic rate and total sleep time.[28] This view states that energy reduction is greater during sleep than during periods of quiet wakefulness and that sleep provides periods of enforced rest, barring the animal from activity for extended periods of time. Endothermic animals exhibit SWS. During NREM sleep, endogenous thermoregulation continues, though functioning at levels below those of wakefulness. Poikilothermic species, on the other hand, do not exhibit clear SWS patterns. It is doubtful, however, that this theory explains the function of sleep in humans. Reduction in metabolism that occurs during sleep is minimal. Although the hypothesis is intriguing, energy conservation theory has been disputed and evidence exists that an increase in sleep time does not correlate with increased metabolic rate.[29,30] It has been shown that there is only an approximately 8 to 10% reduction in metabolic rate during sleep when compared with relaxed wakefulness. This would be insignificant when considering an adult human's basal metabolic expenditure.

Learning Theory

A particularly interesting theory of the function of sleep centers on the role of sleep in the process of learning and memory. A significant body of knowledge exists which suggests that retention of new information depends on activation of some brain function that occurs at a critical period after the registration of this information.[31,32] Two pivotal phases appear to exist. The first one is "consolidation." Medication that causes stimulation of the reticular activating system and cortical excitation during the first 90 seconds after acquisition of new information appears to enhance memory and increase retention. Although the consolidation phase of learning is important, it cannot be considered definitive for fixation of information, since processing continues for a long period of time.

The second critical phase of information processing seems to occur during sleep, specifically REM sleep. Two theories have been proposed, one based on the *passive* hypothesis (unlearning theory) and the other on the *active* hypothesis, which suggests that there are active consolidation mechanisms. An active process is supported by the following facts: Considerable brain activity occurs during this phase of sleep, in which brain oxygen consumption increases, there is an increase in cerebral blood flow, and there is intense activity of cortical and reticular neurons indicating an active, functional process.

Over the past 50 years, the beneficial effects of sleep on the retention of memories acquired during wakefulness have been documented.[33,34] REM sleep appears to have special significance. Despite evidence from animal and human studies, the exact function of REM sleep in childhood development and learning remains unknown. Diverse reasons have been proposed for children's learning difficulties, but no single factor appears to be consistent for all individuals. Most diagnostic and treatment protocols have empirically focused on the child's daytime capabilities.

Theories on the function of REM sleep and dreaming, with which it has a contingent relationship, remain diverse. Facilitation of memory storage, reverse learning, anatomic and functional brain maturation, catecholamine restoration, and others have been postulated.[35] Growing evidence supports the idea that sleep following a learning experience is critical to memory formation. Studies suggest that information acquired during wakefulness is *reactivated* and possibly consolidated during subsequent REM sleep.[36] Several brain areas have been shown to be activated during sequence learning when awake and during subsequent REM sleep.[37] This activation suggests that REM sleep participates in the reprocessing of recent memory traces.[38] Regional cerebral reactivation during post-training REM sleep is not related simply to the acquisition of basic visuomotor skills during prior practice of a serial reaction time task but rather to the implicit acquisition of the stimulus sequence. REM sleep is deeply involved in the reprocessing and optimization of high-order information contained in the material to be learned. Additionally, the level of acquisition of probabilistic rules attained before sleep correlates with an increase in regional cerebral blood flow during subsequent REM sleep. This suggests that post-training cerebral reactivation is modulated by the strength of the memory traces developed during the learning episode.[38]

Interestingly, learning of some perceptual skills has been shown to depend on the plasticity of the visual cortex and to require post-training nocturnal sleep.[39] Sleep-dependent learning of a texture discrimination task can be accomplished in human subjects having only brief (60- to 90-minute) naps containing both NREM sleep and REM sleep.

Newborn infants preferentially orient to face-like patterns at birth, but months of experience with facial observations are required for full face-processing abilities to develop.[40] Models generally assume that the brain areas responsible for newborn orienting responses are not capable of learning and are physically separate from those that later learn from real faces. Newborn face-orienting may be the result of prenatal exposure of a learning system to internally generated input patterns, such as those found in ponto-geniculo-occipital (PGO) waves during active

(REM) sleep. Neonates spend about 18 hours asleep per day, at term, and about 50% of this time is spent in active/REM sleep. Preterm infants spend considerably more time in active sleep. A combination of learning and internal patterns is an efficient way to specify and develop circuitry for facial perceptions.[40] This prenatal learning can account for the newborn preferences for schematic and photographic images of faces, providing a computational explanation for how genetic influences interact with experiences to construct a complex adaptive system.

Sleep loss adversely affects certain types of cognitive processing, particularly associative memory.[41] Long-term potentiation represents a putative cellular basis for learning and memory consolidation. The influence of sleep deprivation has been shown to result in the delay of maximal induction, and the degradation of the maintenance phase of long-term potentiation may represent the sleep deprivation–induced impairment of the underlying neurochemical mechanisms normally responsible for memory acquisition.

Studies relating sleep states to memory processes typically present learning material to participants and then examine recall ability after intervening sleep or sleep deprivation.[42] Most studies have utilized either sleep recordings or sleep deprivation after a learning task. Cueing and positron emission tomography have also been utilized. Data strongly suggest that REM sleep is involved in the efficient memory processing of cognitive procedural material but not declarative material. There are some data, however, which support the contention that SWS or NREM sleep is necessary for declarative memory consolidation. Additionally, the length of the NREM-REM cycle may also be important for declarative memory. Stage 2 NREM sleep may also be involved in memory for motor procedural but not cognitive procedural tasks.[42] After declarative learning tasks, the density of sleep spindles is significantly higher than that with a nonlearning control task and is greatest during the first 90 minutes of sleep.[43] Spindle density also correlates with recall performance both before and after sleep. These findings indicate that spindle activity during NREM sleep is quite sensitive to previous learning experiences.[44]

Flexible cognitive processes are regarded as fundamental to problem solving and creativity. REM sleep has been shown to be associated with creative processes and abstract reasoning, with increased strength of weak associations in cognitive networks.[43] When early and late REM and NREM awakenings are assessed, a dissociation becomes evident, with NREM-awakening task performance becoming more REM-like later in the night but REM-awakening performance remaining constant. The neurophysiology of REM sleep, therefore, represents a brain state more amenable to flexible cognitive processing than that of NREM sleep.

The role of sleep in the development of the CNS and neural circuitry may be extremely important. Kisley and colleagues showed that normal, young infants exhibited significant response suppression.[45] A correlation between increasing age and stronger response suppression was also uncovered, even within an age range restricted to 1 to 4 months. These data suggest that neuronal circuits underlying sensory gating are functional during very early postnatal development.

Minor neurologic and EEG abnormalities have been described in children with "hyperactivity" syndrome.[46] These abnormalities have been associated with specific or global learning difficulties, and the syndrome has previously been described as "minimal cerebral dysfunction." However, neurologic and EEG abnormalities associated with this hyperactivity syndrome have been shown to be nonspecific and variable,[47] resulting in a change of the name of the syndrome to attention deficit hyperactivity disorder (ADHD).

It is noteworthy that of the 15 reading-disabled (dyslexic) children studied by Levinson, 97% revealed evidence of cerebellar-vestibular (C-V) dysfunction. Ninety-six percent of 22 blinded neurologic examinations and 90% of 70 completed electronystagmograms indicated similar C-V dysfunction.[48] Ottenbacher and associates explored the relationship between vestibular function, as measured by duration of postrotatory nystagmus, and human figure–drawing ability in 40 children labeled as learning disabled.[49] Chronologic age and postrotatory nystagmus durations shared significant amounts of variance with human figure–drawing. The variables of IQ and sex were not significant. DeQuiros and Schrager have also identified vestibular dysfunction in some learning-disabled children[50] and described another related syndrome termed "vestibular-oculomotor split," which results in impaired ocular fixation, reduced scanning ability, and poor eye-head coordination.

Despite the evidence that some children with learning disabilities display soft or nonfocal neurologic signs[51] and low scores on tests of visuomotor integration, reading achievement, and ocular scanning,[52] contrary evidence of normal vestibular responses to rotation in dyslexic children has been published. Brown and coworkers measured eye movements provoked by sinusoidal rotation of the subjects at low frequencies.[53] Gain, phase, and asymmetry of the responses were calculated from the eye velocity and stimulus velocity waveforms. There were no differences between the groups in any of the measurements. These results led to the conclusion that "there are no clinically measurable differences in this aspect of vestibular function" in their carefully selected population of dyslexic and control children. However, their conclusions were based on evidence obtained during the waking state. Vestibular nuclei play a major role in the control of eye movements when awake and asleep. If these nuclei are destroyed, eye movements during REM sleep are absent. In a pilot study of four reading-disabled children, a significant difference was found in the mean angular velocity of eye movements during REM sleep when compared with three normal-reading controls.[54]

Correlations exist that associate the phasic events of REMs with C-V control. Pompeiano has shown that lesions of the medial and descending vestibular nuclei in the cat eliminated all phasic inhibition of sensory input, spinal reflexes, and all motor output associated with phasic REM bursts, including eye movements themselves.[55,56] They have also demonstrated that intense, spontaneous discharges from neurons of the vestibular nuclei occur synchronous with the ocular activity of REM sleep. Nystagmus evoked by rotation can be most readily induced during sleep at the time of phasic events of REM sleep[57] and in Wernicke-Korsakoff disease, in which the vestibular nuclei are often damaged and eye movements are absent during REM sleep.[58] These observations partially confirm the influences of vestibular mechanisms on the phasic activity of REM sleep.

An age-related development of phasic inhibition of auditory evoked potentials during the ocular activity of REM sleep and an age-related increase in the duration of the REM bursts have been described in normal subjects.[59] It seems that central vestibular influences underlie these events and that vestibular control of phasic activity follows a developmental maturation schedule.

Considering this evidence, there may be a relationship between the C-V control of REM phasic events and the importance of phasic REM sleep in learning and memory. However, this relationship currently remains a mystery.

A significant body of literature exists supporting a relationship among REM sleep, phasic REM activity, and learning. Sleep patterns in hyperkinetic and normal children were studied by Busby and colleagues.[60] Analysis of sleep pattern variables revealed a significantly longer REM onset latency and greater absolute and relative amounts of movement time for the hyperkinetic group than controls. No other sleep parameter differentiated the groups. Clinical observations of autistic children have suggested that fundamental symptoms of the syndrome of childhood autism involve disturbances of motility and perception. The nature of these disturbances indicates a maturational delay in the development of complex motor patterns and the modulation of sensory input.[59] Sleep studies have provided some evidence for a maturational delay in the differentiation of REM sleep patterns and the development of phasic excitatory and inhibitory mechanisms during REM sleep in these children. These findings implicate a failure of central vestibular control over sensory transmission and motor output during REM sleep. The notation that there is a dysfunction of central vestibular mechanisms underlying the delayed organization and differentiation of the REM sleep state is supported by observations of altered vestibular nystagmus in the waking state in autistic children.[59]

Studies in animals and humans support the importance of REM sleep in learning. Lucero conducted experiments that showed a significant increase in REM sleep duration with respect to controls, a nonsignificant increase in total sleep time, and no changes in SWS duration in animals subjected to consecutive learning experiences.[61] An increase in REM sleep time observed after incremental learning suggests that REM sleep might be involved in the processing of information acquired during wakefulness. It has been postulated that such processing might consist of the transformation of a "labile" program acquired in the learning session into a more "stable" program devoid of superfluous information.

Major evidence regarding the importance of REM sleep in facilitating recall of complex associative information has been documented by Scrima.[62] The beneficial effects of isolated REM and isolated NREM sleep on recall were tested in 10 narcoleptic subjects. The results of complex associative tasks indicated significant differences among three conditions for free recall. Recall was significantly better after isolated REM than after isolated NREM sleep or wakefulness and was significantly better after NREM sleep than after wakefulness. It was concluded that the results were consistent with the proposed neuronal activity correlation theory of Emmons and Simon that REM sleep actively consolidates and/or integrates complex associative information and that NREM sleep passively prevents retroactive interference of recently acquired complex associative information.[63]

Newborn animals and human infants show a greater proportion of REM sleep with respect to total sleep time than adults[64,65] and a progressive decrease in that proportion as growing continues that is paralleled by a decrease in learning ability.[24] Fishbein has shown that REM sleep deprivation, both before and after learning, disrupts primarily long-term memory processes.[66] Evidence has been provided that learning induces a protracted augmentation of paradoxical sleep time, lasting for at least 24 hours.[67] This work, together with previous work, suggests that REM sleep augmentation may be a neurobiologic expression of the long-term process of memory consolidation. Fishbein was able to augment REM sleep using behavioral techniques of learning. Therefore, one psychobiologic function of REM sleep may be to process and maintain information during wakefulness.

Results obtained from nondeprivation studies of animals provide consistent support for the hypothesis that REM sleep is functionally related to learning. Results of studies that have employed multiple training sessions may be interpreted to suggest that either prior REM sleep prepares the organism for subsequent learning or that REM sleep facilitates consolidation and retrieval of prior learning. Given the equivocality of prior REM deprivation literature, the second interpretation seems more reasonable.[68]

Impaired cognitive functioning has been documented in studies on sleep-deprived physicians. In one investigation, cognitive functioning in acutely and chronically sleep-deprived house officers was evaluated.[69] Analysis of data revealed significant deficits in primary mental tasks involving basic rote memory and language and numerical skills, as well as in tasks requiring high-order cognitive functioning and intellectual abilities.

Acquisition of many simple learning tasks in animals is followed by augmentation of REM sleep without any modification of NREM sleep.[31] Augmentation of REM sleep after learning has also been described in human infants.[70] Sleep may be particularly important for RNA and DNA synthesis linked to memory processes. There is some evidence that during sleep, RNA is more actively synthesized, less rapidly degraded, and more slowly transported into the cytoplasm.[71]

As in infants, there is some evidence that REM sleep may increase following learning in older children and adults. Hartman has demonstrated an increase in REM sleep time occurring after days of increased learning, mental stress, and especially demanding events.[72] If learning does cause an increase in REM sleep, brain-damaged patients who are improving should have a higher proportion of REM sleep than those who show no improvement. Following up a group of 9 patients with severe traumatic brain damage, Ron and associates found a correlation between cognition and REM sleep improvement in 7.[73] Greenberg and Dewan compared the percentage of REM sleep in improving and nonimproving aphasic patients and found that the nonimproving patients did, in fact, have less REM.[74] In 32 patients with Down syndrome, phenylketonuria, and other forms of brain damage, Feinberg found a positive correlation between the amount of eye movement during REM sleep and estimates of intellectual function,[10] while in a comparison of 38 normal individuals and 15 brain-damaged patients, it was shown that mentally retarded patients had less REM sleep.[75] Linkage between REM sleep and development of the visual system has been further supported by a recent study by Oksenberg and coworkers.[76] They reported significant adverse changes in the microscopic anatomy of the visual cortex in REM sleep–deprived cats.

In spite of evidence from human and animal studies, the exact function of sleep in the process of learning, memory, and child development is still speculative.

Unlearning Theory

An antithetical hypothesis for the function of REM sleep in learning and memory involves a process of *unlearning*. No single memory center appears to exist in the brain.[77] Many parts of the CNS participate in the representation of a single event. However, localization of memory for a single event generally involves a limited number of neural pathways, and those collections of neurons within which a memory is equivalently represented probably contain a set of no more than a thousand neurons. These interconnected assemblies of cells could store associations.[78,79] If the cells involved in the memory of an event form mutual synapses, regeneration of the activity of the entire neuronal set would occur when part of that event is encountered again. Therefore, Crick and Mitchison proposed that the function of REM sleep is to remove certain undesirable modes of interaction in networks of cells in the cerebral cortex.[80] This would be accomplished during REM sleep by a "reverse learning" mechanism so that the trace in the brain of the unconscious dream can be weakened rather than strengthened by the activity of dreaming. A mathematical and computer model of a network of 30 to 1000 neurons has been developed by Hopfield and colleagues.[81] Their model network has a content-addressable memory or "associative memory" that allows it to learn and store many memories. A particular memory can be evoked in its entirety when the network is stimulated by an adequately sized subpart of the information of that memory. When memories are learned, spurious information is created and can also be evoked. Applying an unlearning process, similar to the learning process but with a reversed sign and starting from a noise input, enhanced the performance of the network in accessing real memories and minimizing spurious ones.

Sleep (in particular REM sleep) may then function to reduce or prevent unwanted, unnoticed, or spurious material acquired during wakefulness. Isolation of the cortex from environmental stimuli may be a necessary feature of the removal of inhibiting and/or competitive stimuli, inappropriate behavior patterns, and overloading of neuronal networks, thus permitting reprogramming and consolidation of more vital material.

Other Hypotheses

The presence of circulating hypnotoxin(s) as possible causes of sleep has received some attention in the literature. These theories hold that during wakefulness there is accumulation of sleep-producing "toxin(s)" which stimulates or results in sleep. Once the toxin(s) has been modified during sleep, awakening occurs. Investigation of many substances, which are claimed to be released subsequent to sleep deprivation, and thalamic stimulation have failed to produce convincing evidence of the accuracy of this theory.[82] Studies of craniopagus and thoracopagus twins reveal independent sleep–wake cycles despite the sharing of circulatory and/or nervous systems.[83]

Sleep may be required for the normal functioning of the motor system and/or skeletal musculature. Muscle aching and change in skeletal muscle enzyme activity have been reported following NREM sleep deprivation.[84] Although the ability to work is not drastically affected by sleep deprivation, physical performance follows definite circadian rhythmicity.[85] Sleep also has a profound effect on certain diseases that affect the motor system, including Parkinson's disease[86] and hereditary progressive dystonia.[87]

Although all theories on the function of sleep have had significant support, there is much conflicting evidence for each theory. The function of sleep may be explained very simply or may be one of the more complex biologic mechanisms known. A unitary explanation of the function of sleep is probably unrealistic. The exact function and purpose of sleep may prove to be a combination or a series of integrations of all proposed hypotheses.

SLEEP DEPRIVATION

Experiments conducted to unravel the meaning and functions of various physiologic processes have involved modification of these systems followed by observations of the consequences of each modification. For many years, research has focused on total sleep deprivation, partial sleep deprivation, and deprivation of various sleep stages in an attempt to identify repercussions.

Total sleep deprivation studies in animals have shown significant deleterious effects. In early experiments, in order to keep animals awake for prolonged periods of time, constant activity was necessary, confounding the results. In 1983, Rechtschaffen and coworkers described an ingenious experimental method that controlled for the stimuli used to keep the animals awake.[88] Experimental and control rats were placed on a platform that rotated and caused awakening only when the experimental animal fell asleep. The activity of the experimental and control animals was kept constant. Experimental animals suffered severe pathologic changes from the sleep deprivation. Changes ranged from a severely debilitated appearance (ungroomed and yellowed fur) to intense neurologic abnormalities (ataxia and motor weakness) and death. Interestingly, there was a loss of EEG amplitude to less than half of normal waking values before the morbidity or mortality of the experimental animals. Necropsy findings included pulmonary edema, atelectasis, gastric ulcerations, gastrointestinal hemorrhage, edema of the limbs, testicular atrophy, scrotal damage, bladder enlargement, hypoplasia of the liver and spleen, and hyperplasia of the adrenal glands (indicating a significant stress response). Body weight decreased in both experimental and control animals but was significantly greater in the experimental, sleep-deprived animals. It is also interesting to note that the animals that ate the most lost the most weight. There was a surprisingly high correlation between the amount of paradoxical (REM) sleep obtained by the experimental animals and the survival time.

In comparison, the effects of total sleep deprivation on human subjects have been remarkably few. Although brief psychotic episodes have been reported in some subjects, long-term psychological effects do not appear to result.[89] The only certain and reproducible effect of total sleep deprivation has been *sleepiness*.

Fatigue, decline in perceptual, cognitive, and psychomotor capabilities, and increasing transient ego-disruptive episodes have been reported by Kales and associates during sleep deprivation.[90] Reality testing was impaired and regressive behavior was noted as the experiment continued. Tests for thought disorders showed shifts in thought processes to a more childlike level of cognition; however, there was no obvious evidence of schizophrenic thinking.

Performance may also be impaired by sleep deprivation. Vigilance and performance on reaction time tests have been shown to be significantly impaired by the loss of as little as one night of sleep.[91] In a study of 44 men participating in a strenuous combat course in Norway, significant impairment was observed in vigilance, reaction time, code testing, and profile of mood state after 24 hours of sleep deprivation. Complaints of symptoms occurred first, and disturbances of senses and behavior followed. Horne and coworkers have reported that after 60 hours of continuous wakefulness, an inherent capacity for signal detection exhibited a stepwise decline during deprivation, falling sharply during the usual sleep time period and leveling out during the daytime.[92] A clear circadian rhythm overlaid the decline due to deprivation. It was concluded that changes in this inherent capacity seem to be consistent with a brain "restitutive" role for sleep.

Significant physiologic changes after total sleep deprivation have been reported. Rebound of stage 4 sleep on the first recovery day and REM rebound on the second and third recovery days were documented by Berger and Oswald in 1962 and Williams and colleagues in 1964.[9,93] After 205 hours of sleep deprivation, Kales and associates reported significant increases in stage 4 sleep and REM sleep and significant decreases in stage 2 sleep.[90] On the first two recovery nights, alterations in REM sleep were noted. There was an increase in REM percentage, appearance of sleep-onset REM (SOREM) periods, a decrease in REM latency, and a decrease in intervals between REM sleep periods. These occurred most dramatically in those subjects who had the greatest psychological disturbances during the deprivation period.

Significant changes in performance and sleep physiology have been documented in subjects only partially deprived of sleep. In 1974, Webb and Agnew reported the results of an experiment conducted on 15 subjects restricted to a regimen of 5½ hours of sleep a night for a period of 60 days.[94] The initial effect was an increase in the total amount of stage 4 sleep. By the fifth week of the experiment, the amount of stage 4 sleep returned to the baseline level. The initial effect on REM sleep was a sharp reduction when compared with the baseline level. During the entire course of the experiment, there was a reduction in REM sleep by 25%. Latency to the onset of stage 4 sleep and latency to the onset of REM sleep were also reduced. Behaviorally, only the Wilkinson Vigilance Task showed a decline in performance associated with continued sleep restriction. Initially, the subjects experienced difficulty with arousal in the morning and felt drowsy during the day, but this did not continue throughout the entire experiment. Mood scales showed no significant changes. It was concluded that the chronic loss of as much as 2.5 hours of sleep per night is not likely to result in major behavioral consequences. However, significant physiologic effects were documented (especially in REM sleep) polysomnographically with partial restriction. Restricting sleep by early morning awakenings generally deprives the subject of REM and stage 2 sleep, usually leaving NREM stage 4 sleep intact. However, recovery night shows a substantial increase in the amount of NREM stage 4 sleep, suggesting that the amount of high-voltage SWS is due to some extent to the preceding total sleep time.[95]

Children differ from adults in their response to acute restriction in sleep. When sleep has been restricted by 4 hours or more, there is a decrease in all stages of sleep (except SWS), a reduction in sleep onset latency, stage 4 latency, and REM latency, and a reduction of wakefulness during the sleep period. Carskadon and coworkers studied the effect of acute, partial restriction of sleep in nine children between the ages of 11 and 13.2 years.[96] These children were permitted to sleep 10 hours on baseline and recovery nights and 4 hours on a single restricted night. No significant differences were found on any performance test. The lack of demonstrable effects may have been because the tests were brief. Wilkinson emphasized that task duration is a major factor in determining a test's sensitivity to sleep loss.[97] On the other hand, significant changes did occur on objective sleep measurements. The multiple sleep latency test showed a significant increase in daytime sleepiness, which persisted into the morning after sleep restriction. This suggested that children were more severely affected by sleep restriction than adults. On polysomnography, the findings were comparable to those in adults, but children did not show recovery rebound of SWS and REM sleep similar to that reported for adults. Although children appear to be able to tolerate a single night of restricted sleep without a decrement in performance of brief tasks, perhaps more prolonged restriction and prolonged tasks similar to those required in school would show decrements. Children seem to require more time to recuperate fully from nocturnal sleep restriction than adults. The extent of daytime sleepiness that occurs is not trivial. With additional nights of partial sleep deprivation, cumulative sleepiness might rapidly become a significant problem. The importance of sleep restriction, daytime sleepiness, and performance of children in school and on their behavior may be greater than previously realized.

In 1972, Dement[98] powerfully described possible outcomes of restricted sleep on wakefulness:

> *"After an excessively long period of wakefulness, the state of sleep becomes preemptive. When we enforce wakefulness, we are probably preventing or minimizing activity in the neural systems that subserve sleep induction and maintenance. As the potency of these systems increase [sic] during the period of their induced inactivity, they may begin to intrude upon wakefulness in an ever more aggressive manner.*
>
> *"The notion of total sleep deprivation could be somewhat illusory, and could result merely in a redistribution of activity in sleep and arousal systems in which NREM sleep would occur in the form of hundreds of microsleeps."*

Microsleep episodes have been well documented in both human and animal studies.[99-101] Kales and colleagues have described disorientation and misperceptions during sleep deprivation that seemed to be associated with "lapses" that become more frequent as deprivation continues.[90] Armington and Mitnick found that sleep deprivation eventually produced brain wave patterns that were more or less continuously at the NREM stage 1 level in subjects who appeared to be behaviorally awake.[99] The most consistent result of modest amounts of sleep loss in humans is the occurrence of these microsleep periods[100] which increase in frequency throughout periods of sleep deprivation. Since gross waking behavior is not affected, these lapses may have significant consequences on performance and its assessment, especially for the school-aged child whose consistent attentiveness is required for success in school. Since the perceptual shutdown can occur before EEG changes are apparent at the outset of sleep under ordinary circumstances, there may be many more such episodes in sleep-deprived subjects than EEG patterns alone would suggest.[98]

PHYLOGENETIC CONSIDERATIONS

Understanding sleep in humans requires some reflection on sleep in other species. Although periods of sluggish activity can be documented in reptiles, it does not appear that physiologic sleep occurs.[102] Although only a relatively small number of mammalian species have been studied, it appears that most, if not all, birds and mammals sleep. Quiescent periods, intervals of reduced responsiveness to environmental stimuli, rapid reversibility of state, specific postures, and characteristic EEG changes have been observed.[103] However, all of these criteria need not be present concomitantly, and quiescence is not always equivalent to inactivity. Ritualistic presleep activity and behaviors occur in many species, including humans. The timing of sleep varies: Some species consolidate sleep into a single period of time, while others distribute sleep throughout a 24-hour continuum.

Sleep in birds is remarkably similar to sleep in mammals. Both demonstrate two distinct types of sleep, with comparable electrophysiologic activity. Major differences appear to be in the pattern of sleep and the greater number of sleep states observed in avian species.[104]

Zepelin and Rechtschaffen studied available sleep data on more than 50 mammalian species.[28] Sleeping patterns were correlated with metabolic rates, gestational periods, and brain weights. Animals with lower metabolic rates tend to sleep less than those with higher metabolic rates. Species that have longer sleep periods tend to exhibit shorter life spans and are smaller in size. Meddis replicated this study in a sample of 65 species and obtained similar results.[105]

NREM-REM cycling appears to be the basic organization of sleep in most species studied. Although the quality and quantity of NREM and REM sleep vary considerably, a regularly patterned series of state changes occurs, with demonstrable slowing of the EEG and the presence of spindling activity.[103] Paradoxical sleep has been recorded in almost all mammalian species studied. Characteristics of this sleep state include desynchronization (activation) of CNS electrical activity, skeletal muscle atonia, periodic twitching, and physiologic instability (especially of the cardiovascular and respiratory systems). Changes in thermoregulation and high arousal thresholds are present. Rhythmic theta activity and PGO spikes are typically seen on EEG during mammalian paradoxical sleep.

Phylogenetic development of REM sleep has been studied by Allison and Van Twyver.[106] It appears to have developed approximately 130 million years ago. Allison and Cicchetti concluded that the volume of REM sleep correlated with lifestyle, risk of predation, and degree of exposure of the sleeping environment.[25]

REM sleep is the preponderant state early in life in most mammals (including humans). Though considered to be ontogenetically primitive, the role of REM sleep in the development of the CNS may be significant. Premature newborn humans spend approximately 90% of their total sleep time in active sleep. This falls rapidly to about 50% by term. A gradual decrease continues throughout the first few years of life to a level of about 20% to 25%. This level remains remarkably constant throughout the remainder of the life cycle.[65]

Jouvet-Mounier and associates have studied the ontogenetic development of sleep in infant cats, rats, and guinea pigs.[107] More than 70 animals underwent electrocortical, electro-ocular, electromyographic, and behavioral monitoring from birth to 50 days of age. REM sleep was the preponderant form of sleep in all of them. Each species varied significantly in the degree of development at birth, with rat pups the most immature, kittens intermediate, and guinea pigs the most mature. Degree of immaturity at birth highly correlated with the amount of paradoxical sleep recorded during the perinatal period. Rat pups exhibited 70% paradoxical sleep at birth, which decreased rapidly almost to adult levels by 30 days of life. A decrease of paradoxical sleep in kittens was considerably slower. Guinea pigs showed the lowest volume of paradoxical sleep (7%); however, this was still approximately double the volume seen in the adult animal. Maturation of SWS is late in comparison with paradoxical sleep, and the time spent in paradoxical sleep and SWS varies during the first postnatal month. These variations are different among species. Newborn kittens have a more highly developed cortex than rat pups.[108] Cortical neurons mature very rapidly and reach the histologic characteristics of adult cortical neurons by the 12th postnatal day, concomitant with the appearance of SWS. In contrast, the cortex of the newborn guinea pig appears histologically the same as that of the adult.[109]

Sleeping dolphins and porpoises are fascinating and of particular ontogenetic interest because of the complexity of the Cetacean CNS. Mukhametov has studied the neurophysiology of sleep in the bottle-nosed dolphin (*Tursiops truncatus*) and the porpoise (*Phocoena phocoena*)[110] and showed that the main characteristics of sleep in these marine mammals are unihemispheric SWS and the apparent absence of paradoxical sleep. EEG characteristics were similar to those typical for the mammalian brain, and three distinct stages can be identified: desynchronization; intermediate synchronization, with sleep spindles, theta activity, and delta waves; and maximal synchronization, with slow waves constituting more than 50% of each recording period. In all dolphins studied, unihemispheric SWS was the main type of sleep recorded. Interestingly, this type of sleep is not found in other mammals. Synchronization of the EEG occurs in one hemisphere, while the opposite hemisphere reveals desynchronization. These cycles of synchrony and desynchrony appear to be independent. Each hemisphere exhibits different amounts of SWS, and deprivation of SWS in one hemisphere does not result in contralateral rebound. Ipsilateral rebound is noted in the SWS-deprived hemisphere only. Mukhametov attempted to identify neurophysiologic and behavioral correlates of paradoxical sleeping in 30 animals of two species and concluded that paradoxical sleep does not appear to be present in the dolphin or porpoise. However, it is very difficult to prove the complete absence of paradoxical sleep, since testing of dolphin fetuses and calves has not yet been possible. It is unknown whether these characteristics represent a phylogenetic, developmental, or adaptive phenomenon. Unraveling the mystery has fascinating teleologic implications.

BEHAVIORAL AND PHYSIOLOGIC CONSIDERATIONS

At first glance, sleep appears to be a simple process, a required part of our 24-hour life cycle. Little attention is paid to the sleeping state, because human lifestyles focus primarily on interactions with the environment and daily fragments of disengagement seem of secondary importance. Time spent in activities not related to goal attainment, pursuit of sustenance, fulfillment, happiness, or success appears to consist of intrusive, unwelcome gaps. However, the importance of these gaps in permitting the individual to function and appropriately interact with the environment during the waking state has only recently been discovered.

Any definition of sleep is complex, both from behavioral and physiologic perspectives. In the simplest terms, it is a reversible disengagement with and unresponsiveness to the external environment, regularly alternating in a circadian manner with engagement and responsiveness. It is now known that this definition is significantly incomplete and simplistic, since sleep is a highly active and complex state.

It seems easy to determine when an individual is sleeping. Behavioral correlates include a recumbent position, closure of the eyelids, quiescence, and diminished responsiveness to external stimuli. These behaviors are fairly consistent among individuals. However, sleep onset requires complex interactions of learned behaviors and physiologic processes. Absence of sudden external stimuli; a suitable, safe, comfortable environment; relaxation of postural muscles; and learned stereotypical behaviors associated with bedtime are required.[111] There is some evidence that rhythmic, monotonous sensory stimulation helps promote sleep.[112] Whether this is behavioral, physiologic, or a combination is speculative.

Physiologically, sleep onset and maintenance are not passive processes. Isolation of the cerebrum from the brainstem and spinal cord (*cerveau isolé*) produces a state indistinguishable from physiologic sleep.[113] A series of exquisite experiments identified neurons of the reticular formation that received collateral input from somatic, visceral, and special sensory pathways and sent ascending projections dorsally and ventrally to the basal forebrain.[114-116] These collections of neurons constitute what is called the *reticular activating system*. Complex projections of neurons from the reticular formation to the posterior hypothalamus-subthalamus, to the basal forebrain, and then to the cortex are responsible for the maintenance of wakefulness.[117]

Although it was initially thought that sleep was the result of a decrease in the activity of this system, brainstem transection experiments resulting in diminished sleep suggested that sleep inducing structures must also be present in the CNS.[118] This sleep inducing structure appeared to be located in the lower brainstem, specifically the dorsal medullary reticular formation and nucleus of the solitary tract. Lesions in this area produced EEG activation in a sleeping animal.[119,120] A sleep facilitation center appears to be present in the rostral hypothalamus,[121] and cortical synchrony can be elicited by stimulation of the midline thalamus.[122] Sleep-inducing neurons are also found in the preoptic area and basal forebrain. Gamma-aminobutyric acid neurons located in the cortex, as well as neurons located in the hypothalamus and basal forebrain, are vital for slow-wave production.[117]

Therefore, sleep onset results from a complex series of events involving changes in levels of somatic, visceral, and special sensory input; active inhibition of neuronal networks that produce cortical desynchronization; and active stimulation of neuronal systems and pathways responsible for cortical synchrony. In addition, the rhythmic organization of these activities is extremely complex and appears to be controlled by neurons located in the suprachiasmatic nucleus.[123] Jouvet described a separate system of neurons located in the upper pons that controlled the induction and manifestations of REM sleep.[124] This system was under the influence of an "oscillator" that was separate (though linked to) that which controlled the rhythmicity of the sleep–wake cycle. According to Hobson, the cholinergic, "REM-on" system of neurons is located primarily in the mesencephalic, medullary, and pontine gigantocellular tegmental fields but may be widespread.[125] Discharges from these neurons are responsible for REM sleep epiphenomena of cortical desynchronization, conjugate eye movements, a decrease in muscle tone by active inhibition of alpha motor neurons, muscular twitching, and cardiorespiratory irregularities. It has also been shown that a self-inhibitory, aminergic, "REM-off" system of neurons, located in the dorsal raphe nuclei, locus coeruleus, and the nucleus parabrachialis lateralis, interacts with the opposing system, resulting in alternations between NREM and REM sleep.

It is clear that the behavioral, neurochemical, and neurophysiologic mechanisms of the sleep–wake cycle and electrophysiologic cycles during sleep itself are complex and intensely integrated. Not all of sleep's characteristics have been elucidated. Further research is needed. Their biological substrate may prove to be simple or reflect extraordinarily complex physiologic processes. The implications for fetal and childhood development may be more significant than our wildest dreams.

References

1. Rechtschaffen A: The function of sleep: Methodological issues. In Drucker-Colin R, Shkurovich M, Sterman MB (eds): The Functions of Sleep. New York, Academic Press, 1979.
2. Moldofsky H: Immunology and sleep. Paper presented at the Association of Professional Sleep Societies, First Annual Meeting, Columbus, Ohio, June 15-20, 1986.
3. Moldofsky H, Lue FA, Davidson JR, Gorczynski R: The effect of 40 hours of wakefulness on immune functions in humans: II. Interleukins-1- and -2-like activities. Sleep Res 1988;17:34.
3a. Irwin M: Effects of sleep and sleep loss on immunity and cytokines. Brain Behav Immun 2002;16:503.
4. Moldofsky H, Lue FA, Davidson JR, Gorczynski R: Disordered diurnal patterns of immune functions in three patients with narcolepsy-cataplexy. Sleep Res 1988;17:223.
5. Sherington CS: Man on His Nature. Cambridge, Cambridge University Press, 1946, p 413.
6. Oswald I: Sleep. Harmondsworth, Middlesex, Penguin Books, 1974.
7. Hartmann E, Orzack MH, Branconnier R: Deficits produced by sleep deprivation: Reversal by d- and l-amphetamine. Sleep Res 1974;3:151.
8. Adam K, Oswald I: Sleep is for tissue restoration. J R Coll Physicians Lond 1977;11:376.

8a. Takahashi M, Arito H: Maintenance of alertness and performance by a brief nap after lunch under prior sleep deficit. Sleep 2000;23:813.

9. Berger RJ, Oswald I: Effects of sleep deprivation on behaviour, subsequent sleep, and dreaming. J Ment Sci 1962;108:457.

10. Feinberg I: The ontogenesis of human sleep and the relationship of sleep variables to intellectual function in the aged. Comp Psychiatry 1968;9:138.

11. Adam K: Body weight correlates with REM sleep. Br Med J 1977;1:813.

12. Sassin JF, Parker DC, Mace JW, et al: Human growth hormone release relation to slow-wave sleep and sleep-waking cycles. Science 1969;165:513.

13. Sassin JF, Frantz AG, Kapen S, et al: The nocturnal rise of human prolactin is dependent on sleep. J Clin Endocrinol Metab 1973;37:436.

14. Boyar RM, Rosenfeld RS, Kapen S, et al: Human puberty: Simultaneous augmented secretion of luteinizing hormone and testosterone during sleep. J Clin Invest 1974;54:609.

15. Weitzman ED, Hellman L: Temporal organization of the 24-hour pattern of the hypothalamic-pituitary axis. In Ferin M, Halberg F, Richart RM, Vanderviele RL (eds): Biorhythms and Human Reproduction. New York, John Wiley, 1974.

16. Valk IM, van der Bosch JSG: Intra-daily variation of the human ulnar length and short term growth—a longitudinal study in eleven boys. Growth 1974;42:107.

17. Griffin SJ, Trinder J: Physical fitness, exercise, and human sleep. Psychophysiology 1978;15:447.

18. Fisher LB: The diurnal mitotic rhythm in the human epidermis. Br J Dermatol 1968;80:75.

19. Finkelstein JW, Roffwarg HP, Boyar RM, et al: Age-related change in the twenty-four hour spontaneous secretion of growth hormone. J Clin Endocrinol Metab 1972;35:665.

20. Jouvet M: The function of dreaming: A neurophysiologist's point of view. In Gazzaniga MS, Blakemore C (eds): Handbook of Psychobiology. New York, Academic Press, 1975.

21. Giuditta A, Neugebauer-Vitale A, Grassi-Zucconi G, et al: Synthesis of brain RNA and DNA during sleep. In Borbely A, Valtax JL (eds): Sleep Mechanisms. Berlin, Springer-Verlag, 1984.

22. Bert J: Sleep in primates under natural conditions and in the laboratory. In Koella WP, Levin P (eds): Sleep 1976: Third European Congress of Sleep Research. Basel, S Karger, 1977.

23. Webb WB: Sleep stage responses of older and younger subjects after sleep deprivation. Electroencephalogr Clin Neurophysiol 1981;52:368.

24. Kovalzon VM: Brain Temperature Variations in ECoG in Free-Swimming Bottle-Nose Dolphins: Sleep 1976: Third European Congress of Sleep Research. Basel, S Karger, 1977.

25. Allison T, Cicchetti DV: Sleep in mammals: Ecological and constitutional correlates. Science 1976;194:732.

26. McGinty DJ, Harper TM, Fairbanks MK: Neuronal unit activity and the control of sleep states. In Weitzman E (ed): Advances in Sleep Research. New York, Spectrum, 1974.

27. Snyder F: Toward an evolutionary theory of dreaming. Am J Psychiatry 1966;123:121.

28. Zepelin H, Rechtschaffen A: Mammalian sleep, longevity, and energy conservation. Brain Behav Evol 1974;10:425.

29. Carpenter AC, Timiras PS: Sleep organization in hypo- and hyperthyroid rats. Neuroendocrinology 1982;34:438.

30. Eastman CI, Rechtschaffen A: Effects of thyroxine on sleep in the rat. Sleep 1979;2:215.

31. Block V, Hennevin E, Leconte P: The phenomenon of paradoxical sleep augmentation after learning: Experimental studies of its characteristics and significance. In Fishbein W (ed): Sleep, Dreams and Memory. Jamaica, NY, Spectrum, 1981.

32. Smith C, Butler S: Paradoxical sleep at selective times following training is necessary for learning. Physiol Behav 1982;29:469.

33. Jenkins J, Dallenbach K: Oblivescence during sleep and waking. Am J Psychol 1924;35:605.

34. VanOrmer EG: Retention after intervals of sleep and waking. Arch Psychol 1932;137:5.

35. Staunton H: The function of dreaming. Rev Neurosci 2001;12:365.

36. Wetzel W, Wagner T, Balschun D: REM sleep enhancement induced by different procedures improves memory retention in rats. Eur J Neurosci 2003;18:2611.

37. Maquet P, Laureys S, Peigneux P., et al: Experience-dependent changes in cerebral activation during human sleep. Nat Neurosci 2000;3:831.

38. Peigneux P, Laureys S, Fuchs S, et al: Learned material content and acquisition level modulate cerebral reactivation during post-training rapid-eye-movement sleep. Neuroimage 2003;20:125.

39. Mednick S, Nakayama K, Stickgold R: Sleep-dependent learning: A nap is as good as a night. Nat Neurosci 2003;6:697.

40. Bednar JA, Mikkulainen R: Learning innate face preferences. Neural Comput 2003;15:1525.

41. Davis CJ, Harding JW, Wright JW: REM sleep deprivation-induced deficits in the latency-to-peak induction and maintenance of long-term

potentiation within the CA1 region of the hippocampus. Brain Res 2003;973:293.

42. Smith C: Sleep states and memory processes in humans: Procedural versus declarative memory systems. Sleep Med Rev 2001;5:491.

43. Walker MP, Liston C, Hobson JA, Stickgold R: Cognitive flexibility across the sleep-wake cycle: REM-sleep enhancement of anagram problem solving. Brain Res Cogn Brain Res 2002;14:317.

44. Gais S, Molle M, Helms K, Born J: Learning-dependent increases in sleep spindle density. J Neurosci 2002;22:6830.

45. Kisley MA, Polk SD, Ross RG, et al: Early postnatal development of sensory gating. Neuroreport 2003;14:693.

46. Carter S, Gold A: The syndrome of minimal cerebral dysfunction. In Barnett MH, Einhorn A (eds): Pediatrics. New York, Appleton-Century-Crofts, 1972.

47. Dykman RA, Ackerman PT, Clements S, et al: Specific learning disabilities: An attentional deficit syndrome. In Myklebust HR (ed): Progress in Learning Disabilities. New York, Grune and Stratton, 1971.

48. Levinson HN: Dyslexia: A Solution to the Riddle. New York, Springer-Verlag, 1980.

49. Ottenbacher K, Abbott C, Haley D, et al: Human figure drawing ability and vestibular processing in learning-disabled children. J Clin Psychol 1984;40:1084.

50. deQuiros JB, Schrager OL: Neuropsychological Fundamentals in Learning Disabilities. San Rafael, Calif, Academic Therapy Press, 1978.

51. Steinberg M, Rendle-Short J: Vestibular dysfunction in young children with minor neurological impairment. Dev Med Child Neurol 1977;19:639.

52. Ottenbacher K, Watson PJ, Short MA, et al: Nystagmus and ocular fixation difficulties in learning-disabled children. Am J Occup Ther 1979;33:717.

53. Brown B, Haegerstrom-Portnoy G, Yingling CD, et al: Dyslexic children have normal vestibular responses to rotation. Arch Neurol 1983;40:370.

54. Sheldon SH, Spire JP, Levy HB: REM sleep eye movements in reading disabled children. Sleep Res 1990;19:34.

55. Pompeiano O: The neurophysiological mechanisms of the postural and motor events during desynchronized sleep. In Kety SS, Evarts EV, Williams HL (eds): Sleep and Altered States of Consciousness. Baltimore, Williams & Wilkins, 1967.

56. Pompeiano O: Mechanisms of sensorimotor integration during sleep. Prog Physiol Psychol 1970;3:1.

57. Reding GR, Fernandez C: Effects of vestibular stimulation during sleep. Electroencephalogr Clin Neurophysiol 1968;24:75.

58. Appenzeller O, Fischer AP Jr: Disturbances of rapid eye movements during sleep in patients with lesions of the nervous system. Electroencephalogr Clin Neurophysiol 1968; 25:29.

59. Ornitz EM: Development of sleep patterns in autistic children. In Clemente CD, Purpura DP, Mayer FE (eds): Sleep and the Maturing Nervous System. New York, Academic Press, 1972.

60. Busby K, Firestone P, Pivik RT: Sleep patterns in hyperkinetic and normal children. Sleep 1981;4:366.

61. Lucero MA: Lengthening of REM sleep duration consecutive to learning in the rat. Brain Res 1979;20:319.

62. Scrima L: Isolated REM sleep facilitates recall of complex associative information. Psychophysiology 1982;19:252.

63. Simon CW, Emmons WH: Responses to material presented during various levels of sleep. J Exp Psychol 1956;51:89.

64. Parmelee AH Jr, Schulz HR, Disbrow MA: Sleep patterns of the newborn. J Pediatr 1961;58:241.

65. Roffwarg HP, Dement WC, Fisher C: Preliminary observations on the sleep patterns in neonates, infants, children, and adults. In Harms E (ed): Problems of Sleep and Dreams in Children. London, Pergamon Press, 1963.

66. Fishbein W: Disruptive effects of rapid eye movement sleep deprivation on long-term memory. Physiol Behav 1971;6:279.

67. Fishbein W, Kastaniotis C, Chattman D: Paradoxical sleep: Prolonged augmentation following learning. Brain Res 1974;71:61.

68. McGrath MJ, Cohen DB: REM sleep facilitation of adaptive waking behavior: A review of the literature. Psychol Bull 1978;85:24.

69. Hawkins MR, Vichick DA, Silsby HD, et al: Sleep and nutritional deprivation and performance of house officers. J Med Educ 1985;60:530.

70. Paul K, Dittrichova J: Sleep patterns following learning in infants. In Levin P, Koella U (eds): Sleep 1974. Basel, S Karger, 1975, p 388.

71. Parkes JD: Sleep and Its Disorders. London, WB Saunders, 1985.

72. Hartman E: The Functions of Sleep. New Haven, Yale University Press, 1976.

73. Ron S, Algom D, Hary D, et al: Time-related changes in the distribution of sleep stages in brain injured patients. Electroencephalogr Clin Neurophysiol 1980;48:432.

74. Greenberg R, Dewan EM: Aphasia and rapid eye movement sleep. Nature 1969;223:183.

75. Feinberg I: Eye movement activity during sleep and intellectual function in mental retardation. Science 1968;159:1256.

76. Oksenberg A, Marks J, Farberk K, et al: Effect of REM sleep deprivation during the critical period of neuroanatomical development of the cat visual system. Sleep Res 1986;15:53.

77. Squire LR: Memory and the Brain. New York, Oxford University Press, 1987.

78. Kohonen T: Associative Memory. New York, Springer-Verlag, 1977.

79. Palm G: Neural Assemblies: An Alternative Approach to Artificial Intelligence. New York, Springer-Verlag, 1982.

80. Crick F, Mitchison G: The function of dream sleep. Nature 1983;304:111.

81. Hopfield JJ, Feinstein DI, Palmer RG: 'Unlearning' has a stabilizing effect in collective memories. Nature 1983;304:158.

82. Kleitman N: Sleep and Wakefulness. Chicago, University of Chicago Press, 1963.

83. Webb WB: The sleep of conjoined twins. Sleep 1978;1:205.

84. Moldofsky H, Scarisbrick P: Induction of neurasthenic musculoskeletal pain syndrome by selective sleep stage deprivation. Psychosom Med 1976;38:35.

85. Nicholson AN, Marks J: Insomnia. Lancaster, MTP, 1983.

86. Marsden CD: 'On-off' phenomenon in Parkinson's disease. In Rinne UK, Klinger M, Stamm G (eds): Parkinson's Disease—Current Progress, Problems and Management. Amsterdam, Elsevier/North Holland, 1980.

87. Segawa M, Hosaka A, Miyagawa F, et al: Hereditary progressive dystonia with marked diurnal fluctuation. Adv Neurol 1976;14:215.

88. Rechtschaffen A, Gilliland MA, Bergmann BM, et al: Physiological correlates of prolonged sleep deprivation in rats. Science 1983;221:182.

89. Passouant P, Popoviciu L, Velok G, et al: [Polygraphic study of narcolepsy during the nycthemeral period.] Rev Neurol (Paris) 1968;118:431.

90. Kales A, Tan TL, Kollar EG, et al: Sleep patterns following 205 hours of sleep deprivation. Psychosom Med 1970;32:189.

91. Glenville M, Broughton R, Wing AM, et al: Effects of sleep deprivation on short duration performance measures compared to the Wilkinson auditory vigilance task. Sleep 1978;1:169.

92. Horne JA, Anderson NR, Wilkinson RT: Effects of sleep deprivation on signal detection measures of vigilance: Implications for sleep function. Sleep 1983;6:347.

93. Williams HL, Hammack JT, Daly RL, et al: Responses to auditory stimulation, sleep loss and the EEG stages of sleep. Electroencephalogr Clin Neurophysiol 1964;16:269.

94. Webb WB, Agnew HW Jr: The effect of a chronic limitation of sleep length. Psychophysiology 1974;11:265.

95. Dement W, Greenberg S: Changes in total amount of stage four sleep as a function of partial sleep deprivation. Electroencephalogr Clin Neurophysiol 1966;20:523.

96. Carskadon MA, Harvey K, Dement WC: Acute restriction of nocturnal sleep in children. Percept Motor Skills 1981;53:103.

97. Wilkinson RT: Sleep Deprivation: Performance tests for partial and selective sleep deprivation. In Apt LE, Riess BF (eds): Progress in Clinical Psychology, vol 8. New York, Grune & Stratton, 1968, pp 28-33.

98. Dement WC: Sleep deprivation and organization of the behavioral states. In Clemente C, Purpura D, Mayer F (eds): Sleep and the Maturing Nervous System. New York, Academic Press, 1972.

99. Armington JC, Mitnick LL: Electroencephalogram and sleep deprivation. J Appl Physiol 1959;14:247.

100. Williams H, Lubin A, Goodnow J: Impaired performance with acute sleep loss. Psychol Monog 1959;73:1.

101. Friedman L, Bergmann BM, Rechtschaffen A: Effects of sleep deprivation on sleepiness, sleep intensity, and subsequent sleep in the rat. Sleep 1979;1:369.

102. Cartwright RD: A Primer on Sleep and Dreaming. Reading, MA, Addison-Wesley, 1978.

103. Zepelin H: Mammalian sleep. In Kryger MH, Roth T, Dement WC (eds): Principles and Practice of Sleep Medicine (3rd ed), Philadelphia, WB Saunders Company, 2000, pp 82-92.

104. Tobler I: Phylogeny of sleep regulation. In Kryger MH, Roth T, Dement WC (eds): Principles and Practice of Sleep Medicine (3rd ed), Philadelphia, WB Saunders Company, 2000, pp 72-81.

105. Meddis R: The evolution of sleep. In Mayes A (ed): Sleep Mechanisms and Function in Humans and Animals: An Evolutionary Perspective. Berkshire, England, Van Nostrand Reinhold (UK), 1983.

106. Allison T, Van Twyver H: The evolution of sleep. Nat Hist 1970;79:56.

107. Jouvet-Mounier D, Astic L, Lacote D: Ontogenesis of the states of sleep in rat, cat, and guinea pig during the first postnatal month. Dev Psychobiol 1970;2:216.

108. Noback CR, Purpura DP: Postnatal ontogenesis of neurons in cat neocortex. J Comp Neurol 1961;117:291.

109. Peters HG, Bademan H: The form and growth of stellate cells in the cortex of the guinea pig. J Anat 1963;97:111-117.

110. Mukhametov LM: Sleep in marine mammals. Exp Brain Res 1984;8:227.

111. Konorski J: Integrative Action of the Brain. Chicago, University of Chicago Press, 1967.

112. Gastaut H, Bert B: Electroencephalographic detection of sleep induced by repetitive sensory stimuli. In Wolstenholme GEW, O'Connor M (eds): On the Nature of Sleep. London, Churchill, 1961, p 260.

113. Bremer F: Quelques proprietes de l'activite electrique du cortex cerebral "isole." CR Soc Biol (Paris) 1935;118:1241.

114. French JD, Magoun HW: Effects of chronic lesions in central cephalic brain stem of monkeys. Arch Neurol Psychiatry 1952;69:591.

115. Lindsley DB, Bowden JW, Magoun HW: Effect upon the EEG of acute injury to the brain stem activating system. Electroencephalogr Clin Neurophysiol 1949;1:475.

116. Moruzzi G: The sleep-waking cycle. Ergeb Physiol 1972;64:1.

117. Jones BE: Basic mechanisms of sleep-wake states. In Kryger MH, Roth T, Dement WC: Principles and Practice of Sleep Medicine. Philadelphia, WB Saunders, 1989, p 121.

118. Barini C, et al: Effects of complete pontine transections of the sleep-wakefulness rhythm: The midpontine pretrigeminal preparation. Arch Ital Biol 1959;97:1.

119. Freemon FR, Salinas-Garcia RF, Ward JW: Sleep patterns in a patient with a brain stem infarction involving the raphe nucleus. Electroencephalogr Clin Neurophysiol 1974;36:657.

120. Westmoreland BF, Klass DW, Sharbrough FW, et al: Alpha-coma. Electroencephalographic, clinical, pathologic, and etiologic correlations. Arch Neurol 1975;32:713.

121. Nauta WJH: Hypothalamic regulation of sleep in rats: An experimental study. J Neurophysiol 1946;9:285.

122. Morison RS, Dempsey EW: A study of thalamocortical relations J Physiol 1942;135:281.

123. Hanada Y, Kawamura H: Sleep-waking electrocorticographic rhythms in chronic cerveau isolé rats. Physiol Behav 1981;26:725.

124. Jouvet M: Paradoxical sleep: A study of its nature and mechanisms. In Himwich WA, Schade JP (eds): Sleep Mechanisms: Progress in Brain Research. Amsterdam, Elsevier, 1965.

125. Hobson JA: The cellular basis of sleep cycle control. Adv Sleep Res 1974;1:217.

Differential Diagnosis of Pediatric Sleep Disorders

2

Meir H. Kryger

Children do not usually complain of sleep problems. An adult, most often a parent or another caregiver, usually initiates the medical evaluation. The major presentations of sleep disorders are insomnia, hypersomnia, and abnormal behaviors during sleep. This chapter will review the differential diagnosis of sleep disorders in children, using as a framework the International Classification of Sleep Disorders.[1]

Insomnia, hypersomnia, and abnormal movements are not simply features of sleep disorders but may provide a clue that an unsuspected medical problem is present. For example, insomnia may be an important clue to the presence of pinworm[2] or iron deficiency[3]. Hypersomnia can be a clue that the tonsils and adenoids are enlarged,[4-6] which may be the cause of cardiac failure.[7]

What Is the Problem? Whose Problem Is It?

Children with sleep disorders seldom bring their disorder to the attention of clinicians directly. Sleep disorders in children are usually suspected because of an observation (for example, of snoring, apnea, behavioral changes) by others. Therefore, the evaluation of a child's sleep must include an interview with the caregiver and a review of the symptoms and behaviors as they affect the patient and the family unit.

Frequently, there is no medical problem at all, but the expectations of the parent or caregiver are inappropriate. For example, a sleepless couple might bring in their 3-month-old child wondering why the child does not sleep through the night and explaining that this is interfering with their own nocturnal sleep. The problem here is

that the parents are not aware of what is normal. Thus, clinicians must know what is normal and what is expected, and they must transmit this to the parents. What is normal in the child can result in a problem for the parents when their work quality suffers as a result of their baby waking up at night.

At times, sleeplessness in a child may be the result of problems in the family (a severe illness in a parent, or marital problems). Thus, in evaluating a child for a sleep disorder, the clinician must ascertain the following: What is the sleep problem? Whose problem is it? What is the cause of the problem?

Children present to clinicians with three types of sleep-related problems. First are the insomnias—disorders of initiating and maintaining sleep; second are the hypersomnias—disorders in which the child sleeps at the wrong time and the wrong place and has excessive sleepiness; and third is abnormal activity or behaviors during sleep. A child may have symptoms that fall into more than one category. This chapter focuses on the most commonly seen disorders.

INSOMNIA

Insomnia is a symptom that reflects a perception, by the patient or the caregiver, that it takes too long to fall asleep or that it is difficult to maintain sleep. Terms such as *sleeplessness, insomnia,* and *restlessness* may be the actual words used. Different people may notice different clinical features. For example, the parent of a child may comment on the child's nocturnal difficulties, whereas the school teacher might notice that the sleep-deprived child falls asleep in class or demonstrates features of hyperactivity.

Children can have disorders in any of the major categories listed in Table 2–1. The clinician

This work was supported by National Institutes of Health grant R01 HL63342-01A1.

Table 2–1. Sleep Disorders in Children

ICD-9-CM	ICD-10-CM	Sleep Disorder (Alternate or Other Commonly Used Name)
Insomnia: Problems Falling Asleep and Staying Asleep*		
307.42	F51.01	Psychophysiological Insomnia (conditioned insomnia)
307.42	F51.02	Paradoxical Insomnia (sleep state misperception)
307.41	F51.03	Adjustment Sleep Disorder (transient insomnia)
307.41	F51.04	Inadequate Sleep Hygiene
780.52	G47.01	Idiopathic Insomnia (childhood onset insomnia)
307.42	F51.05	Behavioral Insomnia of Childhood (sleep onset association disorder)
780.52	G47.09	Insomnia due to other known condition
291.89	F10-19	Insomnia due to substance abuse
995.2	T36-50	Insomnia due to adverse drug effect
307.42	F51.09	Insomnia due to psychiatric/behavioral condition
Sleep-Related Breathing Disorder: EDS and/or Restless Sleep†		
780.51	G47.31	Primary Central Sleep Apnea
770.81	P28.3	Primary Sleep Apnea of Infancy (infant sleep apnea)
780.53	G47.32	Obstructive Sleep Apnea, Pediatric
780.53	G47.0	Sleep-Related Breathing Disorder due to cardiorespiratory disease
780.57	G47.34	Sleep Related Non-obstructive Alveolar Hypoventilation (central alveolar hypoventilation)
780.57	G47.35	Congenital Central Alveolar Hypoventilation Syndrome
Hypersomnia Not Due to a Sleep-Related Breathing Disorder: EDS‡		
347.01	G47.41	Narcolepsy with Cataplexy
347.00	G47.42	Narcolepsy without Cataplexy
780.54	G47.11	Recurrent Hypersomnia (Kleine-Levin syndrome)
780.54	G47.12	Idiopathic Hypersomnia with long sleep time
780.54	G47.13	Idiopathic Hypersomnia without long sleep time
307.44	F51.11	Behaviorally-Induced Insufficient Sleep Syndrome
995.2	F10-19	Other Hypersomnia due to substance abuse
995.2	T36-50	Other Hypersomnia due to the adverse effects of a drug
307.44	F51.19	Hypersomnia due to psychiatric/behavioral condition
Circadian Rhythm Sleep Disorder: EDS and/or Problems Falling Asleep and Staying Asleep§		
PRIMARY		
780.55	G47.21	Delayed sleep phase type (delayed sleep phase syndrome)
780 55	G47.22	Advanced sleep phase type (advanced sleep phase syndrome)
780.55	G47.23	Irregular sleep-wake type
780.55	G47.24	Non-entrained type
780.55	G47.20	Other Primary Circadian Rhythm Sleep Disorder due to a known physiological condition
BEHAVIORALLY INDUCED		
307.45	F51.21	Jet-lag type
307.45	F51.22	Shift-work type
291.89	F10-19	Circadian Rhythm Disorders due to substance abuse
995.2	T36-50	Circadian Rhythm Sleep Disorders due to adverse drug effect
Parasomnia: History of Abnormal Sleep-Related Behavior¶¶		
780.56	G47.51	Confusional Arousals
307.46	F51.3	Sleepwalking
307.46	F51.4	Sleep Terrors
780.56	G47.52	REM Sleep Behavior Disorder, including Parasomnia Overlap Disorder
780 56	G47.53	Recurrent Isolated Sleep Paralysis
307.47	F51.5	Nightmare Disorder

Table 2–1.	Sleep Disorders in Children—Cont'd	
300.15	F44.9	Nocturnal Dissociative Disorder
788.36	N39.44	Sleep-related Enuresis
780.56	G47.59	Parasomnia due to substance abuse
307.47	F51.39	Parasomnia due to psychiatric disorders

Sleep-Related Movement Disorder: Problems Initiating or Maintaining Sleep, Excessive Sleep Movements, or EDS[¶]

333.99	G47.61	Restless Legs Syndrome
780.58	G47.62	Periodic Limb Movement Disorder
780.58	G47.63	Sleep-Related Leg Cramps
780.58	G47.64	Sleep-Related Bruxism
780.58	G47.65	Sleep-Related Rhythmic Movement Disorder (body rocking, head banging)

Isolated Symptoms, Apparently Normal Variants, and Unresolved Issues

307.49	R29.81	Long Sleeper
307.49	R29.81	Short Sleeper
786.09	R06.5	Snoring
307.49	R29.81	Sleeptalking
781.01	R25.8	Sleep Starts, Hypnagogic Jerks
781.01	R25.8	Benign Sleep Myoclonus of Infancy

*See Chapter 11.
†See Chapters 17 to 23.
‡See Chapters 13 to 16.
§See Chapters 8 and 9.
¶¶See Chapters 25 to 27.
¶See Chapter 26.
EDS, excessive daytime sleepiness; ICD-9-CM, International Classification of Diseases, Ninth Edition, Clinical Modification; ICD-10-CM: International Classification of Diseases, Tenth Edition, Clinical Modification.

decides which ones are most likely to be encountered and pursues a diagnosis.

Behavioral and Psychophysiologic Disorders

Some behavioral and psychophysiologic disorders occur in children but not in adults. In limit-setting sleep disorders, for example, caregivers may complain that children make persistent "curtain calls" or refuse to go to sleep. In sleep-onset association disorders, caregivers may complain that the child cries during sleep unless the adult rocks the child or sleeps with the child. The children are either too young to articulate the problem or do not see the behavior as a problem.

Psychiatric Disorders

Children can have almost any of the major psychiatric disorders. Insomnia may be caused by the psychiatric disorder itself[8] or by treatment for the disorder.[9] For example, antidepressants may lead to difficulty in falling asleep or to increased movements during sleep (see "Drug Use and Abuse," later).

Although psychiatric disorders may indeed cause sleep problems, equally important is the potential misdiagnosis of a sleep disorder as a psychiatric disorder[10,11] or even as epilepsy.[12] For example, patients who were initially diagnosed as having schizophrenia have been subsequently found to have narcolepsy.[11] Their very vivid and sometimes frightening hypnagogic hallucinations were misinterpreted to be psychotic hallucinations. Adults with narcolepsy can usually differentiate dreamlike imagery as being "unreal," but children with narcolepsy may be unable to determine whether the hypnagogic hallucinations were "real" (i.e., a hallucination that appeared to be real) or dreams. Similarly, children may be diagnosed as having depression when in fact they have sleepiness that results from a sleep disorder such as one of the movement disorders.

Drug Use and Abuse

A great number of children are being treated with medications that can cause insomnia. These medications might include stimulants (as used for the treatment of attention-deficit/hyperactivity disorder[13]) or antidepressants.[9] The use of alerting illicit drugs must also be assessed.[14] The clinician seeing teenagers should be aware of the illicit drugs being used in the community that might lead to insomnia and other sleep complaints. Thus, if a parent brings a teenager for assessment who has had a personality change and perhaps weight loss, and who has to have clothes laundered frequently because of obvious and increased perspiration, use of drugs such as 3,4-methylenedioxymethamphetamine (MDMA, "Ecstasy") should be considered. Such children may also have restless legs syndrome and insomnia.[15]

Sleep-Induced Respiratory Impairment

Insomnia appears to be a rare manifestation of sleep breathing disorders in children. Caregivers may complain that the child is "restless" and moving a great deal, but insomnia per se is unusual. On the other hand, children with disorders such as asthma, or those with chronic conditions such as cystic fibrosis who may cough a great deal, may have difficulty in initiating and maintaining sleep because of their underlying respiratory disorder.

Movement Disorders

Movement disorders such as restless legs syndrome and periodic movements in sleep occur in children and may cause severe insomnia. As in the adult, the disorder may be secondary—for example, caused by a reduction in iron stores.[3] Surprisingly, other movement disorders—for example, head banging or body rocking (rhythmic sleep disorders)—are less likely to appear with insomnia than might be expected. Patients with the rhythmic sleep disorders are often brought to the physician's attention by a caregiver who is quite concerned about the hazards they believe might be caused by the sometimes vigorous movements.

When a child is suspected or proven to have a movement disorder, especially restless legs syndrome, it is worthwhile to determine whether a reduction in iron stores exists.[3] Serum ferritin, iron, and iron-binding capacity should be measured. A screening complete blood count is not adequate to exclude reduction in iron stores. If reduced levels of iron stores are confirmed, then the source of the iron loss should be determined. Poor diet, blood loss from menses, or blood loss from the gastrointestinal tract should be explored. If gastrointestinal symptoms are present, the clinician should screen for disorders that may cause malabsorption, such as celiac disease.

Disorders of Timing in the Sleep–Wake Cycle

Parents of very young children may believe that a sleep–wake cycle timing problem is present, but frequently this results from unreasonable expectations about the children's sleep—in particular, about when they should be able to sleep through the night.

Teenagers may develop the delayed sleep phase disorder. Patients with this disorder go to bed but are not able to fall asleep until very late. When allowed to sleep in, they will sleep in until lunchtime or later. They have a great deal of difficulty getting out of bed in the morning—for example, to go to school. This diagnosis is really one of exclusion, and it is important that the clinician determine that other causes of difficulty in falling asleep are not present—for example, a movement disorder, the use of stimulants, or playing video games and listening to music late into the night. One should also exclude depression and a pattern of school avoidance.

Children with blindness or neurologic damage may have a timing problem related to their not being able to use the retinohypothalamic pathways to synchronize their sleep–wake cycle to the 24-hour day.[16]

Parasomnias

Sleepwalking, confusional arousals, sleep terrors, and sleeptalking do not necessarily, by themselves, cause insomnia. In fact, they usually do not. However, a child may develop a fear of falling asleep after such an episode has occurred. This can be quite distressing. For example, a child who is known to sleepwalk a great deal may be unable to fall asleep when at a friend's house for fear of having a sleepwalking episode.

Central Nervous System Disorders

Diseases involving the central nervous system may cause insomnia. It is probably prudent to include in this category disorders such as autism, which may result in the child often being awake and active at night.[17,18] As is often the case for childhood sleeping disorders, it is seldom the child who complains of the problem but the caregiver.

HYPERSOMNIA

Disorders of hypersomnia result in excessive sleepiness when the child should be wide awake and alert. Sleepiness has many faces in children, ranging from the inability to stay awake (even falling asleep in school) to what can best be described as hyperactivity and the inability to sit still and focus in school. In some cases, sleepiness is apparent because the child falls asleep at the wrong time and in the wrong place. In other cases, the teacher complains that the child is daydreaming and cannot focus.

Two disorders of excessive daytime sleepiness (EDS) require special attention: those that lead to sleep breathing disorders and those that affect the central nervous system. These disorders are frequently missed by clinicians. Several categories of disorders that cause daytime sleepiness are identical to categories of disorders that are associated with insomnia.

Behavioral and Psychophysiologic Disorders

Any of the disorders that cause insomnia, if they lead to a sufficient loss of nocturnal sleep, can result in daytime sleepiness. Thus, the teenager who falls asleep at 4 AM because of a delayed sleep phase is likely to fall asleep in class and may present with a clinical problem of excessive daytime sleepiness.

Some disorders, however, result in daytime sleepiness even though the child has apparently been in bed and asleep for an acceptable number of hours. Thus, the clinician and the parent should know the normal nocturnal sleep times for children of various ages. The author has evaluated 10-year-old children for EDS whose parents believed it was normal for a child of that age to sleep 7 hours per night, whereas 9 to 11 hours is more appropriate.

Psychiatric Disorders

Several major psychiatric disorders, or the drugs used to treat them, can cause daytime sleepiness. In particular, depression has this effect.

Drug Dependency

The use of licit and illicit drugs must be considered in children with hypersomnias. The clinician should be aware of what drugs are being used in the community.

Sleep-Induced Respiratory Impairment

Obstructive sleep apnea syndrome and its variants lead to excessive daytime sleepiness because of the increased number of arousals during the night. Several issues in children are worth attention. In adults, the main cause of sleep breathing disorders is obesity, but in children it is enlarged tonsils and adenoids. Obese children, however, can develop obstructive sleep apnea syndrome that is indistinguishable from that in adults.[19,20] Arterial hypertension may be caused by sleep apnea in a child.[21] Loud and disruptive snoring in the child with documented daytime sleepiness should be evaluated as a probable case of a sleep breathing disorder. In children, retrognathia and micrognathia can also lead to sleep breathing disorders. Thus, an examination of the upper airway is absolutely critical in the child with excessive daytime sleepiness. Sleepiness in children with obstructive sleep apnea syndrome has been misinterpreted as a feature of depression. Sleep apnea can occur in children of any age.

Sleep breathing abnormalities should be suspected in children if they have the symptoms typically seen in adults (snoring, sleepiness), and it should also be suspected in children with awake hypoventilation, growth retardation, and certain congenital disorders.

Hypoventilation

Children with congenital central hypoventilation syndrome have symptoms that may be similar to those in children with obstructive sleep apnea syndrome.[22-24] Obstructive sleep apnea caused by adenotonsillar hypertrophy may complicate congenital central hypoventilation syndrome[24] and chronic lung diseases. Any sleep breathing disorder that causes hypoventilation may result in pulmonary hypertension, cor pulmonale, and polycythemia.[25,26]

Growth Retardation

Growth retardation may be present in newborns whose mothers had a sleep breathing disorder.[27,28] Growth retardation is a feature of sleep breathing disorders in children of any age.[6,29-32]

Congenital Disorders

Congenital diseases including myopathies,[33,34] muscular dystrophies,[34] neurologic disorders that might affect the system controlling breathing, and disorders resulting in facial skeletal abnormalities or soft tissue abnormalities of the upper airway can all result in sleep breathing disorders.[14,15,35-38]

Movement Disorders

Children with movement disorders may be quite sleepy during the daytime. This is in contrast to adults, in whom excessive daytime sleepiness may not be a prominent symptom with movement disorders.

Disorders of Timing of the Sleep–Wake Pattern

A patient who has non–24-hour sleep–wake syndrome, or the child who is asleep almost all the time or who has a completely random sleep–wake schedule, may have a mass lesion in the central nervous system.

Central Nervous System Abnormality

Just as abnormalities of the central nervous system can lead to insomnia, some also lead to excessive daytime sleepiness. Narcolepsy is a disorder that is frequently missed because most clinicians do not take the time to ask about a patient's sleep. In fact, in some series, it took over 15 years from the onset of symptoms before the diagnosis of narcolepsy was first made.[39] Many patients who are ultimately diagnosed with narcolepsy have previously been diagnosed with a psychiatric condition, frequently depression. Similarly, patients with the obstructive sleep apnea syndrome are often diagnosed with depression.

Some disorders that result in excessive daytime sleepiness because of involvement of the hypothalamic areas of the nervous system also lead to excessive weight gain, which may then cause sleepiness (e.g., obstructive sleep apnea). This may be the situation, for example, in Asperger's syndrome or Kleine-Levin syndrome.

ABNORMAL SLEEP-RELATED BEHAVIORS

Children with abnormal movements and behaviors seldom complain about them. It is usually others who notice the abnormalities, which range from the merely annoying (the chipmunk-like noises of patients with sleep bruxism) to episodes of sleep terrors that are frightening to the observer. Some of these disorders can cause the child a great deal of embarrassment (e.g., sleep enuresis). Although some of the disorders in this category are not serious, they can cause the patient a great deal of distress.

Behavioral or Psychophysiologic Disorders

The parent may complain about a child's wandering at night, making frequent curtain calls, or wanting to sleep in the parental bed. These "disorders" can be disruptive to the family.

Table 2–2. Examples of Complex Syndromes Associated with Sleep Disorders

Syndrome or Disease	Sleep Abnormality
Achondroplasia	Sleep breathing disorders[40,41]
Asperger's syndrome	Hypersomnia, sleep breathing disorders[42-44]
Autism	Insomnia[17,18]
Chiari malformation	Sleep breathing disorder[45]
Down syndrome	Sleep breathing disorders[26,46-49]
Hirschsprung's disease	Sleep breathing disorders[50]
Mucopolysaccharide storage disorders	Sleep breathing disorders[51,52]
Pierre Robin	Sleep breathing disorder[36-38,53]
Prader-Willi	Sleep Breathing disorder[54]
Syringomyelia	Sleep breathing disorder[55]

Movement Disorders

Rhythmic movement disorders (e.g., head-banging) are surprisingly common in children. These disorders are brought to the clinician's attention usually not because of any symptom but because the parent assumes that the sometimes violent movements must be associated with abnormal pathology.

Parasomnias

Parasomnias are extremely common in children. Disorders such as night terrors, sleepwalking, and enuresis can be quite disruptive to the family and cause a great deal of embarrassment for the patient. It is important to differentiate such movements from sleep-related epilepsy (see later).

Central Nervous System Disorders

Severe disorders of the neurologic system, including seizures, may result in abnormal sleep-related behaviors. A sleep behavior that is very stereotypic and almost always the same should alert the clinician to the possibility of a seizure disorder.

SLEEP DISORDERS IN OTHER CLINICAL SYNDROMES

When patients have complex clinical syndromes, a sleep disorder is sometimes overlooked. Table 2–2 gives examples of some complex disorders that have been associated with sleep disorders. Sometimes, treating the sleep disorder can result

in quite substantial clinical improvement. Some clinicians are reluctant to consider a sleep-related diagnosis in patients with, for example, Down syndrome, because of their belief that nothing can be done for sleep disorders in such patients. However, some patients with Down syndrome can do extremely well with treatment for their sleep disorders.

CONCLUSION

Children referred for sleep disorders may not have a sleep disorder at all: the problem may be that the caregiver does not understand normal sleep in children. Some children who are referred for sleep disorders may have a serious condition (e.g., obstructive sleep apnea) that can be treated. If they have a movement disorder caused by an iron deficiency, they can be cured. Children with narcolepsy, on the other hand, will require lifelong management to function normally. Children with sleep disorders require a detailed review of clinical features and a detailed assessment to optimize their management.

References

1. Diagnostic Classification Steering Committee: International Classification of Sleep Disorders: Diagnostic and Coding Manual. Chicago, Ill, American Academy of Sleep Medicine, 2004.
2. St Georgiev V: Chemotherapy of enterobiasis (oxyuriasis). Expert Opin Pharmacother 2001; 2:267-275.
3. Kryger MH, Otake K, Foerster J: Low body stores of iron and restless legs syndrome: A correctable cause of insomnia in adolescents and teenagers. Sleep Med 2002;3:127-132.

4. Lind MG, Lundell BP: Tonsillar hyperplasia in children: A cause of obstructive sleep apneas, CO_2 retention, and retarded growth. Arch Otolaryngol 1982;108:650-654.

5. Mangat D, Orr WC, Smith RO: Sleep apnea, hypersomnolence, and upper airway obstruction secondary to adenotonsillar enlargement. Arch Otolaryngol 1977;103:383-386.

6. Nimubona L, Jokic M, Moreau S, et al: Obstructive sleep apnea syndrome and hypertrophic tonsils in infants [in French]. Arch Pediatr 2000;7:961-964.

7. Ramakrishna S, Ingle VS, Patel S, et al: Reversible cardio-pulmonary changes due to adeno-tonsillar hypertrophy. Int J Pediatr Otorhinolaryngol 2000; 55:203-206.

8. Doghramji PP: Detection of insomnia in primary care. J Clin Psychiatry 2001;62(Suppl 10):18-26.

9. Rosenberg DR, Stewart CM, Fitzgerald KD, et al: Paroxetine open-label treatment of pediatric outpatients with obsessive-compulsive disorder. J Am Acad Child Adolesc Psychiatry 1999; 38:1180-1185.

10. Daniels E, King MA, Smith IE, Shneerson JM: Health-related quality of life in narcolepsy. J Sleep Res 2001;10:75-81.

11. Douglass AB, Hays P, Pazderka F, Russell JM: Florid refractory schizophrenias that turn out to be treatable variants of HLA-associated narcolepsy. J Nerv Ment Dis 1991;179:12-17.

12. Zeman A, Douglas N, Aylward R: Lesson of the week: Narcolepsy mistaken for epilepsy. BMJ 2001; 322:216-218.

13. Efron D, Jarman F, Barker M: Side effects of methylphenidate and dexamphetamine in children with attention deficit hyperactivity disorder: A double-blind, crossover trial. Pediatrics 1997; 100:662-666.

14. Gahlinger PM: Club drugs: MDMA, gamma-hydroxybutyrate (GHB), Rohypnol, and ketamine. Am Fam Physician 2004;69:2619-2626.

15. Vollenweider FX, Gamma A, Liechti M, Huber T: Psychological and cardiovascular effects and short-term sequelae of MDMA ("ecstasy") in MDMA-naive healthy volunteers. Neuropsychopharmacology 1998;19:241-251.

16. Lapierre O, Dumont M: Melatonin treatment of a non-24-hour sleep-wake cycle in a blind retarded child. Biol Psychiatry 1995;38:119-122.

17. Posey DJ, McDougle CJ: The pharmacotherapy of target symptoms associated with autistic disorder and other pervasive developmental disorders. Harv Rev Psychiatry 2000;8:45-63.

18. Richdale AL, Prior MR: The sleep/wake rhythm in children with autism. Eur Child Adolesc Psychiatry 1995;4:175-186.

19. Daniels SR: Obesity in the pediatric patient: Cardiovascular complications. Prog Pediatr Cardiol 2001;12:161-167.

20. Slyper AH: Childhood obesity, adipose tissue distribution, and the pediatric practitioner. Pediatrics 1998;102:e4.

21. Marcus CL, Greene MG, Carroll JL: Blood pressure in children with obstructive sleep apnea. Am J Respir Crit Care Med 1998;157:1098-1103.

22. Silvestri JM, Weese-Mayer DE, Nelson MN: Neuropsychologic abnormalities in children with congenital central hypoventilation syndrome. J Pediatr 1992;120:388-393.

23. Seid AB, Martin PJ, Pransky SM, Kearns DB: Surgical therapy of obstructive sleep apnea in children with severe mental insufficiency. Laryngoscope 1990;100:507-510.

24. Kurz H, Sterniste W, Dremsek P: Resolution of obstructive sleep apnea syndrome after adenoidectomy in congenital central hypoventilation syndrome. Pediatr Pulmonol 1999;27:341-346.

25. Freed D: Pulmonary hypertension in children who snore. Br Med J (Clin Res Ed) 1981;283:231.

26. Levine OR, Simpser M: Alveolar hypoventilation and cor pulmonale associated with chronic airway obstruction in infants with Down syndrome. Clin Pediatr (Phila) 1982;21:25-29.

27. Harding SM: Complications and consequences of obstructive sleep apnea. Curr Opin Pulm Med 2000;6:485-489.

28. Franklin KA, Holmgren PA, Jonsson F, et al: Snoring, pregnancy-induced hypertension, and growth retardation of the fetus. Chest 2000; 117:137-141.

29. Trachtenberg DE, Golemon TB: Office care of the premature infant: Part II. Common medical and surgical problems. Am Fam Physician 1998; 57:2383-2390, 2400-2402.

30. Commare MC, Francois B, Estournet B, Barois A: Ondine's curse: A discussion of five cases. Neuropediatrics 1993;24:313-318.

31. Breton D, Morisseau-Durand MP, Cheron G: Growth retardation and obstructive sleep apnea in infants. Arch Fr Pediatr 1993;50:493-496.

32. Stradling JR, Thomas G, Warley AR, et al: Effect of adenotonsillectomy on nocturnal hypoxaemia, sleep disturbance, and symptoms in snoring children. Lancet 1990;335:249-253.

33. Sasaki M, Takeda M, Kobayashi K, Nonaka I: Respiratory failure in nemaline myopathy. Pediatr Neurol 1997;16:344-346.

34. Khan Y, Heckmatt JZ, Dubowitz V: Sleep studies and supportive ventilatory treatment in patients with congenital muscle disorders. Arch Dis Child 1996;74:195-200.

35. Cohen SR, Ross DA, Burstein FD, et al: Skeletal expansion combined with soft-tissue reduction in the treatment of obstructive sleep apnea in children: Physiologic results. Otolaryngol Head Neck Surg 1998;119:476-485.

36. Kiely JL, Deegan PC, McNicholas WT: Resolution of obstructive sleep apnoea with growth in the Robin sequence. Eur Respir J 1998;12:499-501.

37. Tomaski SM, Zalzal GH, Saal HM: Airway obstruction in the Pierre Robin sequence. Laryngoscope 1995;105:111-114.

38. Reimao R, Papaiz EG, Papaiz LF: Pierre Robin sequence and obstructive sleep apnea. Arq Neuro-psiquiatr 1994;52:554-559.

39. Broughton RJ, Fleming JA, George CF, et al: Randomized, double-blind, placebo-controlled crossover trial of modafinil in the treatment of excessive daytime sleepiness in narcolepsy. Neurology 1997;49:444-451.

40. Tasker RC, Dundas I, Laverty A, et al: Distinct patterns of respiratory difficulty in young children with achondroplasia: A clinical, sleep, and lung function study. Arch Dis Child 1998;79:99-108.

41. Mogayzel PJ Jr, Carroll JL, Loughlin GM, et al: Sleep-disordered breathing in children with achondroplasia. J Pediatr 1998;132:667-671.

42. Godbout R, Bergeron C, Limoges E, et al: A laboratory study of sleep in Asperger's syndrome. Neuroreport 2000;11:127-130.

43. Patzold LM, Richdale AL, Tonge BJ: An investigation into sleep characteristics of children with autism and Asperger's disorder. J Paediatr Child Health 1998;34:528-533.

44. Berthier ML, Santamaria J, Encabo H, Tolosa ES: Recurrent hypersomnia in two adolescent males with Asperger's syndrome. J Am Acad Child Adolesc Psychiatry 1992;31:735-738.

45. Frim DM, Jones D, Goumnerova L: Development of symptomatic Chiari malformation in a child with craniofacial dysmorphism. Pediatr Neurosurg 1990-91;16:228-231.

46. Jacobs IN, Gray RF, Todd NW: Upper airway obstruction in children with Down syndrome. Arch Otolaryngol Head Neck Surg 1996;122:945-950.

47. Hultcrantz E, Svanholm H: Down syndrome and sleep apnea: A therapeutic challenge. Int J Pediatr Otorhinolaryngol 1991;21:263-268.

48. Kasian GF, Duncan WJ, Tyrrell MJ, Oman-Ganes LA: Elective oro-tracheal intubation to diagnose sleep apnea syndrome in children with Down's syndrome and ventricular septal defect. Can J Cardiol 1987;3:2-5.

49. Hoch B, Barth H: Cheyne-Stokes respiration as an additional risk factor for pulmonary hypertension in a boy with trisomy 21 and atrioventricular septal defect. Pediatr Pulmonol 2001;31:261-264.

50. Stern M, Hellwege HH, Gravinghoff L, Lambrecht W: Total aganglionosis of the colon (Hirschsprung's disease) and congenital failure of automatic control of ventilation (Ondine's curse). Acta Paediatr Scand 1981;70:121-124.

51. Kurihara M, Kumagai K, Goto K, et al: Severe type Hunter's syndrome: Polysomnographic and neuropathological study. Neuropediatrics 1992;23:248-256.

52. Semenza GL, Pyeritz RE: Respiratory complications of mucopolysaccharide storage disorders. Medicine (Baltimore) 1988;67:209-219.

53. Clift S, Dahlitz M, Parkes JD: Sleep apnoea in the Prader-Willi syndrome. J Sleep Res 1994;3:121-126.

54. Doshi A, Udwadia Z: Prader-Willi syndrome with sleep disordered breathing: Effect of two years' nocturnal CPAP. Indian J Chest Dis Allied Sci 2001;43:51-53.

55. Pasterkamp H, Cardoso ER, Booth FA: Obstructive sleep apnea leading to increased intracranial pressure in a patient with hydrocephalus and syringomyelia. Chest 1989;95:1064-1067.

Epidemiology of Sleep Disorders during Childhood

3

Judith Owens

NORMAL SLEEP PATTERNS AND BEHAVIOR

Relatively few large-scale epidemiologic studies have been performed to systematically define normal sleep and wakefulness patterns and sleep duration in infants, children, and adolescents. Of those that have examined the issue of what constitutes normal sleep in children in order to better define abnormal or insufficient sleep, most have utilized subjective, parent-report, retrospective, cross-sectional surveys in selected populations. There are even more limited data from studies utilizing more objective methods of measuring sleep quality and duration, such as polysomnography and actigraphy, and many of these studies were conducted prior to the establishment of accepted sleep monitoring and scoring standards.

Descriptions of sleep phenotypes and definitions of normal sleep patterns and requirements must necessarily incorporate the wide range of normal developmental and physical maturational changes across childhood and adolescence. Although cross-sectional studies yield important information regarding sleep in discrete age groups, they do not describe the evolution and persistence of sleep–wake patterns over time, nor do they help to elucidate the complex reciprocal relationship between sleep and cognitive/emotional development from the prenatal period through adolescence.

In general, large epidemiologic studies do support several general trends in normal sleep patterns across childhood:

1. Decreased average 24-hour sleep duration from infancy through adolescence, which involves a decline in both diurnal and nocturnal sleep amounts.[1] In particular, there is a dramatic decline in daytime sleep (scheduled napping) between 18 months and 5 years, with a less marked and more gradual contin-

ued decrease in nocturnal sleep amounts into late adolescence.
2. Increasingly irregular sleep–wake patterns with larger discrepancies between school night and non–school night bedtimes and wake times and increased weekend oversleep from middle childhood through adolescence.
3. A gradual shift to a later bedtime and sleep onset time that begins in middle childhood and accelerates in early to mid adolescence. As with most sleep behaviors, these trends reflect the physiologic/chronobiologic, developmental, and social/environmental changes that occur across childhood.

Also, some evidence suggests that sleep patterns and behaviors in children and adolescents today have changed somewhat from those present in previous generations over time. Several studies have shown not only that average sleep duration decreases across middle childhood and adolescence (in contrast to sleep needs, which do not dramatically decline) but that sleep duration in equivalent age groups has declined over a period of time. This trend appears to be related in school-aged children largely to later bedtimes, and, in adolescents, to earlier sleep offset as well as later sleep onset times.

It is also important to consider the cultural and family context within which sleep behaviors in children occur. For example, cosleeping of infants and parents is a common and accepted practice in many ethnic groups, including African Americans, Hispanics, and Southeast Asians, both in their countries of origin and in the United States. Therefore, the developmental goal of independent self-soothing in infants at bedtime and after night wakings, although clearly associated in a number of studies with fewer subsequent sleep problems in young children, may not be shared by all families. In many traditional societies, sleep is heavily embedded in social practices, and both the sleeping environment and the positioning of sleep periods within the context of other activities is much less solitary and less rigid than in more westernized cultures. The relative value and importance of sleep as a health behavior, the interpretation of problematic versus normal sleep by parents, and the relative acceptability of various treatment strategies (e.g., the cry-it-out approach) for sleep problems are just a few additional examples of sleep issues that are impacted by cultural and family values and practices.

NOSOLOGY

For a variety of reasons, it is often a challenge to operationally define *problematic sleep* in children. The range of sleep behaviors that may be considered normal or pathologic is wide and the definitions are often highly subjective. Researchers have taken a number of approaches to this issue: some use a priori definitions of disturbed or poor sleep (e.g., waking for longer than 30 minutes more than three times a week), whereas others have relied on comparison to normative populations or have based the definition of sleep problems on what the parent subjectively identifies as problematic. Other authors have attempted to incorporate more concrete evidence of daytime sequelae (mood, behavior, academic performance) to define significant sleep problems. Some studies have included reports from other observers, including teachers, to avoid depending solely on parents' expectations for, and tolerance, awareness, and interpretation of, sleep and daytime behaviors. In any event, it is clear that a common nosology in terms of research definitions of sleep disorders in children is lacking and needs to be developed and evaluated to identify and target populations at risk for sleep problems for intervention.

On the other hand, clinically significant sleep problems, like many behavioral problems in childhood, may best be viewed as more loosely occurring along a severity and chronicity continuum that ranges from a transient and self-limited disturbance to a disorder that meets specific diagnostic criteria as outlined in the International Classification of Sleep Disorders (ICSD) and/or the Diagnostic and Statistical Manual of Mental Disorders (DSM-IV). Unlike strict research definitions of sleep problems, the validity of parental

concerns and opinions regarding their child's sleep patterns and behaviors, and the resulting stress on the family, must be considered in defining sleep disturbances in the clinical context. Furthermore, successful treatment of pediatric sleep problems is highly dependent on identification of parental concerns, clarification of mutually acceptable treatment goals, active exploration of opportunities and obstacles, and ongoing communication of issues and concerns.

VARIABLES AFFECTING SLEEP PATTERNS AND BEHAVIORS

The relative prevalence and the various types of sleep problems that occur throughout childhood must also be understood in the context of normal physical and cognitive/emotional phenomena that are occurring at different developmental stages. For example, brief regressions in sleep behaviors often accompany the achievement of motor and cognitive milestones in the first year of life, and increased night-time fears and night wakings in toddlers may be a temporary manifestation of developmentally normal separation anxiety peaking during that stage. Parental recognition and reporting of sleep problems in children also varies across childhood, with parents of infants and toddlers more likely to be aware of sleep concerns than those of school-aged children and adolescents. The very definition of a sleep problem by parents is often highly subjective and is frequently determined by the amount of disruption caused to parents' sleep.

In addition to considering sleep disturbances within a developmental context, a number of other important child, parental, and environmental variables affect the type, relative prevalence, chronicity, and severity of sleep problems. Child variables that may significantly impact sleep include temperament and behavioral style, individual variations in circadian preference, cognitive and language delays, and the presence of comorbid medical and psychiatric conditions. Parental variables include parenting and discipline styles, parents' education level and knowledge of child development, mental health issues (such as maternal depression), family stress, and quality and quantity of parents' sleep. Environmental variables include the physical environment (space, noise, perceived environmental threats to safety, and room and bed sharing), family composition (number, ages, and health status of siblings and extended family members), and lifestyle issues (parental work status and competing priorities for parents' and children's time).

Finally, although many sleep problems in infants and children are transient and self-limited in nature, the common wisdom that all children grow out of sleep problems is not an accurate perception. Certain intrinsic and extrinsic risk factors (such as difficult temperament, chronic illness, neurodevelopmental delays, maternal depression, and family stress) may predispose a given child toward a more chronic sleep disturbance. The persistence of infant sleep problems into early childhood has been documented in a number of studies.

PREVALENCE: SURVEYS OF NORMAL POPULATIONS

The following discussion largely focuses on general sleep problems in children and on non-specific presenting sleep complaints, such as bedtime resistance and night wakings; prevalence data regarding specific sleep disorders such as obstructive sleep apnea syndrome are found in other chapters. A number of studies have examined the prevalence of parent- and child-reported sleep complaints in large samples of children and adolescents; many of these studies have also attempted to further delineate the association between disrupted sleep and behavioral concerns. Most of these studies have utilized broad-based parent-report sleep surveys to assess for a variety of sleep problems, ranging from bedtime resistance to prolonged night wakings to parasomnias.[2,3] There are limitations to these data, including varying definitions of *problem sleep,* difficulty in identifying daytime sleepiness–related behaviors (especially in younger children), and limited information regarding possible confounding factors (e.g., comorbid medical conditions and medication use). Thus, parent reports may over- or underestimate the prevalence of sleep problems. Furthermore, it should be emphasized that parental descriptions of sleep problems are not equivalent to diagnoses of sleep *disorders* made during a clinical evaluation.

Approximately 25% of all children experience some type of sleep problem at some point during childhood. Such problems range from short-term difficulties in falling asleep and night wakings to more serious primary sleep disorders such as obstructive sleep apnea. Studies have reported an overall prevalence of parent-reported sleep problems ranging from 25% to 50% in samples of preschool-aged children to 37% in a community sample of 4 to 10 year olds.[4,5] A more recent study of over 14,000 school-aged children[6] found sleep problems in 20% of 5 year olds and 6% of 11 year olds. Another study found a prevalence of sleeping difficulties in 43% of 8 to 10 year olds.[7] Many studies have examined the self-reported prevalence of sleep problems in adolescents: upwards of 40% of adolescents also have significant sleep complaints,[8] and 12% identified themselves as "chronic poor sleepers."[9]

Studies that have used self-reports of sleep problems from older children have suggested that there may be a discrepancy between parental and child reports, with parents less likely than the children to report sleep onset delays and night wakings. Finally, in studies that have asked health care providers to identify the prevalence of sleep problems seen in their practices, rates of significant difficulties initiating or maintaining sleep across age groups vary, in one recent study making up on average about 3% of all practice visits.[10] In the IMS (Intercontinental Medical Statistics) Health National Disease and Therapeutic Index (NDTI) survey of 2930 office-based practices in the continental United States, which uses diagnostic codes, 0.05% of all pediatric visits were for sleep problems and 0.01% were specifically for insomnia. However, practitioner-identified sleep problems may also underestimate prevalence[11]; for example, in the study by Rona et al.,[6] less than 25% of the school children with sleep problems had consulted a physician.

IMPACT OF SLEEP PROBLEMS

Although a detailed description of the impact of disrupted or insufficient sleep on children's health and well-being is beyond the scope of this chapter, any discussion of the epidemiology of pediatric sleep must underscore the importance of the relationships between sleep problems and mood, performance, and behavior. Many of the studies that have examined these complex relationships have sought to determine how much sleep is needed by infants, children, and teenagers for healthy functioning, and how patterns of growth and development from infancy to adolescence are negatively impacted by insufficient sleep. In general, studies that have examined these relationships have used one of a number of different methodologies:

1. Assessment of effects of experimental sleep restriction on mood, neuropsychological test performance, and observed behavior
2. Evaluation of mood, behavioral, and academic problems in children with clinical sleep disorders (e.g., obstructive sleep apnea syndrome, restless legs syndrome/periodic limb movements during sleep)
3. Examination of the impact of treatment of sleep disorders (pharmacologic, surgical, behavioral) on neurobehavioral measures
4. Identification of behavioral and academic dysfunction in "naturalistic settings," of children identified as poor sleepers or as having inadequate sleep
5. Identification of sleep problems in populations of children with behavioral and academic problems (e.g., attention deficit hyperactivity disorder) compared to normal controls

A number of studies have demonstrated that children for whom parents report sleep complaints are more likely to manifest daytime sleepiness, moodiness, behavioral problems, and school and learning problems.[12] In one recent survey of sleep problems in elementary school–aged children, teachers reported behavioral evidence of significant daytime sleepiness in the classroom setting in 10% of their students.[4] Another study found a significant correlation between early rise times and self-reported difficulties in attention and concentration[13] in fifth graders. Because of their cross-sectional design, however, and the reliance on parental (or self-) report for description of both sleep and behavioral variables in many of these studies, the results must be interpreted cautiously insofar as sleep is considered to be a causal factor.

In similar survey studies, adolescents who reported disturbed or inadequate sleep were also more likely to report subjective sleepiness, mood disturbances, and performance deficits in both social and academic spheres.[14,15] Adolescents may be at increased risk for sleep disturbances and inadequate sleep for a number of biologic, environmental, and psychosocial reasons. The resultant decrease in total sleep time in adolescents has been associated in several studies with poorer grades in school as well as depressed mood, and anxiety. One study[16] that found an overall prevalence of significant sleep problems in about one third of the adolescents surveyed, also reported an increased level of self- and parent-reported externalizing behavioral problems in the sleep-disturbed sample.

Sleep problems are also a significant source of distress for families and may be one of the primary reasons for caregiver stress in families with children who have chronic medical illnesses or severe neurodevelopment delays. Furthermore, the impact of childhood sleep problems is intensified by their direct relationship to the quality and quantity of parents' sleep, particularly if disrupted sleep results in daytime fatigue or mood disturbances and leads to a decreased level of effective parenting. Poor parental sleep has even been implicated as a risk factor for child physical abuse. Successful intervention not only has the effect of improving the sleep of the entire family but may help parents develop behavioral strategies that may generalize for use with daytime behavior problems.

Unlike in adults, however, daytime sleepiness in children may not be characterized by such overt behaviors as yawning and complaining about fatigue but may rather be associated with a host of more subtle or even paradoxical behavioral manifestations (such as increased activity). These range from emotional lability and low frustration tolerance (internalizing behaviors) to neurocognitive deficits to behavioral disinhibition (externalizing behaviors such as increased aggression).[12] In turn, functional deficits in mood, attention, cognition, and behavior may lead to performance deficits in the home, school, and social setting. Objective, reliable, and cost-effective measures of sleepiness and alertness in children are lacking—particularly measures that could be applied to large epidemiologic samples. In addition, subjective self-report data regarding sleepiness are largely unavailable in children, and behavioral manifestations of sleepiness not only vary with age and developmental level but are often not reliably interpreted by parents and other caretakers. Empirical studies involving both normal and sleep-deprived pediatric populations (children with sleep disorders, adolescents) have begun to describe the extent of, and the consequences of, inadequate or disrupted sleep in children.

Studies of sleep in children with primary behavioral and learning problems have further supported an association between sleep and performance impairments. Empirical evidence indicates that children experience significant daytime sleepiness as a result of disturbed or inadequate sleep, and most studies suggest a strong link between sleep disturbance and behavioral problems.

EPIDEMIOLOGY OF SLEEP IN SPECIAL POPULATIONS

Because of the multiple manifestations of poor and insufficient sleep, the clinical symptoms of any primary medical, developmental, or psychiatric disorder are likely to be exacerbated by comorbid sleep problems. Furthermore, sleep problems themselves tend to be more common in those children and adolescents with chronic medical and psychiatric conditions. Improving sleep has the benefit of improving clinical outcome as well.

Sleep disturbances in pediatric special needs populations are extremely common. Significant sleep problems occur in 30% to 80% of children with severe mental retardation and in at least half of children with less severe cognitive impairment; similar estimates in children with autism or pervasive developmental delay are in the 50% to 70% range.[17,18] Significant problems with initiation and maintenance of sleep, shortened sleep duration, irregular sleeping patterns, and early morning waking have been reported in a variety of different neurodevelopmental disorders, including Asperger's syndrome, Angelman's syndrome, Rett's syndrome, Smith-Magenis syndrome, and Williams syndrome. Other studies have suggested that similar rates of sleep problems also occur in both younger and older blind children, with difficulty falling asleep, night wakings, and restless sleep being the most common concerns. These children with pre-existing neurologic abnormalities are also more likely to have sleep problems that are severe, and multiple sleep disorders are likely to occur simultaneously.

Virtually all psychiatric disorders in children may be associated with sleep disruption. Epidemiologic and clinical studies indicate that psychiatric disorders are the most common cause of chronic insomnia. Psychiatric disorders can also be associated with daytime sleepiness, fatigue, abnormal circadian sleep patterns, disturbing dreams and nightmares, and movement disorders during sleep. Growing evidence suggests that primary insomnia (i.e., insomnia with no concurrent psychiatric disorder) is a risk factor for later developing psychiatric conditions, particularly depressive and anxiety disorders.[19]

Several studies have evaluated the prevalence of sleep problems in samples of children and adolescents with a variety of psychiatric disorders.[16,20] The results suggest an increase in a wide range of reported sleep disturbances in these mixed clinical populations, including parasomnias such as nightmares and night terrors, difficulty falling asleep and frequent and prolonged night wakings, sleep-related anxiety symptoms (e.g., fear of the dark), restless sleep, and subjective poor quality of sleep with associated daytime fatigue. Similarly, an association has been reported between DSM psychiatric disorders (including affective disorders, attention deficit hyperactivity disorder, and conduct disorder) and sleep problems in surveys of children and adolescents from the general population.[4] Studies of children with major depressive disorder, for example, have reported a prevalence of insomnia of up to 75% and of severe insomnia of 30%, and sleep onset delay in a third of depressed adolescents, although it should be noted that objective data (e.g., with polysomnography) does not always support these subjective complaints.

Finally, reports of sleep complaints, especially bedtime resistance, refusal to sleep alone, increased night-time fears, and nightmares are common in children who have experienced severely traumatic events (including physical and sexual abuse),[21] and these complaints may also be associated with less dramatic but nonetheless stressful life events such as brief separation from a parent, birth of a sibling, or school transitions.[22] Sleep problems are not universally found in all children experiencing varying degrees of stress, and some authors[21] have suggested that such variables as level of exposure and physical proximity to the traumatic situation, previous exposure, and the opportunity for habituation to the stress may play important roles in either mitigating or exacerbating associated sleep disturbances. Other considerations, such as the age and temperament of the child, and the presence of parental psychopathology, also clearly have an important influence.

Little is currently known about the interaction between sleep disorders and both acute and chronic health conditions (such as asthma, diabetes, and juvenile rheumatoid arthritis), on either a pathophysiologic or behavioral level, although, particularly in chronic pain conditions, these interactions are likely to significantly impact on morbidity and quality of life.[23-26] Much of the information currently available regarding the types of sleep problems that occur in these children comes from studies of adults with chronic medical conditions or from clinical observations. A few recent studies have begun to examine the role of sleep disturbances in sickle cell disease[27] and asthma, two disorders particularly common in high-risk and minority populations. The interaction between sleep and physical and emotional dysfunction in acute and chronic pain conditions, such as burns and juvenile rheumatoid arthritis, has also begun to be explored. Factors such as the impact of hospitalization, family dynamics, underlying disease processes, and concurrent medications are also clearly important to consider in assessing the bidirectional relationship of insomnia and chronic illness in children.

Specific medical conditions that may also have an increased risk of sleep problems include the following:

Allergies: Chronic allergy-mediated rhinitis with nasal congestion and cough, and chronic or frequent sinusitis may be associated with difficulties initiating and maintaining sleep. Atopic dermatitis may cause sleep disruption and fragmentation, difficulty falling asleep, night awakenings, and decreased sleep duration, as a result of frequent scratching and discomfort.

Asthma: Asthma in children has been associated with poorer subjective sleep quality, decreased sleep duration, increased nocturnal wakings with decreased sleep efficiency, and greater daytime sleepiness. The prevalence of sleep problems in children with asthma has been reported to be 60%. Asthma medications may also have adverse effects on sleep; for example, both theophylline and oral corticosteroids may cause significant sleep disruption.

Burns: Children who are severely burned are at particularly high risk for sleep problems, which in turn may have significant adverse effects on their recovery. Difficulty falling asleep, increased arousals, nightmares, and increased daytime sleepiness are common in the acute phase and may persist for up to 1 year after the event.

Headaches: Migraine and tension headaches have been associated with sleep onset and sleep maintenance problems, and migraines have been associated with an increased incidence of sleepwalking. Furthermore, sleep deprivation may trigger headaches in susceptible individuals.

Rheumatologic disorders: Children with juvenile rheumatoid arthritis and with fibromyalgia have been shown to have more frequent night wakings and sleep fragmentation that may be associated with daytime sleepiness.

References

1. Iglowstein I, Jenni O, Molinari L, Largo R: Sleep duration from infancy to adolescence: Reference values and generational trends. Pediatrics 2003; 111:302-307.
2. Owens J, Nobile C, McGuinn M, Spirito A: The children's sleep habits questionnaire: Construction and validation of a sleep survey for school-aged children. Sleep 2000;23:1043-1051.
3. Bruni O, Ottaviano S, Guidetti MR, et al: The sleep disturbance scale for children: Construction and validation of an instrument to evaluate sleep disturbance in childhood and adolescence. J Sleep Res 1996;5:251-261.
4. Blader JC, Koplewicz HS, Abikoff H, Foley C: Sleep problems of elementary school children. A community study. Arch Pediatr Adolesc Med 1997; 151;473-480.
5. Owens J, Spirito A, McGuinn M, Nobile C: Sleep habits and sleep disturbance in school-aged children. J Dev Behav Pediatr 2000;21:27-36.
6. Rona RJ, Li L, Gulliford MC, Chinn S: Disturbed sleep: Effects of sociocultural factors and illness. Arch Dis Child 1998;78:20-25.
7. Kahn A, Van de Merckt C, Rebuffat E, et al: Sleep problems in healthy preadolescents. Pediatrics 1989;84:542-546.
8. Vignau J, Bailly D, Duhamel A, et al: Epidemiologic study of sleep quality and troubles in French secondary school adolescents. J Adolesc Health 1997; 21(5):343-50.
9. Levy D, Gray-Donald K, Leech J, Zvagulis I, Pless IB: Sleep patterns and problems in adolescents. J Adolesc Health Care 1986;7:386-389.
10. Owens J, Rosen C, Mindell J: Medication use in the treatment of pediatric insomnia: Results of a survey of community-based pediatricians. Pediatrics 2003;111:e628-e635.

11. Chervin R, Archbold K, Panahi P, Pituch K: Sleep problems seldom addressed in two general pediatric clinics. Pediatrics 2001;107:1375-1380.

12. Fallone G, Owens J, Deane J: Sleepiness in children and adolescents: Clinical implications. Sleep Med Rev 2002;6:287-306.

13. Epstein R, Hillag N, Lavie P: Starting times of school: Effects on daytime function of fifth-grade students in Israel. Sleep 1998;21:250-256.

14. Wolfson AR, Carskadon MA: Sleep schedules and daytime functioning in adolescents. Child Dev 1998;69:875-887.

15. Giannotti F, Cortesi F: Sleep patterns and daytime functions in adolescents: An epidemiological survey of Italian high-school student population. In Carskadon MA (ed): Adolescent Sleep Patterns: Biological, Social, and Psychological Influences. New York: Cambridge University Press, 2003.

16. Morrison DN, McGee R, Stanton WR: Sleep problems in adolescence. J Am Acad Child Adol Psychiatry 1992;31:94-99.

17. Stores G, Wiggs L: Sleep disturbance in children and adolescents with disorders of development: its significance and management. New York, Cambridge University Press, 2003.

18. Johnson CR: Sleep problems in children with mental retardation and autism. Child Adolesc Psychiatr Clin N Am 1996;5:673-681.

19. Dahl RE, Ryan ND, Matty MK, et al: Sleep onset abnormalities in depressed adolescents. Biol Psychiatry 1996;39:400-410.

20. Price VA, Coates TJ, Thoresen CE: Prevalence and correlates of poor sleep among adolescents. Am J Dis Child 1978;132:583-586.

21. Sadeh A: Stress, trauma, and sleep in children. Child Adolesc Psychiatr Clin N Am 1996;6:685.

22. Field T: Peer separation of children attending new schools. Dev Psychol 1984;20:786.

23. Sadeh A, Horowitz I, Wolach-Benodis L, Wolach B: Sleep and pulmonary function in children with well-controlled stable asthma. Sleep 1998; 21:379-384.

24. Rose M, Sanford A, Thomas C, Opp M: Factors altering the sleep of burned children. Sleep 2001; 24:45-51.

25. Bloom B, Owens J, McGuinn M, et al: Sleep and its relationship to pain, dysfunction and disease activity in juvenile rheumatoid arthritis. J Rheumatol 2002;29:169-173.

26. Lewin D, Dahl R: Importance of sleep in the management of pediatric pain. J Dev Behav Pediatr 1999;20:244-252.

27. Samuels M, Stebbens V, Davies S, et al: Sleep-related upper airway obstruction and hypoxaemia in sickle cell disease. Arch Dis Child 1992; 67:925-929.

Anatomy of Sleep

Stephen H. Sheldon

4

The sleeping and waking states depend on activity in the entire brain, not in particular or independent regions. In general, neural activity in the brainstem diencephalic ascending reticular activating system is responsible for the maintenance of alertness and the waking state. Sleep is a complex, active phenomenon. It is composed of physiologically distinct (but highly synchronized) states, and it cycles at regular intervals. Sleep is not simply a reduction in activity of the reticular activating system; rather, it is generated by many different regions of the central nervous system working together.

This chapter focuses on the various anatomic centers of the central nervous system and their functions in the sleep–wake cycle. Most of the data delineating these areas have been derived from animal lesion experiments. Other data come from observations of signs and symptoms in humans who have suffered from disease or dysfunction of these particular topologic regions of the brain.

THE CORTEX

Sleeping and waking behavior occurs in the absence of the cortex. This has been well documented in animal studies[1-4] and in observations of human newborns with anencephaly and holoprosencephaly.[5] The cortex is involved with the regulation and maintenance of wakefulness by stimulating the ascending reticular activating system, which, in turn, results in a general arousal response (Fig. 4–1). There is some evidence that this cortex–reticular activating system–cortex activation loop may be responsible for the hyperactivity and motor restlessness seen in many children with attention deficit hyperactivity disorder or with syndromes associated with excessive daytime sleepiness. Evidence of increased sleepiness has been documented in a group of children with attention span problems,

hyperactivity, motor restlessness, behavioral difficulties, and school failure.[6] Short mean sleep onset latencies, frequent sleep onsets, numerous microsleep episodes, and pathologically short sleep onset latencies in one or several multiple sleep latency test naps have been documented. Excessive sleep pressure might explain the effect of stimulant medication on decreasing activity, motor restlessness, and improving attention span deficits in some children with attention deficit hyperactivity disorder. By reducing sleepiness, reducing microsleep episodes, and stimulating the cortex, the cortex–reticular activating system–cortex feedback loop may be broken, resulting in improvement of symptoms. Figures 4–2 and 4–3 are schematic representations of the mechanisms involved in slow-wave and rapid eye movement sleep.

Behavioral components of sleep onset may also be under the control of cortical activity. Habits and rituals associated with sleep onset create a relaxed and habitual situation that permits physiologic sleep-onset mechanisms to perform their function. Absence of appropriate and habitual sleep onset associations results in significant sleep onset and maintenance difficulties during early childhood.

Although sleep and wake cycling may be preserved in the absence of the cortex, there is evidence that sleep and wake are dysfunctional in many patients with generalized cortical disease. Some recognizable characteristics remain (e.g., sleep spindles, vertex sharp transients), but architecture may be severely disrupted and, in some cases, no recognizable stages of sleep can be seen.[7-9]

THE CEREBELLUM

The cerebellum is mainly responsible for the control of skeletal musculature, posture, and movement. During sleep, cerebellar activity and

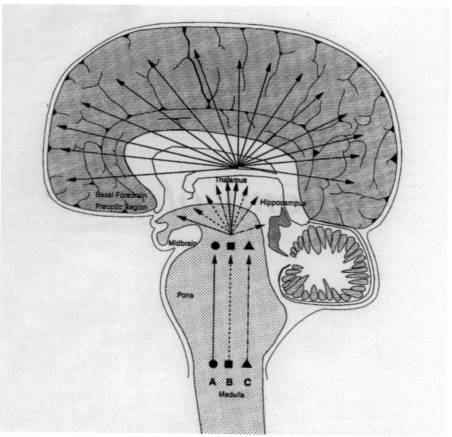

Figure 4–1. Schematic mechanism for generation of wakefulness. *Solid circles A* represent the neurons of the reticular formation. Their major ascending projections into the forebrain proceed along two major routes. The dorsal route terminates in the nonspecific thalamic nuclei, which in turn project in a widespread manner to the cerebral cortex. The ventral route passes through the subthalamus and hypothalamus and continues into the basal forebrain and septum, where neurons in turn project in a widespread manner to the cerebral cortex and hippocampus. *Solid squares B* represent catecholamine neurons of the lower brainstem and locus coeruleus (dorsal pons), which contain norepinephrine, and of the substantia nigra and ventral tegmental area (ventral midbrain), which contain dopamine. The norepinephrine neurons, mainly implicated in processes of cortical activation, project directly and diffusely to the cerebral cortex, as well as to the subcortical way stations. The dopamine neurons, which are predominantly implicated in processes of behavioral activity and responsiveness, project heavily into the basal ganglia and frontal cortex. *Solid triangles C* represent acetylcholine neurons of the brainstem reticular formation (including the laterodorsal and pedunculopontine tegmental nuclei in the dorsal pons and midbrain) and basal forebrain (substantia innominata, diagonal band nuclei, and septum). Cholinergic neurons are implicated in cortical activation and from the brainstem project predominantly to subcortical way stations, including the thalamus, the subthalamus, the hypothalamus, and the basal forebrain and septum. The cholinergic basal forebrain neurons project in a widespread manner to the cerebral cortex and hippocampus. Not shown are other neuronal systems implicated in wakefulness, including histamine neurons located in the posterior hypothalamus, which also project directly to the cerebral cortex. Glutamate neurons located through subcortical structures and in the cerebral cortex are important in the processes of cortical activation and wakefulness. Multiple peptides, such as substance P, corticotropin-releasing factor, thyrotropin-releasing factor, and vasoactive intestinal polypeptide, may be involved in wakefulness and are often colocalized with one of the other primary neurotransmitters, such as norepinephrine and acetylcholine. The neuronal systems implicated in the maintenance of wakefulness may be involved in primary processes of sensory transmission and attention, motor response and activity, and orthosympathetic and neuroendocrine (particularly adrenocorticotropic hormone and thyrotropin-releasing hormone) responses and regulation, by which they may enhance and prolong vigilance and arousal. *(Modified and reproduced with permission from Jones BE: Basic mechanisms of sleep-wake states. In Kryger M, Roth T, Dement WC: Principles and Practice of Sleep Medicine. Philadelphia, WB Saunders, 1989, p 122.)*

feedback may be involved with postural adjustments and body movements, accessory respiratory muscle movements, extraocular muscle movements, and alterations in muscle tone.[10] There is some contribution of the cerebellum to the generation of muscle atonia during sleep,[11,12] but it seems to have little effect on the sleep–wake cycle itself. The cerebellar vermis may also be involved in the generation (or suppression) of sleep spindles, as lesions of this area result in the production of numerous sleep spindles.[13]

THE BASAL GANGLIA

The role of the basal ganglia in the sleep–wake cycle appears to be peripheral. Dopaminergic neurons in the substantia nigra innervate with thousands of synaptic contacts in the striatum.[14] There appears to be little change in the activity of the neurons during wakefulness and during the various stages of sleep (including rapid eye movement sleep).

THE THALAMUS

Animal experiments using low frequency stimulation of the midline thalamic nuclei have resulted in presleep behavior followed by sleep.[15,16] The region that causes this response is very limited, however. Stimulation of the anterior thalamic nuclei has resulted in similar results. The same is not true, however, in humans. The thalamus does not appear to be essential for sleep,[17,18] but it is essential for the production of sleep spindles.[19] Therefore, a thalamic pacemaker may exist that drives cortical neurons and controls electroencephalographic synchronization during non–rapid eye movement sleep.[20] Periodic bursts of high amplitude cortical waves and spindles become more frequent as deeper stages of sleep appear, and they seem to be generated from nonspecific thalamic nuclei through diffuse thalamocortical projections. Areas responsible for driving spindle production appear to be midline and are closely associated to the region where sleep can be promoted in animals by low frequency stimulation.[21]

Sleep spindles and K-complexes are characteristic of the sleeping state and are never seen during wakefulness.[22] The functions of spindles and K-complexes are unknown, but they are thought to have an important function in regulating slow-wave sleep.[23]

THE HYPOTHALAMUS

The posterior, lateral, and medial hypothalamus is the cephalad continuation of the brainstem reticular activating system.[24] Transection at the level of the posterior hypothalamus completely abolishes wakefulness.[25] Posterior hypothalamic lesions generally produce lethargy and sleepiness.[26] Hypersomnia, coma, or changes in circadian rhythmicity are noted in humans, depending on the exact site and extent of the hypothalamic lesion.

FOREBRAIN AND ANTERIOR HYPOTHALAMUS

Basal forebrain areas appear to contain powerful inhibitory and sleep-promoting centers.[27,28] Lesions of the preoptic region have an effect that is opposite to those of the posterior hypothalamus.[29] Insomnia and terminal sleeplessness[30] have resulted from lesions of the anterior hypothalamus and basal forebrain, respectively.[36]

When stimulated, the basal forebrain produces a short sleep onset latency, encephalographic synchronization, and involuntary sleep.[31-33] Lesions of this same area produce insomnia in animals. It is difficult to clearly identify the cell bodies responsible for this phenomenon because this area is quite dense and contains numerous transecting fiber tracts.[34] High frequency stimulation of the thalamus, posterior hypothalamus, and brainstem produces arousal, whereas similar stimulation of the anterior hypothalamus produces rapid sleep onset. With high frequency stimulation of the basal forebrain and low frequency stimulation of the thalamus, presleep behavior, rather than sleep itself, occurs prior to encephalographic synchronization.[35]

BRAINSTEM RETICULAR ACTIVATING SYSTEM

Rather than a single, isolated region in the brainstem, the reticular activating system appears to be diffusely distributed in the medulla and pons, and it extends into the posterior, medial, and lateral hypothalamic regions. Classic experiments by Moruzzi and Magoun[30] revealed that electrical stimulation of a portion of the brainstem resulted in changes on the encephalogram that were identical to those seen upon awakening

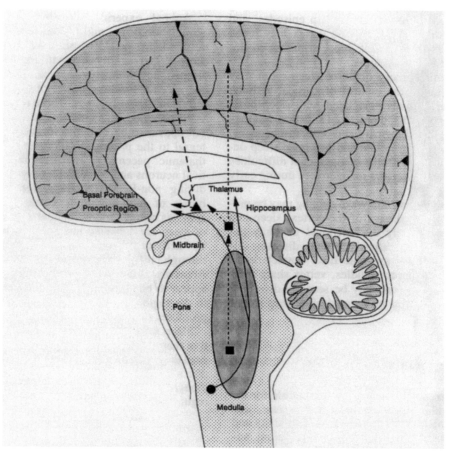

Figure 4–2. Schematic representation of mechanisms generating slow-wave sleep. The *Solid circle* represents neurons of the solitary tract nucleus and adjacent tegmentum, implicated in slow-wave sleep regulation, which project forward into the visceral-limbic forebrain. *Solid squares* represent serotonergic neurons of the brainstem raphe nuclei, which may facilitate the onset of slow-wave sleep and which project forward into the rostral tegmentum, thalamus, subthalamus, hypothalamus, and basal forebrain and also from the midbrain directly to the cortex and hippocampus. The *Solid triangle* represents gamma-aminobutyric acid (GABA) neurons of the hypothalamus and basal forebrain-septum, which project in a widespread manner to the cerebral cortex and hippocampus. These GABAergic neurons are also located in the cerebral cortex, where they are maximally active during slow-wave sleep. Not shown are other neuronal systems implicated in slow wave sleep, including adenosine neurons located in the hypothalamus. Multiple peptides, such as the opiates, alpha-melanocyte–stimulating hormone, and somatostatin, may be involved in slow-wave sleep generation and are often colocalized with one of the other primary neurotransmitters, such as serotonin or GABA. The neuronal systems implicated in the maintenance of slow-wave sleep may be involved in primary processes of sensory inhibition and analgesia, behavioral inhibition, and parasympathetic and neuroendocrine (notably growth hormone) responses and regulation, by which they may facilitate the onset and maintenance of slow wave sleep. *(Modified and reproduced with permission from Jones BE: Basic mechanisms of sleep-wake states. In Kryger M, Roth T, Dement WC: Principles and Practice of Sleep Medicine. Philadelphia, WB Saunders, 1989, p 125.)*

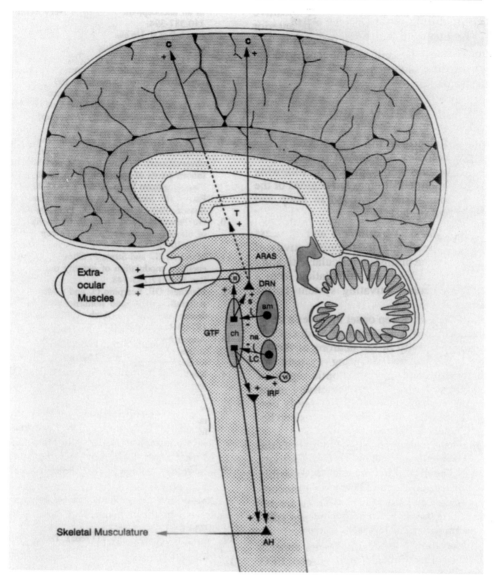

Figure 4–3. Schematic mechanism for the generation of rapid eye movement (REM) sleep. Aminergic (REM-off) neurons located in the dorsal raphe nuclei (serotonergic) and the locus coeruleus (noradrenergic) produce inhibitory postsynaptic potentials on cholinergic (REM-on) neurons located in the mesencephalic, medullary, and pontine gigantocellular tegmental fields. These two systems of neurons continuously interact to produce the alternation between non-REM and REM sleep. Neurons in the gigantocellular tegmental fields produce stimulating postsynaptic potentials to produce the epiphenomena seen during REM sleep. Positive postsynaptic potentials result in conjugate extraocular muscle movement through stimulation of the nuclei of the oculomotor, trochlear, and abducens nuclei. Cortical desynchronization occurs via projections to the thalamus and cortex through the ascending reticular activating system. Muscle atonia is produced by direct stimulation of neurons that produce inhibitory postsynaptic potentials at the level of the anterior horn cell. Intermittent muscle twitches occur through direct stimulation of the anterior horn cells. Not shown are interconnections with the autonomic nervous system that result in the cardiac and respiratory irregularities noted during REM sleep. AH, anterior horn cells; am, aminergic neurons; ARAS, ascending reticular activating system; C, cortex; ch, acetylcholine; DRN, dorsal raphe nuclei; GTF, gigantocellular tegmental fields; IRF, inhibitory reticular formation; LC, locus coeruleus; na, noradrenalin; s, serotonin; T, thalamus; +, stimulating postsynaptic potential; −, inhibitory postsynaptic potential. *(Modified and reproduced with permission from Hobson JA: The cellular basis of sleep cycle control. Adv Sleep Res 1974;1:217-250, and Hauri P: Current Concepts: The Sleep Disorders. Kalamazoo, Mich, Upjohn Company, 1982, p 13.)*

from sleep or during an arousal or an alerting reaction. The area from which encephalographic synchronization occurs runs throughout most of the length of the brainstem in its central core. Electrical stimulation in these regions also results in changes in activity of cortical and thalamic neurons, abolishes thalamic recruiting potentials, has a marked effect on cortical evoked potentials, and significantly affects perception.[11]

Evidence exists that many reticular formation neurons have both cephalad and caudad projections.[33,37] This complex system also appears to have many interneuronal connections with the brainstem deactivating system located in the medullary raphe nuclei.

References

1. Barrett R, Merritt HH, Wolf A: Depression of consciousness as a result of cerebral lesions. Res Publ Assoc Res Nerv Ment Dis 1967;45:241-276.
2. Kleitman N: Sleep and Wakefulness. Chicago, University of Chicago Press, 1963, pp. 241-242.
3. Oswald I: Sleeping and Waking: Physiology and Psychology. Amsterdam, Elsevier, 1962, p 232.
4. Nielson JM, Sedgwick RP: Instincts and emotions in an anencephalic monster. J Nerv Ment Dis 1949;110:387-394.
5. Puech P, Guilly P, Fishgold H, Bounes G: Un cas d'anencephalie hydrocephalique: Étude electroencephalographique. Rev Neurol 1947;79:116-124.
6. Wilkus RJ, Farrell DF: Electrophysiological observations in the classical form of Pelizaeus-Merzbacher disease. Neurology 1976;26:1042-1045.
7. Karacan I, Schneck L, Hinterbuchner LP: The sleep-dream pattern in Tay-Sachs disease (preliminary observations). In Aronson SM, Volk BW (eds): Inborn Errors of Sphingolipid Metabolism. Elmsford, NY, Pergamon Press, 1967, pp 413-421.
8. Parkes JD: Sleep and Its Disorders. Eastbourne, East Sussex, England, WB Saunders, 1985, pp 73-118.
9. Guglielmino S, Strata P: Cerebellum and atonia of the desynchronized phase of sleep. Arch Ital Biol 1971;109:210-217.
10. Marchesi GF, Strata P: Climbing fibers of rat cerebellum: Modulation of activity during sleep. Brain Res 1970;17:145-148.
11. Marchesi GF, Scarpino O, Mauro AM: Studio poligrafico del sonno notturno in pazienti con sindrome cerebellare. Arch Psicol Neurol Psichiat 1977;4:455-472.
12. Anden NE, Fuxe K, Hamberger B, Hokfelt T: A quantitative study on the nigro-striatal dopamine neuron system in the rat. Acta Physiol Scand 1966;67:306-312.
13. Koella WA: Sleep: Its Nature and Physiological Organization. Springfield, Ill, Charles C Thomas, 1967, p 199.
14. Naquet R, Denavit M, Albe-Fessard D: Comparaison entre le role du subthalamus et celui des differentes structures bulbo-mesencephaliques dans le maintien de la vigilance. Electroencephalogr Clin Neurophysiol 1966;20:149-164.
15. Bricolo A: Sleep abnormalities following thalamic stereotactic lesions in man. In Gastaut H, Lugaresi E, Berti-Ceroni G, Coccagna G (eds): The Abnormalities of Sleep in Man. Proceedings of the XVth European Meeting on Electrophysiology, Bologna, 1967, Bologna, Auto Gaggi, 1968, pp 135-138.
16. Purpura DP, Yahr MD (eds): The Thalamus. New York, Colombia University Press, 1966, p 438.
17. Eyzaguirre C, Fidone SJ: Physiology of the Nervous System. Chicago, Year Book Publishers, 1975, pp 343-371.
18. Naitoh P, Antony-Bass V, Muzet A, Ehrhart J: Dynamic relation of sleep spindles and K-complexes to spontaneous phasic arousal in sleeping human subjects. Sleep 1982;5:58-72.
19. Whitlock DG, Aruini A, Moruzzi G: Microelectrode analysis of pyramidal system during transition from sleep to wakefulness. J Neurophysiol 1953;16:414-429.
20. Rossi GF: Electrophysiology of sleep. In Gastaut H, Lugaresi E, Berti-Ceroni G, Coccagna G (eds): The Abnormalities of Sleep in Man. Proceedings of the XVth European Meeting on Electrophysiology, Bologna, 1967, Bologna, Auto Gaggi, 1968, pp 13-23.
21. Ranson SW: Somnolence caused by hypothalamic lesions in the monkey. Arch Neurol Psychiatry 1939;41:1-23.
22. Mitler MM: Toward an animal model of narcolepsy-cataplexy. In Guilleminault C, Dement WC, Passouant P (eds): New York, Spectrum 1976, pp 387-409.
23. von Economo C: Sleep as a problem of localization. J Nerv Ment Dis 1930;71:249-259.
24. Moruzzi G: The sleep-waking cycle. Ergeb Physiol 1972;64:1-165.
25. Sterman M, Fairchild M: Modification of locomotor performance by reticular formation and basal forebrain stimulation in the cat: Evidence for reciprocal systems. Brain Res 1966;2:205-217.
26. Sterman MB, Clemente CD: Forebrain inhibitory mechanisms: Cortical synchronization induced by basal forebrain stimulation. Exp Neurol 1962;6:91-102.
27. McGinty D, Sterman M: Sleep suppression after basal forebrain lesions in the cat. Science 1968;160:1253-1255.

28. Clemente CD, Sterman MB, Wyrwicka W: Forebrain inhibitory mechanisms: Conditioning of basal forebrain induced EEG synchronization and sleep. Exp Neurol 1963;7:404-417.

29. Bremer F: Cerveau isole et physiologie du sommeil. C R Soc Biol 1935;118:1235-1241.

30. Moruzzi G, Magoun HW: Brain stem reticular formation and activation of EEG. Electroencephalogr Clin Neurophysiol 1949;1:455-473.

31. McKeough DM: The Coloring Review of Neuroscience. Boston, Little, Brown, 1982, pp 30-32.

32. Magni F, Willis WD: Identification of reticular formation neurons by intracellular recording. Arch Ital Biol 1963;101:681-702.

33. Jasper HH: Diffuse projection systems: The integrative action of the thalamic reticular system. Electroencephalogr Clin Neurophysiol 1949;1:405-409.

34. Olszewski J, Baxter D: The Cytoarchitecture of the Human Brain Stem. Philadelphia, Lippincott, 1954.

35. Cairns H: Disturbances of consciousness with lesions of the brain stem and diencephalon. Brain 1952;75:109-146.

36. French JD: Brain lesions associated with prolonged unconsciousness. Arch Neurol Psychiatry 1952;68:727-740.

37. Jefferson M: Altered consciousness associated with brain stem lesions. Brain 1952;75:55-67.

Case-Based Analysis of Sleep Problems in Children

Gerald M. Rosen, MD

5

Children with sleep problems will present with variations of four sleep symptoms: difficulties with sleep onset, problems that disrupt sleep, an inability to awaken from sleep at the desired time, and daytime sleepiness. The sleep history is the most important tool for gathering information on sleep symptoms; and BEARS[1] (Bedtime, Excessive daytime sleepiness, Awakenings, Regularity, Snoring) is an easy-to-remember mnemonic device for gathering a history of sleep symptoms. There are many causes for each of these sleep symptoms, and an effective treatment strategy for sleep problems is usually based on a careful analysis of the fundamental causes of the sleep problem, not on the sleep symptom. There are nine major factors important in the control of sleep–wake regulation: circadian, homeostatic, ultradian, developmental, cardiorespiratory, neurologic, psychiatric/behavioral, drugs/alcohol, and other medical problems. These factors form the conceptual foundation necessary to understand sleep problems and to develop effective treatment strategies for solving them. Each of these processes is addressed in depth in a chapter or section (noted in italics and in parentheses) of *Principles and Practice of Pediatric Sleep Medicine,*[2] so only a brief summary will be included here.

Circadian (*Section 4*) rhythms are self-sustaining, nearly 24-hour rhythms, present in all living organisms from single-celled algae to mammals, that allow the organism to anticipate the light–dark cycle, not merely respond to it. In mammals the circadian pacemaker is located in the suprachiasmatic nucleus located in the anterior hypothalamus. The output of the circadian pacemaker modulates the level of alertness; the periodicity of the pacemaker in humans is about 24.2 hours, so it must be corrected each day to remain synchronized with the 24-hour day. This "phase shifting" occurs through numerous zeitgebers, or time cues, which facilitate entrainment. These zeitgebers include clocks, social interactions, meals, and, most importantly, light—the most powerful circadian time cue. The sleep–wake cycle is the most obvious facet of the circadian rhythm, but the output of most other physiologic systems show a circadian pattern of predictable change over the 24-hour day, including: hormone levels (thyroid-stimulating hormone, follicle-stimulating hormone, lutein-stimulating hormone, melatonin, cortisol, antidiuretic hormone), body temperature, gastric acid, intestinal motility, drug metabolism, cardiorespiratory, cellular immunity, and propensity to enter rapid eye movement (REM) and non-rapid eye movement (NREM) sleep. There is a circadian variation in level of alertness, which is independent of the amount of sleep an individual had the night before. Different individuals vary in their circadian phase preferences, preferred sleep time, amplitude of the circadian signal, and duration of the circadian sleep period. Morning types prefer to go to sleep early and awaken early, whereas evening types prefer to go to sleep late and awaken late. Neither is better, just different. An individual's preferred sleep patterns often declare themselves during childhood. During adolescence, whatever the preferred sleep pattern is, there will typically be a phase shift to a later preferred sleep time.

Sleep is also **homeostatically** (*Section 4*) regulated based on the duration of prior wakefulness. EEG delta power (slow-wave activity 0.5-4.0 Hz) is a physiologic index of the sleep homeostatic drive. Sleep duration and timing are largely the result of the interaction and synchronization of the circadian and homeostatic processes. Optimal sleep and wakefulness occur only when these two processes are synchronized.

The **ultradian** (*Section 1*) rhythm is defined by the predictable alternation of wakefulness, NREM sleep, and REM sleep during the sleep period. The ultradian cycles (NREM-REM) are about 60 minutes in early infancy and increase to 90 minutes during early childhood. Since many sleep problems are state specific (i.e., related to wakefulness, REM sleep, NREM sleep), knowing when the specific sleep states are likely to occur during the night and in what intervals is often helpful to understanding what may otherwise be a confusing sleep history. Examples are sleep terrors (slow-wave sleep), obstructive sleep apnea (worse in REM), conditioned arousals in infants (during normal awakenings), and REM sleep behavior disorder (REM sleep).

Important **developmental** (*Section 1*) changes occur in sleep over an individual's lifetime in quantity, percent distribution in various sleep stages, circadian rhythmicity and timing, and consolidation of sleep. At birth, sleep accounts for about one third of the infant's life and does not have a clear circadian pattern. Sleep in the infant is described as quiet (NREM precursor), active (REM precursor), or indeterminate. Active sleep accounts for 50% of the infant's sleep and is the state into which the infant transitions from wakefulness. The ultradian cycles of infants are shorter (see ultradian rhythm earlier). By 3 months of life, a circadian rhythm in the distribution of sleep develops such that the infant begins to sleep more at night and has an established daytime nap schedule; total sleep time decreases to about 15 hours a night; REM and NREM can be scored using adult sleep staging criteria; and REM sleep decreases to about 30% of total sleep time. Total sleep time continues to decrease during childhood as nap duration and frequency decrease, with most children giving up their daytime naps by 5 years of age. Slow-wave sleep is very prominent throughout childhood, and this is likely a factor in some of the common childhood parasomnias, such as sleepwalking and confusional arousals. During adolescence, sleep requirements probably increase, and so does sleepiness. Slow-wave sleep decreases to the adult norms, and REM sleep accounts for about 20% of total sleep time.

Alcohol (*Sections 5 and 14*) and the many other psychoactive prescription and nonprescription **drugs** can have an important impact on wakefulness and sleep, both when they are being taken and while the body is withdrawing from them. Caffeine is a ubiquitous food additive found in many beverages and some foods.

The **cardiorespiratory** (*Section 3*) system undergoes many important changes during sleep: Upper airway resistance increases; central respiratory drive decreases; minute ventilation decreases; during REM sleep, the accessory respiratory muscles—both those that hold the airway open (pharyngeal dilators) and those that can expand the chest (intercostals and scalenes)—are hypotonic; hypoxic and hypercapnic ventilatory responses decrease in NREM sleep and further in REM sleep; cardiac output decreases during sleep; bronchoconstriction increases during sleep in everyone but to a greater extent in patients with asthma, contributing to the common symptom of nocturnal cough; and functional residual capacity decreases (especially in obese individuals asleep in the supine position).

Sleep is fundamentally a **neurologic** (*Section 2*) process controlled by and exclusively for the benefit of the brain, although its precise function is not known. Sleep has withstood the evolutionary test of time and is present as a distinct neurologic process in mammals and birds and as a distinct behavioral process in fish, amphibians, and invertebrates. An increase in parasympathetic tone and a decrease in sympathetic tone (except for phasic increases during REM sleep) are included among the clinically important changes in the neurologic systems of mammals during sleep. Some seizures occur exclusively during sleep (generally NREM). Somatic muscles have decreased tone in NREM sleep and are atonic during REM sleep, which can lead to profound hypoventilation in individuals with neuromuscular diseases associated with muscle weakness. Sleepiness may be a primary neurologic symptom, as it is in narcolepsy, idiopathic hypersomnolence, and Kleine-Levin syndrome, or a secondary neurologic symptom associated with trauma, infection, or tumors of the central nervous system. The dyskinesia of restless legs (typically occurring at bedtime and relieved by movement) is another primary neurologic symptom affecting sleep.

Sleep involves transitions from wakefulness that occur not just at bedtime but also normally at multiple times during the sleep period. **Behavioral** (*Section 9*) issues and **psychiatric** disease that affect an individual's level of arousal (i.e., anxiety, depression, stress, and conditioning factors) can have a profound impact on a child's ability to make these transitions smoothly and quietly.

Many **other medical problems** (*Section 13*) may be associated with sleep disturbance. Any medical problem that leads to pain, pruritis, or inflammation may affect sleep.

The nine physiologic factors just discussed form the pathophysiologic underpinning for all sleep symptoms. The sleep process matrix (Table 5–1) is a tool for organizing and analyzing how these fundamental sleep processes interact with each other and lead to specific sleep symptoms.

As the history of the sleep problem unfolds, the clinician develops hypotheses within each of the nine domains: circadian, homeostatic, ultradian, developmental, cardiorespiratory, neurologic, psychiatric/behavioral, drugs/alcohol, and other medical. A hypothesis is a theory that could explain the problem at hand. At the beginning of an interview, there are usually many hypotheses that may explain the problem. As the patient's story becomes clear, the hypotheses are developed, and questions are formulated, the answers to which will confirm or refute the hypotheses. This process ultimately leads to an analysis and a synthesis of the data, the development of a diagnostic impression, and a treatment plan. This stepwise, sequential process allows complicated clinical cases to be broken down into smaller, more manageable chunks. This model is based on an approach to clinical problem solving described by Dr. Vincent Fulginiti in the book *Pediatric Clinical Problem Solving*.[3]

The following case illustrates the use of this case-based analysis paradigm.

Noah is a 2-year-old boy with frequent nighttime awakenings. He has awakened two to five times a night for the past year, and now that his parents are expecting the birth of their second child, they are bringing Noah in for an evaluation.

This much of the history can be gathered in the first 2 minutes of the interview in response to the question, "What brings you in today?" The remainder of the 1-hour consultation is spent trying to understand what the cause of the problem is and what to do about it. Based on just this amount of information, the clinician develops a number of hypotheses that might explain the problem, as illustrated in the second row of Table 5–1. At this point in the interview, all of these hypotheses are viable explanations for the problem at hand. Clearly, some are more likely than others.

The remainder of the interview is spent confirming or refuting the various hypotheses by gathering the appropriate history. The data gathered in this manner are analyzed and synthesized to form a tentative diagnosis, which leads to a provisional treatment plan. Often, various sleep processes interact with each other to lead to specific sleep symptoms. In Noah's case, the evaluative process led to the diagnosis of a bedtime that is too early and a sleep onset association disorder. However, the story could have ended in several other ways.

This case demonstrates how the case-based sleep process matrix can be used to describe how the various fundamental sleep processes can lead to specific sleep symptoms.

Table 5–1. Sleep Process Matrix for a 2-Year-Old Boy with Sleep Difficulty

	Circadian	Homeostatic	Ultradian	Developmental	Cardio-respiratory	Neurologic	Psychiatric/ Behavioral	Drugs/ Alcohol	Other Medical
Hypotheses	1. Delayed-sleep phase 2. Inappropriate bedtime 3. Irregular sleep schedule	1. Short sleeper 2. Late PM nap	1. Normal awakenings 2. Conditioned awakenings 3. Partial arousals	Separation anxiety	Sleep apnea	1. Seizures 2. RLS/PLMS	1. Sleep onset association disorder 2. Anxiety disorder 3. Family stress	1. Medication side effect 2. Caffeine	1. Eczema 2. GER 3. Otitis media 4. Pain
Data to Gather	1. Timing of sleep onsets, awakenings, naps 2. Light exposure in AM 3. Seasonal variation 4. Family history of phase delay	1. Sleep duration (total) 2. Nap schedule	1. Behavior during awakenings 2. Timing	Other separations	1. Snoring 2. Sleep apnea	1. Neurologic history 2. Growing pains 3. Development	1. Behavior 2. Development 3. Peers 4. How is problem handled and by whom? 5. Marital stress	Medications	ROS

Assessment   Delayed-sleep phase with too-early bedtime/sleep onset association disorder

Treatment
1. Educate parents about circadian influences and normal awakenings at night and the importance of sleep onset associations.
2. Discuss parents' preferred sleep time for child, given that the child sleeps about 11(1/2) hours per night. Schedule wake-up time at 7:30 AM, nap within a window of 1-3 PM, wake up after 3 PM regardless of how long the child has slept.
3. Move bedtime to later. At first begin at 10:30 PM, with bottle and rocking. Put child in the crib (awake but tired) and follow deconditioning protocol so that child can ultimately transition to sleep on his own.

GER, gastroesophageal reflux; RLS/PLMS, restless legs syndrome/periodic limb movements during sleep; ROS, review of systems.

References

1. Mindell JA, Owens JA: A Clinical Guide to Pediatric Sleep: Diagnosis and Management of Sleep Problems. Philadelphia, Lippincott, Williams & Wilkins, 2003.

2. Kryger MH, Roth T, Dement WC: Principles and Practice of Pediatric Sleep Medicine, 3rd ed. Philadelphia, Saunders, 2000.

3. Fulginiti V: Pediatric Clinical Problem Solving. Baltimore, Williams & Wilkins, 1981.

Polysomnography in Infants and Children

Stephen H. Sheldon

6

Polysomnography is the term used to describe a procedure of objective, simultaneous recording of many different physiologic parameters during sleep. Practitioners who treat children with sleep problems should be familiar with the general methods and techniques used in the sleep laboratory. Practical issues such as patient preparation before the study, various methods and systems used to monitor physiologic parameters, and various components of the assessment of the polysomnogram and communication of the results require understanding.

PHYSIOLOGIC PARAMETERS MONITORED DURING SLEEP

Electroencephalogram

Information from the electroencephalogram (EEG) forms the basis for differentiating the stages of sleep. Continuous monitoring of the EEG throughout the night also provides ongoing information about the development and integrity of the central nervous system. Therefore, it is necessary to use standard methods for accurate and reliable recording.

Development of Electroencephalographic Activity in the Fetus

The development of the diencephalon is essential for the establishment of centers that are fundamentally responsible for the control of the sleep–wake cycle and cycling within the sleep state. The diencephalon is prominent during the second month of development; however, it becomes concealed by the greater expansion of adjacent parts of the developing brain. All neuronal impulses that eventually reach the cortex pass through the diencephalon, with the exception of those originating from olfaction. The third

ventricle lies within the diencephalon. A small area in the caudal wall of the third ventricle becomes evaginated during the seventh week of development and forms the pineal body, which in turn eventually becomes conical, solid, and glandular. Melatonin will eventually be secreted by this structure.

After week 7 of gestation, three main regions of the diencephalon can be identified: the epithalamus dorsally, the thalamus laterally, and the hypothalamus ventrally. The thalamus rapidly outgrows the epithalamus, which ultimately becomes a synaptic region for olfactory impulses. Neuronal fibers separate the gray matter of the walls of the thalamus into the various thalamic nuclei. Similarly, the walls of the hypothalamus contain hypothalamic nuclei, the optic chiasm, suprachiasmatic nuclei, and the neural lobe of the stalk and body of the pituitary gland. The hypothalamus eventually becomes the executive region for the regulation of all autonomic activity.

The telencephalon is the most rostral subdivision of the brain. Two lateral outpouchings (evaginations) form the cerebral hemispheres, each containing a lateral ventricle. The cerebral hemispheres first begin to become prominent during week 6 of conceptional age and expand rapidly until they overgrow the diencephalon and mesencephalon during midgestation.

Development of Brain Electrical Activity (Electroencephalogram)

Neuronal electrical activity is essential for cellular migration, dendritic branching, and synaptic facilitation. The development of the EEG consists of the recording of summation potentials at the skin surface from underlying brain tissue. The underlying activity is influenced by distant portions of the central nervous system. The development of the EEG in the fetus, newborn, and child is rapidly changing. Abrupt and striking variations occur between 24 weeks of gestation and 3 months post-term. The appearance of the surface EEG of the premature infant is dependent on postconceptional age.

WEEKS 24 TO 28 OF CONCEPTIONAL AGE

Although some neuronal electrical activity is present before 24 weeks, wakefulness and sleep cannot be clearly differentiated by behavioral or EEG characteristics. At this time, the EEG reveals a *discontinuous* pattern (Fig. 6–1).

Periods of limited electrical activity lasting up to 3 minutes are separated by bursts of activity lasting up to 20 seconds. This activity is typically symmetrical and rhythmic and may be composed of alpha, theta, and delta frequencies. Sharp waves are common at these conceptional ages

and are normal when they are frontal in location or are sporadic in any location. Sharp waves and spikes that are sporadic may be normal up to shortly after 40 weeks of gestation.[1,2] Abnormalities should be considered if the spikes or sharp transients are repetitive or unilateral or occur during the quiescent period of the discontinuous pattern.

WEEKS 28 TO 32 OF CONCEPTIONAL AGE

The previously noted discontinuous activity pattern continues. However, the bursts of activity, as well as the intervals between them, are shortened. Rhythmic delta waves predominate during the bursts. Frequently, 10 to 20 Hz of activity is superimposed on these slow waves and persists until the conceptional term. This fast, superimposed activity comprises what is referred to as *delta brushes* (Fig. 6–2).

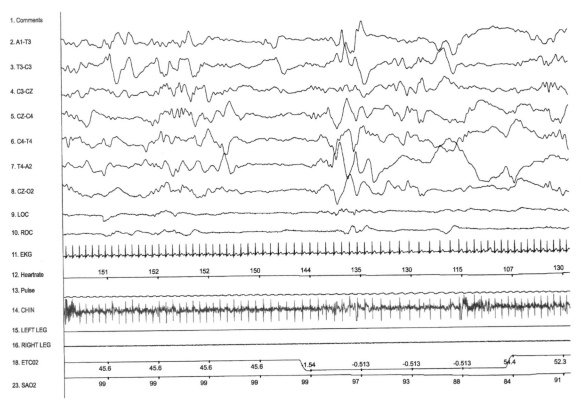

Figure 6–1. Recording of a premature infant with a discontinuous EEG pattern. This 30-second polysomnographic segment represents this pattern, which consists of intermittent bursts of high-voltage, slow-wave activity with somewhat prolonged periods of electrical quiescence between the bursts. The presence of delta brushes depends on the youngster's age. During the periods of relative electrical quiescence, there is a paucity of observable electrical activity.

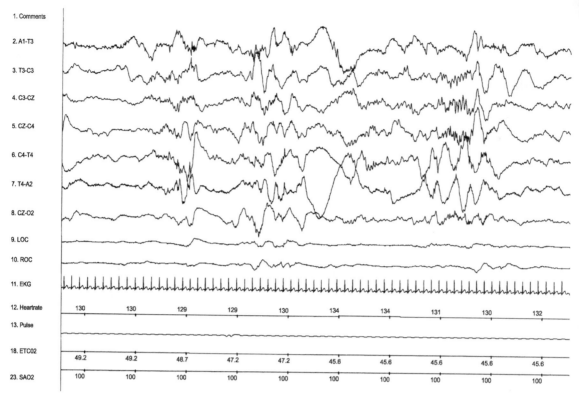

1. Comments	
2. A1-T3	
3. T3-C3	
4. C3-CZ	
5. CZ-C4	
6. C4-T4	
7. T4-A2	
8. CZ-O2	
9. LOC	
10. ROC	
11. EKG	
12. Heartrate	130 130 129 129 130 134 134 131 130 132
13. Pulse	
18. ETC02	49.2 49.2 48.7 47.2 47.2 45.6 45.6 45.6 45.6 45.6
23. SAO2	100 100 100 100 100 100 100 100 100 100

Figure 6–2. Recording of a patient with a discontinuous EEG pattern. Again, this pattern shows high-voltage, slow-wave activity separated by periods of relative electrical quiescence. The electrical activity between bursts is somewhat increased; delta brushes can be seen, and they are of relatively low voltage (10–20 Hz) superimposed on the slow waves during bursts of this activity.

WEEKS 32 TO 36 OF CONCEPTIONAL AGE

Presently, two patterns of EEG may be seen at different times during the recording. The first is the typical discontinuous pattern of slow waves in the range of one to two cycles per second, similar to the previous pattern of a tracé alternant. This pattern is characteristic of quiet sleep. The second EEG pattern is seen during wakefulness and active sleep and consists mainly of continuous, synchronous, rhythmic, and generalized waves of 1 to 2 Hz.

WEEKS 36 TO 40 OF CONCEPTIONAL AGE

As the conceptional term approaches, three EEG patterns can be identified. A quiet sleep pattern of discontinuous activity continues, but the relatively quiescent intervals and slow-wave bursts are persistently shortened. A second pattern consists of continuous irregular waves in the theta and delta frequencies appearing during wakefulness and active sleep. The delta brushes tend to disappear.

A pattern of diffuse, irregular slow waves with an amplitude of less than 50 μV is an alternative to the previous pattern defining wakefulness and active sleep. At the conceptional term, four EEG patterns can be identified.

CONCEPTIONAL TERM TO 3 MONTHS OF AGE

At the conceptional term, the trace-alternant pattern defines quiet sleep (Fig. 6–3). This is a modification of the previous discontinuous pattern and consists of bilateral bursts of high-amplitude slow waves lasting 4 to 5 seconds alternating with periods of low-amplitude activity of a similar duration. During the bursts of slow waves, frontal spikes may appear. The trace-alternant EEG pattern of quiet sleep generally disappears between weeks 3 and 4 of the postconceptional term.

During this developmental period, a new pattern emerges during quiet sleep that appears to represent the continued development of non–rapid

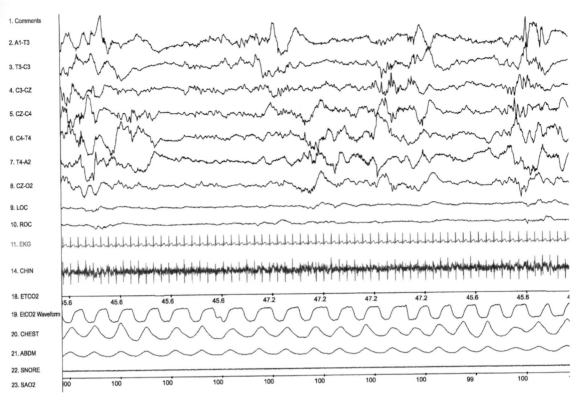

Figure 6–3. Recording of a trace alternant EEG pattern. A trace alternant EEG pattern is a continuation of the development of this discontinuous pattern into a more mature form. There are still bursts of high-voltage, slow-wave electrical activity separated by periods of lower-voltage activity (somewhat relative electrical quiescence compared with the bursts). This EEG pattern is characteristic of quiet sleep (equivalent to non–rapid eye movement [NREM] sleep) in the infant and lasts from about 36 weeks after conceptional term to 44 weeks after conception. Note that respiration during this state is quite monotonous and regular. Heart rate is also very stable and regular, although normal beat-to-beat variability is present.

eye movement (NREM) sleep. Continuous high-amplitude slow waves of 0.5 to 2 Hz appear (Fig. 6–4). They are seen most often in the posterior region of the head. Significantly faster activity of 18 to 25 Hz is often superimposed on this slow-wave activity.

Continuous medium activity is the most common EEG pattern seen during active sleep and wakefulness (Fig. 6–5). This pattern consists mainly of fairly rhythmic waves of 4 to 8 Hz and less than 50 μV. In addition, another pattern occurs during active sleep that consists of continuous low-amplitude, mixed slow waves with superimposed larger delta activity that is either intermittent or continuous.

Sleep–wake transitions are generally rapid during this maturational period. Certain behaviors may continue into sleep (e.g., sucking and swallowing [Fig. 6–6]).

The most consistent behavior correlated with sleep in the newborn is *persistent eye closure.* Infants primarily enter sleep actively. Sleep-onset REM begins to shift to sleep onset through NREM at approximately 3 months of chronologic age. However, sleep-onset REM may continue up to about 6 months of age. Active and quiet sleep periods have cycles of about 45 to 60 minutes. During the conceptional term, approximately half of the total sleep time consists of active sleep and half quiet sleep.

Before 40 weeks of gestation, smooth alterations between active and quiet sleep may be difficult to identify. Mixed-state characteristics are present, and this state is called *indeterminate* sleep.

At this time sleep spindles are poorly defined and shifting, central sharp waves may begin to appear. Synchrony is variable; however, it begins to increase between bursts of the discontinuous

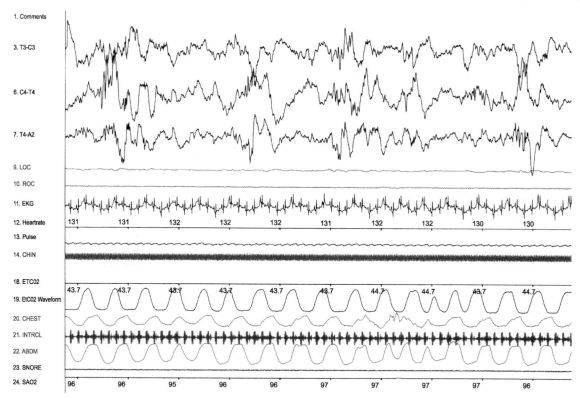

Figure 6–4. Recording of continuous high-voltage activity during quiet sleep. At approximately 44 weeks after conception, the discontinuous pattern begins to disappear and high-voltage, slow-wave activity is noted throughout the record. Again, note that respiration is quite monotonous, which is also characteristic of quiet sleep.

sleep pattern and is nearly completely synchronous by the conceptional term.

During wakefulness and sleep, EEG phenomena may be present that might be considered abnormal in older children. Nonfocal sporadic spikes, frontal sharp transients, anterior slow-wave activity, and transient asymmetries are not considered abnormal in the neonate. However, persistent phenomena (e.g., frequent focal spikes, persistent asymmetry of activity) may be abnormal, especially if they are associated with a history of potential abnormality or physical/behavioral findings that suggest abnormality.

THREE TO 12 MONTHS OF AGE

This period of development of the infant reveals striking maturational changes, as indicated on the EEG. A clear pattern of wakeful activity begins to emerge. Generalized delta and theta activity appears and is often more prominent in the posterior EEG channels. During the first year of life, slow-wave activity during wakefulness becomes more rhythmic and diminishes considerably. From 3 to 5 months of age, theta activity increases in prominence in the central and posterior regions and becomes the dominant waking rhythm after 5 months. The absence of this theta activity at this stage of development may be considered abnormal.[1,2] At 3 months of age, a relatively high voltage (50 to 100 µV or greater) of 3 to 4 Hz of occipital activity is present. By 5 months of age, the frequency increases to about 5 Hz and continues to increase throughout the first year to about 6 to 8 Hz at 12 months of age. The voltage of this activity also decreases by about 25% over this period of time.

During this period of development, sleep-wake transitions are relatively smooth. As the transition begins, the amplitude of waveforms increases and the frequency decreases. Rhythmic and synchronous activity of 75 to 200 µV and 3 to 5 Hz becomes predominant.

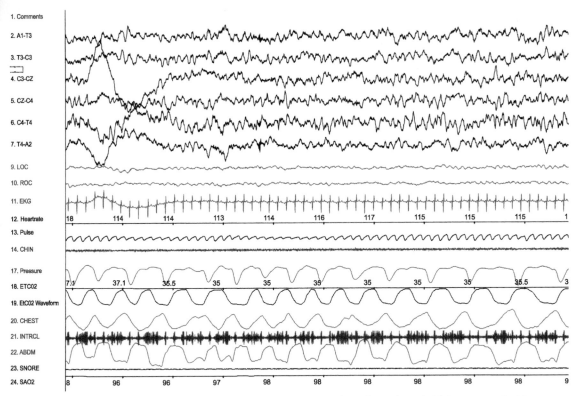

Figure 6–5. Recording of active sleep in the neonate. EEG voltage is moderately high compared with older children and adults, and the frequency is somewhat slower. Note the characteristic morphology of the EEG activity. There is normal beat-to-beat variability in heart rate, and respiration during this state is unstable and variable, with associated brief periods of erratic activity including but not limited to apnea, hypopnea, and tachypnea.

Major changes in the sleep EEG occur over the first year of life. The trace alternant in the newborn is gradually replaced by a continuous slow-wave pattern by 3 months. Clear sleep spindles consisting of waxing and waning and medium-amplitude synchronous waves of about 12 to 14 Hz appear at about 6 to 8 weeks of age. They first appear in the central regions but then expand in distribution. Between 2 and 6 months, sleep spindles assume mature characteristics and appear almost continuously throughout NREM sleep. The complete absence of sleep spindles between 3 and 6 months is most likely abnormal. Before 6 months, sleep spindles may be asymmetrical over the two hemispheres. They slowly become synchronous between 6 and 8 months. The persistence of asymmetrical spindles after 12 months of age may represent a unilateral decrease in the electrical activity of the brain.

Sleep spindles are a ubiquitous phenomenon in the sleep of older children and adults. However, their physiology and the effects of neurologic disorders on their frequency and amplitude are incompletely understood. The differences in spindle frequency may be due to underlying encephalopathy and physiologic differences between partial and generalized epilepsy as well as the possible residual effects of a variety of anticonvulsant medications.[3,4]

Spindle patterns (density, duration, frequency, amplitude, asymmetry, and asynchrony) develop quite rapidly between 1.5 and 3 months of age. This rapid development most likely reflects the developmental changes in thalamocortical structures.[5,6] Spindle expression varies in relation to ascending reticular activating tone, constituting a functionally inhibitory thalamocortical response to neurophysiologic conditions that promote central activation.[1,7] A density of 12 to 14 Hz of

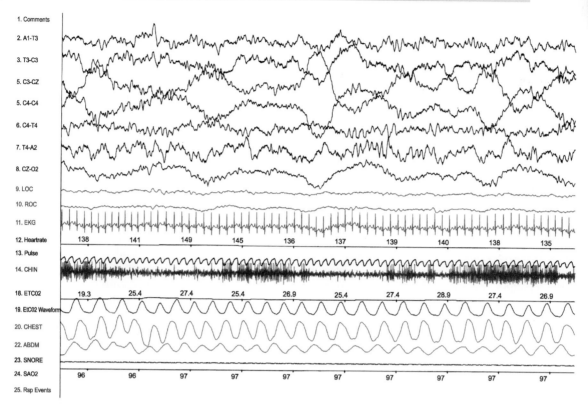

1. Comments
2. A1-T3
3. T3-C3
5. C3-CZ
5. C4-C4
6. C4-T4
7. T4-A2
8. CZ-O2
9. LOC
10. ROC
11. EKG
12. Heartrate   138   141   149   145   136   137   139   140   138   135
13. Pulse
14. CHIN
18. ETCO2   19.3   25.4   27.4   25.4   26.9   25.4   27.4   28.9   27.4   26.9
19. EtCO2 Waveform
20. CHEST
22. ABDM
23. SNORE
24. SAO2   96   96   97   97   97   97   97   97   97   97
25. Rsp Events

Figure 6–6. Recording of a sucking artifact. Non-nutritive sucking is common in infants and small children. The sucking artifact is often seen on the chin muscle electromyogram (EMG) when the youngster is sucking on a pacifier or bottle. This sucking behavior can persist into transitional sleep and may be seen in other sleep stages. Chin muscle EMG in this 30-second epoch reveals periodic and episodic crescendos of muscle activity that at times are rhythmic. There may appear to be changes in airflow during this time, since the sensor (either a thermistor or cannula) can be moved by the flange of the pacifier either deeper into the air stream or out of the air stream. In the assessment of nasal airflow, care must be taken when the baby is sucking on a pacifier. A physiologic consequence of the change in airflow must be apparent for an abnormal respiratory event to be considered in the presence of a sucking artifact.

activity is greater in stage 2 than slow-wave sleep.[5,6] Three months of age appears to be a significant juncture in the maturational process. Sleep spindle evolution seems to be an accurate reflection of the significant maturation of central nervous system processes and the resulting behaviors that occur at 10 to 12 weeks of age and in the development of NREM states and slow-wave sleep. Concordance between the quantitative aspects and nocturnal organization of individualization of slow-wave sleep in infants occurs from about 4.5 months of age.[5,6]

At 3 months of age, clear differentiation of NREM sleep states by EEG criteria is quite difficult. However, by 6 months, NREM sleep can typically be differentiated into three distinct states

(stages 1 and 2 and slow-wave sleep), and the EEG takes on a more mature pattern. Although rudimentary-vertex sharp transients and K-complexes can be identified in the neonatal period, they typically appear for the first time between 5 and 6 months of age. Vertex waves are generally seen during the lighter stages of sleep (stages 1 and 2), are of high amplitude (up to 250 μV) and negative polarity, and last less than 200 msec. K-complexes are similar to vertex waves but are considerably slower (lasting at least 0.5 second). K-complexes are often followed by a sleep spindle and have a wide distribution about the vertex. Both vertex waves and K-complexes can occur in short bursts or appear spontaneously or may occur in response to a sudden sensory stimulus.

The EEG during REM sleep also undergoes significant changes, with a decrease in the amplitude and a slight increase in and mixture of frequencies. Sawtooth waves appear, and the electrical pattern gradually begins to resemble a more mature, relatively low-voltage, mixed-frequency pattern. By 3 to 5 months of age the percentage of REM sleep decreases, constituting about 40% of the total sleep time. By the end of the first year of life, REM sleep equals about 30% of the total sleep time.

Changes During Early and Middle Childhood

Slow, consistent, and continuous changes occur during this period of development. However, these changes are more subtle, evolve over a longer period of time, and become more consistent and reproducible.

Waking rhythms with the eyes closed increase gradually from about 5 to 7 Hz of relatively high-voltage activity to the typical sinusoidal 8- to 12-Hz frequency of low–to–medium voltage activity characteristic of the adult pattern. They are most prominent over the occipital regions of the head. These developing alpha rhythms are characteristic of relaxed wakefulness with the eyes closed. It is easily attenuated with eye opening, focusing attention, or increased vigilance. Well developed alpha activity is present in most normal children by 8 years of age. The amplitude of alpha activity gradually increases during early and middle childhood but remains at a relatively low to moderate amplitude during puberty, adolescence, and adulthood.[1,2]

Transitional sleep patterns of drowsiness can be identified after 1 to 2 years of age. This sleep-wake transition becomes more mature and alpha activity diffuses and becomes admixed, with slower, mixed-frequency activity. Brief microsleep episodes occur and become more frequent during drowsiness and transitional sleep (stage 1). These microsleep episodes become longer and consolidate, alpha activity disappears from the EEG, muscle tone may decrease slightly, and slow-rolling eye movements are clearly evident.

Slow, high-voltage activity, which is very prominent during infancy and early childhood, decreases significantly throughout early and middle childhood. Diffuse, synchronous theta activity is very prominent between the ages of 1 and 4 years. This activity begins to diminish after the age of 4 years, and by 5 to 6 years of age alpha activity is about equally prominent. After 6 years of age, alpha activity becomes the predominant waking rhythm. However, hypersynchronous theta activity (Fig. 6–7) during stage 1 and early stage 2 sleep is very common during this phase of development. Indeed, even a theta–delta pattern (Fig. 6–8) can frequently be identified during slow-wave sleep in some children.

All stages of sleep are easily discernible during middle childhood. NREM sleep states can be clearly differentiated and become more similar to adult stages 1 to 4. Although the frequencies are somewhat slower in children and gradually increase to those in adults, the most striking difference is in the higher amplitude of waveforms at all frequencies until puberty, where a more adult pattern is notable. From early through middle childhood, the structure of sleep as recorded on the EEG also assumes a more mature adult characteristic.[3,8] During later infancy, sleep cycles last about 40 to 50 minutes. This cycle length increases gradually to about 60 minutes by 18 to 24 months and to 90 minutes by 5 years of age. The EEG activity of REM sleep also assumes adult characteristics and is cycled regularly with NREM sleep. After 3 months of age, most infants will shift from entering sleep through the REM pattern to entering sleep through the NREM pattern. This transition is generally complete by about 6 to 8 months of age. The percentage of REM sleep also gradually continues to decrease, from 50% at the conceptional term to 30% by 1 to 2 years and to 20 to 25% by 3 to 5 years of age.

The standard *International 10-20 System* allows for symmetrical, reproducible lead placement; comparison of EEGs from the same patient and from different patients; and recordings from the same or different laboratories (Fig. 6–9, A-C). Improper electrode placement on the scalp can lead to problems with the overall validity, evaluation, and scoring of sleep stages.

Sleep stage scoring has been standardized using a limited, referential EEG montage. In most sleep laboratories, a central recording site (C3 or C4) is coupled with a referential site (usually the opposite earlobe or mastoid process). Although only one channel of the EEG is necessary for identification of the NREM stages in adults,

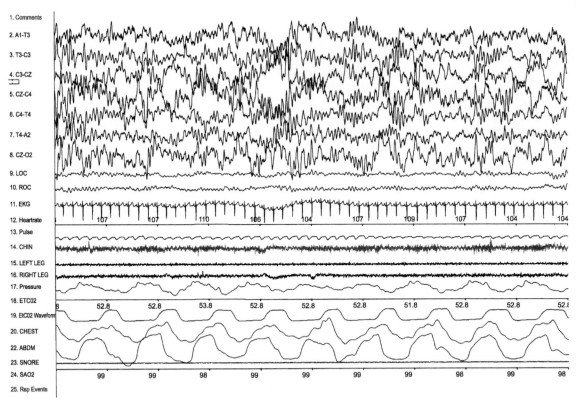

Figure 6–7. Recording of hypersynchronous theta activity in stage 2 sleep. This is a 30-second epoch recorded from a 3-year-old child. Note the predominance of theta activity in this EEG. A slow background and theta preponderance can be seen in toddlers, making the scoring of these epochs for sleep stage difficult. However, in this epoch, transients that suggest K-complexes and slow spindle-like activity can be seen. Therefore, this epoch was scored as stage 2 sleep. Coincidentally, there is a mild snoring artifact noted on the chin muscle EMG, and the end-tidal CO_2 is quite elevated. The persistence of this pattern of respiration might be indicative of alveolar hypoventilation, which may be characteristically obstructive. Full assessment of the complete polysomnogram would be required.

many laboratories use more comprehensive derivations to obtain a more complete EEG assessment. The addition of an occipital recording channel is helpful in demonstrating alpha activity in older children. A coronal or parasagittal bipolar montage may be helpful in identifying nocturnal seizure disorders. A complete EEG montage and recording strategy may be used to assist in the localization of abnormal EEG activity.

Electro-Oculogram

The recording of eye movements during sleep provides important information regarding the identification of a sleep state. Fixation of the eyes on exogenous stimuli follows a clear developmental course. Visual fixation on a single patterned stimulus has been recorded in premature newborns as early as week 30 of conceptional age.[2,5] The corneal reflection technique has permitted determination of the waking states (crying, quiet wakefulness, and drowsiness). Younger infants seem to spend more time in drowsiness, whereas older infants spend more time in quiet wakefulness as determined by fixation. Fixation time during quiet wakefulness increases with increasing gestational age, and fixation occurs more frequently in quiet wakefulness than drowsiness.

Measuring eye movements to determine the state of wakefulness has been overshadowed by the electro-oculogram (EOG) in determining a sleep state. The evaluation of eye movements during sleep is clearly required for the determination of the REM sleep state.

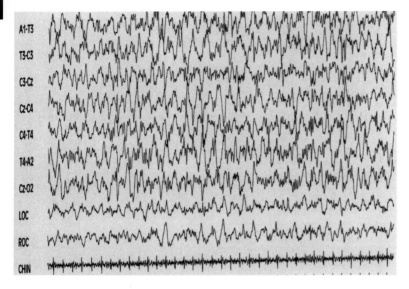

Figure 6-8. Recording of theta-delta sleep. Theta activity in toddlers and small children can predominate and be seen throughout the record. This 30-second epoch depicts theta–delta sleep, in which there is considerable theta activity superimposed on delta activity during slow-wave sleep.

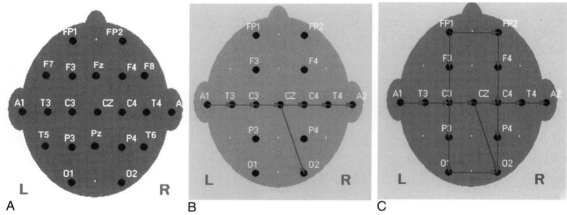

Figure 6–9. A, International 10-20 System of EEG electrode placement. This system allows for symmetrical, reproducible lead placement within and between subjects. It provides for the comparison of EEGs from the same patient and from different patients and the comparison of recordings from the same or different laboratories. From top to bottom, the standard EEG layout begins on the left side and progresses to the right side and begins at the front of the head and progresses to the back of the head. L, left; R, right. **B,** Bipolar transcoronal electrode array. The montage consists of A1-T3, T3-C3, C3-CZ, CZ-C4, C4-T4, and T4-A2. There is also an occipital channel (CZ-O2). This electrode array is standard in some laboratories. It provides greater information than the traditional referential layout of a polysomnogram, since it can differentiate between sharp waves and spikes that may be epileptic in nature and the vertices of sharp waves. It can also provide information regarding hemispheric differences in electrical activity. L, left; R, right. **C,** Expanded transcoronal and parasagittal electrode array. It consists of the transcoronal array *and* additional electrodes over the right and left hemispheres that can more accurately localize questionable electrical activity as anterior or posterior. Nonetheless, the gold standard for the EEG is a complete International 10-20 System electrode array that can accurately identify and diagnose abnormal electrical activity.

The eye is a functional dipole, with the cornea being 75 to 100 µV positive compared with the retina. By using EOG techniques, conjugate and nonconjugate eye movements can be recorded with the eyelids closed. Recording electrodes are conventionally placed at the outer canthus of each eye and offset from the horizontal plane by approximately 0.5 to 1.0 cm. These distances may be modified depending on the size of the infant. Offsetting the electrodes from the horizontal plane (one above and one below) is crucial for the identification of vertical and oblique eye movements.

Eye movements occur in saccades during wakefulness and in saccadic bursts during active sleep. Slow-rolling and dysconjugate eye movements can occur during quiet wakefulness, drowsiness, and sleep–wake transitions and in certain medical/surgical abnormalities (e.g., extraocular muscle paralysis, brainstem anatomic abnormalities, disorders that affect the cranial nerves). Since retinal development in premature infants involves migration of the vasculature from the region surrounding the optic disc toward the periphery as well as the development of central control of eye movements, the EOG may reveal both saccadic and dysconjugate eye movements in younger premature infants. Since the characteristics of the electromyogram (EMG) may not be as reliable as the EEG and EOG, the identification of REM sleep requires a characteristic EEG pattern and the presence of at least *some* saccadic eye movements.

The development of clear conjugate eye movements during wakefulness depends to a great extent on the stage of retinal development and the maturational level of fixation. However, the saccadic eye movements during sleep do not require retinal development or conscious fixation. Control may be mediated through a number of different but interrelated central neurologic mechanisms that include, but are not limited to, cerebral and cerebellar cortical and subcortical development, oculomotor/trochlear/abducens nuclei development, and the maturation of central vestibular nuclei. The development of the vestibular system is important for fixation during wakefulness and ocular saccades during active sleep.[1,8]

Ocular movements have been identified by traditional visual inspection of saccades beneath the closed eyelid. This technique may have specific limitations, especially in the sleep laboratory. EOG is considerably more reliable and cost-effective, and eye movements can be identified by post hoc inspection of the polysomnographic recording. Unfortunately, the specific limitations of EOG are present in smaller infants. The eyes of premature neonates present weaker dipoles, and there may be considerable difficulty with subjective analysis. In an attempt to resolve these obstacles, automated methods for the analysis of REMs during active sleep in infants has been described.[3,9] Computer analysis of slope and amplitude threshold criteria have been performed. Digital filtering is used to improve the effectiveness, identification, and quantification of ocular movements. The method has been shown to be highly reliable and useful in differentiating between tonic and phasic states during active sleep. This differentiation of REM sleep into two distinct states by the presence or absence of phasic muscle and extraocular muscle activity may hold specific significance for the evaluation of studies of sleep-related cardiorespiratory physiology during infancy. In healthy adults, the different physiologic characteristics of tonic and phasic REMs can be clearly identified.[5,10] This may also be true of infants.

Dream-related and non–dream-related ocular movements occur in both humans and animals.[7,11] It appears that only high-amplitude REMs and eye movements occurring in bursts have any possibility of corresponding to visual images. Intense REMs during sleep have been investigated as a possible indication of a delay in the neural development of infants.[8,12] Becker and Thoman evaluated the occurrence of "REM storms" in first-born infants from the second through the fifth postnatal week and again at 3, 6, and 12 months of age. The amount of REMs within each 10-second interval of active sleep was rated on a scale based on the frequency and intensity of eye movements. Bayley scales of mental development were administered to the cohort of infants at 12 months of age. A significant negative correlation was found between the frequency of REM storms and Bayley scores. By 6 months of age, REM storms seemed to express dysfunction or delay in the development of central inhibitory feedback control for sleep organization and phasic sleep-related activities.

Although few studies exist in infants and children, eye movement density has been shown to be significantly decreased during the second and third REM periods after a night of complete and partial sleep deprivation. The rebound of slow-wave sleep is generally confined to the first NREM sleep period and increases in activity amplitude of 0.05 to 3 Hz.

Piezoelectric strain gauge transducers have also been used to evaluate eye movements during sleep.[10,13] These sensors have been shown to be highly sensitive to fine microtremor activity during wakefulness. This micronystagmoid activity diminishes during NREM sleep and increases during REM sleep. It is very intriguing to note that microtremor ocular activity also increases after the presentation of an auditory stimulus to subjects during NREM sleep. Similar increased microtremor activity also occurs with the appearance of K-complexes in the EEG.

Electromyogram and Movement Activity During Sleep

Although EMG activity during sleep can be assessed using any number of skeletal muscle groups, it has become customary to record muscle tone from the chin. Certain sleep disorders (e.g., bruxism, REM sleep behavior disorder) may present with unusual muscle activity that can be recorded by surface EMG. Additional information may be provided regarding the patient's sleep–wake behavior, permitting quantification of arousal responses and movements during sleep.

In general, three recording electrodes are applied to the chin, although a recording is obtained from only two. The extra electrode is placed to provide a backup in the event an electrode becomes displaced during the recording. Electrodes filled with electroconductive cream are taped to the skin in the submental region. This procedure effectively records the activity of superficial muscles as well as the genioglossus muscle.

EMG activity from other muscles (e.g., anterior tibial) may be simultaneously recorded for the evaluation of abnormal or paroxysmal movements during sleep.

Body movements are characteristic of the sleep state. Both short-wave sleep and REM sleep generally end with a body movement or abrupt increase in chin muscle EMG activity. The next sleep cycle follows.

Intermittent body movements frequently occur during sleep without a significant change in the state or beginning of a new sleep cycle. These movements without a state change involve both brief phasic activity lasting less than 6 seconds and gross slower body movements (squirming) lasting longer than 6 seconds. Maturation of this skeletal muscle activity also follows a regular and predictable pattern. During wakefulness, gross motor and fine motor activities form the basis for half of the developmental screening test. Maturation of gross motor, fine motor, and phasic muscle movements during sleep may also be a sensitive marker of neurologic development.

During quiet wakefulness, random muscle activity usually does not occur. However, a wide range of elementary and complex motor activities are known to occur during sleep. Minute, random electrical activity constitutes the basic physiologic condition of the skeletal muscles during sleep.[11] In NREM sleep, minute, random motor activity decreases considerably when compared with the quiet waking state. During REM sleep, there is a sudden increase in isolated motor unit action potentials. Particular structural features of the anterior tibial muscle make it seemingly the most active muscle during sleep,[11] and monitoring of the anterior tibial EMG activity during sleep is recommended during nocturnal polysomnography in all neonates, infants, children, adolescents, and adults.

Although a significant decrease in the number of body position shifts occurs during sleep across the life cycle,[12,15] in middle childhood there do not appear to be differences in the number and frequency of major body movements and position shifts in normal youngsters. During early childhood, there appears to be an increase in the duration of maintenance of body position and in the number of periods of more than 30 minutes of positional immobility. In middle childhood, prone, supine, and lateral positions occupy equal proportions of the sleep period. Sleeping in the prone position is characteristically abandoned as maturation continues.

Characteristic body and muscle movements in premature newborns and term neonates during quiet sleep appear similar to startle (Moro's) reflexes, generalized phasic movements,[14] and a tonic increase in submental muscle activity. In contrast to the total simultaneous pattern of motor activity seen during quiet sleep, active sleep is characterized by a more uncoordinated and localized pattern of movements such as generalized phasic movements, localized tonic activity, localized phasic activity, and brief clonic muscle activity. With increasing conceptional age, there is a decrease in the occurrence of the startle reflex, generalized phasic movements, and localized phasic movements. Localized tonic activity tends to remain constant with increasing conceptional age. The differences in decreasing tendencies among these movements may indicate the variation in maturational changes for different parts of the central nervous system.[13]

The degree of phasic activity during sleep may reflect the maturity of the developing brainstem. Dissociation of sleep-related phasic motor phenomena may hold special clinical significance for some infants.[14,16] On the other hand, the types of skeletal muscle movement show specific developmental relationships with respect to conceptional age. Fukumoto and colleagues[17] described the ontogenetic evolution of three types of movement: gross, localized , and phasic (twitches lasting less than 0.5 second). All body movement parameters decreased in frequency with maturation. Interestingly, each type of movement behavior showed a fairly specific and individual time course. The earliest decrease between week 30 of conceptional age and 18 months of chronologic age occurs in phasic activity, which takes place relatively early in the development of the infant. Localized movements decrease in frequency next, and gross movement continues unchanged until a basal level is reached at approximately 9 to 13 months of postnatal age. The number of epochs without body movements increases steadily until about 8 months of age.

Gross, localized, and phasic movements are controlled by the central nervous system at different organizational levels. Phasic activity is more ontogenetically simple and decreases early during maturation. Gross movements are quite complex and require a greater degree of central nervous system integration. Therefore, these types of movement are correlated with the maturational processes of the central nervous system and provide an additional window and indicator of normal and abnormal development. The evaluation of these types of movement during polysomnography can provide an additional assessment when coupled with traditional developmental appraisals.

The evolution of movements and specific spontaneous behaviors during sleep in neonates has been reported by Meyers.[18] The frequency distribution of time intervals between spontaneous behaviors showed that movements were typically spaced closely in time. However, none of these spontaneous motor activities occur with a set interval between successive behaviors. Spontaneous muscle activity in the sleeping neonate conforms to a single pattern of temporal organization regardless of the specific movement displayed or the state of sleep. The pattern approximates a systematic alternation of periods of increasing and decreasing intervals between successive behaviors.

When clear NREM states can be identified, body movements reveal a clear state-dependent relationship.[19] A continuum of movements can be demonstrated with decreasing frequency, respectively, among wakefulness, stage 1 (transitional sleep), REM sleep, stage 2 (NREM), and slow-wave sleep. The relative frequency of body movements seems to be regulated by state-dependent mechanisms, and body movements may be a reliable measure of the development and organizational maturation of sleep state differentiation, particularly if the time base is long enough. When the maturational progression of these states does not follow the expected developmental pattern, support for the diagnosis of a delay in maturation of the central nervous system may be considered. Prolonged, uninterrupted sleep states without body movements or position change might indicate abnormal development of the arousal response and constitute a subtle indication of an underlying central nervous system control abnormality.

Body position may have a significant effect on sleep state organization and might suggest that the central vestibular system contributes to the development and organization of a state. Hashimoto and coworkers studied the contribution of the prone and supine body positions to both physiologic and behavioral correlates during sleep in neonates.[16,20] Quiet sleep occupied a greater percentage of the total sleep time when the newborn was in the prone rather than the supine position. Gross movements and phasic muscle activity were also less frequently observed in the prone position, although there was no difference in localized movements between the two body positions. Predictably, since there was an increase in quiet sleep, respiration was more regular in the prone position. Interestingly, the pulse rate during quiet sleep was higher in this position.

The type and frequency of body movements during sleep may provide significantly useful information regarding the integrity of the central nervous system in term newborns. Hakamoda and associates[17,21] studied body movements in term newborns with significant illnesses or malformations such as perinatal asphyxia, purulent meningitis, meconium aspiration syndrome, gastrointestinal bleeding, porencephaly, and hydranencephaly. Newborns who had recovered from transient vomiting were also evaluated and used as a comparison group. Generalized body movements, localized tonic movements, and generalized phasic movements were evaluated. Patients with minimally depressed background EEG activity showed an increase in generalized movements and localized tonic movements during quiet sleep. On the other hand, hydrancephalic infants showed an increase in generalized phasic movements in active and quiet sleep and a profound decrease in generalized movements during sleep when EEG abnormalities were markedly severe. The absence of or a significant decrease in generalized body movements or an increase in generalized phasic muscle activity might indicate a very poor prognosis for particular infants. On the other hand, the presence of localized tonic movements (even in small amounts) suggests the preservation of cortical function.

Spontaneous body movements and behaviors appear to be controlled by an interaction of endogenous rhythms that do not appear to run independently.[18,22] Instead, a system of interaction between endogenous oscillations exists. By 2 weeks of age, an ultradian 3- to 4-hour cycle can easily be identified. This cycle is typically related to feeding patterns and may be controlled by hypothalamic mechanisms and metabolic requirements. A 50-minute basic rest and activity cycle (BRAC), originally described by Kleitman,[23] can be identified, and a circadian cycle is present at about 8 to 12 weeks of age.

The BRAC appears to trigger sensory and motor mechanisms characterizing both of the phases of enhanced stereotypical motor activity

during the day and night in children with developmental disabilities and associated stereotypical behaviors during wakefulness and sleep.[18,22] The peak frequency of stereotypical behaviors seems to follow the same mean REM-to-REM interval on consecutive nights.

New methods of the digital and statistical analysis of EEG, EMG, and EOG activity have the potential to describe the structural and temporal characteristics of tonic electrophysiologic activity during sleep.[20,24] Three components can be identified: slow-fast, hemispheric shift, and ocular movement activation. Cycles of tonic electrophysiologic activity, which are both slower and faster than the typical 90-minute ultradian rhythm of sleep states, can be identified by the use of these components in older children and adults.

Activity monitoring accelerometry can also provide significant information regarding disturbed sleep in infants and children. First, the monitoring of sleep states by actigraphy is generally consistent with polysomnography when assessing certain parameters of sleep and the sleep–wake cycle in children. Sadeh and colleagues have described actigraphic sleep–wake scoring in sleep-disturbed children compared with a control group of healthy children.[25] Movements measured actigraphically that are characteristic of wakefulness lasting longer than 5 minutes were significantly greater in the sleep-disturbed group of children, clearly showing poorer sleep quality in this group (12 to 18 months of age). Sleep measurements showed significant night-to-night stability in both groups. The stability of specific measurements and their age trends were different between the groups. These data clearly showed that the measurement of body movements during sleep at home could discriminate between sleep-disturbed and healthy children with a highly correct assignment rate.

Other motor disorders of childhood have significant sleep-related correlates and motor behaviors that can be monitored and assessed polysomnographically. Gadoth and coworkers studied sleep-related body movements and periodic limb movements in unrelated patients with L-dopa–responsive, hereditary, progressive dystonia. Also studied were their unaffected family members.[26] All patients with dystonia had an increase in major body movements during REM sleep. Most unaffected parents and siblings had similar REM-related body movements, periodic limb movements, or both. Therefore, a common mechanism for the dystonia, body movements, and periodic limb movements may exist, and a causative relationship between these two motor phenomena during sleep seems to be implied.

Electrocardiogram Activity

At least one channel of the polysomnogram is dedicated to recording the patient's electrocardiogram (ECG). Cardiac activity is generally monitored for rate and rhythm, since only a limited, single channel is used. Only relative information about cardiac electrical function is provided by polysomnography, and clinical conclusions regarding a patient's ECG is generally not possible. If a comprehensive evaluation of cardiac activity is necessary, Holter monitoring may be added to the recording strategy.

The anatomy and function of the fetal cardiovascular system differ profoundly from those of extrauterine life. Although the right and left heart function in parallel during fetal life, immediately after birth the right and left sides function in series. Anatomic and physiologic changes in the respiratory and cardiac systems occur immediately at birth. Alveolar fluid within the lung is expressed and absorbed, being replaced immediately with air. Pressure changes and oxygenation result in closure of the ductus arteriosus and ventricular and atrioseptal communicating channels, isolating the pulmonary and systemic circulation.

Heart rate generally decreases during natural sleep and is about 4 to 8 beats per minute slower when the heart rate during quiet wakefulness is compared with quiet sleep.[3,27] During tonic periods of REM sleep, a decrease in rate of approximately 8% less than that for quiet wakefulness has been reported. A reduction in heart rate during sleep appears to parallel sleep-related alterations in blood pressure.[5,28] In addition, heart rate variability is clearly greater in REM sleep than in slow-wave sleep.[7,29] Although there is a significant decrease in heart rate during tonic periods of REM sleep, heart rate is also significantly influenced by phasic activity during REM sleep.[8,30] During the phasic activity of REM sleep, there are clear episodes of short-lasting tachycardia followed occasionally by a brief rebound

bradycardia before a return to baseline levels. Variations in heart rate differ significantly according to the sleep state. Before week 37 of gestational age, the sequential curves of heart rate show periodic variations present in both active and quiet sleep.[9,31] After 37 weeks, slow periodic variations are still present in active sleep but superimposed by fast variations synchronous with respiratory cycles. Fast variations prevail in quiet sleep.

In newborns suffering from pathologic conditions (medical or surgical), less variability associated with respiration is seen with prematurity, young age at recording, and hypercapnia. However, this diminished respiratory-related variation in heart rate can be very transient. Pronounced variations similar to those in babies without abnormalities are observed in two thirds of the patients with or without ventilatory assistance.[9,31] The periodicity of heart rate and respiration varies during sleep in newborn babies.[10,32] The period durations obtained by power spectral analysis showed two maximums. In many cases the cycles of respiration and heart rate were not identical. It has been shown that newborns have two separate cycles with different period durations. The shorter cycle probably originates from fetal life; the longer one represents the development of a more mature periodicity. In studying respiration and heart rate variation in normal infants during quiet sleep over the first year of life, Litscher and associates showed that both the respiratory rate during quiet sleep and respiratory variability decrease with age.[11,33] A comparison of the cardiorespiratory data from the first and last quiet sleep periods showed no significant differences within any of the age groups studied.

VanGeijn and colleagues studied heart rate as an indicator of the sleep state in newborn infants.[13,34] During quiet sleep, the R-R interval length was longer, the long-term irregularity index lower, and the interval-difference index higher than those found during the immediately preceding or following active sleep. For nonconsecutive quiet and active sleep states, a maximum separation was obtained and, with discriminant function analysis, correctly classified in 93% of quiet and active sleep epochs. These data have specific implications for the identification of the sleep state in the fetus without the need for antepartum invasive monitoring.

Heart rate and its variability can be affected by medications. In one study by Gabriel and Albani, it was demonstrated that the amount of active sleep, as well as the incidence of apnea and/or cardiac slowing occurring predominantly during active sleep, was decreased at therapeutic levels of phenobarbital.[35] With declining serum drug levels, active sleep showed a rebound effect; at the same time, apnea and/or cardiac slowing relapsed. These findings tend to confirm the fact that neonatal apnea is facilitated by active sleep-inhibitory brain mechanisms and these mechanisms have significant effects not only on the respiratory system but also on the cardiovascular system.

Beat-to-beat variability in heart rate has been used as an index of the integrity of the autonomic nervous system in early infancy. Mazza and coworkers have shown that the beat-to-beat heart rate variability during active sleep and quiet sleep correlated very well with the instantaneous heart rate (R-R interval).[36] The correlation coefficient was .49 to .92 in quiet sleep and .50 to .03 in active sleep. Regression analysis supported a linear approximation of the beat-to-beat heart rate variability to the instantaneous heart rate over the range investigated. The slopes of these linear functions were similar in both active sleep and quiet sleep for infants from birth to 4 months of age.[15,36]

The assessment of vagal tone may be a significant method of assessing the periodic variation in heart rate associated with respiration (respiratory sinus arrhythmia). Arendt and associates studied vagal tone in 20 full-term infants and found that the heart period and its variability were highly correlated with vagal tone.[37] Variation in vagal tone among sleep states was also detected. Repeated assessments revealed that the average vagal tone values collected for the same sleep state were not significantly correlated across successive days. This short-term variability both among and within individuals does not support the notion that a single assessment of vagal tone can be used by itself to identify infants at risk for sudden unexpected death during sleep or predict a neurodevelopmental outcome. However, successive assessments might provide a greater degree of information.

In older infants and children, heart rate reveals significant respiratory modulation. This is referred to as a normal sinus arrhythmia (see Fig. 6–2). However, in newborn infants the respiratory modulation of heart rate is variable.

Particular types of heart rate variation are enhanced during periods of slow heart rate and diminished when heart rate is high. Shechtman and Harper have shown that the maturational patterns of heart rate, based on the correlation of heart rate variations, were strongly influenced by the sleep–wake state and were dissimilar to those previously reported for the correlation between cardiac and respiratory measures.[38] Their findings suggest dissimilar developmental patterns for autonomic and somatic motor systems and include a discontinuity in autonomic development at approximately 1 month of age. They speculated that these trends reflected a change in the nature of sleep states as forebrain connections develop.

State-dependent variations also occur over the first year of life. Litscher and colleagues performed spectral analysis of breathing and heart rate patterns during the first and last episodes of quiet sleep recorded over an 8-hour all-night period on 19 infants at 6 weeks, 6 months, and 1 year of age.[33] A total of 43 recordings were analyzed. Their results demonstrated that the respiratory rate decreases during quiet sleep and the respiratory variability decreases with age. Calculations of heart rate in beats per minute and heart rate variability (%) revealed a slowing of heart rate and an increase in variability. A comparison of the cardiorespiratory data from the first and last quiet sleep periods showed no significant differences within any one of these age groups.

When Haddad and coworkers studied the state dependence of the QT interval in normal infants at 2 weeks, 1 month, 2 months, 3 months, and 4 months of life, they found that the QT index (defined as the QT interval divided by the square root of the R-R interval) was significantly greater during quiet sleep than REM sleep. This significant difference was present in all age groups studied.[19,39]

Cardiac output is also coupled to heart rate during wakefulness. However, cardiac output is only slightly decreased during slow-wave sleep.[3,18,27,40] A decrease in cardiac output is more significantly pronounced during the tonic REM state, its average being about 9% less than that during quiet wakefulness. Changes in cardiac output are not accompanied by changes in stroke volume, which tends to remain constant during quiet wakefulness, slow-wave sleep, and REM sleep.

Blood pressure also varies significantly between quiet wakefulness and sleep. There is a relatively modest decrease in blood pressure during NREM sleep (approximately 14 mm Hg).[7,29] It decreases to an even greater extent during tonic REM sleep. Blood pressure variation during REM sleep is complex and notable. Periods of relative hypotension are interrupted by brief, sharp increases in mean arterial pressure.[8,30] Oscillations in blood pressure appear to be related to the phasic phenomena of REM sleep. Blood pressure increases appear to occur shortly before or after the onset of bursts of phasic activity (e.g., eye movements, phasic muscle twitches).

Abnormalities and intercurrent medical conditions can affect the variability and state dependence of heart rate and contribute to arrhythmias. Fagioli and colleagues have shown that there is a high frequency of sinus pauses in malnourished infants.[19,41] This arrhythmia was identified mainly during quiet sleep. After the nutritional rehabilitation of the infants studied, there was a dramatic reduction in the frequency of these sinus pauses. They concluded that the large number of sinus pauses seen in infants suffering from severe malnutrition may reflect a disturbance of neurovegetative regulation that is intensified by sleep-related physiologic changes.

Cardiac and other cardiovascular variations during sleep in newborns, infants, and children are complex and appear to hold particular and consequential clinical relevance. Phasic excitation of the heart and vascular changes in the coronary, systemic, and cerebral circulations may profoundly influence the course of other medical conditions in the fragile child.

Respiratory Activity

Three respiratory parameters are typically monitored during polysomnographic assessment: nasal/oral airflow, respiratory effort, and oxygen saturation. The recording of nasal and oral airflow is most commonly accomplished by the placement of thermistors or thermocouples in the stream of air. This method of recording airflow is simple, comfortable, and highly reliable for most patients but can be imprecise due to positional factors and may require the technician to frequently adjust the sensors and alter the amplifier sensitivity. Pneumotachograph recording is less commonly used, requires the patient to wear a large facemask during sleep, and may be impractical for many patients.

Respiratory effort may be measured with strain gauges, chest wall impedance, intercostal EMG, inductance plethysmography, and pneumatic transducers. All of these methods provide reliable information regarding the patient's breathing by monitoring movement of the chest and abdomen. In children and adults the least restrictive methods are preferable, largely because they minimize discomfort and promote compliance with the all-night procedure.

Pulse oximetry is the standard for noninvasive, continuous monitoring of arterial oxygen saturation. The probe may be placed on an earlobe, finger, toe, or foot (in the younger infant). Using spectrophotoelectric principles for recording, the pulse oximeter circumvents the complications associated with the transcutaneous measurement of the partial pressure of oxygen or the use of an indwelling arterial catheter. It provides reliable information regarding respiratory function and highly correlates with simultaneous blood gas determinations.

Anterior Tibial EMG Activity

If periodic leg movements during sleep or nocturnal myoclonus is suspected, EMGs from the left and right anterior tibial muscles are recorded. Two surface electrodes are taped approximately 3 cm apart on each leg to monitor leg muscle activity during the sleep period. Leg muscle EMG can also provide additional information about limb and body movements during the recording period.

Audio-Video Monitoring

Continuous audio and video monitoring and recording of the patient during the sleep period can provide significant details about underlying sleep-related pathology. Somnambulistic episodes can be chronicled, seizure activity can be documented, and some symptoms of sleep apnea (e.g., loud snoring) can be recorded. Continuous monitoring also provides a necessary safety function as well as detailed observational data about the patient's sleeping positions at the time of abnormal physiologic events.

POLYSOMNOGRAPHIC TECHNIQUES

Neonatal and Infant Monitoring

Indications for Study and Common Usage

- Suspected apnea of prematurity
- Suspected apnea of infancy
- Suspected severe gastroesophageal reflux with or without aspiration
- Evaluation of some children who have suffered apparently life-threatening events
- Suspected seizure disorder
- Presence of major morphologic abnormalities, especially those that involve congenital malformations of the head, face, mouth, tongue, neck, and/or chest (e.g., Pierre Robin syndrome, Treacher Collins syndrome, Beckwith's syndrome)
- Suspected central hypoventilation syndrome
- Congenital neuromuscular disorders associated with generalized hypotonia
- Metabolic/genetic disorders associated with hypotonia and/or abnormalities of the head and neck
- Postoperative evaluation of infants who have undergone surgery of the face, mouth, and/or neck (e.g., status/post–cleft palate repair)
- Other (individualized indications that depend on the infant's presenting problem)

Potential Future Usage

- Evaluation of development and/or maturation of the central nervous system.
- Evaluation of long-term prognosis for the "new morbidity" (New morbidity includes entities such as learning disabilities, behavioral abnormalities, and isolated developmental delays.)
- Evaluation of the acute neurophysiologic status of infants suffering from intrauterine drug exposure
- Prognosis of the intrauterine drug–exposed infant
- Evaluation of the developmental and neurologic outcomes of many other congenital and acquired abnormalities (e.g., infants who are status/post-intraventricular hemorrhage)
- Objective neurophysiologic evaluation of infants with low 5-minute APGAR scores

Equipment Recommended: Standard/Elective

Standard Polygraph and Standard EEG Electrode Array

EEG: CHOICE OF MONTAGE

Raw data monopolar recordings are standard for all patients. Two montages might be elected in the evaluation of the neonate. A single scoring channel is inadequate for comprehensive polysomnographic analysis of the neonate or child. The two standard electrode arrays are shown in Table 6–1.

The standard transcoronal electrode array is used in children under 2 years of age unless otherwise indicated by physician order. In small and premature infants, a double-distance electrode array may be used. The standard-distance transcoronal and parasaggital electrode array is used in all children over 2 years of age unless otherwise indicated.

EMG

Standard chin muscle EMG should be used for identification of the sleep state. In addition, the optional limb-surface EMG (e.g., bilateral, upper and lower extremities) might be used to identify phasic activity and limb movements.

EOG

Standard EOG activity may be monitored using two electrodes placed 1 cm lateral to the outer canthi of each eye and offset from the horizontal by 1 cm. Eye movement during the neonatal period is often nonconjugate. This must be taken into consideration in the evaluation of the EOG.

Wrapping the infant's head in a soft, self-adhering bandage is usually recommended. This protects the electrodes against displacement. If the head is wrapped loosely, a sweat artifact is usually avoided.

Recording of Respiratory Movements and Function

Respiratory Effort

Respiratory effort should be measured and/or monitored by inductive plethysmography or piezocrystal belts. Chest effort and abdominal

Table 6–1. Standard Electrode Arrays			
Standard-Distance Transcoronal Montage	**Standard-Distance Bitemporal Montage**		
A1-T3	1. FP1-F7	9. A1-T3	
T3-C3	2. F7-T3	10. T3-C3	
C3-CZ	3. T3-T5	11. C3-CZ	
CZ-C4	4. T5-O1	12. CZ-C4	
C4-T4	5. FP2-F8	13. C4-T4	
T4-A2	6. F8-T4	14. T4-A2	
CZ-O2	7. T4-T6	15. CZ-O2	
C4-A1 or C3-A2	8. T6-O2		

movement are recorded on separate channels and calibrated in phase when the child is awake, assuming there is no respiratory distress during the waking state. Measuring respiratory effort by means of only the chest wall and abdominal impedance has poor sensitivity and specificity and should be avoided. In addition to the assessment of continuous changes in chest and abdominal circumference (or volume with plethysmography), intercostal EMG is also used to evaluate respiratory effort. This is an indirect measurement of diaphragmatic muscle activity. Electrodes are placed in the fifth intercostal space in the anterior axillary line and calibrated to record diaphragmatic as well as intercostal muscle activity.

Nasal/Oral Airflow

Airflow is best measured and/or monitored by nasal pressure transduction and continuous monitoring of the capnography waveform. Thermistor application has been the standard technique in adult laboratories but might not be as sensitive a measure of airflow as pressure is in children.

Although the phenomenon is not universal, newborn infants are typically obligate nasal breathers. The measurement of nasal airflow alone may be adequate for most studies. The measurement of end-tidal CO_2 is a highly accurate method of determining airflow at the nose and mouth. Side-stream analysis of end-tidal CO_2 is conducted on all patients. Waveforms are recorded, and a running 10-second average is also recorded on all patients. A split-lumen cannula is used for measuring both nasal/oral pressure and end-tidal CO_2. When supplemental oxygen is required, the nasal pressure lumen is abandoned and supplemental oxygen provided, leaving the end-tidal CO_2 lumen for recording the capnography waveform. There is a 3-second sampling delay when measuring side-stream end-tidal CO_2; therefore, analysis and the categorization of occlusive and partially occlusive respiratory events, as well as central respiratory pause, must take this sampling delay into account.

Hemoglobin-Oxygen Saturation

Continuous monitoring of SaO_2 by pulse oximetry is standard in all neonatal polysomnographic procedures. In the sick neonate and/or the premature infant, the infant's blood pH and temperature should be known in order to accurately assess oxygen saturation during the study. In addition, it is important to be aware of the P50 (position of the hemoglobin-oxygen dissociation curve) for fetal hemoglobin for accurate monitoring and assessment.

Optional Parameters

$TcPO_2$ and $TcPCO_2$ may be continuously or intermittently monitored during the study. These parameters will be individually ordered when needed. However, the complication rate (burns) from the heated probes is significantly greater than that seen with continuous monitoring of SaO_2. Therefore, these methods should be reserved only for certain circumstances and individualized for each patient. The probe site should be relocated every hour when continuous monitoring is required. Transesophageal pressure may also be monitored and is highly sensitive and specific for increasing nadirs of negative intrathoracic pressure in the high upper airway resistance syndrome.

Measurement of Heart Rate and Rhythm

Continuous monitoring of heart rate and rhythm may be accomplished by using standard ECG lead II placement. Alternatively, an electrode may be placed in the middle of the chest (midsternal region) and referenced to A1 or A2. The rate should be determined by the frequency of QRS complexes and the fast Fourier transformation of the R-R interval, and beat-to-beat variability should be evaluated by the comparison of R-R intervals and assessed during wakefulness, quiet sleep, and active sleep.

Movement

Movement may be monitored by limb EMG (upper and lower); direct observations by the technician, with his/her notations on the record; and/or video recording. Actigraphy may also be considered for monitoring activity. Behavioral observations and notations are significant and important during neonatal and infant polysomnography.

Standard Duration of the Study

Polysomnograms should last a minimum of 6 hours but optimally 8 hours. The timing of the studies is also important. They should be conducted during the late evening and early morning hours (e.g., 10:00 PM to 6:00 AM).

Description

A polysomnogram consists of the continuous nocturnal monitoring of the EEG (bipolar transcoronal and parasaggital electrode array), EOG (left outer and right outer canthus), chin muscle EMG, left and right anterior tibial muscle EMG, lead II ECG, instantaneous heart rate (R-R interval by flicker fusion threshold analysis), nasal/oral airflow by capnography and pressure transduction, end-tidal CO_2 trend by capnometry, chest and abdominal wall respiratory movement by piezocrystal belts, body position, upper

respiratory tract sound by sonography, and oxygen saturation by pulse oximetry. Continuous pulse volume is measured by using finger plethysmography. The record is scored and evaluated according to the accepted criteria of Rechtschaffen and Kales for children over 6 months of age[42] or Anders, Parmalee, and Emdee for children younger than 6 months of age.[43] Analysis is conducted in 30-second epochs; all epochs of the recording are analyzed.

ARCHITECTURE

The analysis of sleep structure throughout the night is known as its architecture. Sleep latency is the time from lights out to sleep onset. REM latency is the time from sleep onset to the first REM sleep period. WASO means "wake after sleep onset." Sleep efficiency is calculated by dividing the WASO by the total sleep time. The sleep state percentages for the entire recording are also reported. Laboratory effects may result in a somewhat longer sleep latency period than at home and a slight decrease in REM sleep.

ELECTROENCEPHALOGRAM

There is a comprehensive screening EEG electrode array. It is not a diagnostic EEG recording.

CHIN ELECTROMYOGRAM

The submental muscles are continuously evaluated for a snore artifact and/or bruxism. The genioglossus muscle is the principal muscle being recorded.

ANTERIOR TIBIAL MUSCLE ELECTROMYOGRAM

The continuous recording of the EMG of the left and right anterior tibial muscle is analyzed for periodic and/or episodic limb movements and restless legs syndrome as well as phasic muscle activity during REM sleep.

ELECTROCARDIOGRAM

The continuous recording of lead II is assessed for rhythm, rate, and abnormalities that may be associated with central or obstructive respiratory events.

RESPIRATORY ANALYSIS

The comprehensive evaluation of sleep-related respiratory status is conducted. The number of occlusive (apneas) and partially occlusive (hypopneas) respiratory events is provided.

Significant central apneas, hypopneas, and/or periodic breathing are reported in the Impression. The average length of each is calculated. The apnea index represents the total number of apneas divided by the total sleep time. The A + H index represents the total number of apneas plus hypopneas per hour of sleep. The REM RDI represents the respiratory disturbance index (total number of apneas plus hypopneas) during REM sleep only. Baseline and nadir SaO_2 are reported, as are baseline and maximum end-tidal CO_2.

OTHER CONSIDERATIONS

Several other issues are important in understanding the processes of polysomnography. These issues include patient preparation by the practitioner for the sleep study, patient safety, and the physical layout of the laboratory.

Patient Preparation

The proper preparation of the patient for the study will alleviate anxiety about the procedure and increase patient compliance. Before the study, the practitioner should discuss with the patient the reason for the testing, the procedures that will be used, and what the patient can expect from the laboratory staff. Directly addressing these issues will help alleviate the anxiety associated with sleeping in a strange laboratory environment and will result in a more representative night's sleep. The extra effort and additional time with younger patients and their families can significantly ease tension. Most laboratories will permit a tour of the facilities before the study to familiarize the child with the equipment that will be used. Parents are also encouraged to spend the night in the laboratory with their child.

Patients and their families often feel that the placement of multiple electrodes, sensors, and monitoring equipment will interfere with sleep. Although the potential exists, experience shows that children (and adults) sleep quite well in the laboratory, and the sleep recorded is generally representative of the patient's typical sleep physiology. However, there may be a discrepancy in the measurement of sleep between the first night in the laboratory and consecutive nights. On occasion, two or more nights of polysomnography may be required for an accurate assessment of the presenting problem. This can frequently be anticipated from historical information before the study night, and many sleep laboratories will require a clinical evaluation in the sleep center before the investigation. The staff of the sleep center can determine the appropriate polysomnographic montage and the number of nights required for an accurate diagnosis to be made.

Patient Safety

The safety of the patient is of primary importance within the sleep laboratory. Because the patient is connected to complex electrical equipment, the potential for exposure to incoming electrical currents and shock hazards is minimized by compulsive attention to the inspection and maintenance of the recording apparatus. A single electrical ground is affixed to the patient. If more than one is used, the creation of a "ground loop" is greatly enhanced.

It is necessary for the technician to continuously observe the patient throughout the entire recording period. Patients may require prompt medical attention during the course of the sleep study, and the laboratory staff is prepared for these situations. Therefore, the technicians remain vigilant with the patient and recording throughout the entire study period.

Sleep Laboratory Environment

Although sleep laboratories differ markedly in layout, design, and decoration, they generally consist of one or more bedrooms for monitoring patients, an adjacent control room, a restroom, and a storage area. To reduce the probability of one patient disturbing the sleep of another, each patient is provided with a private room. Ideally, the sleep rooms simulate a home environment, are painted a neutral color, and are light and sound attenuated. The rooms are always easily accessible to the technician. Some laboratories have separate patient preparation rooms. The supplies needed for patient setup can be kept in this area and patients will be able to relax and attempt to sleep in the bedroom. Furthermore, efficiency can be maximized because additional time-consuming "cleanup" procedures can be performed in areas other than the sleep room.

The control room is large enough to accommodate the equipment required for all recordings and should be safe and comfortable for the technician. In addition, the room must be constructed in a manner that minimizes electrical interference and artifact intrusion. Since polysomnographic records consist of voluminous pages of data, an adjacent reading and storage room is helpful.

The design of sleep laboratories is geared toward both patient comfort and safety and the technician's needs. With the appropriate management strategies, the physical laboratory environment can ensure efficient patient care and accurate, reproducible recordings.

References

1. Bowersox SS, Kaitin KI, Dement WC: EEG spindle activity as a function of age: Relationship to sleep continuity. Brain Res 1985;334:303-308.

2. Spehlmann R: EEG Primer. Amsterdam, Elsevier, 1981.

3. Willis J, Schiffman R, Rosman NP, et al: Asymmetries of sleep spindles and beta activity in pediatric EEG. Clin Electroencephalogr 1990; 21:48-50.

4. Drake ME Jr, Pakalnis A, Padamadan H, et al: Sleep spindles in epilepsy. Clin Electroencephalogr 1991;22:144-149.

5. Orem J, Barnes CD: Physiology in Sleep. New York, Academic Press, 1980.

6. Louis J, Zhang JX, Revol M, et al: Ontogenesis of nocturnal organization of sleep spindles: A longitudinal study during the first 6 months of life. Electroencephalogr Clin Neurophysiol 1992;83: 289-296.

7. Soh K, Morita Y, Sei H: Relationship between eye movements and oneiric behavior in cats. Physiol Behav 1992;52:553-558.

8. Becker PT, Thoman EB: Rapid eye movement storms in infants: Rate of occurrence at 6 months predicts mental development at 1 year. Science 1981;212:1415-1416.

9. Feinberg I, Baker T, Leder R, March JD: Response of delta (0-3 Hz) EEG and eye movement density to a night with 100 minutes of sleep. Sleep 1988;11:473-487.

10. Coakley D, Williams R, Morris J: Minute eye movement during sleep. Electroencephalogr Clin Neurophysiol 1979;47:126-131.

11. Askenasy JJ, Yahr MD: Different laws govern motor activity in sleep than in wakefulness. J Neural Transm Gen Sect 1990;79:103-111.

12. DeKoninck J, Lorrain D, Gagnon P: Sleep positions and position shifts in five age groups: An ontogenetic picture. Sleep 1992;15:143-149.

13. Hakamada S, Watanabe K, Hara K, Miyazaki S: Development of the motor behavior during sleep in newborn infants. Brain Dev 1981;3:345-350.

14. Kohyama J, Watanabe S, Iwakawa Y: Phasic sleep components in infants with cyanosis during feeding. Pediatr Neurol 1991;7:200-204.

15. DeKoninck J, Lorrain D, Gagnon P: Sleep positions and position shifts in five age groups: An ontogenetic picture. Sleep 1992;15:143-149.

16. Kohyama J, Watanabe S, Iwakawa Y: Phasic sleep components in infants with cyanosis during feeding. Pediatr Neurol 1991;7:200-204.

17. Fukumoto M, Mochizuki N, Takeishi M, et al: Studies of body movements during night sleep in infancy. Brain Dev 1981;3:37-43.

18. Myers A: Organization of spontaneous behaviors of sleeping neonates. Percept Mot Skills 1977;45:791-794.

19. Wilde-Frenz J, Schulz H: Rate and distribution of body movements during sleep in humans. Percept Mot Skills 1983;56:275-283.

20. Hashimoto T, Hiura K, Endo S, et al: Postural effects on behavioral states of newborn infants—a sleep polygraphic study. Brain Dev 1983;5:286-291.

21. Hakamada S, Watanabe K, Hara K, et al: Body movements during sleep in full-term newborn infants. Brain Dev 1982;4:51-55.

22. Meier-Koll A, Fels T, Kofler B, et al: Basic rest activity cycle and stereotyped behavior of a mentally defective child. Neuropadiatrie 1977;8: 172-180.

23. Kleitman N: Sleep and Wakefulness. Chicago, University of Chicago Press, 1963.

24. Sussman P, Moffitt A, Hoffmann R, et al: The description of structural and temporal characteristics of tonic electrophysiological activity during sleep. Waking-Sleeping 1979;3:279-290.

25. Sadeh A, Lavie P, Scher A, et al: Actigraphic home-monitoring sleep-disturbed and control infants and young children: A new method for pediatric assessment of sleep-wake patterns. Pediatrics 1991;87:494-499.

26. Gadoth N, Costeff H, Harel S, Lavie P: Motor abnormalities during sleep in patients with childhood hereditary progressive dystonia, and their unaffected family members. Sleep 1989;12: 233-238.

27. Mancia G, Baccelli G, Adams DB, Zanchetti A: Vasomotor regulation during sleep in the cat. Am J Physiol 1971;220:1086-1093.

28. Sheldon SH, Spire JP, Levy HB: Pediatric Sleep Medicine. Philadelphia, WB Saunders, 1992.

29. Guazzi M, Zanchetti A: Blood pressure and heart rate during natural sleep of the cat and their regulation by carotid sinus and aortic reflexes. Arch Ital Biol 1965;103:789-817.

30. Gassel MM, Ghelarducci B, Marchiafava PL, Pompeiano O: Phasic changes in blood pressure and heart rate during the rapid eye movement episodes of desynchronized sleep in unrestrained cats. Arch Ital Biol 1964;102:530-544.

31. Radvanyi MF; Morel-Kahn F: Sleep and heart rate variations in premature and full term babies. Neuropadiatrie 1976;7:302-312.

32. Baust W, Gagel J: The development of periodicity of heart rate and respiration in newborn babies. Neuropadiatrie 1977;8:387-396.

33. Litscher G, Pfurtscheller G, Bes F, Poiseau E: Respiration and heart rate variation in normal infants during quiet sleep in the first year of life. Klin Padiatr 1993;205:170-175.

34. VanGeijn HP, Jongsma HW, deHaan J, et al: Heart rate as an indicator of the behavioral state: Studies in the newborn infant and prospects for fetal heart rate monitors. Am J Obstet Gynecol 1980; 136:1061-1066.

35. Gabriel M, Albani M: Rapid eye movement sleep, apnea, and cardiac slowing influenced by phenobarbital administration in the neonate. Pediatrics 1977;60:426-430.

36. Mazza NM, Epstein MA, Haddad GG, et al: Relation of beat-to-beat variability to heart rate in normal sleeping infants. Pediatr Res 1980;14:232-235.

37. Arendt RE, Halpern LF, MacLean WE Jr, Youngquist GA: The properties of V in newborns across repeated measures. Dev Psychobiol 1991; 24:91-101.

38. Schechtman VL; Harper RH: Minute-by-minute association of heart rate variation with basal heart rate in developing infants. Sleep 1993;16:23-30.

39. Haddad GG, Krongrad E, Epstein RA, et.al.: Effect of sleep state on the QT interval in normal infants. Pediatr Res 1979;13:139-141.

40. Kumazawa T, Baccelli G, Guazzi M, et al: Hemodynamic patterns during desynchronized sleep in intact cats and cats with sinoaortic deafferentation. Circ Res 1969;24:923-927.

41. Fagioli I, Salzarulo P, Salomon F, Ricour C: Sinus pauses in early human malnutrition during waking and sleeping. Neuropediatrics 1983;14:43-46.

42. Rechtschaffen A, Kales A (eds): A Manual of Standardized Terminology, Techniques and Scoring System for Sleep Stages of Human Subjects. Los Angeles, BIS/BRI, UCLA, 1968.

43. Anders T, Emde R, Parmelee A (eds): A Manual of Standardized Terminology, Techniqued and Criteria for Scoring of States of Sleep and Wakefulness in Newborn Infants. Los Angeles, UCLA Brain Information Service, NINDS Neurological Information Network, 1971.

Physiologic Variations during Sleep in Children

Stephen H. Sheldon

7

The physiology of the human organism has been extensively studied, and many functions are clearly understood. Responses of organ systems in various states of health and disease are well known during the waking state. For many years, function during the sleeping state had been assumed to parallel that of waking. In 1963, Nathaniel Kleitman published his historic volume, *Sleep and Wakefulness*.[1] Kleitman proposed that physiologic processes vary according to state; that organ systems function and interrelate differently asleep and awake. Since then, several major texts describing human physiology during sleep have been published.[2] Over the past 40 years, it has become clear that focusing on the functioning of the human organism in health and disease states only during periods of wakefulness provides limited insight on which to base many therapeutic regimens. If organ systems function differently during the sleeping state, the response to disease processes will also vary between states.

This chapter focuses on specific variations in the function of organ systems during the sleeping state that may affect the response to disease processes and the efficacy of therapeutic regimens. Specific changes in the central nervous system, temperature regulation, and the endocrine, cardiovascular, and respiratory systems are discussed.

CEREBRAL BLOOD FLOW DURING SLEEP

Consistency of cerebral blood flow (CBF) during sleep depends on alterations in cerebral vascular resistance. Upper and lower limits of autoregulation are not fixed: they vary with the chemical environment, metabolic needs, and neurogenic input.[3] Data regarding CBF in humans are limited because of difficulties in measurement. However, in 1981, Meyer and coworkers[4] developed a noninvasive method for estimating local

and regional blood flow in the brain and opened the door for other investigators to study the effect of blood flow variations in the intact human central nervous system.

Animal experiments have revealed significant variations in CBF during sleep. There appears to be a significant decrease in CBF during non–rapid eye movement (NREM) sleep and a profound increase during rapid eye movement (REM) sleep. In general, cerebral vasodilatation occurs during sleep.[5] Response to state change is, however, heterogeneous, with different regions of the brain exhibiting different magnitudes of alteration. Additionally, differences exist in blood flow between slow-wave sleep (SWS) and paradoxical sleep (REM).[6] Townsend[7] found a consistent decrease in CBF during SWS, with an overall average decrease of 10%. During REM sleep, there was a significant increase in blood flow, with an overall increase of approximately 8% over the baseline state.

The exact mechanisms responsible for variations in CBF during sleep are unknown. It has been suggested, however, that changes may be in response to variations in metabolic rates of cerebral tissue during various stages of sleep. Brain temperature decreases in NREM sleep and increases in REM sleep.[8] This REM sleep–related increase is attributed to increased blood flow and increased metabolic rate during this stage. Neuronal activity in many central nervous system regions is higher during REM sleep than during NREM sleep, and this increased activity may be responsible for the increased metabolic rate.[9] In addition, there appears to be a neurogenic component to the control of CBF during sleep.[10] Meyer and Toyoda have suggested that the variation in CBF during different stages of sleep is a function of neurogenic control.[11]

During REM sleep, local blood flow has been shown to increase in the rhombencephalon, whereas blood flow in the mesencephalon decreases.[12] Cortical blood flow has been noted to increase by 30% to 50% in REM sleep when compared with SWS.[8] Larger differences are seen in the brainstem. White matter and cortex show the least alteration. During REM sleep, phasic oscillations in blood flow have been observed and appear to correlate with bursts of phasic activity (e.g., twitches, eye movements). During SWS, oscillations are not as dramatic or as consistent.[12]

Intrinsic regulation of CBF during wakefulness and sleep is significantly affected by the chemical environment (Table 7–1). Although CBF is dramatically altered by changes in arterial carbon dioxide tension ($PaCO_2$), moderate changes do not appear to be associated with significant variation in cerebral circulation during sleep.[13] When $PaCO_2$ disturbances occur, extravascular pH appears to be an important variable.[14]

Cerebral metabolic rate and CBF seem to be insensitive to alterations in the arterial oxygen tension (PaO_2) within the physiologic range.[8] If the arterial PaO_2 is lowered to below about 50 mm Hg, CBF begins to increase precipitously in response to the hypoxia.[15] Hypoventilation seen during sleep in normal subjects results in a progressive decrease in oxygen saturation (SaO_2). In a study reported by Doust and Schneider,[16] a decrease in SaO_2 from 96% during wakefulness to 87% during SWS was seen in normal subjects.

Intracranial pressure also reveals sleep-related changes. There is little variation of intracranial pressure from the waking state as the subject enters NREM sleep.[17] During REM sleep, however, large intracranial pressure (ICP) waves occur that are almost double the steady state pressure. In most individuals, these ICP waves are of little clinical significance. However, in patients with little ICP reserve, small increases during sleep may result in depressed neuronal function.

BODY TEMPERATURE REGULATION DURING SLEEP

Core body temperature exhibits a highly stable circadian rhythmicity and has been used as a major marker for other endogenous rhythms. As the night progresses, core body temperature falls and reaches its nadir during the early morning hours. During REM sleep, however, core temperature increases approximately 0.2° C.

Homeothermic temperature regulation is characteristic of mammals. Interestingly, animal experiments have shown that during REM sleep, body temperature follows environmental temperature, increasing as the ambient temperature increases, decreasing as the ambient temperature decreases. Return to NREM sleep is accompanied by a rise in core temperature to homeostatic levels. This positive correlation of variation of body temperature with environmental temperature during REM sleep suggests a shift toward poikilothermy (i.e., thermoregulatory mechanisms are depressed). On the other hand, a negative correlation exists during NREM sleep, indicating that thermoregulation remains intact during this state.[18]

Sweating and shivering are major temperature-regulating mechanisms during wakefulness (Table 7–2). Significant variations are seen in both functions during sleep. Sweating remains intact during NREM sleep in neutral or warm environments,[19] but it is notably absent during REM sleep.[20] Similarly, shivering and thermoregulatory vasomotor activity, which occur during wakefulness and NREM sleep, are not present (or are significantly depressed) during REM sleep. It has been shown that absence of shivering during REM sleep results from mechanisms

Table 7–1. **Physiologic Variations in the Central Nervous System during Wake and Sleep**

Parameter	Wake	Slow-Wave Sleep	REM Sleep
Blood flow	Neurogenic and chemical control	Heterogeneous changes	Increased 30%-50% Phasic oscillations
Brain temperature	Related to metabolic rate	Decreased	Increased
Intracranial pressure	Relatively stable	Relatively stable	Increased Phasic oscillations

Table 7–2.   Physiologic Variations in Temperature Regulation during Wake and Sleep

Parameter	Wake	Slow-Wave Sleep	REM Sleep
Regulation	Homeothermic	Homeothermic	Variable
			Varies positively with environmental temperature
Sweating	Present	Present	Relatively absent
Vasomotor activity	Present	Present	Relatively absent
Shivering	Present	Present	Absent

other than muscle atonia associated with this state. Animals lesioned in the pontine tegmentum (which results in abolition of REM atonia) still do not shiver during REM sleep.[21]

The diaphragm is normally unaffected by generalized skeletal muscle inhibition during REM sleep, but it does not show increased activity (i.e., tachypnea) to warming or cooling. Cooling of the hypothalamus during NREM sleep in animals results in increased oxygen consumption and metabolic heat production, but neither cooling nor heating of the hypothalamus during REM sleep results in a thermoregulatory response.[22] These data support the assumption that hypothalamic thermoregulation is significantly decreased or absent during REM sleep.

ENDOCRINE VARIATIONS DURING SLEEP

The effects of sleep on hormone secretion are outlined in Table 7–3.

Growth Hormone

In prepubertal children, secretion of growth hormone (GH) is clearly coupled with sleep onset. It peaks early in the first third of the night during SWS and is secreted exclusively during sleep.[23] During puberty and throughout adolescence, the pattern of secretion of GH is modified from the prepubertal paradigm. Several minor peaks occur throughout the day, although GH still reaches its maximal concentration during sleep. Shifting of

Table 7–3.   Effects of Sleep on Hormone Secretion

Hormone	Normal Sleep Phase Peak and/or Trough	Effect of Shifted Phase	Sleep Dependency
Growth hormone	Secreted at sleep onset Peaks early in sleep period	Secretion time follows the shift in sleep phase.	Yes
Prolactin	Secreted 30-90 min after sleep onset Peaks in the early morning hours	Secretion time follows the shift in sleep phase.	Yes
Thyroid-stimulating hormone	Peaks in the early evening Declines more gradually across the sleep period	There is no significant change in secretion. Sleep appears to modulate (inhibit) secretion.	No
Luteinizing hormone	Rises during sleep in prepubertal children Secondary peaks occur during wake during puberty.	There is a shift in secretion that follows the shift in sleep phase.	Yes
Follicle-stimulating hormone	Sleep-related rise in secretion occurs.	There is a shift in secretion that follows the shift in sleep phase.	Yes
Cortisol	Peaks at the end of the sleep period Nadir occurs early in the sleep period.	There is no significant change in secretion. Sleep appears to modulate (inhibit) secretion.	No No

the sleep phase to times of day other than the normal sleep period is accompanied by shifts in the timing of secretion of GH.[24,25] A 180-degree reversal of sleep phase results in a 180-degree shift in peak secretion of GH. This sleep-associated release of GH has been related to Jouvet's theory of monoaminergic sleep systems. Agreement rests in observations that NREM sleep and hypothalamic releasing factors are both triggered by the same serotonergic neurons in the raphe nuclei of the brainstem.[26]

Prolactin

Under basal conditions, prolactin rhythmically peaks each night. As with GH, summits are almost entirely restricted to the sleep interval and are clearly coupled to the sleeping state.[27] Prolactin levels generally increase 30 to 90 minutes after sleep onset and reach maximal levels in the early morning hours.[20] Prolactin secretion also occurs during daytime naps and remains coupled to sleep after acute sleep–wake phase reversals. This sleep-related pattern of secretion is present from late puberty to old age and persists during pregnancy, when higher levels of prolactin are secreted. Although prolactin and GH secretion are both connected to the sleeping state, peaks of each hormone are not coincident. In contrast to the adolescent and adult GH rhythm, the prolactin peak during sleep appears to be the only major aligned episode of release across 24 hours.[28]

Cortisol

Like core body temperature, cortisol follows a clear, well-established, consistent circadian rhythm; it has also been used as a phase reference point for other endogenous rhythms.[29] Maximal cortisol secretion generally occurs at the end of the sleep period, and its nadir is located early in the sleep period. Manipulation of the timing of sleep does not dramatically change adrenocorticotropic hormone–cortisol secretion as it does GH and prolactin, and its rhythm is most likely independent of sleep itself, controlled by a different endogenous oscillator. A reduction in plasma cortisol concentration seems to occur regardless of the timing of the sleep period.[26] This suggests that cortisol secretion and the rhythm of the sleep–wake cycle are independent. Sleep appears to only modulate the release of cortisol, inhibiting rather than controlling secretion.

Thyroid-Stimulating Hormone

Daily maximums of thyroid-stimulating hormone (TSH) secretion are seen to rhythmically recur each evening and precede the onset of sleep.[30] The TSH peak begins in the early evening and then declines across the sleep phase. This sleep-associated decline in TSH suggests that sleep is almost as important a determinant of the locus of the maximum TSH rhythm as it is for GH and prolactin. However, with shifts in the sleep phase, the rise in TSH levels appears to be coupled to clock time rather than sleep period. Changing the timing of the sleep period reveals that inhibition of TSH secretion occurs with sleep, although the rise to peak of this hormone is still synchronized to clock time. Therefore, sleep appears to truncate the circadian secretory episode of TSH.[26]

Luteinizing Hormone

Luteinizing hormone (LH) has been shown to drive male testosterone production by the Leydig cells of the testes, and it exhibits sleep-related rhythmicity during puberty.[31-33] However, these sleep-associated changes in LH secretion and testosterone production have been shown to occur prior to Tanner stage 2.[34] LH increases during sleep seems to be responsible for initiation of pubertal changes. LH surges are followed momentarily by elevations in plasma testosterone levels, which, in turn, induce the changes in secondary sexual characteristics seen during this stage of development.[32,35] As boys traverse puberty, enhanced episodic release of LH and testosterone occur during wakefulness until Tanner stage 5 is reached. At this time, an adult pattern of equivalent pulse height of LH secretion across the sleep cycle occurs.[32] Change of sleep phase results in a corresponding change in LH and testosterone activity. Testosterone levels peak during sleep in the adult in spite of a weakened or absent nocturnal rise in LH activity.[20]

Follicle-Stimulating Hormone

Follicle-stimulating hormone (FSH) follows a pattern similar to that of LH. Increases in LH occur at sleep onset, and wakefulness appears to inhibit LH and FSH secretion. The delay of sleep or the acute reversal of the sleep–wake cycle results in corresponding changes in FSH activity patterns. Pubertal girls show sleep-coupled release of LH and FSH during sleep.[20] Estradiol levels, however, do not increase until 10 to 14 hours later. Cycling women do not show sleep-related release, but there may be inhibition of LH secretion 2 to 3 hours after sleep onset.

CARDIOVASCULAR VARIATIONS DURING SLEEP

The physiologic variations in the cardiovascular system during wake and sleep are outlined in Table 7–4.

Heart Rate

Heart rate is generally reduced during natural sleep in most animal species. When compared with quiet wake (QW), the effect of synchronized (NREM) sleep on heart rate is a slight decrease in heart rate of 4 to 8 beats per minute.[36] During REM sleep, a decrease in rate of 17 beats per minute (approximately 8% less than the mean for QW) has been noted. Reduction in heart rate during sleep appears to parallel sleep-related alterations in blood pressure, in that the variation is more pronounced during REM sleep, and heart rate variability is clearly greater in REM sleep than in NREM SWS.[37]

Heart rate is also significantly influenced by phasic phenomena of REM.[38] During bursts of rapid eye movements and body movements, there are clear episodes of short-lasting tachycardia, followed occasionally by a rebound brief bradycardia before return to baseline levels.

Cardiac output is generally coupled to heart rate during wakefulness. During sleep, however, cardiac output has been shown to be only slightly reduced during SWS when compared with the waking state.[36,39] Reduction in cardiac output becomes more pronounced, however, during the tonic REM state, its average then being about 9% less than during QW. Changes in cardiac output are not accompanied by changes in stroke volume, which tends to remain constant during QW, SWS, and REM cycles.

Blood Pressure

Extended studies of laboratory animals have revealed a moderate, but significant decrease in blood pressure (approximately 14 mm Hg) during NREM sleep when compared with QW.[37] A more significant fall has been shown to occur during REM sleep (approximately 25 mm Hg). Changes in blood pressure are more complex and variable during REM sleep than during NREM sleep. Brief sharp increases in mean arterial pressure occur, which are superimposed on relatively hypotensive values. These oscillations in blood pressure appear to be related to brief excitatory somatomotor phenomena that are typical of REM sleep. Blood pressure rise begins with, or occurs shortly following, the onset of bursts of rapid eye movements and muscle twitches.[38]

Table 7–4.	Physiologic Variations in the Cardiovascular System during Sleep		
Parameter	**Waking**	**Slow-Wave Sleep**	**REM Sleep**
Heart rate	Variable Dependent on activity	Mildly decreased compared to wake	Variable Decrease with phasic increases
Cardiac output	Variable Dependent on activity	Mildly decreased compared to wake	Mildly decreased compared to wake and SWS
Blood pressure	Variable Dependent on activity	Mildly decreased compared to wake	Decreased compared to SWS and wake Phasic elevation
Peripheral vasomotor activity	Variable Dependent on activity	Mild vasodilation	Vasodilation with periods of phasic vasoconstriction

REM, rapid eye movement; SWS, slow-wave sleep.

Two types of blood pressure changes in desynchronized sleep occur in the cat. First, a tonic blood pressure alteration takes place, consisting of hypotension lasting throughout the desynchronized sleep episode. Second, there are frequent phasic pressure changes, which consist of brief blood pressure rises that occur simultaneously with other phasic phenomena.[40]

Marked, brief cutaneous vasoconstriction occurs concomitantly with phasic events during REM sleep.[20] Other regional vasoconstriction takes place as well. For example, there is a significantly reduced urine volume production during REM sleep, which is considered to be the result of a reduced renal blood flow during this state. A central inhibitory influence on vasoconstriction, which is present during REM sleep, has been shown to be potentiated by sinoaortic denervation.[20] Vasoconstriction normally seen in the iliac artery during REM sleep is converted to vasodilatation. Surprisingly, the buffering action of the sinoaortic nerve depends more on chemoreceptive reflexes than on baroreceptor reflexes. The baroreflexes are diminished during REM sleep in the cat, and this variation may be necessary to maintain homeostasis.

Cardiovascular variations during sleep hold specific and significant clinical relevance. Phasic excitation of the heart and coronary circulation may precipitate decreased coronary artery blood flow and precipitate myocardial infarction (or other myocardial dysfunction) during REM sleep. Nowlin and coworkers reported that nocturnal exacerbations of angina generally occur during REM sleep.[41] As early as 1923, MacWilliams reported that deaths from cardiac disorders occur more frequently during sleep than wakefulness.[42] Most deaths were found to occur around 05:00 to 06:00, a time when sleep consists primarily of the REM state.

RESPIRATORY VARIATIONS DURING SLEEP

Well-defined changes in respiratory patterns occur during sleep (Table 7–5). These alterations result in modification of ventilatory control, blood-gas and respiratory patterns, and regulatory responses to changes that are significantly different than in the waking state.

In general, hypoventilation occurs during sleep in the normal individual. During SWS, there is a slight decrease in minute ventilation. A change in metabolic rate is demonstrated by a decrease in oxygen uptake and an increase in carbon dioxide production by approximately 10% to 20%.[43] Subsequently, a change in ventilatory control also occurs, as alveolar ventilation falls more than expected in response to these metabolic changes.[44] Consequently, the partial pressure of CO_2 increases during SWS.

One of the most striking features of breathing during SWS is its monotonous regularity and lack of breath-to-breath variability. Respiratory rate is slightly lower and the tidal volume is slightly greater in SWS than in wakefulness.[45,46] All major indices of respiratory function appear to be in a stable state during this time. In con-

Table 7–5. Physiologic Variations in the Respiratory System during Sleep

Parameter	Waking	Slow-Wave Sleep	REM Sleep
Minute ventilation	Varies with activity	Mildly decreased	Variable
Respiratory Rate	Varies with activity	Mildly decreased	Variable
$Paco_2$	Stable	Mildly increased	Increased
Pao_2	Stable	Mildly decreased	Decreased
Hypercapnic ventilatory response	Sensitive to elevation in carbon dioxide	Mildly decreased response	Decreased to a greater extent when compared to wake and SWS
Hypoxic ventilatory response	Sensitive to decreases in oxygen tension	Mildly decreased response	Decreased to a greater extent when compared to wake and SWS

$Paco_2$, arterial carbon dioxide tension; Pao_2, arterial oxygen tension; REM, rapid eye movement; SWS, slow-wave sleep.

trast, during REM sleep, significant irregularity is noted. Irregularities in respiratory patterns were part of the original description of REM sleep by Aserinsky and Kleitman in 1953.[47] These irregularities of respiration and rapid breathing patterns associated with REM sleep have been subsequently confirmed in studies in human infants, human adults, and other species,[48-50] and as seen with cardiovascular changes, there is a significant temporal relationship to the phasic components of REM sleep.[48,51,52]

Respiratory changes seen in REM sleep appear to be secondary to internally activated neural events.[53] This is consistent with the powerful REM sleep–coupled neural influences on other systems, which apparently arise from the brainstem.

The neonate (in particular the premature newborn) exhibits irregular breathing patterns. Breath-to-breath variability and long episodes of periodic breathing occur.[54,55] Periodic breathing patterns in premature infants occur during wake, quiet sleep, and active sleep. Although present during quiet sleep, periodic breathing is significantly increased during REM sleep.[56] During quiet sleep, periodic breathing appears to be quite regular: breathing and apneic intervals are of similar durations. These intervals are, on the other hand, quite irregular during active sleep.[57] The cause of periodic breathing is unknown, but many investigators believe that it depends on oscillations in blood gases during sleep.[58]

REM atonia, which affects almost all skeletal muscles, also affects muscles involved in respiration. The diaphragm, however, maintains its activity during REM sleep, but intercostal muscles and muscles of the upper airway are significantly hypotonic or atonic during this stage.[20] Decrease in muscle tone of the accessory muscles of respiration results in hypoventilation and/or upper airway occlusion. Neonates and infants appear to be particularly susceptible to intercostal muscle hypotonia resulting in rib cage collapse and "see-saw" respiratory efforts (paradoxical respiration).

Mucociliary clearance of pulmonary secretions is reduced during sleep. The cough reflex is significantly suppressed during NREM and REM sleep, and the presence of coughing appears to depend on arousal from sleep.[59] Decreased clearance of secretions becomes clinically significant in patients with pathologic states that involve increased mucous production (e.g., asthma). Sleep architecture is frequently disrupted by numerous arousals, perhaps to assist in clearance of these pulmonary secretions. In addition, respiratory tract smooth muscle tone is also affected by sleep. There is a decrease in this tone in NREM sleep when compared with wakefulness. Tone continues to decrease in tonic REM sleep; however, there is a phasic increase superimposed on this decrease during bursts of rapid eye movements.[20]

During wakefulness, the newborn infant responds to hypoxia in a manner different from that of older children and adults.[60] At lowered Pa_{O_2}, a biphasic response is seen, with an initial period of hyperventilation followed by a fall in ventilation to a level below the baseline. A similar response curve is noted during REM sleep, but the initial hyperventilatory response is less dramatic. During NREM sleep, hyperventilation is noted and sustained, without the fall seen in the other two states.

Ventilatory response to hypoxemia is decreased during NREM sleep (compared with wakefulness) in adult men. In contrast, the responses during NREM and during wakefulness are similar in women. The reason for this sex differentiation is unknown.[61-63] During REM sleep, the ventilatory response to hypoxia is below that of NREM sleep in both males and females.

Ventilatory response to hypercapnia is depressed during sleep in the adult human.[64] The slope of the ventilatory–CO_2 response curve falls during NREM sleep when compared with wakefulness.[65-67] This decrease in response from wakefulness to NREM sleep has been reported to be approximately 50%.[68,69] This change does not appear to occur in females.[70] Hypercapnic response appears to be lowest in REM sleep when compared with wakefulness and NREM. The mean hypercapnic response during REM sleep seems to be approximately 28% lower than in the other two states.[68,70,71]

In transient or semi–steady state experiments in human neonates, hypercapnic ventilatory response differs from in the adult. Studies indicate that there is no difference in the ventilatory response to CO_2 between active and quiet sleep.[72-75] Using rebreathing techniques, however, a lower response in REM sleep is suggested,[60,76] and the hypercapnic response is lower in preterm neonates than in term infants.[77]

SKELETAL MUSCLE ACTIVITY VARIATIONS DURING SLEEP

As early as 1894, a reduction in spinal reflexes and loss of patellar reflex activity during sleep was noted.[78] These observations have been systematically confirmed. Hodes and Dement[79] documented a decrease in spinal reflexes during sleep, and a decrease in body motility associated with the progression into SWS was corroborated by Rohmer and coworkers.[80]

Skeletal muscle activity and spinal cord reflex activity are diminished to their greatest extent during REM sleep.[79,81] Periodically occurring twitches and muscular tremors of the face and limbs frequently occur during this stage of sleep.[82] Progressive relaxation of the skeletal musculature and attenuation of reflexes are most prominently seen during REM sleep. During REM sleep, periodic bursts of excitatory activity break through the generalized tonic inhibition. Hyperpolarization of the intracellular membrane is correlated with active inhibition of the motor neuron at the spinal level.[83] Stimulation of neurons in the pons (specifically in the nucleus pontis oralis) results in different peripheral effects depending on whether the subject is awake, in NREM sleep, or in the REM sleep state. During wakefulness, stimulation of these neurons results in excitatory postsynaptic potential generation. During REM sleep, however, inhibitory postsynaptic potentials are recognized. Thus, membrane potentials are reversed depending on the state of arousal. There appears to be a neuronal gate that opens specifically during REM sleep. In addition, coactivation of facilitative and inhibitory neuronal activity explains the twitches and jerks accompanying REM sleep.

Major body movements are strongly related to the stage of sleep, with the rate of body movements progressively decreasing from waking, through stage 1, REM sleep, and stage 2, to SWS.[84] Although body movements occur during all stages of sleep, they are most frequent during REM sleep and least frequent during SWS.[85] Within a single night's sleep, the number of body movements can vary considerably (from 70 to 200 movements).[86]

VARIATIONS IN GENITOURINARY FUNCTION DURING SLEEP

Changes in renal function occur during sleep and are characterized by a decrease in urine volume and an increase in urine osmolality.[87] These changes generally occur in conjunction with REM sleep, but they appear to be more related to decrease in regional blood flow and not primarily mediated by REM-related antidiuretic hormone release (though a nocturnal peak in vasopressin secretion can be demonstrated).[88] In addition to renal conservation of water during sleep, excretion of sodium chloride is reduced during this state.

Penile tumescence occurs during REM sleep in children and adult males.[89-92] The most striking amount of nocturnal penile tumescence episodes occur in the prepubertal and pubertal years, gradually declining in frequency throughout the later years of life. A similar phenomenon appears to occur in females during REM sleep. Most evidence for this phenomenon stems from similarities between phasic shifts of vaginal vascular blood flow and penile blood flow during REM sleep. Karacan and coworkers[93] reported clitoral erections in three women during REM sleep. Abel and coworkers[94] documented increases in relative pulse pressure within the vagina during REM sleep.

VARIATIONS IN GASTROINTESTINAL FUNCTION DURING SLEEP

It has been shown that physiologic activity during sleep is not homogeneous. It varies as a function of the stage of sleep as well as the time of night. Parasympathetic activity seems to dominate NREM sleep, and sympathetic activity dominates REM sleep.[95]

Gastrointestinal function is extrinsically and intrinsically modified during sleep. Finch and coworkers[96] demonstrated that gastroduodenal motility during sleep shows a strong relationship with body movements and with sleep stage changes. Although there appear to be no statistically significant relationships between gastric acid secretion and stages of sleep,[97] a circadian variation of secretion is seen, with peaks occurring about 02:00. There appears to be a lack of inhibition of gastric acid secretion during sleep in patients with duodenal ulcers. It is speculated that epigastric pain during sleep in duodenal ulcer patients may be more related to the prolonged fast associated with sleep than to factors associated with gastric acid secretion.[98]

Swallowing and esophageal function are important determinants of gastroesophageal reflux during sleep. Swallowing is significantly suppressed during sleep.[99] This suppression of swallowing is most noticeable during SWS, and refluxed gastric contents maintain mucosal contact for longer periods of time. Acid contact and prolonged acid clearance is considered to be the prime factor in the development of esophagitis in patients with gastroesophageal reflux.[100]

Salivary flow, another important determinant of acid clearance, nearly ceases during sleep.[101] Body position also appears to play an important role in acid clearance, with supine positions associated with markedly prolonged esophageal acid clearance.[100]

Orr and coworkers[99] documented that sleep impairs esophageal acid clearance in both normal subjects and patients with esophagitis. However, patients with esophagitis took a significantly longer time for acid clearance even during waking hours. This is especially noteworthy, as most gastroesophageal reflux occurred during arousals from sleep in this study, as well as in a study of spontaneous gastroesophageal reflux in normal subjects.[102] These data clearly implicate defective acid clearance as a major determinant in the pathogenesis of esophageal inflammation in patients with gastroesophageal reflux. Few data are available regarding esophageal motility and acid clearance during sleep in the infant with significant gastroesophageal reflux.

References

1. Kleitman N: Sleep and Wakefulness. Chicago, University of Chicago Press, 1963.
2. Orem J, Barnes CD: Physiology in Sleep. New York, Academic Press, 1980.
3. Ekstrom-Jodal, Haggendal E, Linder LE, Nilsson NJ: Cerebral blood flow autoregulation at high arterial pressures and different levels of carbon dioxide tension in dogs. Eur Neurol 1971-72;6:6-10.
4. Meyer JS, Hayman LA, Amano T, et al: Mapping local blood flow of human brain by CT scanning during stable xenon inhalation. Stroke 1981;12:426-436.
5. Bridges TH, Clark K, Yahr MD, et al: Plethysmographic studies of the cerebral circulation: Evidence for cranial nerve vasomotor activity. J Clin Invest 1958;37: 763-772.
6. Reivich M, Isaacs G, Evarts E, Kety S: The effects of slow-wave sleep and REM sleep on regional blood flow in cats. J Neurochem 1968;15:301-306.
7. Townsend RE, Prinz PN, Obrist WD: Human cerebral blood flow during sleep and waking. J Appl Physiol 1973;35:620-625.
8. Greenberg JH: Sleep and the cerebral circulation. In Orem J, Barnes CD (eds): Physiology in Sleep. New York, Academic Press, 1980, pp 57-95.
9. Reivich M: Blood flow and metabolism couple in the brain. In Plum F (ed): Brain Dysfunction in Metabolic Disorders. New York, Raven Press, 1974, pp 125-140.
10. Perves MJ: The Physiology of the Cerebral Circulation. London, Cambridge University Press, 1972.
11. Meyer JS, Toyoda M: Studies of rapid changes in cerebral circulation and metabolism during arousal and rapid eye movement sleep in human subjects with cerebrovascular disease. In Zulch KJ (ed): Cerebral Circulation and Stroke. New York, Springer-Verlag, 1971, pp 156-163.
12. Baust W: Local blood flow in different regions of the brain-stem during natural sleep and arousal. Electroencephalogr Clin Neurophysiol 1967;22: 365-372.
13. Alexander SC, Cohen PJ, Wollman H, et al: Cerebral carbohydrate metabolism during hypocarbia in man: Studies during nitrous oxide anesthesia. Anesthesiology 1965;26:624-632.
14. Wahl M, Deetjen P, Thurau K, et al: Micropuncture evaluation of importance of perivascular pH for the arteriolar diameter on the brain surface. Pflugers Arch 1970;316:152-163.
15. Kogure K, Scheinberg P, Reinmuth OM, et al: Mechanism of cerebral vasodilatation in hypoxia. J Appl Physiol 1970;29:223-229.
16. Doust LJW, Schneider RA: Studies on the physiology of awareness: Anoxia and the levels of sleep. Br Med J 1952;1:449-455.
17. Gucer G, Viernstein LJ: Intracranial pressure in the normal monkey while awake and asleep. J Neurosurg 1979;51:206-210.
18. Parmeggiani PL, Franzini C, Lenzi P, Cianci T: Temperature changes in cats sleeping at different environmental temperatures. Brain Res 1971;33: 397-404.
19. Henane R, Buguet A, Roussel B, Bittel J: Variations in evaporation and body temperatures during sleep in man. J Appl Physiol 1977;42:50-55.
20. Orem J, Keeling J: A compendium of physiology in sleep. In Orem J, Barnes CD: Physiology in Sleep. New York, Academic Press, 1980, pp 315-335.

21. Hendricks JC, Bowker RM, Morrison AR: Functional characteristics of cats with pontine lesions during sleep and wakefulness and their usefulness for sleep research. In Koella WP, Levin P (eds): Sleep 1976. Basel, Karger, 1977, pp 207-210.

22. Parmeggiani PL, Agnati LF, Zamboni G, Cianci T: Hypothalamic temperature during sleep cycles at different ambient temperatures. Electroencephalogr Clin Neurophysiol 1975;38:589-596.

23. Parker DC, et al: Rhythmicities in human growth hormone concentration in plasma. In Krieger DT (ed): Endocrine Rhythms. New York, Raven Press, 1979, pp 143-173.

24. Parker DC, Rossman LG: Physiology of human growth hormone release in sleep. In Scow RO (ed): Endocrinology. Amsterdam, Exerpta Medica, 1973, pp 655-660.

25. Parker DC, Rossman LG: Sleep-wake cycle and human growth hormone, prolactin and luteinizing hormone. In Raiti S (ed): Advances in Human Growth Hormone Research. Washington, DC, U.S. Government Printing Office, 1974, pp 294-312.

26. Parker DC, et al: Endocrine rhythms across sleep-wake cycles in normal young men under basal state conditions. In Orem J, Barnes CD (eds): Physiology in Sleep. New York, Academic Press, 1980, pp 145-179.

27. Parker DC, Rossman LG, Vander Laan EF: Sleep-related, nychthermeral and briefly episodic variation in human plasma prolactin concentrations. J Clin Endocrinol Metab 1973;36:1119-1124.

28. Sassin JF, Frantz AG, Weitzman ED, Kapen S: Human prolactin: 24-hour pattern with increased release during sleep. Science 1972;177:1205-1207.

29. Aschoff J: Circadian rhythms: General features and endocrinological aspects. In Krieger D (ed): Endocrine Rhythms. New York, Raven Press, 1979, pp 1-61.

30. Parker DC, Pekary AE, Hershman JM: Effect of normal and reversed sleep-wake cycles upon nyctohemeral rhythmicity of plasma thyrotropin: Evidence suggestive of an inhibitory influence in sleep. J Clin Endocrinol Metab 1976;43:318-329.

31. Boyar R, Finkelstein J, Roffwarg H, et al: Synchronization of augmented luteinizing hormone with sleep during puberty. N Engl J Med 1972;287:582-586.

32. Parker DC, Judd HL, Rossman LG, Yen SS: Pubertal sleep-wake patterns of episodic LH, FSH, and testosterone release in twin boys. J Clin Endocrinol Metab 1975;40:1099-1109.

33. Kapen S, Boyar RM, Finkelstein JW, et al: Effect of sleep-wake cycle reversal on luteinizing hormone secretory pattern in puberty. J Clin Endocrinol Metab 1974;39:293-299.

34. Judd HL, Parker DC, Yen SSC: Sleep-wake patterns of LH and testosterone release in prepubertal boys. J Clin Endocrinol Metab 1977;44:865-869.

35. Judd HL, Parker DC, Siler TM, Yen SS: The nocturnal rise of plasma testosterone in pubertal boys. J Clin Endocrinol Metab 1974;38:710-713.

36. Mancia G, Baccelli G, Adams DB, Zanchetti A: Vasomotor regulation during sleep in the cat. Am J Physiol 1971;220:1086-1093.

37. Guazzi M, Zanchetti A: Blood pressure and heart rate during natural sleep of the cat and their regulation by carotid sinus and aortic reflexes. Arch Ital Biol 1965;103:789-817.

38. Gassel MM, Ghelarducci B, Marchiafava PL, Pompeiano O: Phasic changes in blood pressure and heart rate during the rapid eye movement episodes of desynchronized sleep in unrestrained cats. Arch Ital Biol 1964;102:530-544.

39. Kumazawa T, Baccelli G, Guazzi M, et al: Hemodynamic patterns during desynchronized sleep in intact cats and cats with sino-atrial deafferentation. Circ Res 1969;24:923-937.

40. Mancia, G, Zanchetti, A: Cardiovascular regulation during sleep. In Orem J, Barnes CD: Physiology in Sleep. New York, Academic Press, 1980, pp 1-55.

41. Nowlin JB, Troyer WG Jr, Collins WS, et al: The association of nocturnal angina pectoris with dreaming. Ann Intern Med 1965;63:1040-1046.

42. MacWilliam JA: Blood pressure and heart action in sleep and dreams: Their relation to haemorrhages, angina and sudden death. Br Med J 1923;22:1196-1200.

43. Phillipson EA, Murphy E, Kozar LF: Regulation of respiration in sleeping dogs. J Appl Physiol 1976;40:688-693.

44. Sullivan CE: Breathing in sleep. In Orem J, Barnes CD (eds): Physiology in Sleep. New York, Academic Press, 1980, pp 213-272.

45. Orem J, Netick A, Dement WC: Breathing during sleep and wakefulness in the cat. Resp Physiol 1977;30:265-269.

46. Lugaresi E, et al: Breathing during sleep in man in normal and pathological conditions. In Fitzgerald H, Gautier H, Lahiri S (eds): The regulation of Respiration during Sleep and Anesthesia. New York, Plenum, 1978, pp 35-45.

47. Aserinsky E, Kleitman N: Regularly occurring periods of eye motility, and concomitant phenomena, during sleep. Science 1953;118:273-274.

48. Phillipson EA, Kozar LF, Murphy E: Respiratory load compensation in awake and sleeping dogs. J Appl Physiol 1976;40:895-902.

49. Snyder F, Hobson JA, Morrison DF and Goldfrank F: Changes in respiration, heart rate, and systolic blood pressure in human sleep. J Appl Physiol 1964;19:417-422.

50. Snyder F: Autonomic nervous system manifestations during sleep and dreaming. In Kety SS, Evarts EV, Williams HL: Sleep and Altered States of Consciousness. Baltimore, Williams & Wilkins, 1967, pp 469-487.

51. Aserinsky E: Periodic respiratory pattern occurring in conjunction with eye movements during sleep. Science 1965;150:763-766.

52. Baust W, Holzbach E, Zechlin O: Phasic changes in heart rate and respiration correlated with PGO-spike activity during REM sleep. Pflugers Arch 1972;331:113-123.

53. Pompeiano O: The neurophysiological mechanisms of the postural and motor events during desynchronized sleep. In Ketty SS, Evarts EV, Williams HL (eds): Sleep and Altered States of Consciousness. Baltimore, Williams & Wilkins, 1967, pp 351-423.

54. Rigatto H, Brady JP: Periodic breathing and apnea in preterm infants: I. Evidence for hypoventilation possibly due to central respiratory depression. Pediatrics 1972;50:202.

55. Rigatto H, Brady JP: Periodic breathing and apnea in preterm infants: II. Hypoxia as a primary event. Pediatrics 1975;55:604.

56. Rigatto H, Kalapesi Z, Leahy FN, et al: Ventilatory response to 100% and 15% O_2 during wakefulness and sleep in preterm infants. Early Hum Dev 1982;7:1.

57. Rigatto H: Control of breathing during sleep in the fetus and neonate. In Kryger MH, Roth T, Dement WC (eds): Principles and Practice of Sleep Medicine. Philadelphia, WB Saunders, 1989, pp 237-248.

58. Waggener TB, Stark AR, Cohlan BA, Frantz ID 3rd: Apnea duration is related to ventilatory oscillation characteristics in newborn infants. J Appl Physiol 1984;57:536.

59. Bateman JRM, Clarke SW, Pavia D, Sheahan NF: Reduction in clearance of secretions from the human lung during sleep. J Physiol 1978;284:55P.

60. Rigatto H: Control of ventilation in the newborn. Annu Rev Physiol 1984;46:661-674.

61. White DP, Douglas NJ, Pickett CK, et al: Hypoxic ventilatory response during sleep in normal premenopausal women. Am Rev Respir Dis 1982;126:530-533.

62. Douglas NJ, White DP, Weil JV, et al: Hypoxic ventilatory response decreases during sleep in normal men. Am Rev Resp Dis 1982;125:286-289.

63. Hedemark LL, Kronenberg RS: Ventilatory and heart rate response to hypoxia and hypercapnia during sleep in adults. J Appl Physiol 1982;53:307-312.

64. Douglas NJ: Control of ventilation during sleep. Clin Chest Med 1985;6:563.

65. Birchfield RI, Sieker HO, Heyman A: Alterations in respiratory functions during natural sleep. J Lab Clin Med 1959;54:216-222.

66. Douglas NJ, White DP, Pickett CK, et al: Respiration during sleep in normal man. Thorax 1982;37:840-844.

67. Gothe B, Altose MD, Goldman MD, Cherniack NS: Effects of quiet sleep on resting and CO_2-stimulated breathing in humans. J Appl Physiol 1981;50:724-730.

68. Bulow K: Respiration and wakefulness in man. Acta Physiol Scand 1963;59(Suppl 209):1-110.

69. Douglas NJ, White DP, Weil JV, et al: Hypercapnic ventilatory response in sleeping adults. Am Rev Resp Dis 1982;126:758-762.

70. Berthon-Jones M, Sullivan CE: Ventilation and arousal response to hypercapnia in normal sleeping adults. J Appl Physiol 1984;57:59-67.

71. White DP: Occlusion pressure and ventilation during sleep in normal humans. J Appl Physiol 1986;61:1279-1287.

72. Anderson JV Jr, Martin RJ, Abboud EF, et al: Transient ventilatory response to CO_2 as a function of sleep state in full-term infants. J Appl Physiol 1983;54:1482-1488.

73. Davi M, Sankaran K, Maccallum M, et al: The effect of sleep state on chest distortion and on the ventilatory response to CO_2 in neonates. Pediatr Res 1979;13:982-986.

74. Haddad GG, Leistner HL, Epstein RA, et al: CO_2-induced changes in ventilation and ventilatory pattern in normal sleeping infants. J Appl Physiol 1980;48:684-688.

75. Rigatto H, Kalapesi Z, Leahy FN: Chemical control of respiratory frequency and tidal volume during sleep in preterm infants. Respir Physiol 1980;41:117-125.

76. Honma Y, Wilkes D, Bryan MH, Bryan AC: Rib cage and abdominal contributions to ventilatory response to CO_2 in infants. J Appl Physiol 1984;56:1211-1216.

77. Moriette G, Van Reempts P, Moore M, et al: The effect of rebreathing CO_2 on ventilation and diaphragmatic electromyography in newborn infants. Respir Physiol 1985;62:387-397.

78. Tarchanoff J: Quelques observations sur le sommeil. Arch Ital Biol 1894;21:318-321.

79. Hodes R, Dement WC: Depression of electrically induced reflexes ("H" reflexes) in man during low voltage EEG sleep. Electroencephalogr Clin Neurophysiol 1964;17:617-629.

80. Rohmer F, et al: La motilité spontanée, la fréquence cardiaque et la fréquence respiratoire au cours du sommeil chez l'homme normal: Leurs relations avec les manifestations electroencephalographiques et la profondeur du sommeil.

In La Société d'Electroencephalographie et de Neurophysiologie Clinique de Langue Française (eds): Le Sommeil de Nuit Normal et Pathologique, Études Electroencephalographiques. Paris, La Société d'Electroencephalographie et de Neurophysiologie Clinique de Langue Française, 1965, pp 192-207.

81. Jacobson A, Kales A, Lehmann D, Hoedemaker FS: Muscle tonus in human subjects during sleep and dreaming. Exp Neurol 1964;10:418-424.

82. Baldridge BJ, Whitman RM, Kramer M: The concurrence of fine muscle activity and rapid eye movements during sleep. Psychosom Med 1965;27:19-26.

83. Chandler SH, Nakamura Y, Chase MH: Intracellular analysis of synaptic potentials induced in trigeminal jaw-closer motoneurons by pontomesencephalic reticular stimulation during sleep and wakefulness. J Neurophysiol 1980;44:372-382.

84. Wilde-Frenz J, Schulz H: Rate and distribution of body movements during sleep in humans. Percept Mot Skills 1983;56:275-283.

85. Oswald I, Berger RJ, Jaramillo RA, et al: Melancholia and barbiturates: A controlled EEG and eye-movement study of sleep. Br J Psychiatry 1963;109:66-78.

86. Gardner R, Grossman WL: Normal motor patterns in sleep in man. In Weitzman ED (ed): Advances in Sleep Research, vol 2. New York, Spectrum, 1975, pp 67-107.

87. Mandell A, et al: Dreaming sleep in man: Changes in urine volume and osmolality. Science 1966;151:1558-1560.

88. Rubin RT, Poland RE, Gouin PR, Tower BB: Secretion of hormones influencing water and electrolyte balance (antidiuretic hormone, aldosterone, prolactin) during sleep in normal adult men. Psychosom Med 1978;40:44-59.

89. Halverson H: Genital and sphincter behavior on the male infant. J Gen Psychol 1940;56:95-136.

90. Ohlmeyer P, Brilmayer H, Hullstrung H: Periodische vorgange im Schlaf. Pflugers Arch 1944;248:559-560.

91. Fisher C, Gross J, Zuch J: Cycle of penile erections synchronous with dreaming (REM) sleep: Preliminary report. Arch Gen Psychiatry 1965;12:29-45.

92. Karacan I, Williams RL, Thornby JI, Salis PJ: Sleep-related penile tumescence as a function of age. Am J Psychiatry 1975;132:932-937.

93. Karacan I, Rosenblum A, Williams R: The clitoral erection cycle during sleep. Psychophysiology 1970;7:338.

94. Abel GG, Murphy WD, Becker JV, Bitar A: Women's vaginal responses during REM sleep. J Sex Marital Ther 1979;5:5-14.

95. Snyder F, Hobson JA, Morrison DF, Goldfrank F: Changes in respiration, heart rate, and systolic pressure in human sleep. J Appl Physiol 1964;19:417.

96. Finch PM, Ingram DM, Henstridge JD, Catchpole BN: Relationship of fasting gastroduodenal motility to the sleep cycle. Gastroenterology 1982;83: 605-612.

97. Orr W, Hall WH, Stahl ML, et al: Sleep patterns and gastric acid secretion in duodenal ulcer disease. Arch Intern Med 1976;136:655-660.

98. Orr W, Robinson M: The sleeping gut. Med Clin North Am 1981;65:1359-1376.

99. Orr W, Robinson M, Johnson L: Acid clearance during sleep in the pathogenesis of reflux esophagitis. Dig Dis Sci 1981;26:423-427.

100. Johnson LF, DeMeester TR, Haggitt RC: Esophageal epithelial response to gastroesophageal reflux: A quantitative study. Am J Dig Dis 1978;23:498-509.

101. Helm JF, Dodds WJ, Riedel DF, et al: Determinants of esophageal acid clearance in normal subjects. Gastroenterology 1980;78:1181.

102. Dent J, Dodds WJ, Friedman RH, et al: Mechanism of gastroesophageal reflux in recumbent asymptomatic human subjects. J Clin Invest 1980;65:256-257.

Chronobiology of Sleep in Children 8

John H. Herman

A circadian rhythm is defined as an intrinsic bio-logic rhythm with a periodicity (peak-to-peak duration) of approximately 24 hours. Circadian rhythms are a basic property of higher life forms, including plants and animals. In mammals, cir-cadian rhythms are coupled to the timing of sleep and wakefulness. Circadian rhythms undergo a developmental course, from their beginnings in utero to adult expression. This chapter describes basic properties of circadian rhythms and then reviews some of their fundamental properties as they develop during childhood. Animal studies are employed to illustrate findings that are appli-cable to infants and children.

Entrainment of the fetus to day and night begins in utero as a passive response to maternal melatonin secretion. In the perinatal period, vari-ous expressions of an endogenous circadian pace-maker neuroanatomic structure (including the suprachiasmatic nucleus, the pineal body, and their connections to the retina) develop sequentially, resulting in the successive appearance of circadian rhythms of melatonin secretion, temperature, wakefulness, and sleep. Circadian rhythms are fully expressed within the first 6 months of life.

In the infant and young child, the timing of light exposure controls the timing of melatonin secretion and consequently the timing of sleep. In early childhood and in preadolescent children, the phase relationship of the child's circadian rhythm to environmental light and darkness is variable. The hour at which the child is awak-ened, the timing and brightness of artificial light-ing after sunset and before sunrise, the timing of exercise, the child's feeding schedule, and the timing of social interactions might each influence the child's timing of sleep propensity. The num-ber of hours of darkness (less than 3 lux) to which the child is exposed may influence the duration of the child's melatonin secretion and the number of hours that the child sleeps.

It is becoming increasingly clear that sleep quality impacts human development. Both the hours at which a child sleeps and the duration of sleep appear to be modifiable. Beginning in utero, and continuing through childhood, envi-ronmental and social activities are capable of influencing the timing and duration of sleep.

THE CIRCADIAN RHYTHM SYSTEM: BASIC PROPERTIES

The duration of daylight changes continually. The magnitude of change from the shortest to the longest day of the year is directly dependent on latitude. The farther one is from the equator, the greater the change from shortest day to longest day. Without artificial light, human and mam-malian ancestors were in synchrony with changes in photoperiod (day length) that varied from greater than to less than 12 hours. The circadian rhythm system must be viewed as having the capacity to track continually changing times of light exposure, including changing times of sun-rise and of sunset.

In contrast to sleep homeostasis, in which sleep drive increases with increased awake time, the body's internal clock mechanism, or circadian rhythm, exhibits a cyclical tendency that is mostly independent of prior wakefulness—this is the circadian rhythm of sleep propensity.[1] Thus, a child or adolescent may be unable to begin nocturnal sleep at a desired hour despite sleep-ing little on previous weekday nights and exhibiting daytime sleepiness during school hours. For example, a child with a 9 PM bedtime might remain awake until midnight. Biologic markers of circadian rhythms, such as the daily rise and fall in core body temperature, continue in the absence of normal social, lighting, or other time cues. Each individual possesses a precise internal clock, the periodicity of which can be "unmasked" in various types of laboratory protocols. This clock typically has a peak-to-peak cycle duration of approximately 24.1 to 24.3 hours.[2,3]

Period Length

The duration of the circadian rhythm (Fig. 8–1), sometimes referred to as period length, or tau, appears to be a genetically heritable property of the suprachiasmatic nucleus (SCN). Period length (see Fig. 8–1A) is measured from one cycle's temperature minimum to the next, or from the onset of melatonin secretion on consecutive days, in experimental conditions that eliminate environmental influences.[4] The SCN contains an autonomous circadian pacemaker. It is the site of generation of circadian rhythmicity. Metabolic and electrical activity rhythms in the SCN have been observed in vivo, and the SCN maintains rhythmicity in vitro. A transplanted SCN from a donor can restore circadian function after the destruction of a host's SCN. Single SCN "clock cells" exhibit independent firing-rate rhythms. The proteins responsible for rhythmicity within the SCN have been identified in circadian mutants (tau mutant hamsters and Clock mutant mice). These mutants have enabled the isolation of so-called clock genes.[5]

Amplitude

The amplitude of the circadian rhythm—that is, the change in a measured parameter from nadir to peak (acrophase)—is an estimate of the biologic capacity to oscillate every day from deep sleep to intense alertness. The amplitude of the circadian rhythm appears to be minimal at birth and to attain adult levels within the first year of life, as measured by melatonin or temperature. Figure 8–1B shows the effects of constant routine (such as staying in bed under conditions of continuous dim illumination for 24 hours) on damping circadian rhythm amplitude. Factors such as exercise and a constant bed and wake-up time do not affect the amplitude of the circadian rhythm.[6]

Phase

The phase of a circadian rhythm refers to the relationship between the internal timekeeping

mechanism and the environmental time. Ideally, core temperature drops and sleepiness occurs at the desired hour of sleep, and body temperature is rising and an individual feels rested at the desired hour of awakening. This is referred to as being "in phase." Phase advance refers to the internal clock's being set early with respect to environmental time, and phase delay refers to the internal clock's being set late with respect to environmental time (Fig. 8–1C). The tendency for

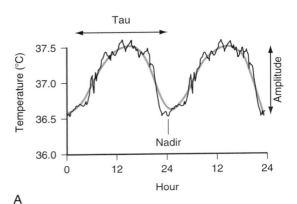

A

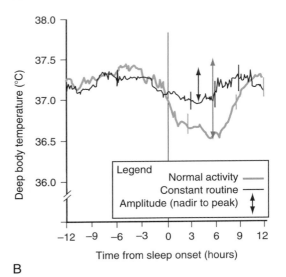

B

Figure 8–1. Properties of a single cycle of the circadian rhythm. **A,** One cycle of the circadian rhythm of temperature drawn twice to illustrate the duration of the circadian rhythm (tau, or τ), here measured from succeeding temperature nadirs, and the amplitude of the circadian rhythm, in this case, temperature difference from apogee to nadir. **B,** The amplitude of the circadian rhythm is reduced by the subject remaining in bed for 24 hours (constant routine, CR) compared to the amplitude of temperature from peak to nadir when the subject is engaged in normal waking activity.

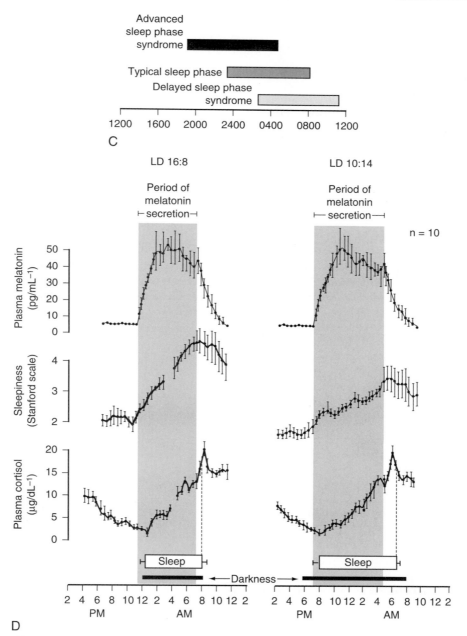

Figure 8–1. cont'd—C, Phase of circadian rhythm refers to the relationship of the internal clock to environmental timing of light and dark, the *top bar* illustrates advanced sleep-phase syndrome (sleep from 7:00 PM to 5:00 AM), the *middle bar* illustrates normal phase timing (sleep from 11:00 PM to 8:00 AM), and the *bottom bar* illustrates delayed sleep phase syndrome (sleep from 2:30 AM to 11:00 AM). **D,** The relative duration of biological day to biological night changes as the light-to-dark ratio is changed from 16 hours of light and 8 hours of darkness *(left, black bar)* to 10 hours of light and 14 hours of darkness *(right, black bar),* resulting in an increased duration of melatonin secretion *(top),* delayed cortisol secretion *(middle),* and increased duration of temperature suppression *(bottom).* (A and C, redrawn from Baker SK, Zee PC: Circadian disorders of the sleep wake cycle. In Kryger M, Roth T, Dement W (eds): Principles and Practice of Sleep Medicine, 3rd ed. Philadelphia, WB Saunders, 2000, pp 607, 610; D redrawn from Wehr TA, Aeschbach D, Duncan WC: Evidence for a biological dawn and dusk in the human circadian timing system. J Physiol 2001;535:937-951.)

phase to be delayed appears to increase from childhood to adolescence.[7]

Morningness–Eveningness Preference and Phase

The duration of an individual's circadian rhythm is correlated with "owl" versus "lark" behavior (referred to as morningness versus eveningness): the longer the period length, the greater the owl tendencies. Evening types (owls) have a later onset of melatonin secretion, their morning temperature rise is later, and they wake up later than do morning types. Dropping temperature is related to sleep onset and rising temperature is correlated with preferred wake-up time.[8] Individuals who are maximally alert in the morning have an earlier peak in circadian temperature than do individuals who are most alert

in the evening. Individuals with morning preference have a greater change in temperature from nadir to peak. These lark types awaken and begin sleep earlier than individuals with evening preference.[9] The phase of temperature and melatonin secretion can be predicted fairly accurately by having an individual maintain a sleep log for several weeks, even with irregular sleep times.[10] With the approach of adolescence, circadian phase shifts to a later hour, as does an increase in evening preference for activities. This occurs at about age 12 to 13 years.[11]

Biological Day and Biological Night

A property of any waveform is the proportion of the wave cycle during which values are above the mean as opposed to below the mean. From the perspective of circadian rhythms, this

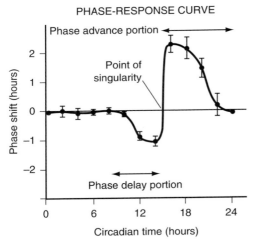

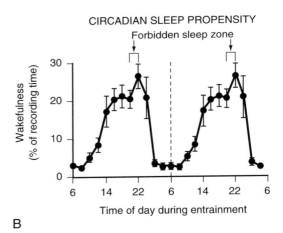

A   B

Figure 8–2. A, The phase-response curve to light (in Syrian hamsters) showing the change in the phase of the circadian rhythm in response to exposure to light at different times. The phase-response curve shows no phase-shifting effect of light during the circadian hours of normal light exposure (typically, the hours of daylight). Exposure to light *before* the moment of singularity results in a maximal phase-delaying effect during the hours of normal darkness (negative numbers). Exposure to light *after* the moment of singularity results in a maximal phase-advancing effect during the hours of normal darkness (positive numbers). A person's circadian time must be known to predict whether the response to bright light will have a phase-advancing or a phase-delaying effect. Point of singularity: the time at which light exposure (or another zeitgeber) switches from having a phase-advancing to a phase-delaying effect on the circadian rhythm. **B,** Circadian sleep propensity double-plotted for one circadian cycle, showing the forbidden sleep zone (a brief time period typically preceding sleep onset), during which sleep is least likely to occur during the circadian day. (A, redrawn from Takahashi JS, Zatz M: Regulation of circadian rhythmicity. Science 1998;2178:1104-1111; B, redrawn from Dijk D-J, Czeisler CA: Contribution of the circadian pacemaker and the sleep homeostat to sleep propensity, sleep structure, electroencephalographic slow waves and sleep spindle activity in humans. J Neurosci 1995;15:3526-3538.)

refers to the ratio of biological day (above the mean) to biological night (below the mean). Figure 8–1D displays two different lengths of environmental light and dark: a 16-hour light period followed by an 8-hour dark period (on the left) and a 10-hour light period followed by 14 hours of darkness (on the right). At latitudes both north and south of the equator, half the year has day length greater than night length. This means that environmental night is greater than 12 hours for half of the year in almost every country, a situation that was far more behaviorally significant before the invention of indoor light, beginning with candles. Figure 8–1D shows that the duration of biological night can change in response to changing durations of environmental night length, including a lengthening in the duration of melatonin secretion.[12]

The capacity to increase the duration of biological night is a critical factor in appreciating the flexibility of the human sleep–wake cycle.

Contemporary humans, in essence, attempt to exist year round on a schedule similar to a short summer night.[13]

Implicit in the description of long versus short biological nights is the hypothesis that there is one switch (entrained to dusk) for the beginning of biological night, and a second switch (entrained to dawn) for the beginning of biological day (Fig. 8–3).[13] The end of biological night does not occur at a set time after its beginning, and the time of awakening is not a constant interval after dim-light melatonin onset (DLMO). Instead, the switches for biological night and day are capable of tracking changing environmental day lengths.[9] This is referred to as a two-oscillator model.[14] The duration of sleep, temperature suppression, and cortisol suppression each increases as biological nights lengthen. The concept of a flexible (within limits) biological night has significant implications for human development.

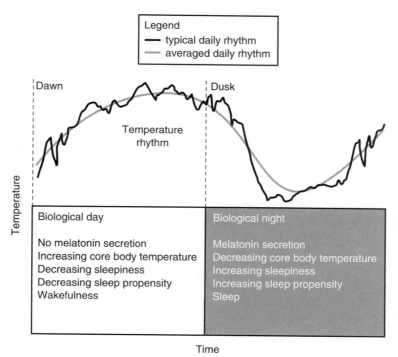

Figure 8–3. Biological day coincides with the environmental time from dawn to dusk, and in diurnal species, including humans, it exhibits qualities compatible with alertness and activity. In diurnal species, biological night, which coincides with darkness, is compatible with rest and immobility. The durations of biological day and biological night are responsive to changes in the duration of daylight as it varies from less than 12 to greater than 12 hours, depending on latitude and season. (Redrawn from Wehr TA, Aeschbach D, Duncan WC: Evidence for a biological dawn and dusk in the human circadian timing system. J Physiol 2001;535:937-951.)

Consolidated Sleep Period

Optimal sleep is one manifestation of biological night. The timing of biological night and an increased sleep propensity (sleepiness) are initiated by the beginning of darkness, or dusk, which is signaled from the retina to the SCN via the retinal hypothalamic pathway (Fig. 8–4). Dusk permits the expression of melatonin (i.e., DLMO) by the pineal body, and it begins the nocturnal phase of the circadian rhythm, or biological night. This includes a drop in core body temperature, which reaches a nadir approximately 2 hours prior to habitual wake-up time (see Figs. 8–1A and Fig. 8–3), and a concomitant decrease in glucose utilization,[15] urinary metabolism, and appetite. After the temperature begins its nightly drop and serum melatonin begins its rise, sleep propensity increases rapidly and the consolidated period of nocturnal sleep begins (see Fig 8–3).[16]

Rate of Change from Biological Day to Biological Night

Human circadian rhythms have traditionally been represented graphically as a plot of core body temperature or melatonin secretory levels averaged from several subjects. The resulting plot of mean values resembles a sine wave (Figs. 8–3 and 8–5A) that is similar to a frequency histogram recording electrophysiologically from SCN neurons.[17] However, if melatonin secretory profiles are measured consecutively, time-locked to melatonin onset or offset, the resulting waveform resembles more of a square wave, with a rapid transition from biological day to biological night, as shown in Figure 8–5B.[8] This rapid transition is consistent with experimental findings in constant-routine protocols of a brief sleep "gate," before which sleep is unlikely to occur and after which sleep is likely to occur.[18] As day changes to night, the output of the SCN switches an organism from one mode of functioning, in which it is interactive with its environment, to another, in which it is nonresponsive and immobile.[13]

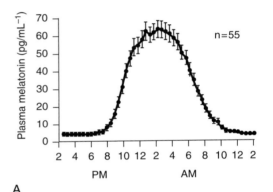

A

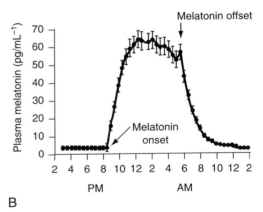

B

Figure 8–5. **A,** Melatonin secretory profile derived from averaging serum levels of melatonin. The result is a sinusoidal waveform with a periodicity of approximately 24 hours. **B,** Plotted values are derived from averaging forward and backward from each subject's time-locked melatonin onset and offset. B reveals melatonin as an on-or-off switch, demarcating the onset of biological night and the onset of biological day. (Redrawn from Wehr TA, Aeschbach D, Duncan WC. Evidence for a biological dawn and dusk in the human circadian timing system. J Physiol 2001;535:937-951.)

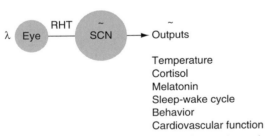

Figure 8–4. The input to the suprachiasmatic nuclei (SCN) is via special retinal receptors that form a synaptic connection to the retinohypothalamic tract, which carries light information to the SCN. These light receptors do not form synaptic connections with the optic nerve, and they transmit no visual information to the CNS visual processing centers. Therefore, conscious light perception and SCN input are via distinct pathways; if either is destroyed, the other can remain fully functional. (From Rivkees S: Mechanisms and clinical significance of circadian rhythms in children. Curr Opin Pediatr 2001; 13:352-357.)

Point of Singularity

Each cycle of a circadian rhythm has an acrophase and a nadir (see Fig. 8–1D). The circadian nadir is significant: it is near the minimum of body temperature. Before this time, light has a phase-delaying effect, and after this time, light has a phase-advancing effect[19] (see Fig. 8–2A). Sometimes referred to as the point of singularity, the circadian nadir is coincident with the beginning of the rises of core body temperature, cortisol secretion, and the proportion of sleep occupied by rapid eye movement sleep. Exposure to bright light centered at the point of singularity significantly reduces the amplitude of core body temperature, plasma cortisol secretion, and melatonin secretion.[20]

Forbidden Sleep Zone

The "forbidden sleep zone" immediately precedes the onset of biological night. This is the time at which sleep is least likely to occur during a circadian cycle (see Fig. 8–2B). This 1- to 3-hour period is well established in human adults and adolescents. Because the forbidden sleep zone precedes the normal hour of sleep, many individuals with delayed sleep phase have difficulty advancing their hour of sleep despite sleep deprivation and daytime sleepiness.[21,22] Although forbidden sleep zones have not been studied in children, they appear to be particularly robust, as even children who are sleepy enough to fall asleep in school are not able to begin nighttime sleep at an earlier hour.

Circadian Outputs

An extremely large number of biologic, behavioral, cognitive, and emotional factors demonstrate consistent and predictable circadian rhythms. Core body temperature (see Fig. 8–1A), hormone secretion, and cell metabolism are among the better-known biologic parameters that demonstrate a circadian rhythm.[23] Human performance is well documented to demonstrate a circadian rhythm, and a variety of measures of cognitive skills show circadian changes in performance. Mood and emotions also follow predictable circadian patterns.[24,25] It is currently believed that most of our organs contain their own clock mechanisms, and that each of these maintains a synchronous relationship with the body's master clock via outputs from the SCN.[26]

Phase Shifts

Only disrupted phase, and no other aspect of the circadian rhythm, is considered a circadian sleep disorder. The phase of the circadian rhythm is synchronized with environmental time by a variety of zeitgebers (or time givers, and thus clock setters), principally bright light, but also including the timing of sleep and the timing of social contacts. Suitably timed exposures to bright light result in large shifts in the circadian phase.[27] In contrast to bright light (and melatonin), most other factors have only weak and inconsistent effects in shifting circadian phase.[28]

The phase-shifting effect of bright light (or any other zeitgeber) requires not only that it be delivered at a suitable time (see Fig. 8–2A), for sufficient duration, and at necessary intensity, but also that the individual not be exposed to light at times where the phase-shifting effect would be in the opposite direction.[29] For example, exposure to bright light during normal hours of morning sleep (after the point of singularity) will not result in a phase advance unless darkness is present during the earlier (evening) time interval to which sleep is to be phase advanced.

It appears that both light of ordinary room intensity[30,31] and daytime napping[32] are capable of inducing a small phase shift. These so-called weak zeitgebers[33] have been demonstrated to change circadian phase under conditions of constant routine, an experimental technique that eliminates all stimuli that would interfere with a phase shift. It is not clear how effective weak zeitgebers would be in shifting circadian rhythms under normal conditions.

Melatonin

Melatonin is secreted by the pineal gland during darkness, and the timing of its secretion appears to be under the control of the SCN.[34] Melatonin is sometimes referred to as the hormone of darkness. The endogenous rhythm of melatonin secretion is entrained by the light–dark cycle.[35] Light is able to both suppress and entrain melatonin production.[34] The normal timing of sleep is tightly coupled to the melatonin secretory profile. Melatonin is associated with sleep in diurnal mammals and with waking in nocturnal animals.

Melatonin administration and light exposure shift circadian phase in opposite directions. Thus, melatonin administration before DLMO results in a phase advance, and melatonin administration after the morning melatonin offset results in a phase delay. The phase-response curve to melatonin is similar to the phase-response curve to light but in the opposite direction.[36,37] Melatonin is more effective in altering the timing of circadian rhythms than that it is as a hypnotic.[38] The administration of exogenous melatonin alters the timing of endogenous melatonin secretion on subsequent days.[39]

In a constant-routine experimental paradigm, in which sleep is permitted for only 10 minutes, followed by 20 minutes of forced wakefulness for multiple 24-hour periods, sleep occurs only during intervals that coincide with melatonin secretion (greater than 10 pg/mL has been suggested as a minimal sleep-inducing melatonin level[4]). During intervals when melatonin is not secreted, sleep does not occur.[40]

The nocturnal onset of melatonin secretion is time-locked in humans to the opening of the nocturnal sleep gate: as melatonin secretory levels increase, body temperature falls. In a variety of free-running conditions, sleep occurs only when body temperature is dropping or low. These findings suggest that melatonin participates in sleep–wake regulation in humans.[18]

Masking

The environment exerts influences that keep an individual entrained with local day and night. These are exogenous influences that "mask" the body's endogenous circadian rhythm. Masking is so universally present that the body's circadian rhythm may be observed only under extremely controlled experimental conditions that eliminate the multiple zeitgebers of everyday life that keep all of us entrained. The timing of bright and dim light exposure, social activities, exercise, and meals all induce a masking effect.[41] Some degree of masking is occurring continually in all mammals whose endogenous circadian rhythm is not precisely 24 hours, as environmental zeitgebers synchronize circadian rhythms with the local hours of light and darkness.

Entrainment

Entrainment refers to an individual's hours of biological day and biological night being in synchrony, or in phase, with environmental day and night. Entrainment of circadian rhythms to an environmental schedule appears to be accomplished by a variety of factors, many of which have already been discussed: bright or dim light, social schedule, melatonin,[42,43] social activities,[44] and exercise.[45] Bright light induces greater entrainment than dim light; specifically, exposure to bright light induces a greater evening drop and morning rise in core body temperature. Daytime exposure to bright light also results in an advance in the circadian rhythm of body temperature compared to dim light.[46] These findings suggest that both dim and bright light entrain an organism to environmental phase, or time, but that bright light further enhances entrainment by inducing a greater amplitude of the temperature rhythm and an earlier rise in core body temperature. These findings suggest that children and adolescents with sleep initiation problems would benefit from daytime bright light exposure.

Effect of Indoor Light on Phase

The light of dawn (an average of 155 lux, similar to indoor lighting) is sufficient to induce a phase advance in normal subjects. It is also sufficient to prevent phase delay in subjects living in constant dim illumination.[47] Subjects kept in constant dim light (as opposed to timed indoor light) for 21 days who had knowledge of clock time and who had social cues in a group setting demonstrated free-running circadian rhythms, with a periodicity of 24{1/4} hours in melatonin and temperature rhythms.[48] This study shows that normal individuals may not be able to remain entrained to environmental time in the absence of timed light as a zeitgeber. Ordinary room light is capable of shifting the rhythms of temperature, melatonin,[49] and cortisol, indicating that the master circadian pacemaker has shifted in response to indoor light.[15,31] Both temperature and hour of sleep shifted to the earlier phase, indicating a change in the output of the master clock, similar to results observed in studies using bright light. It has also been shown that the timing of exposure to normal room light modulates the effect of bright light on circadian phase, such as room light exposure during biological night, including television sets and computer monitors. This suggests that even in the presence of normally timed bright light, indoor light after or before normal daylight hours may induce a phase shift in the circadian rhythm.[50] These studies collectively indicate that indoor room light is sufficient to continually exert weak influences on circadian rhythms, but that it is insufficient to abruptly switch rhythms to a vastly altered sleep–wake schedule.

Resetting Circadian Time in Children

The phase-response curve (PRC), or the degree to which the circadian rhythm will be advanced or delayed, is based on the time at which bright light or melatonin is administered. Typically, the advance or delay of the circadian system is measured in the number of minutes that the circadian temperature nadir is advanced or delayed.

Timing of Light

The PRC shows that there is virtually no change in circadian rhythms (for example, timing of the temperature nadir) induced by exposure to light during the middle of the circadian "day"; on the other hand, there is maximal responsiveness when exposure occurs immediately before or after the temperature nadir.[51] Other investigators have found that under certain experimental conditions, light delivered at any time during the circadian day had a slight phase-shifting effect.[50] At about the time of the temperature minimum (point of singularity), a switch is thrown, and at this point light changes from having a phase-delaying to a phase-advancing effect: immediately before the temperature minimum, light has its maximal phase-delaying effect, and immediately after the temperature minimum, light has its maximal phase-advancing effect.[52]

Intensity of Light

The intensity of the light greatly influences the magnitude of the response, with bright light (about 5000 to 10,000 lux) having a much greater effect than normal room light (100 to 200 lux). Even dim light (less than 100 lux) might have a slight effect on shifting circadian rhythms.[53] The timing of sleep and darkness is as important as the timing of the bright light.[54]

A homologous phase-response relationship probably exists for melatonin and circadian rhythms, in which melatonin has the opposite effect of light: evening melatonin would advance the circadian rhythm and morning melatonin would exert a phase-delaying effect.[22] A single dose of melatonin properly timed is capable of advancing the human circadian clock.[55] In subjects living in constant dim light for a month, melatonin administered 2 hours before the temperature acrophase had a maximal effect on advancing the circadian rhythm.[34] Melatonin synthesis normally begins about the hour of sunset; in indoor-living humans, it typically begins to be present in plasma shortly after sunset (about 8 PM to 9 PM) and gradually rises to a peak about 3 AM to 4 AM, followed by a decline in plasma concentration to near zero by 9 AM. Both DLMO and melatonin offset have been found to be as reliable as core body temperature in estimating circadian rhythms.[3]

DEVELOPMENT OF CIRCADIAN RHYTHMS

In Utero and in the Neonatal Period

Some aspects of circadian rhythm appear to begin in utero in mammalian species. The mature circadian rhythm system requires connections from a fully functioning SCN to retinal inputs and to multiple targeted outputs. The circadian system is not fully functional at birth in most mammalian species. However, circadian rhythms begin in utero as the fetus becomes entrained to the mother's rhythm. From the standpoint of the fetus, this is an exogenous rhythm, externally imposed by factors such as maternal temperature or melatonin, prior to the development of the fetus's own fully developed SCN. In mammals, maternal melatonin and the maternal circadian temperature cycle convey information about environmental time. In some species, the retinohypothalamic tract transmits light information to the fetal SCN in utero, which is capable of becoming entrained to environmental light shortly prior to birth. However, light appears to be a less potent entraining factor in utero than maternal melatonin secretion.[56]

The Suprachiasmatic Nucleus

Neurogenesis of the SCN occurs 3 to 5 days before birth in rats and hamsters, respectively.[57,58] If a pregnant hamster is injected with melatonin the day before delivery, after weaning (on day of life 20) the midpoint of the pups' subjective *night* will coincide with the time of the injection. If the pregnant hamster is injected with a dopamine agonist, after weaning the midpoint of the pups' subjective *day* will coincide with the time of the injection. This demonstrates that dopamine and melatonin either are, or mimic, maternal entraining signals that represent day and night.[59,60]

The responsiveness of a pup's circadian clock to melatonin and dopamine agonist injections is gone by day 4 of life, replaced by an equally robust response to light (subjective night in rodents) and darkness (subjective day in rodents).[61] If two groups of pregnant hamsters are injected with a dopamine agonist 12 hours apart, the circadian rhythms of the two groups will be 12 hours out of synch on the day of weaning, demonstrating that the prenatal dopamine agonist set the phase of the offspring's circadian rhythms.[60] In rats, at about the same time—the end of the first week of life for the rat pup—the SCN develops the ability to be entrained by light. At this time, the circadian rhythm of N-acetyltransferase first appears.

The human SCN develops early in gestation, and circadian rhythms are present in the fetus and newborn. The circadian system seems to be functional in human fetal life and can receive circadian inputs through the mother.[62]

Uniqueness of SCN Tissue

For the lateral geniculate nucleus (LGN) to develop normally, afferents from the retina must innervate LGN cells during development. In visual deprivation studies, LGN hypertrophy results from interruption of retinal afferent fibers. Visual input from the retina is crucial in cell development and neural arborization in the LGN, as in most other CNS structures that are part of a sensory system. In contrast, there is no evidence that afferents from the retinohypothalamic tract, the raphe, or the intrageniculate nucleus influence the development of the SCN. Lesioning afferent fibers does not result in SCN hypotrophy. No other tissue takes on pacemaker properties if the SCN is enucleated early in development.[63,64]

Pacemaker properties of SCN cells are intrinsic: SCN fetal tissue develops its intrinsic rhythmicity even if transplanted to a totally different environment, such as the anterior chamber of an adult eye.[65] Fetal SCN tissue may be minced prior to transplantation, destroying specific spatial relationships, yet intrinsic rhythmicity develops normally.[66]

Role of Melatonin in Development

When the fetus's SCN begins to function, melatonin from the mother is probably the principal factor entraining it to the prevailing light–dark cycle.[67] Even when a pregnant mother is kept in constant light, the mother's rhythm and the rhythms of her offspring demonstrate a consistent phase relationship with each other.[68] This indicates that entrainment of the newborn to its mother results from intrauterine factors, especially when environmental zeitgebers are absent.

Nonphotic Zeitgebers in Development

In the absence of light cues for day and night, social contact may act as an entraining factor in developing mammals. Mice born and raised to the age of weaning in constant lighting conditions remain entrained to their mother's circadian rhythm. The mouse pup's daily onset of wheel running (nighttime) is entrained to the mother's termination of nursing, and therefore, the pups time of wheel running coincides with the mother's absence. In constant lighting conditions, the mother's return is taken by the pups as their rest time and her absence as their wake time.[67]

The newborn's temperature and melatonin secretory rhythms are in phase with environmental night and day, probably resulting from infant–mother synchronization. Feeding and rest–activity synchronization to mother and environment develop rapidly during the neonatal period.

In the First Year of Life

From birth to 6 months, the human infant develops robust circadian rhythms. The retinohypothalamic tract is present in humans before birth, and plasma melatonin demonstrates a rhythm influenced by light within the first 2 days after birth.[69] Human rhythms are in phase with their environment when they appear, suggesting entrainment that precedes the ability to measure them. The SCN may be functioning before birth in humans but may not yet have developed output-entraining mechanisms. Human fetal rhythms are entrained to those of the mother, and the probable synchronizing substance is melatonin.[70] The human fetus shows a rhythm in heart rate and fetal movement activity that is also circadian.[71]

A weak circadian rhythm, showing newborn-mother entrainment, is observable in 24-hour consecutive plots of the infant's tympanic membrane temperature during days of life 1 to 14.[72] This implies that some degree of entrainment of the circadian rhythm of temperature has occurred in utero in the human fetus. If a human infant is exposed to only sunlight (no incandescent or florescent light) for the first 6 months of life, the sequential development of behavioral and physiologic properties of the infant's circadian rhythm become evident.[72] The circadian rhythm of temperature appears first, soon after birth, and becomes statistically significant within 1 week. Most apparent in 24-hour temperature plots of the first 2 weeks of life are a morning increase and an evening fall in temperature. The wake circadian rhythm appears soon after, attaining significance at day 45, approximately the same time that increased melatonin concentration begins to occur at sunset (DLMO, defined as salivary concentration greater than 20 pg/mL, equivalent to adult levels).[72]

The circadian rhythm of sleep appears last, attaining significance after day 56. Ninety- to 120-minute zones of sustained wakefulness first appear in the second month of life, after awakening and prior to sleep onset (forbidden sleep zone). The infant's nocturnal sleep-onset is coupled to sunset before day 60, and subsequently it is coupled to family bedtime, giving evidence of initial photic entrainment followed by social entrainment. Even in the absence of artificial light after sunset, the infant's sleep onset time tracks the family's schedule, as the infant remains awake for 1 to 3 hours every night in darkness.[72] Actigraphy monitoring of rest–activity cycles in the 3-week-old human infant also shows a circadian rhythm.[73]

Before sleep or wake demonstrates a circadian rhythm, the infant's morning awakening appears to become entrained to the rise in body temperature, and the two appear to remain coupled. Morning entrainment of awakening to rising body temperature appears to precede the coupling of sleep onset to sunset; dawn is a more powerful zeitgeber than dusk. A coupling of sleep onset to evening darkness first appears on a consistent basis during week 7 of life. A proclivity for sleep to occur during the night and wake to occur during the day is present in the first weeks of life as well. By week 14, the infant has developed a wake maintenance zone beginning at sunset and continuing for 1 to 3 hours.[72]

By 6 months of life, the human infant, when exposed only to sunlight, is entrained to both it and the social rhythm of the household. Maintenance of wakefulness zones are apparent as the infant remains awake after sunset.[72] Just as the organization of sleep stages attains adult criteria by age 6 months,[74] the human circadian rhythm displays period, amplitude, and phase activity at 6 months of age that are similar to these elements in adult human circadian rhythms. It appears that circadian rhythms are one of the earliest maturing physiologic-behavioral systems.

In the Preschool Child

Little research is available on the preschool child's circadian rhythms, probably because this is a period when aberrations and idiosyncrasies are more readily tolerated due to the absence of social scheduling requirements. It appears that preschool children are behaviorally similar to preadolescents, who are relatively phase advanced compared to adolescents.[75] The preschool child frequently becomes entrained to maternal or familial rhythms before becoming synchronized with a school schedule.

In the School-Aged Child

Remaining awake later on weekends and sleeping to a later hour has a phase-delaying effect, making it more difficult for the school-aged child to initiate sleep on Sunday night and to awaken on Monday morning.[76] This effect (remaining awake later and subsequent phase delay) may be greater over extended school vacations. During preadolescence in most children, sleep gradually becomes more delayed with respect to biological night, resulting in a propensity to initiate sleep and awaken at a later hour despite little change in tau, or period length. Adolescents are better able to sleep after their body temperature rises and to remain awake after body temperature falls than younger children.[77]

Carskadon and colleagues[2] measured the circadian rhythm duration of 12- to 15-year-olds by having them follow a 28-hour day for 12 consecutive days. They were in dim light for two thirds of the 28 hours (waking period) then in darkness the remaining third of the time (sleep period). Because the human circadian clock is unable to synchronize to the 28-hour schedule, the timing of sleep and waking become "uncoupled" from the body's temperature and melatonin rhythm. In this protocol, measurement of the time from one temperature or melatonin peak to the next indicates the unmasked cycle length of the body's clock. The circadian rhythm duration of both temperature and melatonin was found to be 24.3 hours, longer than 24 hours, but similar to that found in older individuals.[2] This study demonstrates that the age-related, adolescent "night owl" propensity, or tendency toward delayed sleep and awakening, does not result from a longer adolescent clock cycle but must be caused by other factors, such as the timing of sleepiness with respect to the circadian temperature cycle.[7]

Another study found that 10th grade and 3rd grade children sleep the same number of hours on weekends, about 9{1/4} hours, but the bedtimes and wake-up times of older children are 2 hours later than those of younger children. This indicates that the biological clock of the late adolescent is set 2 hours later than that of the younger child, and that sleep need has not changed significantly from early childhood to adolescence.[75]

CONCLUSIONS

Circadian rhythms in humans develop in utero, under control of maternal melatonin early in gestation, and later under control of the fetus' developing SCN. Light suppresses the secretion of melatonin, a hormone that is secreted in darkness and is related to biological night in humans. Melatonin levels are higher at approximately the time when sleep occurs. The pacemaker system (anatomically centered in the SCN) receives information about the presence of light, which suppresses melatonin secretion, from the retina. The timing of the pregnant mother's exposure to light affects her secretory melatonin levels and those of the fetus. If the mother's light exposure during the later portion of gestation is restricted to daytime hours, this could increase the likelihood that the newborn will first express a sleep-wake pattern in synchrony with environmental light and dark.

Circadian rhythms of some aspects of human physiology are present at birth. A sleep–wake circadian rhythm that is quite robust emerges in the first 6 months of life, including the hour at which sleep begins and ends. The history of an individual's recent light exposure determines a specific time at which the circadian clock permits sleep to begin (biological night) and as well as a time at which an individual is likely to awaken (biological day).

The greater the proportion of the 24-hour period that is occupied by darkness (biological night), the longer is the duration of melatonin secretion, which is associated with an increase in the number of hours of sleep. Thus, both the circadian rhythm (timing) of sleep and the homeostasis (amount) of sleep are influenced by light exposure. Data from healthy human subjects suggest that sleep time increases if the duration of environmental night (dark period) is increased. The same data suggest that sleep time decreases if the duration of environmental night is decreased. Humans are biologically and behaviorally equipped to accommodate to long nights in winter and short nights in summer.

The timing of biologic rhythms is also partially under the control of factors other than light, especially if exposure to bright light is curtailed. The timing of social and family activities may influence the timing of sleep. Thus, regular timing of family activities, including meals and bedtimes, is likely to facilitate the development of more regular rhythms in a human infant, child, or adolescent.

Indoor light can be disruptive to sleep. We possess a circadian mechanism that has not adapted to the variety of light- and sound-emitting devices that may be present in many households during the hours of night. The presence of indoor light allows each family (or individual) to select its hours of darkness (and quiet), a phenomenon that could be detrimental to the optimal expression of sleep in children. In effect, artificial light enables the contraction of environmental night, possibly decreasing a child's total hours of sleep.

A family's timing of activities and their hours of light exposure influence when and how much a child sleeps throughout development. The encroachment of (artificial) daytime into hours historically reserved for sleep has unknown influences on human development, as this is a recent phenomenon from a biologic perspective.

References

1. Dijk DJ, Czeisler CA: Contribution of the circadian pacemaker and the sleep homeostat to sleep propensity, sleep structure, electroencephalographic slow waves and sleep spindle activity in humans. J Neurosci 1995;15:3526-3538.
2. Carskadon MA, Labyak SE, Acebo C, Seifer R: Intrinsic circadian period of adolescent humans measured in conditions of forced desynchrony. Neurosci Lett 1999;260:129-132.
3. Czeisler CA, Duffy JF, Shanahan TL, et al: Stability, precision, and near-24-hour period of the human circadian pacemaker. Science 1999;284:2177-2181.
4. Lewy AJ, Cutler NL, Sack RL: The endogenous melatonin profile as a marker for circadian phase position. J Biol Rhythms 1999;14:227-236.
5. Weaver DR: The suprachiasmatic nucleus: A 25-year retrospective. J Biol Rhythms 1998;13:100-112.
6. Waterhouse J, Minors D, Folkard S, et al: Lack of evidence that feedback from lifestyle alters the amplitude of the circadian pacemaker in humans. Chronobiol Int 1999;16:93-107.
7. Carskadon MA, Vieira C, Acebo C: Association between puberty and delayed phase preference. Sleep 1993;16:258-262.
8. Duffy JF, Rimmer DW, Czeisler CA: Association of intrinsic circadian period with morningness-eveningness, usual wake time, and circadian phase. Behav Neurosci 2001;115:895-899.
9. Horne JA, Ostberg O: A self-assessment questionnaire to determine morningness-eveningness in human circadian rhythms. Int J Chronobiol 1976;4:97-110.
10. Martin SK, Eastman CI: Sleep logs of young adults with self-selected sleep times predict the dim light melatonin onset. Chronobiol Int 2002;19:695-707.
11. Shinkoda H, Matsumoto K, Park YM, Nagashima H: Sleep-wake habits of schoolchildren according to grade. Psychiatry Clin Neurosci 2000;54:287-289.
12. Wehr TA, Aeschbach D, Duncan WC: Evidence for a biological dawn and dusk in the human circadian timing system. J Physiol 2001;535:937-951.
13. Wehr T: The impact of changes in nightlength (scotoperiod) on human sleep. In Turek FW, Zee PC (eds): Regulation of Sleep and Circadian Rhythms. New York, Marcel Dekker, 1999, pp 263-285.
14. Pittendrigh CS, Daan S: A functional analysis of circadian pacemakers in nocturnal rodents: V. Pacemaker structure: A clock for all seasons. J Comp Physiol A 1976;106:333-355.
15. Braun AR, Balkin TJ, Wesenten NJ, et al: Regional cerebral blood flow throughout the sleep-wake cycle: An $H_2(15)O$ PET study. Brain 1997;120:1173-1197.
16. Krauchi K, Wirz-Justice A: Circadian clues to sleep onset mechanisms. Neuropsychopharmacology 2001;25:S92-96.
17. Zhang L: New electrophysiological approaches to the suprachiasmatic circadian pacemaker. Bol Estud Med Biol 1994;42:31-36.
18. Shochat T, Luboshitzky R, Lavie P: Nocturnal melatonin onset is phase locked to the primary sleep gate. Am J Physiol 1997;273:R364-370.
19. Czeisler CA, Wright KP: Influence of light on circadian rhythmicity in humans. In Turek FW, Zee PC (eds): Regulation of Sleep and Circadian Rhythms. New York, Marcel Dekker, 1999, pp 149-180.
20. Jewett ME, Kronauer RE, Czeisler CA: Light-induced suppression of endogenous circadian amplitude in humans. Nature 1991;350:59-62.
21. Folkard S, Barton J: Does the "forbidden zone" for sleep onset influence morning shift sleep duration? Ergonomics 1993;36:85-91.
22. Lavie P: Ultrashort sleep-waking schedule: III. "Gates" and "forbidden zones" for sleep. Electroencephalogr Clin Neurophysiol 1986;63:414-425.
23. Porkka-Heiskanen T, Stenberg D: Cellular and molecular mechanisms of sleep. In Turek FW, Zee PC (eds): Regulation of Sleep and Circadian Rhythms. New York, Marcel Dekker, 1999, pp 287-307.
24. Wood C, Magnello ME: Diurnal changes in perceptions of energy and mood: J R Soc Med 1992;85:191-194.
25. Boivin DB, Czeisler CA, Dijk D, et al: Complex interactions of the sleep-wake cycle and circadian phase modulates mood in healthy subjects. Arch Gen Psychiatry 1997;54:145-152.
26. Yamazaki S, Numano R, Abe M, et al: Resetting central and peripheral circadian oscillators in transgenic rats. Science 2000;288:682-685.
27. Minors DS, Waterhouse JM, Wirz-Justice A: A human phase-response curve to light. Neurosci Lett 1991;133:36-40.

28. Duffy JF, Kronauer RE, Czeisler CA: Phase-shifting human circadian rhythms: Influence of sleep timing, social contact and light exposure. J Physiol 1996;495:289-297.

29. Mitchell PJ, Hoese EK, Liu L, et al: Conflicting bright light exposure during night shifts impedes circadian adaptation. J Biol Rhythms 1997;12:5-15.

30. Boivin DB, Czeisler CA: Resetting of circadian melatonin and cortisol rhythms in humans by ordinary room light. Neuroreport 1998;9:779-782.

31. Waterhouse J, Minors D, Folkard S, et al: Light of domestic intensity produces phase shifts of the circadian oscillator in humans. Neurosci Lett 1998;245:97-100.

32. Buxton OM, L'Hermite-Baleriaux M, Turek FW, van Cauter E: Daytime naps in darkness phase shift the human circadian rhythms of melatonin and thyrotropin secretion. Am J Physiol Regul Integr Comp Physiol 2000;278:R373-382.

33. Minors DS, Waterhouse JM: Deriving a "phase response curve" from adjustment to simulated time zone transitions. J Biol Rhythms 1994;9:275-282.

34. Geoffriau M, Brun J, Chazot G, Claustrat B: The physiology and pharmacology of melatonin in humans. Horm Res 1998;49:136-141.

35. Reiter RJ: Pineal melatonin: Cell biology of its synthesis and of its physiological interactions. Endocr Rev 1991;12:151-179.

36. Lewy AJ, Ahmed S, Sack RL: Phase shifting the human circadian clock using melatonin. Behav Brain Res 1996;73:131-134.

37. Lewy AJ, Ahmed S, Jackson JM, Sack RL: Melatonin shifts human circadian rhythms according to a phase-response curve. Chronobiol Int 1992; 9:380-392.

38. Turek WF, Czeisler CA: Role of melatonin in the regulation of sleep. In Turek FW, Zee PC (eds): Regulation of Sleep and Circadian Rhythms. New York, Marcel Dekker, 1999, pp 181-195.

39. Zaidan R, Geoffriau M, Brun J, et al: Melatonin is able to influence its secretion in humans: Description of a phase-response curve. Neuroendocrinology 1994;60:105-112.

40. Lavie P: Melatonin: Role in gating nocturnal rise in sleep propensity. J Biol Rhythms 1997;12:657-665.

41. Dijk D-J, Edgar DM: Circadian and homeostatic control of wakefulness and sleep, in the regulation of sleep. In Turek FW, Zee PC (eds): Regulation of Sleep and Circadian Rhythms. New York, Marcel Dekker, 1999, pp 111-147.

42. Lockley SW, Skene DJ, James K, et al: Melatonin administration can entrain the free-running circadian system of blind subjects. J Endocrinol 2000; 164:1-6.

43. Arendt J: Complex effects of melatonin. Therapie 1998;53:479-488.

44. Klerman EB, Rimmer DW, Dijk DJ, et al: Nonphotic entrainment of the human circadian pacemaker. Am J Physiol 1998;274:991-996.

45. Baehr EK, Fogg LF, Eastman CI: Intermittent bright light and exercise to entrain human circadian rhythms to night work. Am J Physiol 1999; 277:1598-1604.

46. Park SJ, Tokura H: Effects of different light intensities during the daytime on circadian rhythm of core temperature in humans. Appl Human Sci 1998;17:253-257.

47. Danilenko KV, Wirz-Justice A, Krauchi K, et al: The human circadian pacemaker can see by the dawn's early light. J Biol Rhythms 2000;15:437-446.

48. Middleton B, Arendt J, Stone BM: Human circadian rhythms in constant dim light (8 lux) with knowledge of clock time. J Sleep Res 1996;5:69-76.

49. Brainard GC, Rollag MD, Hanifin JP: Photic regulation of melatonin in humans: Ocular and neural signal transduction. J Biol Rhythms 1997;12:537-546.

50. Jewett ME, Rimmer DW, Duffy JF, et al: Human circadian pacemaker is sensitive to light throughout subjective day without evidence of transients. Am J Physiol 1997;273:R1800-1809.

51. Takahashi JS, Zatz M: Regulation of circadian rhythmicity. Science 1982;4565:1104-1111.

52. Jewett ME, Kronauer RE, Czeisler CA: Phase-amplitude resetting of the human circadian pacemaker via bright light: A further analysis. J Biol Rhythms 1994;9:295-314.

53. Boivin DB, Duffy JF, Kronauer RE, et al. Dose-response relationships for resetting of human circadian clock by light. Nature 1996;379: 540-542.

54. Mitchell PJ, Hoese EK, Liu L, et al: Conflicting bright light exposure during night shifts impedes circadian adaptation. J Biol Rhythms 1997;12:5-15.

55. Lewy AJ, Sack RL: Exogenous melatonin's phase-shifting effects on the endogenous melatonin profile in sighted humans: A brief review and critique of the literature. J Biol Rhythms 1997; 12:588-594.

56. Weaver DR, Reppert SM: Direct in utero perception of light by the mammalian fetus. Brain Res Dev Brain Res 1989;47:151-155.

57. Altman J, Bayer SA: Development of the diencephalon in the rat: III. Ontogeny of the specialized ventricular linings of the hypothalamic third ventricle. J Comp Neurol 1978;182:995-1015.

58. Altman J, Bayer SA: Time of origin of neurons of the rat superior colliculus in relation to other components of the visual and visuomotor pathways. Exp Brain Res 1981;42:424-434.

59. Viswanathan N, Davis FC: Single prenatal injections of melatonin or the D1-dopamine receptor agonist SKF 38393 to pregnant hamsters sets the

offspring's circadian rhythms to phases 180 degrees apart. J Comp Physiol [A] 1997;180:339-346.

60. Viswanathan N, Weaver DR, Reppert SM, Davis FC: Entrainment of the fetal hamster circadian pacemaker by prenatal injections of the dopamine agonist SKF 38393. J Neurosci 1994;14:5393-5398.

61. Weaver DR, Reppert SM: Definition of the developmental transition from dopaminergic to photic regulation of c-*fos* gene expression in the rat suprachiasmatic nucleus. Brain Res Mol Brain Res 1995;33:136-148.

62. Seron-Ferre M, Torres-Farfan C, Forcelledo ML, Valenzuela GJ: The development of circadian rhythms in the fetus and neonate. Semin Perinatol 2001;25:363-370.

63. Mosko S, Moore RY: Retinohypothalamic tract development: Alteration of suprachiasmatic lesions in the neonatal rat. Brain Res 1979;174:1-15.

64. Mosko S, Moore RY: Neonatal suprachiasmatic nucleus ablation: Absence of functional and morphological plasticity. Proc Natl Acad Sci 1978;75: 6243-6246.

65. Roberts MH, Bernstein MF, Moore RY: Differentiation of the suprachiasmatic nucleus in fetal rat anterior hypothalamic transplants. Dev Brain Res 1987;32:59-66.

66. Wiegand SJ, Gash, DM: Organization and efferent connections of transplanted suprachiasmatic nuclei. J Comp Neurol 1988;267:562-579.

67. Reppert SM: Interaction between the circadian clocks of mother and fetus. CIBA Found Symp 1995;183:198-207.

68. Viswanathan N: Maternal entrainment in the circadian activity rhythm of laboratory mouse (C57BL/6J). Physiol Behav 1999;68:157-162.

69. Rivkees SA, Hofman PL, Fortman J: Newborn primate infants are entrained by low intensity lighting. Proc Natl Acad Sci 1997;94:292-297.

70. Stark RI, Daniel SS: Circadian rhythm of vasopressin levels in cerebrospinal fluid of the fetus: Effect of continuous light. Endocrinology 1989;124:3095-3101.

71. Patrick, J, Campbell K, Carmichael L, et al: Patterns of gross fetal body movement over 24-hour observation intervals during the last 10 weeks of pregnancy. Am J Obstet Gynecol 1982;142:363-371.

72. McGraw K, Hoffmann R, Harker C, Herman JH: The development of circadian rhythms in a human infant. Sleep 1999;22:303-310.

73. Nishihara K, Horiuchi S, Eto H, Uchida S: The development of infants' circadian rest-activity rhythm and mothers' rhythm. Physiol Behav 2002;77:91-98.

74. Rechtschaffen A, Kales A (eds): A Manual for Sleep Stages of Human Subjects: A Manual of Standardized Terminology: Techniques and Scoring System, Los Angeles, UCLA Brain Information Service/Brain Research Institute, 1968.

75. Israel DN, Ancoli-Israel S: Sleep and rhythms in tenth vs third graders. Sleep 2000;23(Suppl 2): A197.

76. Yang CM, Spielman AJ, Martinez E, et al: The effects of delayed weekend sleep schedule on subjective sleepiness and cognitive functioning. Sleep 1998;21(Suppl):202.

77. Dijk DJ, Duffy JF: Circadian regulation of human sleep and age-related changes in its timing, consolidation and EEG characteristics. Ann Med 1999;31:130-140.

Circadian Rhythm Disorders: Diagnosis and Treatment

9

John H. Herman

Circadian rhythm disorders are characterized by normal sleep quantity and quality at the wrong time, as dictated by societal or familial demands. The circadian pacemaker may be delayed or advanced with respect to the desired hour of sleep, or clock time and circadian time may be out of phase. This may result at least partly from a genetic propensity when a parent suffers from the same symptoms or propensity. The phase delay or advance is typically aggravated by the child being exposed to light at the wrong time and not exposed to light at the right time. The wrong time to be exposed to light is shortly before or during the desired hours of sleep. The right time to be exposed to light is during the desired hours of waking.

Some Consequences

Circadian rhythm disorders are frequently associated with daytime sleepiness. The struggles that occur when a child is unable to fall asleep until an inappropriately late hour may have features in common with sleep onset association disorder or sleep phobia. Children who are sleep deprived secondary to a circadian rhythm disorder frequently have symptoms similar to those of attention deficit hyperactivity disorder (ADHD). Circadian rhythm disorders commonly lead to sleep deprivation during the night and sleepiness during the day at school.

Biologic Clocks and Circadian Rhythms

All individuals possess inherent circadian rhythms of greater or less than 24 hours, with the vast majority longer than 24 hours (Fig. 9–1). Circadian rhythms are entrained to be in phase with environmental time by "zeitgebers," or time cues, mainly light but also including activity

schedules,[1] exercise, and other environmental factors.[2] Circadian rhythms develop during infancy and are robust by 1 year of age.[2] Individuals with circadian rhythm disorders have failed to properly entrain to environmental zeitgebers and are either phase delayed (delayed sleep phase syndrome [DSPS]) or phase advanced (advanced sleep phase syndrome [ASPS]) (Fig. 9–2). Some individuals "free-run" with respect to environmental time, and their hour of sleep moves progressively later or earlier, going in and out of synchrony with the expected hour of sleep (non–24-hour sleep–wake disorder). It is suspected that individuals with longer genetic circadian rhythms might require stronger zeitgebers to remain in phase with environmental time, and this might explain why both heredity and environment are components of circadian rhythm disorders. Also, motivation appears to be a factor, and certain individuals with psychiatric or behavioral symptomatology appear to be more likely to become phase delayed or advanced. It is difficult to parse the genetic, environmental, behavioral, and psychiatric contributions to a child's circadian rhythm disorder.

Forbidden Sleep Zone

The "forbidden sleep zone" immediately precedes the onset of biologic night. This is the time at which sleep is least likely to occur during a circadian cycle.[3] This 1- to 3-hour period is well established in human adults and adolescents. Since the forbidden sleep zone precedes the normal hour of sleep, many adolescents with delayed sleep phase seem unable to advance their hour of sleep despite sleep deprivation and daytime sleepiness. Although forbidden sleep zones have not been studied in children, they appear to be particularly robust, as many children who fall asleep in school

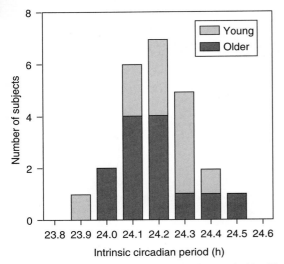

Figure 9–1. Duration of circadian rhythm period in 25 adults who participated in a constant routine protocol designed to reveal the intrinsic period length. Half were younger and half older adults. Note that over 90% of the subjects had period lengths greater than 24 hours. (From Dijk DJ, Duffy JF, Czeisler CA: Contribution of circadian physiology and sleep homeostasis to age-related changes in human sleep. Chronobiol Int 2000;17:285-311.)

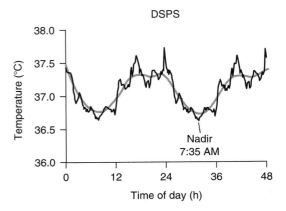

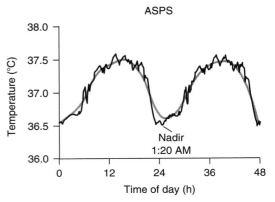

Figure 9–2. Illustrations of the temperature curves of individuals with delayed sleep phase syndrome (DSPS) (temperature nadir for DSPS at 7:35 AM and for advanced sleep phase syndrome [ASPS] at 1:20 AM). The temperature minimum is approximately 5-6 hours after sleep onset in an 8-hour sleeper. From these temperature minimums, a sleep period from 2:00 to 10:00 AM can be predicted for the DSPS illustration and from 8:00 PM to 4:00 AM for the ASPS illustration. The timing of the temperature nadir must be estimated when timing the administration of bright light in treating DSPS or ASPS.

are not able to begin night-time sleep at an earlier hour.

Prevalence

Circadian rhythm disorders appear in at least 10% of children. DSPS alone affects 5 to 10% of adolescents but may appear in children as young as those who are just starting school.[4] ASPS is seen less frequently but also appears at the age of starting school. Non–24-hour circadian rhythm is relatively rare and appears in adolescents. Some evidence suggests that more males than females display DSPS.

Differential Diagnosis

A careful history is essential to distinguish circadian rhythm disorders from other sleep disorders. The hallmark of circadian rhythm disorders is that when the child is permitted to sleep on his or her desired schedule, sleep is normal and daytime sleepiness rapidly subsides. Circadian rhythm disorders should be distinguished from primary insomnia, settling disorders, generalized anxiety disorders, mood disorders, attention deficit disor-

der (ADD)/ADHD, restless legs/periodic limb movements, and obstructive sleep apnea syndrome (Table 9–1). School avoidance/refusal may be confused with DSPS.

DELAYED SLEEP PHASE SYNDROME

DSPS is a disorder in which the major sleep episode is delayed significantly and persistently, typically by 1 or more hours beyond the desired bedtime, in children or adolescents. Bedtime and

Table 9-1. Differential Diagnosis of Delayed Sleep Phase Syndrome (DSPS)

Symptom	DSPS	Primary Insomnia	Settling Disorder	Anxiety	Mood Disorder	ADD/ADHD	RLS/PLMD	OSAS
				Syndrome				
Bedtime struggles	Usual	Unusual but may be seen	Usual unless parent present	Usual, bedtime may be phobia	Usual	Usual	Rare, child typically sleepy	Rare, child typically sleepy
Difficulty initiating sleep	Always, essential for diagnosis	Usual or disrupted sleep	Usual unless parent present	Usual	Usual	Rare, sleep is normal	Usual	Rare
Disrupted sleep at random times	Never	Usual	Usual	Usual	Usual	Rare, sleep is normal	Usual	Usual due to respiratory arousals
Disrupted sleep at fixed times	Never	Rare	Usual	Never	Never	Never	Never, awakenings in first half of night	Never
Sleeping late on weekends	Always	Rare	Rare, frequent naps	Rare, overactive waking system	Usual	Usual	Usual	Usual, sleep rebound
Awakening struggles	Usual	Rare, may follow poor sleep	Rare	Rare, typically compliant child	Usual, wish to isolate	Usual	Rare	Usual, sleep non-refreshing
Excessive daytime sleepiness	Usual	Rare	Rare	Rare	Usual	Rare	Usual	Usual
Complaints of fatigue	Usual	Usual	Rare	Rare	Usual	Rare	Usual	Usual
Attentional/ hyperactivity symptoms	Usual due to sleep loss	Usual due to poor sleep quality	Usual due to poor sleep quality	Rare	Usual due to mood disorder	Always	Usual due to poor sleep quality	Usual due to poor sleep quality

ADD/ADHD attention deficit disorder/attention deficit hyperactivity disorder; OSAS, obstructive sleep apnea syndrome; RLS/PLMD, restless legs syndrome/periodic limb movement disorder.

awakening become issues for them. Children appear to be less tolerant of sleep deprivation than adults, and a 1-hour delay in sleep onset may result in pathologic symptoms.

Presenting Complaints

The presenting complaints are listed below.

- Bedtime struggles or difficulty awakening at the desired time
- Complaints of insomnia at bedtime and/or excessive sleepiness in the morning
- Inability to wake up at the desired time
- Falling asleep at school or being too sleepy in the morning to participate in normal activities
- Symptoms consistent with behavioral dysregulation, ADHD, or depression
- Preferring to not eat breakfast and being hungry at or close to bedtime

Diagnostic Criteria

The criteria below are similar to those described in the *International Classification of Sleep Disorders, Revised: Diagnostic and Coding Manual* and are required for diagnosis.

- The sleep pattern is significantly delayed, typically by more than 1 hour.
- There is an inability to fall asleep at the desired clock time and an inability to awaken spontaneously at the desired time of awakening.
- This sleep pattern has been present for at least one month.
- Normal quality and quantity of sleep are observed when the child can sleep on his or her desired schedule.
- Children with DSPS sleep later on weekends and holidays.
- They report less daytime sleepiness on weekends, when they awaken spontaneously at a later hour.
- No other sleep or psychiatric disorder is present that could explain the patient's symptoms.
- The delayed phase is not the result of social preference or an overloaded school, social activity, or work schedule.

Family Dynamics

In DSPS, both the child and the parents are usually perplexed that he or she cannot fall asleep more quickly. Frequently, family disputes erupt around bedtime and awakening time. Control battles ensue. Parents' efforts to advance the timing of their child's sleep onset by earlier bedtime, extra alarm clocks, relaxation techniques, and sleeping pills are not successful. The hour of sleep and waking become the center of family conflicts. When other behavioral or psychiatric syndromes are present in the child or family members, the child's sleep habits become flashpoints for disputes. Sometimes the family dynamics must be addressed before DSPS in a child can be treated. If the other family members are sleeping to a late hour on non-workdays, the child may have no resources for dealing with DSPS.

Interpersonal Dynamics

Patients with DSPS, especially adolescents, typically are "night owls" or "night people" and say they feel and function best and are more alert during the late evening and night hours. Children with DSPS nap more frequently during school days, complain of daytime sleepiness, have more attention problems, poorer school achievement, and more injuries and are more emotionally upset than the other children.[5] DSPS may become a "lifestyle" in some children whose identities become enmeshed with late-night activities, such as phone calls, Internet interaction, and chat rooms. Late-night children often become close friends. Children who awaken and retire at an earlier hour are viewed with condescension by cliques of night owls. In some instances DSPS becomes ingrained, and the child may pursue a career that involves or permits late-night activity, such as writing, software, or the service or entertainment sector. The earlier in life DSPS is treated, the less resistance is typically encountered.

Coexistence with Psychiatric/Behavioral Symptoms

ADHD, oppositional symptoms, conduct disorder, aggressive symptoms, and symptoms of depression appear frequently in many but not all children with DSPS (see Table 9–1).[6] In some instances DSPS leads to chronic sleep deprivation, which may aggravate underlying psychopathologic tendencies in a child.[7] When psychiatric symptoms and DSPS are present conjointly, it is important to establish whether the psychiatric symptoms are present independent of the DSPS or only occur with it.[8] For example, on weekends or holidays, when the child sleeps until spontaneous awakening, do psychiatric symptoms lessen? If the psychiatric symptoms and DSPS coexist temporarily, it is best to treat the DSPS before addressing the psychiatric symptoms. If the psychiatric symptoms are present regardless of prior sleep, then treating both the psychiatric symptoms and the DSPS concurrently might be warranted.

Age of Onset

DSPS may be encountered in young children. Frequently, a child's late hours of sleep become problematic only with the start of school. Many DSPS patients report that their difficulties began after a summer vacation. After a summer of sleeping late, these children find it impossible to sleep on a normal schedule when school resumes. Adolescence appears to be the most common period of life for the onset of DSPS.

Evaluation

The following factors are considered in the evaluation of children for DSPS.

- Usually have one parent with DSPS symptoms or night owl preference
- Typically accomplish tasks such as homework best at a later hour
- Feel best at or near bedtime
- Experience academic, emotional, and behavioral problems during morning hours
- Must be evaluated for substance abuse
- Should be evaluated for depression, ADHD, school refusal, conduct disorder, oppositional defiant disorder, and anxiety disorders
- In some cases it is necessary for the family to maintain a diary of bedtime, time of sleep onset, and wake-up time for a minimum of two weeks and as long as 1 month to establish a pattern.
- May describe their sleep habits significantly differently from the way their parents portray them
- Tend to cover windows to block out sunlight
- Watch TV or computer monitors near or after the desired bedtime

Singular Significance of Sunday Night

Sunday night bedtime is frequently the major flashpoint for school aged children. Many children with DSPS awaken and retire at a considerably later hour on weekends, effectively "moving" to a more westward time zone. Sunday night the child is expected to return to a weekday schedule (or move east) and finds it impossible. Late-night sleep onset is followed by a battle when the child must awaken for school Monday morning, and the week is off to a bad start, frequently with behavioral, emotional, and familial conflicts followed by disruptive behavior, hyperactivity, distractibility, failure to attend, and learning problems in school.

In adolescents, failure to cooperate with a plan to reschedule their sleep may be a sign of clinical depression or oppositional defiant symptoms. Adolescence is a particularly vulnerable life stage for the development of this syndrome: For some children, adolescence, with increased autonomy and noncompliance, becomes synonymous with DSPS.

TREATMENT OPTIONS FOR DELAYED SLEEP PHASE SYNDROME

The various options for the treatment of DSPS are discussed below. They are also summarized in Table 9–2 along with a summary of additional therapeutic interventions useful in the treatment of other causes of sleep onset insomnia.

Establishing the Patient's Temperature Nadir

The nadir of core body temperature, or the minimum temperature in the circadian cycle, typically occurs about two thirds of the way through the sleep cycle. A child who begins sleep at 9:00 PM and spontaneously awakens at 7:00 AM on weekends typically has a temperature minimum at approximately 3:00 to 4:00 AM. It is crucial to establish the timing of the temperature minimum, also known as the point of singularity, as light administered before the minimum causes a *phase delay,* or results in sleep occurring later, and light administered after the minimum causes a *phase advance,* or results in sleep occurring earlier (see Fig. 9–2). The timing of the temperature nadir may best be established by a careful history of when the child or adolescent prefers to begin sleep and to awaken, which may require keeping a diary. Sometimes the child's preferred hour of sleep onset is as late as 4:00 AM and their preferred hour of awakening is remarkably late, such as 2:00 PM. Such children might have a core body temperature minimum at as late as 11:00 AM. Therefore, exposure to light before 10:00 AM will cause a further phase delay and not the expected phase advance.

Phase Shifting: A Family System Approach

Moving a child's propensity to sleep is called phase advance when shifting to an earlier hour and phase delay when shifting to a later hour. The child and the family first must understand the basic principles behind the child's inability to sleep at a desired time. This may be more difficult than expected when one or more family members believe the problem to be essentially behavioral.

Nevertheless, behavioral issues frequently overlay circadian rhythm disorders. The entire family and the patient must be motivated to undergo the phase shift. Resistance may arise from a variety of areas, as one or more family members may be invested in the child's propensity to sleep late, such as a parent who sleeps until noon on weekends. Expectations must be explored. The family and child must comprehend that this may be a lifelong issue that will affect the child long after he or she leaves the home of origin. This may be the first time that someone has said to the child, "After you are grown up and no longer live with your parents, this may continue to be an issue that you will have to cope with on your own."

The child must be encouraged to "own" the problem, or take responsibility for it. The parents must be convinced that the root of the problem is not intentional defiance. Children should be encouraged to set their own alarms and wake up on their own. Parents must recognize that the less involved they are with their child's awakening, the more the child may assume responsibility.

Sleep Hygiene

The treatment of DSPS must begin with ensuring good sleep hygiene if manipulations with light and melatonin are to be effective. Instructions for good sleep hygiene include the following:

- Sleep only when sleepy. If a child is not sleepy, reading in bed with a dim light might be an option for some families. This reduces the time the child is struggling with initiating sleep.
- If the child can't fall asleep within 20 minutes, allow him or her to do something boring until the child feels sleepy. The child should not be exposed to bright light after bedtime.

- Minimize the child's naps. This will optimize the probability that the child will be tired at bedtime. If the child requires a nap, allow less than 1 hour of sleep, before 3:00 PM if possible. Lights should remain on during naps.
- The child must adhere to approximately the same wake-up time and bedtime 7 days a week. Other children might be able to sleep late on weekends and still fall asleep earlier on Sunday night, but the hallmark of children with DSPS is that they can't. Children with the same wake-up time every morning will be more stable emotionally and less oppositional in the morning than children who sleep late on weekends.
- A quiet time with minimal light and less activity should precede bedtime. Television and computer monitors should be avoided. Maximizing active playing and exercise is recommended to help you sleep well, but the timing of the workout is important. Exercising in the morning or early afternoon will not interfere with sleep.
- Every child deserves a consistent bedtime. As much as a child might protest, a set bedtime, similar to a home-cooked meal, is appreciated by the child as a basic component of good parenting.
- Develop sleep rituals for your child. Children's sleep is enhanced by rituals, such as reading stories, quiet games, a drink, or just chatting. Having a set time for bathing and getting into pajamas helps a child prepare for sleep. It is important to give your child cues that it is time to slow down and prepare for sleep.
- Allow your child to use his or her bed only for sleeping. Refrain from permitting your child to use the bed to watch TV, do homework, or use the computer. The child then knows that when it is time to go to bed, it is time to sleep.
- Avoid all foods or beverages with caffeine after lunch. This includes chocolate and many beverages with caffeine as an additive. Coffee, tea, cola, cocoa, chocolate, and some prescription and nonprescription drugs contain caffeine.
- Some children benefit from a light snack before bed. For these children, if their stomachs are too empty, it can interfere with sleep. However, if your child eats a heavy meal before bedtime, this can interfere as well. Dairy products and turkey contain tryptophan, which acts as a natural sleep inducer. A warm glass of milk is sometimes recommended probably because of its tryptophan content.

- Give your child a hot bath 90 minutes before bedtime. A hot bath will raise your body temperature, but it is the drop in body temperature that may leave you feeling sleepy.
- Make sure your child's bed and bedroom are quiet and comfortable. A hot room can be uncomfortable. A cooler room along with enough blankets to stay warm is recommended. Too many blankets can overheat a child even in a cold room.
- Use sunlight to set your child's biologic clock. As soon as your child gets up in the morning, have him or her play in sunlight, preferably outside.

Bright-Light Therapy

Bright-light therapy should include control of light and dark exposures across the whole day. The following list of therapeutic components illustrates this point.

- The patient with DSPS should use bright-light exposure early in the morning and avoid light after the hour of sunset as much as possible.[9] The light of dawn is extremely important in entraining circadian rhythms[10] in children as well as adults.[11] Such control of light exposure should produce a phase advance. One to 2 hours outdoors or indoors in early morning direct sunlight or (if rising before sunrise in the early morning) in front of a light box that emits 2500 lux will usually produce a phase advance in a few days.
- Parents and patient are encouraged to remove coverings from windows and to place the child's bed where the most direct sunlight will be present.
- Children are encouraged not to cover their heads with blankets and to face the light when sleeping.
- If possible, parents are encouraged to move their child to a bedroom facing east or south, with morning-light exposure.
- Avoid light after sunset as much as possible, as even ordinary indoor light may affect a child's circadian rhythm.[12]
- Bright light is more effective when it is experienced in conjunction with active play or exercise.[13]

Bright-Light Box

If a family is considering purchasing a bright-light box, encourage them to go to one of several web sites that show illustrations of products. Frequently, a portable unit that can be placed next to the child as he or she goes through morning routines, does homework, reads, or is next to a video monitor is preferable. Instructions for each unit must be followed to allow the correct amount of light exposure, as light intensity decreases as a function of the square of the distance. The child should not look directly at the light. If he or she has an adverse reaction to the light box, increase the distance. Some children become irritable or exhibit other symptoms of hypomania when exposed to bright morning light. In such cases, light exposure should be stopped or the duration decreased until hypomanic symptoms subside.

Melatonin

Melatonin has been shown to be effective as a hypnotic in children,[14,15] but there is more evidence that it is effective in altering sleep phase.[16] Various studies show it to be effective in the treatment of DSPS.[17] It is a hormone secreted by the pineal gland associated with body temperature drop and lowered metabolism. Melatonin administered 1 hour before the desired time of sleep onset will advance the timing of sleep if given in conjunction with the blocking of light exposure.[18] Many adolescents may be insufficiently motivated to expose themselves to early morning sunlight or a bright-light box but may be willing to take melatonin. Ideally, melatonin before the hour of sleep is administered in conjunction with early morning bright light. A physiologic level of melatonin is achieved with a dose of less than 1 mg. In children, it is best to begin with 1 mg and proceed to 3 mg if this is ineffective. Melatonin may be administered for a few weeks during phase shifting and reintroduced if phase delay symptoms recur.

Advancing Bedtime

Along with the administration of morning light and/or evening melatonin, bedtime is typically advanced 15 minutes per day, as is the time of melatonin administration. If the child has difficulty falling asleep on a given night, bedtime should not be further advanced until sleep onset is less than 30 minutes after bedtime.

Chronotherapy

Chronotherapy is a behavioral technique that systematically delays bedtime, following the

Table 9–2.   Various Therapeutic Interventions for Syndromes Presenting with Sleep Onset Insomnia

Treatment	DSPS	Primary Insomnia	Settling Disorder	Anxiety	Mood Disorder	ADD/ADHD	RLS/PLMD	OSAS
Behavioral interventions	Always employed	May be helpful	Always employed	Helpful	Helpful	Helpful	Rarely helpful	Never
Relaxation techniques	May be helpful as secondary treatment	Helpful	Rarely helpful	Helpful	May be helpful	May be helpful as secondary treatment	Rarely helpful	Rarely helpful
Morning bright-light treatment	First-line treatment along with PM darkness	Rarely helpful	Rarely helpful	Rarely helpful	May be helpful, especially SADS	If DSPS, may be helpful	Rarely helpful	Never
More structured bedtime and awakening time	Always	Helpful	Always employed	May be helpful, especially routines	May be helpful, especially routines	May be helpful, especially routines	Never, awakenings typically occur in first half of night	Rarely helpful
Melatonin	Helpful	May be helpful	Rarely helpful	Rarely helpful	Rarely helpful	Rarely helpful	Rarely helpful	Rarely helpful, always treat OSA first
Hypnotics	Never	May be helpful	Never	Rarely helpful	Rarely helpful	Never	May be helpful	Never
SSRIs	Never	Never	Never	May be helpful	Helpful	Rarely helpful	Never	Never
5-HT-2A antagonists	Never	Rarely helpful	Never	May be helpful	May be helpful	Rarely helpful	May be helpful	Rarely helpful, always treat OSA first
Stimulants	Never	Never	Never	Never	Never	Helpful only if true ADHD	Never	Rarely helpful, always treat OSA first
Psychotherapy	Rarely helpful	Helpful	May be helpful	Helpful	Helpful	May be helpful	Never	Never

ADD/ADHD attention deficit disorder/attention deficit hyperactivity disorder; DSPS, delayed sleep phase syndrome; 5-HT, serotonin; OSAS, obstructive sleep apnea syndrome; RLS/PLMS, restless legs syndrome/periodic limb movement disorder; SADS, seasonal affective disorder syndrome; SSRIs, selective serotonin reuptake inhibitors.

natural tendency of human biology. Bedtime is delayed by 3-hour increments each day, establishing a 27-hour day. The procedure is maintained until the desired bedtime is reached (e.g., 9:00 PM), at which point the child is properly entrained. This approach is favored by adolescents who are extreme night owls and who therefore are delighted at the concept of a later bedtime and wake-up time. It is difficult to administer, as a parent typically must be present to oversee the temporarily unusual sleep and wake-up times, such as 12:00 noon to 8:00 PM. However, schedule normalization takes no more than a week.

Successful Phase Advance Therapy

The first sign that the light and/or melatonin are having their desired effect is an earlier hour of sleep onset and fewer struggles with morning awakening. This is often followed by a report from the parents that the child's morning appetite has increased.

Maintenance Phase

Once the desired sleep schedule is attained, the next problem is its maintenance. When adolescents with DSPS stay up late studying, socializing, or engaging in other activities, it is probable that they will be drawn back to sleeping late. A strategy must be determined in advance for counteracting this tendency. Frequently, the adolescent agrees that he or she may remain awake late at times but must arise and be in sunlight relatively early. Parents need to be vigilant that weekends, school holidays, or summer vacations do not result in a return of phase delay.

ADVANCED SLEEP PHASE SYNDROME

ASPS is a disorder in which the major sleep episode is advanced in relation to the desired clock time, which results in symptoms of compelling evening sleepiness, an early sleep onset, and an awakening that is earlier than that desired.

The following indications show the symptomatology of ASPS.

- Inability to stay awake until the desired bedtime or inability to remain asleep until the desired time of awakening. Children and ado-

lescents with ASPS fall asleep doing homework, at social events, immediately after dinner, or before dinner if it is at a late hour.
- Symptoms are present for at least 3 months.
- When not required to remain awake until the later bedtime, patients will have a habitual sleep period that is of normal quality and duration; with a sleep onset earlier than that desired, they will awaken spontaneously earlier than desired, and they will maintain stable entrainment to a 24-hour sleep–wake pattern.

The major complaint may concern the inability to stay awake in the evening, early morning insomnia, or both.

Unlike other sleep maintenance disorders, the early morning awakening occurs after undisturbed sleep. Unlike other causes of excessive sleepiness, daytime school or activities early in the day are not affected by sleepiness. This problem becomes apparent in children and adolescents when social and academic activities stretch into the evening hours. The evening activities are cut short by the need to retire much earlier than the social norm.

Typical sleep onset times are as early as 5:00 to 6:00 PM but no later than 8:00 PM, and wake-up times can be as early as 1:00 to 3:00 AM but no later than 5:00 AM. These sleep onset and wake-up times occur despite the family's best efforts to delay sleep to later hours.

There can be negative personal or social consequences to children and adolescents when their peers are engaged in evening activities and the patient avoids them due to early sleep. Frequently, this interferes with family functions such as going out for dinner.

Attempts to delay sleep onset to a later time may result in embarrassment due to falling asleep during social gatherings.

If a child or adolescent with ASPS is continually forced to stay up later for social or vocational reasons, the early awakening aspect of the syndrome could lead to chronic sleep deprivation, daytime sleepiness, or napping.

Epidemiology

ASPS is more likely to appear in children who have one parent or grandparent with ASPS tendencies, which may not be sufficiently severe to be syndromic. Similar to narcolepsy, the gene and gene product responsible for ASPS have been identified.[19]

Differential Diagnosis

ASPS should be differentiated from other disorders producing early evening sleepiness, such as obstructive sleep apnea, disrupted nocturnal sleep, chronic sleep deprivation, and narcolepsy. Sometimes the early morning awakening is mistakenly thought to be indicative of depressive illness. Like DSPS patients, ASPS patients have no intrinsic sleep abnormalities; they report that sleep itself is restful and restorative.

Treatment

ASPS is treated with chronotherapy or bright-light therapy. Chronotherapy would involve a systematic delay of bedtime until the desired time is achieved. Bright-light therapy would involve inducing a phase delay, with the light exposure in the early evening. There are limited data about the effectiveness of bright-light therapy for ASPS.

NON–24-HOUR SLEEP–WAKE DISORDER

This condition can occur when the intrinsic period of the circadian pacemaker free-runs with respect to the 24-hour day. Alternatively, children's and adolescents' self-selected exposure to artificial light may drive the circadian pacemaker to a schedule longer than 24 hours. Affected children are not able to maintain a stable phase relationship with the 24-hour day. Parents initially report that their child's sleep behavior is completely random and has no pattern. Only by maintaining a sleep log for 2 to 6 weeks is it possible to "smooth out" aberrations and estimate the circadian periodicity. These children are then typically revealed to have an incremental pattern of successive delays in sleep onsets and wake times (free-running), progressing in and out of phase with local time. When the child's endogenous rhythm is out of phase with the family and school, both insomnia and excessive daytime sleepiness are present. Conversely, when the child's endogenous rhythm is in phase with home and school, symptoms remit. The intervals between symptomatic periods may last several weeks to several months. Blind individuals unable to perceive any light are particularly susceptible to this disorder.

Treatment

Melatonin administration has been reported to improve the timing of sleep in non–24-hour sleep–wake disorder, especially in the blind. Begin at 3 mg 1 hour before the desired hour of sleep onset. Once a patient is entrained, melatonin may be lowered to 1 mg. The patient should be in as much light and as active as possible during the intended wake period and in conditions of dark, quiet, and bedrest during the intended sleep period. In nonblind individuals, exposure to the light of dawn or a bright-light box at the time of dawn may be essential to maintain entrainment.

CONCLUSIONS

Circadian rhythm disorders are fairly common in children and frequently masquerade as other sleep disorders, most notably insomnia and daytime sleepiness. Many children have been evaluated extensively from a medical perspective before they are referred to a sleep specialist. For the most part, an in-depth interview including the child and caretakers is sufficient to establish the diagnosis of circadian rhythm disorder. In many cases a 1-week to 1-month diary is essential to make the diagnosis, especially when the family describes the child's sleep as "chaotic" and not following any pattern. In almost every case, a sleep diary that is collected over a sufficient period of time will reveal an underlying pattern of when sleep occurs.

Frequently, a second disorder coexists along with the circadian rhythm disorder, such as depression, an anxiety disorder, obstructive sleep apnea, or restless legs syndrome/periodic limb movement disorders. In some instances polysomnography is required to establish the severity of a coexisting disorder, and it should be treated before the circadian rhythm disorder can be addressed. Treating obstructive sleep apnea first, for example, will make it much easier for a child to comply with changing his or her sleep schedule. In some instances, for example in a child with a psychiatric disorder, correcting the circadian rhythm disorder can alleviate symptoms of depression or anxiety. To cite another example, it is well known that early morning bright light has an antidepressant effect in some individuals. Children with phase delay syndrome and anxiety symptoms frequently become very anxious about their inability to initiate sleep. The correction of DSPS may exert an anxiolytic effect in such children.

Discussions with children and their families about circadian rhythm disorders are frequently profound, as the sleep disorder specialist informs the child about symptoms that may continue throughout his or her life and offers suggestions for treatment strategies to address them. It is extremely rewarding when diagnosing and treating a circadian rhythm disorder in a child with only bright-light therapy and sometimes melatonin results in an enormous improvement in the child's quality of life.

References

1. Klerman EB, Rimmer DW, Dijk DJ, et al: Nonphotic entrainment of the human circadian pacemaker. Am J Physiol 1998;274:R991-R996.
2. Rivkees SA: Mechanisms and clinical significance of circadian rhythms in children. Curr Opin Pediatr 2001;13:352-357.
3. Lavie P: Ultrashort sleep-waking schedule: III. 'Gates' and 'forbidden zones' for sleep. Electroencephalogr Clin Neurophysiol 1986; 63: 414-425.
4. Mindell JA, Owens JA: A Clinical Guide to Pediatric Sleep: Diagnosis and Management of Sleep Problems. Philadelphia, Lippincott, Williams & Williams, 2003.
5. Giannotti F, Cortesi F, Sebastiani T, Ottaviano S: Circadian preference, sleep and daytime behaviour in adolescence. J Sleep Res 2002;11:191-199.
6. Cardinali DP: The human body circadian: How the biologic clock influences sleep and emotion. Neuroendocrinol Lett 2000;21:9-15.
7. Dahl RE, Lewin DS: Pathways to adolescent health sleep regulation and behavior. J Adolesc Health 2002;31(Suppl 6):175-184.
8. Kayumov L, Zhdanova IV, Shapiro CM: Melatonin, sleep, and circadian rhythm disorders. Semin Clin Neuropsychiatry 2000;5:44-55.
9. Lafrance C, Dumont M, Lesperance P, Lambert C: Daytime vigilance after morning bright light exposure in volunteers subjected to sleep restriction. Physiol Behav 1998;63:803-810.
10. Danilenko KV, Wirz-Justice A, Krauchi K, et al: The human circadian pacemaker can see by the dawn's early light. J Biol Rhythms 2000;15:437-446.
11. Clodore M, Foret J, Benoit O, et al: Psychophysiological effects of early morning bright light exposure in young adults. Psychoneuroendocrinology 1990;15:193-205.
12. Boivin DB, Czeisler CA: Resetting of circadian melatonin and cortisol rhythms in humans by ordinary room light. Neuroreport 1998;9:779-782.
13. Baehr EK, Fogg LF, Eastman CI: Intermittent bright light and exercise to entrain human circadian rhythms to night work. Am J Physiol 1999;277:R1598-R1604.
14. Ivanenko A, Crabtree VM, Tauman R, Gozal D: Melatonin in children and adolescents with insomnia: A retrospective study. Clin Pediatr (Phila) 2003;42:51-58.
15. Pires M, Benedito-Silva A, Pinto L, et al: Acute effects of low doses of melatonin on the sleep of young healthy subjects. J Pineal Res 2001;31:326-332.
16. Sack RL, Lewy AJ, Hughes RJ: Use of melatonin for sleep and circadian rhythm disorders. Ann Med 1998;30:115-121.
17. Dagan Y, Yovel I, Hallis D, et al: Evaluating the role of melatonin in the long-term treatment of delayed sleep phase syndrome (DSPS). Chronobiol Int 1998;15:181-190.
18. Garcia J, Rosen G, Mahowald M: Circadian rhythms and circadian rhythm disorders in children and adolescents. Semin Pediatr Neurol 2001;8:229-240.
19. Reid KJ, Chang AM, Dubocovich ML, et al: Familial advanced sleep phase syndrome. Arch Neurol 2001;58:1089-1094.

S

Sleep and Colic

Marc Weissbluth

10

The hypothesis that colic might be a sleep disorder caused by developmental or biologic factors within the child[1] was based on the natural history of colic and links between colic, sleeping problems, and difficult temperament.[2,3] Only retrospectively obtained data obtained from parents' reports supported the hypothesis.[4] It was also suggested that "postcolic" sleep problems occur after 3 or 4 months of age because some parents experienced difficulty in establishing age-appropriate sleep routines.[1] Recent research utilizing more objective measures has provided prospectively obtained data associating colic with sleep problems.

NATURAL HISTORY OF COLIC

Wessel and coworkers[5] diagnosed as colicky an infant "who, otherwise healthy and well-fed, had paroxysms of irritability, fussing or crying lasting for a total of more than 3 hours a day and occurring on more than 3 days in any 1 week . . . and . . . the paroxysms continued to recur for more than 3 weeks." The criterion "more than 3 weeks" was added because nannies left families after about 3 weeks of crying. He thought that nannies knew that if babies cried for more than 3 weeks, then the crying would continue. The mothers, now alone caring for their babies at night, came to his pediatric office after 3 weeks complaining that their children were always crying (M. A. Wessel, personal communication, 2002). About 26% of infants in their study had colic. Illingworth[6] defined colic as "violent rhythmical, screaming attacks which did not stop when the infants were picked up, and for which no cause, such as underfeeding, could be found." Together, they studied about 150 infants.

The *age of onset* of these behaviors is characteristic. Wessel and colleagues and Illingworth found that the attacks were absent during the first few days but were present in 80% of affected infants by 2 weeks and about 100% by 3 weeks. The attacks begin in premature babies shortly after the expected due date, regardless of their gestational age at birth. The *time of day* when these behaviors occur is another characteristic. During the first month, crying appears to occur randomly, but later it occurs predominantly in the evening hours. In 80% of infants, the attacks start between 5 and 8 PM and end by 12 PM. For 12% of infants, the attacks start between 7 and 10 PM and end by 2 AM. In only 8% are the attacks randomly distributed throughout the day and night. The *age of termination* of these spells is also characteristic. They disappear by 2 months of age in 50% of infants, by 2-3 months of age in 30%, and by 3-4 months of age in 10%. Using Wessel's criteria, the infant's *behavioral state* was observed to be associated with colicky behavior.[2] In 84% of colicky infants, the crying spells begin when they are awake, in 8% they start when asleep, and in 8% they occur under variable conditions. When the crying spell ends, 83% of the infants fall asleep.

As there are other definitions of colic, data from different studies may not be comparable. Some studies claim to use Wessel's criteria but exclude "fussing" or exclude the criterion of "more than 3 weeks." The problem with excluding the 3-week criterion is that an extremely high prevalence rate may result. For example, in Wessel's study, 49% of infants would have been diagnosed with colic without that criterion. Reijneveld and coworkers[7] showed that even small differences between definitions of colic based on the duration of crying result in large changes in prevalence rates, and they concluded that different definitions of colic could not be compared because they mostly identified different infants. Their study excluded "fussing" from the definition of colic, but they recommended that future studies should define colic using the duration of both crying and fussing, plus the amount of parental distress. This is an important point, because it is now known that fussing, as opposed to crying, is a major part of colicky behavior,[8] and parental distress over colic may be a major factor in producing postcolic sleep problems.[9] Because of this concern of comparability, this chapter includes the definitions of colic utilized by different researchers.

Studies of colic are also difficult to compare because they have been performed at different ages. Finally, small sample sizes and modest group differences have led researchers to different interpretations of the clinical significance of data from a single study.

ETIOLOGY

A recent study showed that colicky infants, defined as crying or fussing for at least 3 hours per day for a minimum of 3 days per week, had higher urinary levels of 5-hydroxy indoleacetic acid, a metabolite of serotonin.[10] This supported the hypothesis that some temporal and behavioral features of colic might be caused by a serotonin–melatonin counterbalancing system involving the gastrointestinal smooth muscles.[11] Concentrations of serotonin are high in infants during the first month of life, and after 3 months they decline. Immediately after delivery, concentrations of serotonin show a circadian rhythm with highest levels at night. Melatonin is derived transplacentally from the mother; concentrations are high in infants immediately after birth, they fall rapidly to extremely low levels within several days, they increase slightly between 1 and 3 months, and only after 3 months is there an abrupt increase in melatonin concentrations, with a circadian rhythm that demonstrates higher concentrations at night.

Serotonin and melatonin have opposite effects on intestinal smooth muscle: serotonin causes contraction and melatonin causes relaxation. Animal studies show that serotonin potency causing intestinal smooth muscle contraction is much greater in the neonatal period than at older ages. It was hypothesized that in some infants, the balance between circulating serotonin concentrations and intestinal smooth muscle sensitivity to serotonin might lead to painful gastrointestinal cramps in the evening when serotonin concentrations are highest. The high nocturnal melatonin concentration antagonizes the contraction induced by serotonin on intestinal smooth muscle.

Alternatively, independent of the action of melatonin and serotonin on intestinal smooth muscle, their effects might be mediated by the developing central nervous system. For example, the occurrence of pineal melatonin rhythmicity is coincident with consolidation of night sleep.

In a study that defined colic as fussing or crying for 3 or more hours on each of 3 successive days, it was observed that colicky infants had a blunted rhythm in cortisol production compared with control infants.[12] The control infants exhibited a clear and marked daily rhythm in cortisol that was not observed in the colicky infants. However, the level of cortisol production averaged over the day was similar for both groups. Additionally, researchers in this study (who were blind to the colic status) coded behavioral measures from videotapes and arrived at the same conclusion as many other studies: the crying of these infants was not caused by differences in handling by the mother, and the colic was not simply a maternal perception.

Maternal smoking was evaluated as a cause in one study, where colic was defined as more than 3 hours of crying per day for more than 3 days a week or more than 1.5 hours of crying per day in 6 of 7 days. Maternal smoking occurred twice as often among infants with colic.[13] In contrast, food hypersensitivity has not been linked to infantile colic.[14]

CRYING

Some degree of irritability, fussing, or crying is universal; crying for "unknown reasons" occurs in all babies.[15] Brazelton[16] reported that the median duration of crying was 1.75 hours during the second week, with a gradual increase to 2.75 hours at 6 weeks, followed by a decrease in crying thereafter to 1 hour or less by 12 weeks of age. The fussiest infants, whom he called "colicky," cried 2 to 4 hours per day every day, and their crying also increased between 6 and 8 weeks of age. The distress experienced by parents over their inability to deal with this crying cannot be overstated. Recent data have shown infant homicides to increase after the second week and to peak at the eighth week, and Paulozzi and Sells[17] concluded that the "peak in risk in week 8 might reflect the peak in the daily duration of crying among normal infants between weeks 6 and 8."

In studies of crying in infants, there are no clear discontinuities in measurements of irritability, fussing, or crying, whether by direct observation in hospital nurseries, by voice-activated tape recordings in homes, or by parent diaries. Thus, colic appears to represent an extreme amount of normally occurring and unexplained crying or fussing present in all healthy babies.

Because the spells of irritability, fussing, or crying are universal, differing only in degree between infants, because the occurrence of spells is related to postconceptual age and independent of parenting practices, and because the behaviors exhibit state specificity and a circadian rhythm, it is reasonable to think that these behaviors reflect normal physiologic processes. An example is the normal physiologic processes involving the development of arousal–inhibitory or wake–sleep control mechanisms. In all babies, the consolidation of night sleep develops during the second month (when the peak of crying occurs), and this periodic alternation of sleep and wake states is well developed by 3 to 4 months of age (when colic ends).

FUSSING

Recent research has shown that persistent low-intensity fussing, rather than intense crying, characterizes infants diagnosed as having colic.[8] In fact, the title of Wessel's paper[5] was "Paroxysmal fussing in infants, sometimes called 'colic.' " Fussing is not a well-defined behavior, and although not defined in Wessel's paper, it is usually described as an unsettled, agitated, wakeful state that would lead to crying if ignored by parents. Because sucking is soothing to infants, some parents misattribute the fussing state to hunger and vigorously attempt to feed their baby. These parents may misinterpret their infants as having a growth spurt at 6 weeks because they appeared to be hungry all the time, especially in the evening. They do not view their child as fussy. Even if the time spent feeding their infants at night to prevent crying is more

than 3 additional hours a day, on more than 3 days a week, for more than 3 weeks, parents do not view them as colicky because there is a paucity of crying. Over a 34-month period, at newborn visits, I routinely questioned every new parent who joined my general pediatric practice whether their child fulfilled Wessel's exact diagnostic criteria for colic. All families had been followed since the child's birth and received counseling regarding the normal development of crying or fussing. There were 118 colicky infants out of 747 (16%). However, the vast majority of infants had little or no crying. Instead, they fulfilled Wessel's criteria because they had long and frequent bouts of fussing, which did not lead to crying because of intensive parental intervention.

In one study, fussing was defined by "Your baby is unsettled, irritable, or fractious and may be vocalizing but not continuously crying" and crying was defined as "periods of prolonged distressed vocalizations" (see p. 2530 of St. James-Roberts and Plewis[8]). This study is noteworthy because it supports previous research that showed that between 2 to 6 weeks, there is predominately an increase in fussing, not crying. Furthermore, fussing and sleeping, but notably, not crying, were found to be stable individual characteristics from 6 weeks to 9 months of age. The amount of crying during the first 3 months did not predict crying behavior at 9 months. More pointedly, and in agreement with another study,[9] "high amounts of early crying do not make it highly probable that an infant will . . . have sleeping problems at 9 months of age" (see p. 2538 of St. James-Roberts and Plewis[8]).

COLIC AND SLEEP

Kirjavainen and associates[18] made the diagnosis of colic if infants exhibited "intensive crying (despite consoling efforts) for 3 hours or more a day, on 3 or more days a week" and were otherwise healthy and thriving. Parents kept a daily diary, and night-time sleep onset was defined as the time when the first 15-minute episode occurred after 9 PM. Sleep recordings were performed only at night between 9 PM and 7 AM. At about 4.5 weeks, the total sleep time from the diary was significantly shorter in the colic group (12.7 versus 14.5 hours/day, $P < .001$). Although colicky infants slept less than the control group throughout the 24-hour record, the most dramatic decrease in sleep between the groups occurred at night between 6 PM and 6 AM. The diary data showed that by *6 months* of age, the colicky infants slept slightly less than the noncolicky infants, but the group differences were not significant. The first polygraph recording was performed when the infants were about *9 weeks* old. There were no differences between the groups in the night recordings in sleep characteristics. A subgroup analysis was performed on 11 colicky infants whose diary data were closest to the polygraph data, to take into account the delay between the diaries and the recordings. In this older subgroup of colicky infants, the total sleep time was increased (from 12.7 to 13.2 hours/day). The second polygraphic recordings were performed at about *30 weeks* of age, and again there were no differences in sleep characteristics between the infants formerly with and without colic. Also, at this age, the formerly colicky infants had fewer nocturnal arousals.

This study by Kirjavainen and associates[18] of 15 colicky infants showed clearly that among infants with colic, parent diary data showed shorter total sleep times compared with the age-matched control group at *4.5 weeks,* but that by *9 weeks,* there were no group differences in polygraphic data obtained during the night. Also, this report suggests that over time, between the ages of 5 and 9 weeks, sleep duration in colicky infants increases. On the basis of only the polygraphic data, the authors concluded that infantile colic was not associated with a sleep disorder.

The enormous day-to-day variability in infant colicky behavior noted in this study (J. Kirjavainen, personal communication, 2002) has been noted in another study.[2] This variability makes it difficult to interpret the results derived from a single night-time polygraphic study. In addition, every child, including Kirjavainen's son, had poorer sleep quality (more awakenings, shorter sleep duration) in the laboratory than at home. The day-to-day variability and a laboratory effect may have masked group differences.

St. James-Roberts and colleagues used the term *persistent criers* to describe colicky infants, because their amount of fussing or crying exceeded 3 hours per day most days in a week, and the term *moderate criers* for those who usu-

ally fussed or cried for 30 minutes or less per 6 hour period of the day.[19] Utilizing diaries that had been validated with concurrent 24-hour audio recordings, the colicky infants, at *6 weeks* of age, slept significantly less than noncolicky infants (12.5 versus 13.8 hours/day). There were no group differences regarding time spent awake or time spent feeding. Colicky infants slept less throughout the 24-hour diary record. Unlike other studies,[12,18] the clearest group differences for sleep were in the daytime. In fact, there were no significant group differences regarding sleep at night (between midnight and 6:00 AM). Additionally, at night, there were no statistically significant group differences for crying or fussing behavior. The clearest group differences for crying or fussing behavior were in the daytime. The groups were similar in the timing and duration of the infant's longest sleep period. This analysis of sleep cycle maturation led to the conclusion that the "chief difference between them lies in amounts of daytime fuss/crying and sleeping, rather than in the diurnal organization of sleep and waking behavior" (from p. 148 of St. James-Roberts et al.[19]). Additionally, at *6 weeks* of age, substantial negative correlations between amounts of fuss/crying and sleeping were observed in both groups. Because the authors observed no deficit in wakefulness, only sleeping, they felt that there was a specific trade-off between fussing or crying and sleep, "rather than a more global disturbance of infant behavioral states" (from p. 150 of St. James-Roberts et al.[19]). The researchers concluded that persistent crying is associated with a sleep deficit.

Utilizing sensors embedded within a mattress to continuously monitor body movements and respiratory patterns, a prospective study of 20 colicky infants, who cried an average of at least 2.5 hours per day, showed that at 7 and *13 weeks* of age, they slept less than control infants. The colicky infants had more difficulty falling asleep, were more easily disturbed, and had less quiet, deep sleep.[20]

At about *8 weeks* of age, utilizing diary data previously validated by audio taping, infants were diagnosed with colic if they had fussing or crying for 3 hours or more on each of 3 days during a 3-day study.[12] Per 24 hours, the colicky infants slept significantly less (11.8 versus 14.0 hours per day). The colicky infants slept less during the day, evening, and night; however, the difference in sleeping between the colicky infants was significant only during the night-time. Crying and sleeping showed a significant negative correlation in the colicky infants but not in the control infants. White and colleagues[12] concluded that colic might be associated with a disruption or delay in the establishment of the circadian rhythm of sleep–wake activity. At *4 months* of age, a prospective study showed that the mean total sleep duration, based on parental reports, of 48 infants who had had colic, based on Wessel's exact definition, was 13.9 ± 2.2 hours.[2]

In my general pediatric practice, where at every visit all parents receive anticipatory advice regarding sleep hygiene, the parents of colicky infants describe the development of early bed-times, self-soothing at night-time sleep onset, longer night sleep periods, fewer night awaken-ings, and regular, longer naps later than the par-ents of noncolicky infants describe them. This suggests that colic may be associated with a delay in maturation of sleep–wake control mech-anisms. However, the data show that by *6, 8,* and *12 months,* there are no significant differences between colicky and control groups regarding duration of night sleep,[18,21] although night wak-ing has been reported to be more common at *4, 8,* and *12 months* in infants who previously had colic.[4,21] This might be interpreted as a slightly delayed maturation of normal nocturnal sleep duration coupled with a more persistent impair-ment of the learned ability to return to sleep unassisted during a naturally occurring noctur-nal arousal from sleep.

COLIC AND WAKEFULNESS

Parents of colicky infants often report that day-time sleep periods are extremely irregular and brief. Also, some parents of colicky infants describe a dramatic increase in daytime wakeful-ness and sometimes a temporary but complete cessation of napping when their infants approached their peak fussiness at age 6 weeks. It has been suggested that, before 3 to 4 months of age, the period of inconsolability in the evening hours (when the infant cries and cannot sleep) might reflect periods of high arousal sim-ilar to the circadian forbidden zone (from p. 77 of Weissbluth[22]). In adults, the forbidden zone is a period during which sleep onset and prolonged

consolidated and restorative sleep states do not easily occur. In this context, it might be more appropriate to describe colic not as a disorder of impaired sleep but as a disorder of excessive wakefulness in the evening. This view is sup-ported by recent polygraph investigations show-ing that in infants, a circadian forbidden zone does exist between 5 PM and 8 PM.[23]

COLIC AND TEMPERAMENT

Studies evaluating colic and temperament are difficult to compare because of different ages of infants studied, small sample sizes (often with null findings), small but statistically significant group differences, different temperament-assess-ment instruments, comparisons between tem-perament ratings and global impressions of temperament, and possible measurement bias resulting from reliance on parental reports for both crying and temperament.

Temperament characteristics of mood, inten-sity, adaptability, and approach/withdrawal ten-dency are statistically related, and infants who were described as negative in mood, intense, slowly adaptable, and withdrawing were diag-nosed as having difficult temperaments because they were difficult for parents to manage. These infants were also observed to be irregular in all bodily functions. When parents performed a temperament assessment at *2 weeks* of age and a 24-hour behavior diary at *6 weeks* of age, it was observed that more difficult temperaments at 2 weeks predicted an increased frequency and duration of crying and fussing at 6 weeks.[24] Although statistically significant, the author thought it was a weak association and concluded that "early infant temperament predisposes to early crying and fussing but is of limited use as a clinical predictor"(from p. 514 of Barr[24]). However, recent research utilizing a more com-prehensive assessment of infant temperament found the association between early infant tem-perament and later infant crying to be more robust. At *4 weeks* of age, infants who were more difficult in general, more intense, and less dis-tractible (consolable) cried more during their *second month* of life than other infants.[25]

Another prospective study of infants defined colic as paroxysmal crying that is difficult to console and lasts for 3 or more hours a day dur-ing 3 or more days a week.[21] Temperament assessments were done at the ages of 3 and 12 months. At 3 months, the colicky infants were more intense, less persistent, less distractible, and more negative in their mood. However, at 12 months, ratings on the temperament questionnaire showed no group differences between the colicky infants and the control group, but the general impression of the mothers of the colicky group was that they were more difficult (23% versus 5%).

Infants who had colic, using Wessel's criteria, are significantly more likely to have a difficult temperament than noncolicky babies when the temperament assessment is performed at 4 months of age.[2] Furthermore, this progression occurs even when colic is successfully treated with dicyclomine hydrochloride,[2] an atropinic drug that may act centrally in the nervous system to relax gastrointestinal smooth muscle. Similar results were observed in babies who cried more than 3 hours per day: when behavioral management significantly reduced evening fussing and crying, this successful treatment had no effect on temperament ratings, and the infants were still described by their parents as difficult.[26] These results suggest that congenital factors, not colic-induced parental distress or fatigue, cause increased crying or fussing behavior during the first 3 to 4 months and subsequently lead to an assessment of difficult temperament at age 3 to 4 months.

Colic does not appear to be an expression of a permanently difficult temperament. In one study of only 10 colicky infants, in which colic was defined as cry bouts occurring more than 3 hours per day more than 3 times per week, subsequent measurements of temperament at 5 and 10 months did not show group differences between formerly colicky and noncolicky infants.[27]

SLEEP AND TEMPERAMENT

Continuous recordings of sleep patterns in the second day of life were correlated with temperament assessments at 8 months. It was observed that infants with the most extreme values on all sleep variables were more likely to have difficult temperaments.[28]

Temperament assessments performed at a mean age of 3.6 months showed an association between problems of sleep–wake organization, difficult temperament, and extreme crying.[29]

These babies were selected for persistent crying and were compared with babies with no current crying problem. Mothers of crying infants scored high on depression, anxiety, exhaustion, anger, adverse childhood memories, and marital distress. The authors concluded that factors related to parental care, although they did not cause persistent crying, did function to maintain or exacerbate the behavior. The persistence of parental factors may explain why at 1 year there are reported to be more difficulty in communication, more unresolved conflicts, more dissatisfaction, and greater lack of empathy in families with a colicky infant[30] and after 4 years, formerly colicky children have been reported to be more negative in mood on temperament assessments.[31]

In a study of 60 5-month-old infants, the infants rated as difficult had mean sleep times substantially less than the infants rated as easy (12.3 ± 1.5 versus 15.6 ± 1.6 hours; $P < .001$).[3] Although nine infant temperament characteristics were measured, only five were used to establish the temperament diagnosis of difficult. Four of these (mood, adaptability, rhythmicity, and approach/withdrawal tendency) were highly significantly correlated negatively with total sleep duration. No significant correlations occurred with the remaining temperament characteristics. Because the temperament characteristic "mood" relates to crying or fussing behavior, some authors describe the association between colic and difficult temperament as an artifact (from p. 43 of Barr and Gunnar[32]). However, mood is only one of the five temperament characteristics comprising the difficult temperament.

When the original study of 60 5-month-old infants was extended to include 105 infants, those with difficult temperaments slept 12.8 hours and those with easy temperaments slept 14.9 hours.[33] This observation was subsequently confirmed in another ethnic group with different parenting practices.[34] It thus appears that infants who have a difficult temperament have briefer total sleep durations when assessed at 4 to 5 months of age.

Support for an association between sleep and temperament is also based on a study in which objective measures of sleep–wake organization, derived from time-lapse video recordings, were compared with parental perceptions of infant temperament at 6 months of age.[35] The authors state, "Infants considered (temperamentally) easy have longer sleep periods and spend less time out of the crib for caretaking interventions during the night" (from p. 769 of Keener et al.[35]). However, the authors' analysis also led them to the conclusion that night waking is caused by environmental rather that biologic factors. Thus, this study has been cited as not supporting a general association between temperament and sleep–wake patterns.[36] It should be noted that the increased time out of the crib for temperamentally more difficult children at 6 months corresponds to the observation that increased night waking occurs in formerly colicky infants at 4, 8, and 12 months.[9,21]

Utilizing a computerized movement detector, it was observed that for 12-month-old children, those with the temperament trait of increased rhythmicity went to sleep earlier and had longer sleep durations,[37] and by 18 months of age, there was again the observation that both subjective and objective measures of improved sleep were associated with easier temperament assessments.[38] The authors correctly state that it is unclear whether the association is a biologic continuity between daytime temperament features and night-time sleeping, or whether the influence of the child's sleep behavior affects the mother's perceptions or ratings on temperament assessment instruments.[38]

The same 60 infants who were evaluated at 4 months of age[3] were restudied at 3 years.[39] Again, temperamentally easy children had longer sleep durations compared with children with more difficult temperaments. However, there was no individual stability of temperament or sleep duration between the ages of 4 months and 3 years. Thus, temperament ratings and associated sleep patterns at age 4 months do not predict temperament or sleep patterns at 3 years.

POSTCOLIC SLEEP

A retrospective study of 141 infants *between 4 and 8 months* of age from middle-class families showed that the history of colic, using Wessel's exact definition, significantly covaried with the parent's judgment that night waking was a current problem.[4] The frequency of awakening was a problem in 76% of infants, the duration of awakenings was a problem in 8%, and both frequency and duration were a problem in 16%. The frequency of night awakenings significantly correlated positively with the duration of night awakenings. Other studies also reported more night waking at 8 and 12 months[21] and ages 14 to 18 months[40] in postcolic children. Among infants who had had colic, the total sleep duration was less than among those who had not had colic (13.5 ± 0.3 versus 14.3 ± 0.2 hours, respectively; $P < .05$).[4]

Group differences in sleep duration between colicky and noncolicky infants, and between easy and difficult infants were observed to generally decrease over time.[41] Data obtained even during the first 4 months support a trend toward normalization.[20] For example, in one study, infants were diagnosed as irritable if crying occurred an average of at least 2.5 hours per day at 1 month of age. The irritable infants slept less, but over the 3-month study period, differences between the two groups diminished as the amount of crying subsided. Also, the irritable infants "spent less time in the content-awake or quiet-alert state that is optimal for parent-infant interaction" (from p. 8 of Keefe et al.[20]).

Some studies suggest that both infant irritability and sleep deficits are moderately stable individual characteristics during the first year of life or beyond.[8,9,40] One study showed that children with colic had more sleeping problems and the families exhibited more distress than a control group at age 3 years.[41] The trend of decreasing group differences with increasing age between colicky and noncolicky infants with regard to sleep, taken together with the normal polygraph recordings of colicky infants at 9 weeks of age, suggests that it is parenting practices, not biologic factors, that contribute to enduring sleep problems beyond 9 weeks of age.

As previously reported,[42] it may be difficult for parents of formerly colicky infants to eliminate frequent night awakenings and to lengthen sleep durations after those infants are 4 months old. Parents, because they are fatigued, may unintentionally become inconsistent and irregular in their responses to their infant. It cannot be overemphasized that "parents are never truly prepared for the degree to which the babies' sleep–wake patterns will dominate and completely disrupt their daily activities" (from p. 390 of Parmelee[43]). They may become overindulgent and oversolicitous regarding night awakenings and fail to appreciate that they are inadvertently depriving their child of the opportunity to learn how to fall asleep unassisted. Some mothers have difficulty separating from their child, especially at night, and other mothers have a tendency toward depression that might be aggravated by the fatigue from struggling to cope with a colicky infant. In either case, simplistic suggestions to help the child sleep better often fail to motivate a change in parental behavior. If the child fails to learn to fall asleep unassisted, the result is sleep fragmentation or sleep deprivation driven by intermittent positive parental reinforcement. This causes fatigue-driven fussiness long after the colic has resolved, which ultimately creates a sleep-deprived family.

Support for this view has come from research on infants at *5 months* of age who were followed to *56 months* of age. Wolke and Meyer[9] showed that "long crying duration and [the parents] having felt distressed about crying during the first *5 months* were significant predictors of night waking problems at *20 months*" (p. 198 [italics mine]) but not at *56 months*. In particular, later sleep problems are mainly related to the comorbidity of crying with sleep problems at *5 months* rather than to crying problems alone. Sleep problems at *5 months* remained the best predictor of sleep problems (especially night waking) at *20 months*. These authors concluded that postcolic "sleep problems are likely to be due to a failure of the parents to establish and maintain regular sleep schedules. . . . This conclusion *does not* blame parents for sleep difficulties: rather, it recognizes why many parents adopt strategies to deal with night waking in the least conflictual manner by night feeding or co-sleeping. This may be especially true of parents who are dealing with a temperamentally more difficult infant" (from p. 203 of Wolke and Meyer[9]). The authors also concluded that postcolic sleeping problems are not caused simply by increased crying per se but appear to be the consequence of associated infant sleeping problems and altered care-taking patterns for dealing with night waking in infancy.

Bates and associates recently evaluated the interaction between family stress, family management, disrupted child sleep patterns (variability in amounts of sleep, variability in bedtime, and lateness of bedtime), and preschool adjustment in children about 5 years old.[44] Children with disrupted sleep did not adjust well in preschool, and, in this analysis, disrupted sleep directly caused the behavior problems. These authors did not find any evidence that family stress or family management problems caused both disrupted sleep and behavior problems. They concluded that "sleep irregularity accounted for variation in (behavioral) adjustment independently of variation in family stress and family management" (from p. 70 of Bates et al.[44]). Interestingly, in support of their conclusion that disrupted sleep and not family stress was the main cause of behavioral problems, they observed that "in clinical treatment of young oppositional children, we have seen some spectacular improvements in manageability associated with the parents instituting a more adequate schedule of sleep for their children. Our clinical impression in these cases was that the changes were too rapid to be accounted for by other changes, such as in parental discipline tactics" (from p. 71 of Bates et al.[44]). The senior author agrees with my hypothesis that sleep modulates temperament and that "parenting responses to (sleep) issues would be involved in the continuity/discontinuity of temperament. . . . If parents make the effort to manage their kids' sleep schedules consistently, I would think that over years they are going to see less difficult and unmanageable behavior" (J. E. Bates, personal communication, 2002).

In a recent report, 64 children who had had, as infants, "persistent crying" (defined as fussing or crying more than 3 hours on 3 days in the week) were studied at 8 to 10 years of age.[45] The authors concluded that they were at risk for hyperactivity problems and academic difficulties. In addition, at 8 to 10 years of age, the previous persistent criers took longer to fall asleep, suggesting to the senior author that "they were less effective in controlling their own behavioural state to fall asleep" (D. Wolke, personal communication, 2002).

Therefore, it appears that increased crying or fussing behavior alone in infancy does not directly cause later sleep problems. Although the postcolicky child's family may be stressed, it appears that it is the failure to establish age-appropriate sleep hygiene that specifically leads to later disrupted sleep and behavioral problems.

SUMMARY AND DISCUSSION

Different definitions of colic and different ages of infants at the time of the study make it difficult to come to firm conclusions. During the first 4 months, colicky infants, by definition, exhibit more crying or fussing behavior. Data from parent diaries obtained at 4.5, 6, 7, and 8 weeks of age show that colicky infants sleep less than noncolicky infants (about 12 to 12.5 hours versus about 14 to 14.5 hours),[8,12,18,20] but there is disagreement over whether the decreased sleep occurs predominately during the day or night hours. By 9 weeks of age, polygraphic data do not show group differences in sleeping between colicky and noncolicky infants. Although group differences in sleeping duration between infants who had had colic and infants who had not been colicky were present even at 4 months of age,[4] these differences disappear by 6 to 8 months.[18,21] This raises the suggestion that parenting practices might be especially important in affecting sleep patterns after 9 weeks, especially regarding the development of a night waking habit. Also, by 6 months of age, researchers are more apt to view parents as contributing to sleeping problems,[35] especially night waking.

There appears to be agreement that infant crying alone does not predict the development of sleep problems.[8,9] Rather, the comorbidity of crying plus parental distress at 5 months, or of crying plus sleep problems at 5 months, predicts night waking at 20 months but not at 56 months.

Temperament assessments rely on parental reports, which often raises questions about how much the assessments reflect parental perceptions as opposed to objective descriptions of behavioral styles in children. At 2 and 4 weeks of age, infant difficultness predicted increased crying or fussing at about 6 weeks of age.[24,25] Infants with colic are more likely to have a difficult temperament when assessed at 4 months of age[2] but not at 12 months.[21] A difficult temperament is associated, at many ages, with problems in sleeping, such as shorter sleep durations and night waking, but this association is not predictive of later sleep problems. At 4 to 5 months of age, infants with a difficult temperament have total sleep durations of about 13 hours as opposed to about 15 hours for infants with an easy temperament.

The association of difficult temperament and sleeping problems during and shortly after age 4 months occurs despite successful treatment of colic. This suggests that crying or fussing behavior does not simply cause a measurement bias that makes parents imagine their children both to be difficult and to not sleep well. My impression is that it is exactly those parents with the willingness and resources to invest heavily in soothing during periods of fussing who are able to prevent some of the fussing that would otherwise escalate into crying, thus preventing some postcolic sleep problems. On the other hand, some parents are unable to manage severe infant fussing and become overwhelmed by the crying. Or perhaps they feel that because they cannot influence their child's crying behavior during the first few months, they also cannot influence their child's sleeping habits later.

It is important to help parents of postcolicky infants establish healthy sleep habits. Some of these children have difficulty falling asleep and staying asleep. At about 4 months, they have not developed self-soothing skills, perhaps because parents had invested constant soothing to prevent fussiness from developing into crying, or perhaps because inability to self-soothe is in fact an integral component of colic. A successful intervention effort to help families cope with infant crying during colic reduces parental distress. Continued education about age-appropriate sleep hygiene after colic ends is likely to prevent sleep problems from persisting beyond 4 months. Unsuccessful intervention and education increases the likelihood that temperament issues, family stress, and sleeping problems will persist beyond 4 months.

LINKS BETWEEN COLIC, SLEEP, AND TEMPERAMENT: AN ALTERNATIVE VIEW

The previous discussion assumes that individual differences in the neurologic maturation of sleep–wake control mechanisms, and the ability to regulate state (or self-soothe) are the primary determinants of how much fussiness, crying, and sleeping occur in babies during the first 4 months. Parenting practices during the first 4 months were ascribed a secondary role that develops in reaction to infant fussiness and crying. After 4 months, parenting practices were considered to be more important in maintaining sleep problems. An alternative view is that parenting practices do indeed make a major contribution to the outcome during the first 4 months of life.

This analysis is based on data from an outcome study using Wessel's exact definition of colic and data on temperament at 4 months of age,[2] an analysis of sleep and temperament at about 4 months of age,[3] and an assumption that the difficult temperament at about 4 months represents an overtired behavioral style. Certainly, the natural history of crying and fussy behavior (age of onset, age of cessation, evening time of occurrence, and occurrence mainly during the first 3 or 4 months with a peak at about 6 weeks) and its occurrence in all cultures strongly argue for biologic factors regarding etiology. However, the possibility remains that the severity (or intensity) and the duration of these behaviors are influenced by parenting practices. For example, infants in traditional or tribal cultures that practice constant holding and frequent breast-feeding may have less fussiness or crying. Also, the videotape studies that show no differences between parenting behaviors for colicky and noncolicky infants might reflect either an observation period that is too short, a too-small sample size, or extra effort on the part of the parent, motivated by the presence of video cameras in the home during the study.

Consider a balance between the baby's disposition to express distress and the parent's capability to soothe the baby. Not only do babies vary in their expression of fussing or crying behavior but also parents vary in their capability to soothe. Factors that affect parents' ability to soothe fussiness and crying and to promote their baby's sleep, and that might influence the outcome over the first few months, include the following:

1. Father involvement versus absent father
2. Agreements or disagreements between mother and father regarding child rearing, such as breast-feeding versus bottle-feeding or crib versus family bed
3. Absence or presence of marital discord or intimacy issues between wife and husband
4. Absence or presence of baby blues or postpartum depression
5. Absence or presence of other children requiring attention
6. Ease or difficulty of breast-feeding
7. Absence or presence of medical problems in child, mother, father, or other children
8. Number of bedrooms in the home
9. Presence or absence of relatives, friends, or neighbors to help
10. Help or interference from grandparents
11. Ability or inability to afford housekeeping help
12. Ability or inability to afford childcare help
13. Absence or presence of financial pressures, such as for mother to return to work soon

For example, assuming that 20% of infants have colic, consider three groups of children who developed along different paths:

A. In a cohort of 20 infants with colic, about 75%, or 15 infants, will not have a difficult temperament at 4 months of age.[2] At 4 months of age, these children will have an easier temperament and sleep longer than other children. The colic will have resolved. These children may have had a milder form of colic, or their parents may have vast resources for soothing.
B. In the same cohort of 20 infants with colic, about 25%, or five infants, will have a difficult temperament at 4 months of age and sleep less than other children.[2] At 4 months of age, the discrete spells of evening fussing or crying will be less well defined, but the disposition to express distress at any time will persist because these children remain overtired. Therefore, they will tend to be at their worst at the end of the day when they are most overtired. I call this fatigue-driven fussiness. These children may have had a more severe form of colic, or their parents may have limited resources for soothing.
C. Among 80 noncolicky infants, about 5%, or four infants, will have a difficult temperament at 4 months of age and resemble those infants in group B: they sleep less than other children, they are overtired, and they fuss and cry, especially at the end of the day. The parents of these children may have limited resources for soothing, or they may allow their child to become overtired by skipping naps, allowing too late a bedtime, or contributing to fragmented night sleep by giving too much attention at night. Alternatively, circumstances beyond the parents' control, such as extensive and necessary traveling, interfere with establishing sleep routines.

Therefore, at 4 months of age, there are nine infants who are overtired and who fuss or cry more than other children. The five (56%) from group B had colic and the four (44%) from group C did not have colic. These percentages are in close agreement with a recent study of colicky infants, in which colic was defined as "paroxysms of irritability, fussing, or crying lasting for 3 or more hours in any 1 day and occurring on 3 or more days in any 1 week" (from Clifford et al., p. 1184[46]). Mothers who participated, compared with mothers who declined or dropped out of the study, were more likely to be married, to have completed more formal education, to have a higher family income, to have higher levels of social support and lower levels of anxiety and depression, to breast-feed, and to be nonsmokers. The researchers described three groups of infants. In their first group, colic resolved by 3 months of age in 86% of infants, similar to group A (75%). In their second group, at 3 months of age, there were 35 children with colic, of whom 18 (51%) had colic at 6 weeks of age, similar to group B (56%). The authors referred to these children as having "persistent colic." In their third group, at 3 months of age, there were also 17 children (49%) with colic but they did not have colic at 6 weeks of age, similar to group C (44%). The authors referred to this group of infants as having "latent distress." They did not publish data comparing the mothers of infants with "persistent colic" versus "latent distress."

Although the authors[46] suspected that the persistent colic occurred in the 18 infants because of "a persistent mother-infant distress syndrome," they noted that colic "does not result in lasting effects to maternal mental health." However, they acknowledged that their results regarding the effects of colic on maternal health might be different in other populations "with different access to resources that may ease the burden of caring for a fussy infant . . . (who might not) be able to seek respite when they felt overwhelmed . . . (or did not have) adequate resources to buffer the effects of their infants' colic (p. 1186-1187)." The reason that I object to the term *mother-infant distress syndrome* is that it puts undue blame on mothers, when fathers, marriage, family, and financial concerns may play an equal if not greater role in the family's ability to soothe a baby. In fact, one recent study showed dysfunctional interactions between the colicky baby and the father to be much greater than between the colicky baby and the mother.[47]

After 4 months of age, it is my impression that the persistence of limited resources for soothing usually causes a continuation of sleeping problems and parental distress. However, intervention can correct the sleep problems and alleviate some of the parental distress. An improvement in parenting practices regarding sleep produces rapid and dramatic improvement in sleeping and behavior in children from group C, but the improvement in children from group B is much slower and more incremental. This is most likely because the infants from group B and their parents are more overtired, the children have been more consistently parent-soothed, and there may be lingering biologic delays in the development of sleep consolidation and nap rhythms.

The clinician should be aware of the social resources available to a family, because lack of these resources interferes with the parents' ability to soothe their child and help their child sleep. Clear identification of the social strengths and weaknesses in the family's support system permits a more individualized intervention program.

References

1. Weissbluth M: Crybabies: Coping with Colic, What To Do When Baby Won't Stop Crying. New York, Arbor House, 1984, pp 66-79, 131-146.
2. Weissbluth M, Christoffel KK, Davis AT: Treatment of infantile colic with dicyclomine hydrochloride. J Pediatr 1984;6:951-955.
3. Weissbluth M: Sleep duration and infant temperament. J Pediatr 1981;99:817-819.
4. Weissbluth M, Davis AT, Poncher J: Night waking in 4- to 8-month-old infants. J Pediatr 1984;104:477-480.
5. Wessel MA, Cobb JC, Jackson EB, et al: Paroxysmal fussing in infancy, sometimes called "colic." Pediatrics 1954;14:421-435.
6. Illingworth RS: Three-months' colic. Arch Dis Child 1954;29:165-172.
7. Reijneveld SA, Brugman E, Hirasing RA: Excessive infant crying: The impact of varying definitions. Pediatrics 2001;108:893-897.
8. St. James-Roberts I, Plewis I: Individual differences, daily fluctuations, and developmental changes in amounts of infant waking, fussing, crying, feeding, and sleeping. Child Dev 1996;67:2527-2540.
9. Wolke D, Meyer R: Co-morbidity of crying and feeding problems with sleeping problems in infancy: Concurrent and predictive associations. Early Dev Parenting 1995;4:191-207.
10. Kurtoglu S, Uzum K, Hallac IK, Coskun A: 5 Hydroxy-3-indole acetic acid levels in infantile colic: Is serotoninergic tonus responsible for this problem? Acta Paediatr 1997;86:764-765.

11. Weissbluth L, Weissbluth M: Infant colic: The effect of serotonin and melatonin circadian rhythms on intestinal smooth muscle. Med Hypotheses 1992;39;164-167.

12. White BP, Gunnar MR, Larson MC, et al: Behavioral and physiological responsivity, sleep, and patterns of daily cortisol production in infants with and without colic. Child Dev 2000; 71:862-877.

13. Sondergaard C, Henriksen TB, Orbel C, Wisborg K: Smoking during pregnancy and infantile colic. Pediatrics 2001;108:342-346.

14. Hill DJ, Hosking CS: Infantile colic and food hypersensitivity. J Pediatr Gastroenterol Nutr 2000;30:S67-S76.

15. Aldrich CA, Sung C, Knop C: The crying of newly born babies: 1. The community phase. J Pediatr 1945;26:313-326.

16. Brazelton TG: Crying in infancy. Pediatrics 1962; 29:40-47.

17. Paulozzi L, Sells M: Variation in homicide risk during infancy—United States, 1989-1998. MMWR Morb Mortal Rep 2002;51:187-189.

18. Kirjavainen J, Kirjavainen T, Huhtala V, et al: Infants with colic have a normal sleep structure at 2 and 7 months of age. J Pediatr 2001;138:218-223.

19. St. James-Roberts I, Conroy S, Hurry J: Links between infant crying and sleep-waking at six weeks of age. Early Child Dev 1997;48:143-152.

20. Keefe MR, Kotzer AM, Froese-Fretz A, Curtin M: A longitudinal comparison of irritable and nonirritable infants. Nurs Res 1996;45:4-9.

21. Lehtonen L, Korhonen T, Korvenranta H: Temperament and sleeping patterns in colicky infants during the first year of life. J Dev Behav Pediatr 1994;15:416-420.

22. Weissbluth M: Colic. In Ferber R, Kryger MH (eds): Principles and Practice of Sleep Medicine in the Child. Philadelphia, WB Saunders, 1995, pp 75-78.

23. Giganti F, Fagioli I, Ficca G, Salzarulo P: Polygraphic investigation of 24-h waking distribution in infants. Physiol Behav 2001;73:621-624.

24. Barr RG: Feeding and temperament as determinants of early infant crying/fussing behavior. Pediatrics 1989;84:514-521.

25. Blum NJ, Taubman B, Tretina L, Heyward RY: Maternal ratings of infant intensity and distractibility: Relationship with crying during the second month of life. Arch Pediatr Adolesc Med 2002;156:286-290.

26. Wolke D, Gray P, Meyer R: Excessive infant crying: A controlled study of mothers helping mothers. Pediatrics 1994;94:322-332.

27. Stifter CA, Braungart J: Infant colic: A transient condition with no apparent effects. J Appl Dev Psychol 1992;13:447-462.

28. Novosad C, Freudigman K, Thoman EB: Sleep patterns in newborns and temperament at eight months: a preliminary study. J Dev Behav Pediatr 1999;20:99-105.

29. Papousek M, von Hofacker N: Persistent crying in early infancy: A non-trivial condition of risk for the developing mother-infant relationship. Child Care Health Dev 1998;24:395-424.

30. Raiha H, Lehtonen L, Korhonen T, Korvenranta H: Family life 1 year after infantile colic. Arch Pediatr Adolesc Med 1996;150:1032-1036.

31. Canivet C, Jakobsson I, Hagander B: Infantile colic: Follow-up at four years of age—Still more "emotional." Acta Paediatr 2000;89:1-2.

32. Barr RG, Gunnar M: Colic: The 'Transient Responsivity' Hypothesis. In Barr RG, Hopkins B, Green JA (eds): Crying as a Sign, a Symptom, and a Signal. Series: Clinics in Developmental Medicine, vol 152, Cambridge: Cambridge University Press, 2000, pp 42-44.

33. Weissbluth M, Liu K: Sleep patterns, attention span, and infant temperament. J Dev Behav Pediatr 1983;4:34-36.

34. Weissbluth M: Chinese-American infant temperament and sleep duration: An ethnic comparison. Dev Behav Pediatr 1982;3:99-102.

35. Keener MA, Zeanah CH, Anders TF: Infant temperament, sleep organization, and nighttime parental interventions. Pediatrics 1988;81:762-771.

36. Anders TF, Sadeh A, Appareddy V: Normal sleep in neonates and children. In Ferber R, Kryger M (eds): Principles and Practice of Sleep Medicine in the Child. Philadelphia, WB Saunders, 1995, p 15.

37. Scher A, Tirosh E, Lavie P: The relationship between sleep and temperament revisited: Evidence for 12-month-olds—A research note. J Child Psychol Psychiatry 1998;39:785-788.

38. Scher A, Epstein R, Sadeh A, et al: Toddlers' sleep and temperament: Reporting bias or a valid link—A research note. J Child Psychol Psychiatry 1992;33:1249-1254.

39. Weissbluth M: Sleep duration, temperament, and Conners' ratings of three-year-old children. J Dev Behav Pediatr 1984;5:120-123.

40. Stahlberg M-R: Infantile colic: Occurrence and risk factors. Eur J Pediatr 1984;143:108-111.

41. Rautava P, Lehtonen L, Helenius H, Sillanpaa M: Infantile colic: Child and family three years later. Pediatrics 1995;96:43-47.

42. Weissbluth M: Sleep and the colicky infant. In Guilleminault C (ed): Sleep and Its Disorders in Children. New York, Raven Press, 1987, pp 129-140.

43. Parmelee AH Jr: Remarks on receiving the C. Anderson Aldrich Award. Pediatrics 1977;59: 389-395.

44. Bates JE, Viken RJ, Alexander DB, et al: Sleep and adjustment in preschool children: Sleep diary reports by mothers relate to behavior reports by teachers. Child Dev 2002;73:62-74.

45. Wolke D, Rizzo P, Woods S: Persistent infant crying and hyperactive problems in middle childhood. Pediatrics 2002;109:1054-1060.

46. Clifford TJ, Campbell MD, Speechley KN, Gorodzinsky F: Sequelae of infant colic: Evidence of transient distress and absence of lasting effects on maternal mental health. Arch Pediatr Adolesc Med 2002;156:1183-1188.

47. Raiha H, Lehtonen L, Huhtala V, et al: Excessive crying infant in the family: Mother-infant, father-infant, and mother-father interaction. Child Care Health Dev 2002;28:419-429.

Disorders of Initiating and Maintaining Sleep

Stephen H. Sheldon

11

Sleeplessness is one of the most frequent complaints presented to the sleep practitioner, since the entire family is affected by a child who cannot sleep at night. Symptoms of sleep deprivation may be identified in one or all members of the family. It is not unusual for a worn, haggard, frustrated parent to seek help for a child who appears happy, active, alert, and well rested.

Sleeplessness appears to be a final common pathway for a heterogeneous group of disorders that may have many etiologies. Underlying causes may be chronophysiologic, medical, psychological, social/environmental, or a combination of factors. Indeed, considerable overlap exists among underlying conditions. Some children may have no difficulty falling asleep but are unable to maintain continuity of sleep throughout the night, resulting in multiple nocturnal awakenings. Other children may have significant difficulty falling asleep at a prescribed time but, once asleep, will sleep throughout the night. Still others may suffer from both difficulty settling and night-time awakenings.

The typical connotation of the term "insomnia" does not appear to be applicable to sleepless children. The underlying causes of disorders of initiating and maintaining sleep (DIMS) during childhood appear to be considerably different from those of insomnia in adults, and different approaches to diagnosis and therapy are required.

Sleep onset and maintenance require appropriate interaction between biologic and psychological determinants. When one or more of these factors are disrupted or dysfunctional, sleeplessness results. Disorders of partial arousal from sleep stages and sleep–wake transition disorders (such as sleepwalking and night terrors) are discussed in Chapter 9.

To appropriately manage these problems, accurate diagnosis is essential. This chapter focuses on the epidemiology, clinical presentation, diagnostic features, differential diagnosis, and management paradigms for DIMS in childhood.

GENERAL CONSIDERATIONS

The problem of sleeplessness during childhood does not appear to be solely neurodevelopmental. Instead, sleeplessness reflects a pattern of interaction between physiologic and behavioral variables.[1] Interactions between the parent and the child at times of sleep transition are important. Parents display a wide variety of normal responses to their sleeping infant, and these responses change as the infant ages. Under normal circumstances, parents frequently respond to a signaling (crying) infant during the first few months of life. With older infants, parental intervention usually involves occasional checks during sleep. It is interesting to note that during the first two thirds of the first year of life, when infants are undergoing rapid neurodevelopmental changes and entrainment to appropriate sleep–wake cycles, almost half of all infants are already asleep when placed in the crib.[2]

As the infant ages, sleeplessness may contribute to significant parental anxiety, anger, fear, feelings of helplessness, and feelings of hopelessness. Parental concerns focus not only on the child's difficulties sleeping but also on their own sleeplessness. Prolonged night-time awakenings should be thought of as being derived from an interaction between the child's temperamental predisposition for awakening at night and other factors of health, development, and parental management.[3] The concerns of parents may be justified. Recent studies in adults have suggested that short sleep duration is related to increased morbidity.[4] During childhood, a lack of sleep seems to significantly affect school performance. A study of 9000 children with superior school performance[5] and higher test scores on intelligence tests[6] were associated with a longer duration of night-time sleep.

Despite nocturnal awakenings, it is rare for children less than 5-years of age to suffer from significant sleep deprivation. Young infants and toddlers sleep when necessary at any place or time. Although the parents are often concerned that a child awakening at night might be sleep deprived, it is not usually the case. Problems arise when social and educational demands are juxtaposed with sleep demands.[7]

The parents of older children often consider the total sleep time that is affected by television viewing in the evening. Weissbluth and colleagues have shown that total sleep time is the same today as it was 60 years ago.[8] Television viewing has had minimal or no effect on daytime or evening sleep in children 5 years of age or older. Although girls sleep slightly longer than boys at night, there appears to be no sex difference for daytime sleep or television viewing. The sex difference in total nocturnal sleep time is also seen in adults. Though there was no change in total sleep time, increased television viewing correlated with consistently decreased scores on standardized tests for reading, written expression, and mathematics.[8]

INCIDENCE AND PREVALENCE

Brief awakenings at night are normal in children and adults. Most often the individual turns over, immediately falls back asleep, and does not recall the arousal.[7] Studies of incidence and prevalence of night-time awakening in the pediatric population have been limited because of their subjective nature, relying on parental reports and questionnaires. Despite the limitations of this method of investigation, the frequency of sleeplessness during childhood seems high. Bax has shown that nocturnal awakenings during the first 5 years of life approximate 20% in the 0- to 2-year-old age group. There seems to be a slight decline in 3- to 4-year-old children, but the problem is still common in 10% of 4- to 5-year-old children.[7] Of the children exhibiting nocturnal awakenings at 12 months of age, 40% still experienced them at 18 months. Forty percent of children who were still awakening at 18 months continued to awaken at 2 years (but not necessarily the same 40%). When children awakening

at 18 months were studied, 54% were still awakening at 2 years and 23% at 3 years of age. At 5 years nocturnal awakening still occurred, though less significantly and less frequently after school entry.

In another study by Jenkins and associates, night-time awakening was reported in 23% of children at 1 year, 24% at 18 months, and 14% at 3 years of age.[9] Richman and coworkers showed that at 3 years of age, 13% of children have problems settling and 14 percent awaken at night.[10]

Inherent difficulties are present in the evaluation of data collected by parental reports and questionnaires, since night-time awakenings are noted only if the child is fussy and requires attention. Periods of quiet wakefulness during normal sleep hours are missed. To overcome this problem, Anders longitudinally videotaped parent and baby interactions during normal sleep periods.[11] *Settling* was defined as sleeping without removal from the crib between midnight and 5:00 AM for at least 4 weeks and night-time awakening as an arousal during that time at least once weekly for 4 weeks. A simple awakening occurred when the baby awoke after being asleep and then returned to sleep without fussing or being removed from the crib. A complex awakening occurred when the baby awoke after being asleep and then fussed and was removed from the crib. Sixty percent of 2-month-old infants and 62% of 9-month-old infants were initially placed in their cribs awake. Seventy percent of the males were placed in their cribs awake, compared with 50% of the females. There was also a difference between sexes in the time the infants were placed in their cribs. Females at 2 and 9 months of age were placed in their cribs between 8:00 and 9:00 PM and removed at 7:00 and 8:00 AM. Males at 2 months were placed in their cribs between 7:00 and 10:00 PM and removed at 6:00 and 8:00 AM. Males at 9 months were placed in their cribs between 7:00 and 9:00 PM and removed at 6:00 and 8:00 AM. Average sleep onset latency for the group of infants placed in their cribs awake was 27.5 minutes for 2-month-olds and 16.4 minutes for 9-month-olds. Two thirds of the infants who were placed in their cribs awake entered *active* sleep first. This correlated well with polysomnographic studies that showed active sleep-onset REM (rapid eye movement) during infancy.[12] Half of the awakenings for those at 2 and 9 months of age were simple and half were complex. The length of simple awakenings was 9 minutes for those at 2 and 9 months and tended to be more prominent as morning approached. Complex awakenings lasted longer and the duration changed with age, being 75 minutes for 2-month-olds and 24 minutes for 9-month-olds.[11] At 2 months of age, complex awakenings occurred predominantly between midnight and 6:00 AM. Females seemed to awaken more regularly between 3:00 and 6:00 AM. At 9 months, males demonstrated 2 peaks of complex awakening. The first peak occurred between 9:00 PM and midnight and the second between 3:00 and 6:00 PM. Females remained more regular, with a single peak between 3:00 and 6:00 AM.

Moore and Ucko reported that 50% of the infants who had settled successfully awakened again at night when they were 7 to 12 months of age.[13] Most parents and child health care practitioners will attest to the presence of this second peak of nocturnal awakenings. The etiology may be developmentally or physiologically based, however, night-time awakenings during this time may also be secondary to shifts and stresses in the environment.[13]

BEHAVIORAL CHARACTERISTICS, TEMPERAMENT, AND NIGHT-TIME AWAKENING

Zuckerman and colleagues conducted a longitudinal study of night-time awakening based on interviews with 308 parents.[14] For infants at 8 months of age, 10% of the mothers reported that their babies awoke three or more times per night, 8% reported that their babies took an hour or longer to settle after awakening, and 5% complained that their own sleep was severely disrupted by the child; 18% reported at least one of these problems. By 3 years of age, 29% of the children enrolled in the study had difficulty settling and/or staying asleep. Of the children with sleep problems at 8 months of age, 41% still had a problem sleeping at 3 years of age, compared with only 26% of the children without a sleeping problem at 8 months of age who developed a problem by 3 years of age. In this study, children with persistent sleep problems were more likely to have behavior problems, especially tantrums and behavior management problems, than those without persistent sleep problems. On the other hand, children with sleep problems were not more likely to have fears, anxiety, or other behavior problems as measured by the Behavior Screening Questionnaire.

Some evidence exists that there is a temperamental predisposition to night-time awakening. If this is true, the evaluation of the sleepless child requires a broader perspective. In a private pediatric practice, 25% of 60 randomly selected patients between 1 and 12 months of age suffered from night-time awakenings, which correlated significantly with temperamental characteristics of low sensory threshold .[3]

To determine if common sleep disturbances in young children, such as night-time awakening and bedtime struggles, tend to persist; if they are related to environmental stress factors and are accompanied by other behavioral problems; and if their persistence is related to other factors, Kataria and associates studied 60 children between the ages of 15 and 48 months.[15] The mothers were interviewed at the beginning of the investigation and after a period of 3 years. The children identified with sleep disorders were compared with those without sleep disorders. Forty-two percent of the children studied had disturbed sleep at the initial interview, and 84% of these children had persistence of the sleep disturbance after 3 years. The persistence of the sleep disorder had a significant relationship with the increased frequency of stress factors in the environment. Other generalized behavior difficulties were present in 30% of sleep-disturbed children and 19% of non–sleep-disturbed children. The latter finding is not statistically significant. Cosleeping (sleeping with a parent or sibling) was noted more frequently in sleep-disturbed children (34%) than in non–sleep-disturbed children (16%). Twenty percent of the mothers at the initial interview and 30% of the mothers at the 3-year followup perceived their children's sleep disturbances as stressful to them and to their family life. They concluded that early identification of the child with a sleep disturbance and timely intervention would help both the child and the family.

It is apparent that settling problems, night-time awakenings, or a combination of both seriously disrupt family life in many instances and lead to fatigue, irritability, the limitation of the parents' activities, and, on occasion, marital strain.[16] Night-time awakening is undoubtably a trigger for child abuse on some occasions, and the symptoms of difficulty settling and night-time awakening should be taken seriously by the practitioner.[7] Stress and depression, which are common in parents with young children, are often made worse by a lack of sleep. Parents who themselves have not slept cannot think rationally about ways of coping with their child's night-time awakenings.

Stress in the home is frequently associated with poor sleeping at night. Marital discord, separation, divorce, financial or professional difficulties, parental affective illness, medical disorders, death, family, move, school entry or change, toilet training, and the birth of a new sibling may all contribute.[1] A cry certainly is a powerful biologic signal. It is indeed difficult to ignore, whether the response is positive or negative.

Although night-time awakening and settling problems have medical, biologic, and psychosocial underpinnings, some consider these symptoms to be a conditioned reflex. Wilkes has stated the following:

> "The child wakes, cries, the mother intervenes with loving attention and a drink; the child repeats his crying nightly and each time is quickly rewarded. With such regular reinforcement, the reflex is soon established."[17]

However, this proposition is too simplistic when considering DIMS, since a combination of interactions among many variables contribute to the final common pathway of sleeplessness.

In contrast to sleep duration in older children, adolescents, and adults (which appears to be related to mental and physical health status and environmental and social factors), sleep duration in infancy seems determined primarily by neurologic maturation and to some degree by temperament. Weissbluth compared infant temperament characteristics with total sleep duration and found that 4 of the 5 infant temperament characteristics (mood, adaptability, rhythmicity, and approach/withdrawal) that are used to establish temperament diagnoses of *easy* or *difficult* were highly negatively correlated with total sleep duration.[18]

There appear to be consistent patterns of behavior in babies. Some children are definitely more quiet and less active than others. Therefore, a consideration of the baby's personality may be important in the assessment of the sleep disorder.[3,19] Persistent sleep problems have been shown

to be associated with increased rates of temper tantrums and generally greater difficulty in managing the child's behavior at 3 years of age. This suggests that persistent sleep problems are a part of more pervasive behavioral difficulties between the parent and child involving limits and boundaries.[14]

Sensory thresholds, defined as the levels of extrinsic stimulation required to evoke a discernible response,[3] may also be important in evaluating the child's behavior and sleep problems. A low sensory threshold may partially explain problems such as teething and sleeplessness. In Carey's study, the distribution of the temperament syndrome revealed that 76% were easy or intermediate low and 24% were intermediate high or difficult. Of the 15 infants who awoke at night, 13 had low sensory thresholds.[3] There are two theoretical mechanisms of how low sensory threshold contributes to night-time awakening. First, a greater response to stimuli during the day makes infants more arousable at night. Second, the infant may generally be more responsive to internal and external stimuli at night.

However, great care must be taken in evaluating infant temperament and sleep problems. Oberklaid and coworkers have shown that toddler temperament ratings differ according to sex, age, social class, and cultural contexts. Future temperament norms may need to specify the characteristics of the group of children from which they were derived to allow for more valid comparisons.[20]

After 3 to 4 months of age, a major feature of a child's difficult temperament is the proclivity to cry and fuss in many situations.[21] Infants beyond this age range who cry excessively also tend to have irregular sleep or sleep patterns characterized by frequent awakenings.[22] Also, it appears that in the age range of 3 to 18 months, infants who cry more at any time during the day and night are also more likely to cry during sleep–wake transitions.

COSLEEPING

Cosleeping (sharing a bed with another individual) is common in many cultures. Concerns about the suffocation of children and night-time awakenings appear to be unfounded.[7] It is often recommended for the infant to sleep in a separate room soon after birth to avoid contamination of the sleep–wake transition with the need for a parent to be present in order to fall asleep. Parents are often concerned that putting the child in a separate room at night may result in feelings of inattentiveness to the child's needs. However, Bax reports that parents often become *more* attentive to their child when the sleeping environments are separated. A cry from a distant bedroom easily wakes up the parent to respond to the child's needs.[7] Loudspeaker systems and intercom units have been marketed to ensure this arousal response in the parent. These techniques appear to conflict with the contention that cosleeping is not detrimental. However, it is interesting to note that Bax reported 68% of the children with sleep problems to have experienced cosleeping, compared with 22% of those without sleep problems.

The prevalence and correlations of sleeping in the parental bed among healthy children between 6 months and 4 years of age were studied by Lozoff and colleagues.[23] In this cross section of families in a large U.S. city, cosleeping was a routine practice in 35% of white and 70% of black families. Cosleeping in both racial groups was associated with approaches to sleep management at bedtime that emphasized parental involvement and body contact. Cosleeping children were significantly more likely to fall asleep out of bed and to have adult company and body contact at bedtime. Among white families only, cosleeping was associated with the older child, lower level of parental education, less professional training, increased family stress, a more ambivalent maternal attitude toward the child, and disruptive sleep problems for the child.

Objective evidence of cosleeping resulting in sleep disruption has been reported by Monroe.[24] Couples who were good sleepers and habitually slept together were studied polysomnographically when they slept together and apart. When the couple slept apart, more slow-wave sleep and less REM sleep were identified. This seems to indicate a rebound of slow-wave sleep similar to that seen in sleep-deprived subjects. It was concluded that sleeping together may be good for marital bliss, but sleeping apart eliminated disturbances of sleep when partners change positions. Similar studies have not been performed in children.

Breast-feeding may be associated with a concurrent mother-infant adaptation that involves frequent night-time awakenings. However, when a mother stops breast-feeding, the rate of sleep problems among breast-fed children at 8 months of age is the same as that for children whose mothers never breast-fed.[14] Breast-feeding and ethnic differences may not be linked to persistent sleep problems because these characteristics may be associated with different child-rearing expectations and behaviors.[25] Night-time awakening during infancy is considered to be a normal occurrence in some cultures, especially when children sleep with their parents.

EVALUATION OF THE SLEEPLESS CHILD

The evaluation of the sleepless child should be approached in the same manner as that for any other clinical problem. Evaluation begins with a comprehensive medical, developmental, and behavioral history. The physical exam should be comprehensive, paying special attention to developmental landmarks and the central nervous system (CNS).[7]

Parents will usually seek help for the problem only if the child's sleeplessness has resulted in parental sleeplessness or fear that the child is becoming significantly sleep deprived. It is clear that unless the clinician takes the initiative to obtain a *comprehensive sleep history* during the normal course of well-child care and health maintenance, problems will often be missed. Persistent night-time awakenings have been frequently ascribed to parental mismanagement of nocturnal arousals. Appropriate attention should be paid to the methods with which the parents have responded to their sleepless child in the past. The following questions may elucidate significant aspects of the patient's history and provide insight into sleep patterns and habits.

1. What is the normal evening bedtime?
2. What specific activities are performed during a period of 2 hours immediately before bedtime?
3. How long does it normally take the child to fall asleep?
4. If it takes the child longer than 30 minutes to fall asleep, what does the child do during the period of time from lights out to sleep onset? What are the parents' responses to these behaviors?

5. What steps have the parents/caretakers taken to assist the child in falling asleep?

6. Is the child permitted to fall asleep somewhere other than in his/her own bed and bedroom?

7. Exactly what associations does the child require in order to fall asleep (e.g., stuffed animal, special toy, pacifier, bottle, being held, watching television, night-light)?

8. After sleep onset, does the child awaken? For how long? At what times? How many times per night?

9. If the child awakens at night, what interventions are required for the child to fall back asleep?

10. Does the child exhibit any unusual behaviors or movements during sleep? Does the child walk in his/her sleep? Bang his/her head? Wake suddenly with a piercing scream? Jerk his/her legs? Grind his/her teeth?

11. Does the child snore? Is the snoring mild, moderate, or severe? Does the child snore every night?

12. What time does the child awaken in the morning? Does the child awaken spontaneously, or is the child awakened by a clock? Parent? Sibling? Is it difficult to wake up the child? How does the child feel on awakening? Grumpy? Happy? Tired?

13. At what time during the day is the child the most active and alert? The most tired and cranky?

14. Does the child nap during the day? How many times each day? At what times?

15. Does the child exhibit any unusual behaviors during daytime naps?

16. Where does the child nap? Are the same sleep associations present for the child during daytime naps?

A sleep diary or sleep log maintained for a period of 2 weeks is of great assistance in analyzing children's sleep problems. The diary provides more objective longitudinal evidence of sleep patterns and a baseline from which to compare the progress and success of treatment regimens. By keeping the sleep diary during the course of treatment, clear evidence of change is provided for the parents and practitioner.

Despite parental concern that their child is being sleep deprived because of difficulty settling and/or night-time awakening, this is usually not the case. If the child remains active, alert, and playful during normal waking hours, the volume of sleep during the previous 24 hours is most likely appropriate.[7] On the other hand, parental sleep deprivation is most often real. The treatment of the child's sleep problem will most likely result in resolution of the parents' sleep problems.

GENERAL CONCEPTS ON THE MANAGEMENT OF CHILDHOOD DISORDERS OF INITIATING AND MAINTAINING SLEEP

A variety of solutions to sleep onset and maintenance problems have been suggested, and there have been significant contradictory recommendations regarding optimal management. No single approach appears to be universally effective. Recommendations have included attention to night-time rituals, firm handling, letting the child "cry it out," the use of hypnotics and sedatives, general support and sympathy, and different combinations of these.[16] Many are appropriate, but some are not. For example, Wilkes[17] has described a method for deconditioning night-time awakenings in one night.

"The child cries. Father stamps in, flings down the side of the cot, and slaps him once. But firmly, he flings up the cot side, and stamps out, slamming the door behind him (locking it with older children). The child screams and shouts for hour after hour until, depending on his strength and determination, eventually he subsides in a lather of sweat and exhaustion."

Obviously, this method of treatment goes against most acceptable methods and may result in numerous difficulties in addition to problems with sleep.

The behavioral methods of treatment have been used successfully in the management of childhood psychological and behavioral problems. However, a behavioral approach may not be appropriate for all problems related to sleeplessness. This approach requires careful analysis of the individual problem and the establishment and resulting gradual attainment of the specific goals of treatment. Emphasis should be placed on removing the factors that reinforce the problem and planning a replacement or substitution with appropriate behaviors. Many sleep problems will resolve spontaneously, and time is always on one's side in the management of many sleep disorders.[7] Simple behavioral procedures may occupy the parents' attention long enough that a spontaneous remission may occur in the interim.

Night-time awakenings and settling problems are very often interactional in nature, affecting the entire family and not merely the child. Therefore, the management of the problem should be directed at the family and not just the child. In many circumstances, the best method of treatment is habit training (behavior modification) and attention to the principles of sleep hygiene (Table 11–1). If there is failure to respond, some recommend the short-term use of sedation.[3] It is thought that a short-term course of a hypnotic or sedative may alter the infant's arousal threshold enough to facilitate the learning of a more acceptable sleep pattern. However, there are many conflicting opinions, and it is thought by many that medication rarely has a place in the management of most sleep disorders.

Changes in the physical sleeping environment may cause dramatic changes in sleep patterns. Children who experience a persistent problem with sleeplessness may sleep well at a grandparent's home only to have the symptoms return in their own home environment. This is frequently irritating to young parents, who may feel insecure about their role.[7] Appropriate support and management of the entire family are essential during these times.

According to Bax,[7] the short-term use of chloral hydrate or Phenergan may be necessary. In these situations, it is important to start with an adequate dose and be weaned quickly from the medication. This method seems more efficacious than starting with small doses and increasing them until the desired effect is achieved. The latter method may be accompanied by increasing tolerance to the medication, and larger doses may be required.

During any behavioral management regimen, parents must be warned that the child's sleep problem may appear to worsen for a few days at the beginning of treatment. This characteristic frequently results in the abandonment of the treatment protocol if there is no adequate warning, support, and reassurance. When there is improvement, it tends to happen quickly.

Jones and Verduyn[16] reported that 53% of children's sleep problems resolved completely by means of a behavioral approach. Thirty-seven percent more showed partial resolution, and 10% were unchanged at the end of the treatment

Table 11–1. **Principles of Sleep Hygiene in Childhood**
The child's bedroom should be dark and quiet.
Bedtime routines should be strictly enforced.
The time of morning awakening should be firmly and consistently structured.
Bedroom temperatures should be kept comfortably cool (<75° F).
Environmental noise should be minimized as much as possible. Background music and/or white noise may inhibit extraneous noise.
Children should not go to bed hungry and may have a snack before bedtime.
Excessive fluids before bedtime may result in bladder distention and arousal and disrupt sleep.
Children should learn to fall asleep alone (i.e., without their parents' presence in the room).
Vigorous activity should be avoided before bedtime.
A bath is often a stimulating activity for children. If bedtime struggles are present after the child's bath, it may be moved to the morning or separated from the child's bedtime by at least 2 hours.
Methylxanthine-containing beverages and food (e.g., caffeinated beverages/colas, tea, chocolate) should be avoided for several hours before bedtime.
Parents should read the labels on all over-the-counter and prescription medications. Some medications contain alcohol or caffeine and may disrupt sleep.
Naps should be developmentally appropriate. Brief naps may be refreshing, but prolonged naps or napping too frequently may result in significant accumulation of sleep during the day and make it more difficult to fall asleep at night.

Modified with permission from Sheldon SH, Spire JP, Levy HB: Pediatric Sleep Medicine. Philadelphia, WB Saunders, 1992, p 76.

regimen. Maternal psychiatric history was not related to the outcome. The success of sleeping through the night remained unchanged at 6-month followup. It is important to note that the problem was less likely to resolve when marital discord was present. Response was best when both parents were persuaded to attend sessions with the physicians. Consistency and persistency are imperative in management, and cooperation between the parents during treatment regimens will result in the more rapid and complete resolution of symptoms.

BEHAVIORAL AND/OR CONDITIONED FACTORS CAUSING SLEEPLESSNESS

Disorder of Sleep Onset Associations

It has been pointed out in Chapter 1 that brief nocturnal awakenings are normal, especially during transitions between REM and non-REM sleep. These brief arousals may serve an important survival function. The sleeping environment may be checked and the body repositioned. Bedclothes may be adjusted to the sleeper's comfort. The return to sleep is most often rapid, and the short arousal is not remembered. However, if the sleeping environment has changed, returning to sleep may be difficult and the individual may become fully alert.

Sleep onset occurs through complex behavioral and physiologic interactions. First, the body must be physiologically ready for sleep at its appropriate position in the circadian cycle. A series of bedtime rituals follow. On retiring, a pillow might be fluffed and covers or blankets positioned. Other factors may also be required, such as a night-light, soft music, television, and/or the presence of a bed partner. Without these behavioral rituals, sleep onset may be difficult. In other words, we *learn* to fall asleep in a particular manner, and this learned behavior is repeated night after night. When these *sleep onset associations* are absent, falling asleep may be troublesome.

Children learn to fall asleep in the same manner. Certain conditions must be present to ease the transition. The child may require a particular bedroom, lying in a certain crib or bed, and holding a favorite stuffed animal or special blanket.[1,26]

These conditions are usually present all night. Being held and rocked, the presence of television, being read a story, and pacifier suckling may not be present all night. After a normal arousal, it may be hard for the child to return to sleep, since the child has not learned to fall asleep on his/her own without these associations. Ferber persuasively states the importance of these associations as follows:

> *"Thus the problem is not one of abnormal wakings but one of difficulty in falling back to sleep. And the difficulty arises because of the child's particular associations with falling asleep."*[26]

A disorder of sleep onset associations occurs most commonly in infants and toddlers. The older the child, the more control s/he has over the environment and the less likely s/he is to require associations that are not present within the sleep environment during nocturnal arousals. Association problems become less significant after the age of 4 years, although they may occasionally persist into adolescence.

Clinical Presentation and Diagnosis

The usual complaint is one of prolonged nighttime awakenings. Settling may not be of concern to the parents, since associations may be present early in the evening. During the night, the child may fuss significantly until s/he is removed from the crib or bed, permitted to sleep in the parents' bed, held, or rocked. Daytime sleepiness is most often not present, although the parents may be significantly sleep deprived from chronically responding to their child's nocturnal crying. The time of settling is usually normal. The review of a sleep diary usually reveals normal sleep onset latency time and frequent, prolonged nocturnal arousals. Total sleep is usually normal, the timing of the major sleep period is normal, and the morning wake-up time is usually normal. Parents often report that the child rapidly returns to sleep if given a bottle. The volume of fluid consumed by the youngster during these nocturnal feedings is usually small. For the breast-fed infant, sleep returns quickly once nursing begins and the nocturnal feedings are perceived by the mother to be different from the daytime feedings. These characteristics help differentiate association problems from disorders of excessive nocturnal fluids. Physiologic processes controlling the sleep–wake cycle can be assumed to be functioning normally if the child sleeps well while being held or rocked. If there is significant dysfunction of the central mechanisms controlling sleep, the child will not sleep well under any circumstances. The physical exam is usually normal. A rapid return to sleep when habitual associations are reestablished helps differentiate normal from abnormal arousals and determine the diagnosis of disordered sleep onset associations as the problem.

Treatment

Treatment is straightforward. The child must learn to make the transition from wakefulness to sleep without expecting participation of the parent. Success rates are high if parents are given sufficient support. Relearning usually takes less than 1 week.[26]

The child must learn to fall asleep alone and under conditions that can be easily reestablished after normal nocturnal arousals. Bedtime rituals should not be stimulating or require ongoing activity or parental participation. Holding, rocking, nursing, and pacifier suckling should be discontinued. The child should be placed in the crib or bed alone and should learn to fall asleep by himself/herself.

Two basic principles must be followed. The parents must be *consistent* in reestablishing appropriate sleep onset associations and *persistent* with the regimen. The following paradigm is usually rapidly successful if the parents are consistent and persistent. For some families, sleepless nights may seem worse for the first day or two of treatment. Therefore, the treatment regimen should begin on days when parental sleeplessness will not affect their performance the next day. Although some degree of crying should be expected during the beginning of the treatment phase, it is usually kept to a minimum by *gradually* establishing appropriate sleep onset associations. Letting the child "cry it out" will usually maintain crying at its maximum and often results in parental frustration and treatment failure.

1. The first night

   - The child should be placed in the crib or bed with only those association objects that will be present during normal nocturnal awakenings.

   - The room should be dark (although a small night-light may be used), quiet, and at a comfortable temperature. A room that is too hot or cold will tend to inhibit sleep. When the room temperature cannot be controlled, the child should be dressed appropriately for the ambient temperature.

   - The parent may soothe and comfort the child until s/he is lying down quietly. Allowing some crying will rarely result in psychological trauma to the child and is often more difficult for the parent.

   - Once the child is quiet in the bed or crib, the parent should leave the room.

   - If the child begins to cry, the parents should allow it for a short period of time. The exact time should be developmentally appropriate; however, a period of at least 1 to 2 minutes (according to a clock or a stopwatch) should elapse before the parent first responds.

   - The parent may then return to the room to comfort the child; however, *the child should not be removed from the crib or bed.* The parent may remain in the room quietly soothing the child until s/he lies back down in the crib or bed and is quiet, at which time the parent should leave the room.

   - If and when the child begins to cry again, the parent should wait slightly longer before responding (a period of 2 to 3 minutes is usually appropriate) and repeat the immediately preceding step.

   - The above process should be repeated (keeping the wait–response period at 2 to 3 minutes on the first night) until the child is sleeping.

   - On the first night, this process of cry–wait–respond may last for several hours before the child falls asleep. Parents must be warned that this might occur. It is important that they be supported and reassured that the process will be successful if they are persistent and consistent with the regimen. If they give up and remove the child from the crib or bed on the first or second night of management, a treatment failure is likely. It is also important to involve all caretakers in the treatment program so that sharing responsibilities may occur and consistency be assured.

2. The second night

   - Treatment on the second night is similar to that on the first; however, the wait–response period may be lengthened to 2 to 4 minutes for the first and 5 minutes for subsequent waiting times. If the child is beginning to calm down at the end of the wait–response time, it is usually better to wait slightly longer to see if the child settles on his/her own.

- Parental interventions should be *supportive*. The child should know that the parent is *understanding* and is nearby .
- Parents must not exhibit anger or frustration or escalate these feelings as the night progresses.

3. Subsequent nights

- Treatment on subsequent nights should parallel that on the first two nights.
- However, by the third night improvement is usually seen. Night-time awakenings are usually shorter, loud crying may be replaced with mild whimpering, and a return to sleep without parental intervention occurs.
- Nocturnal arousals may still occur, but crying does not. The child has learned to fall back asleep on his/her own without parental assistance.

During the course of management, parents should record progress in a sleep diary. This is important for the parents and practitioner so that improvement can be documented. During the course of treatment, follow-up visits should occur at weekly intervals. The sleep diaries should be evaluated at each visit. Once the child is falling asleep on his/her own, s/he will most often continue to sleep well. Occasional disruptions might occur, especially during times when the usual regimen is altered (e.g., vacations, birthdays, holidays). The parental response to and management of these intermittent sleep disruptions will determine whether or not they will persist. If the disruption is managed in a manner consistent with that for the original regimen, rapid resolution will occur and the child will continue to sleep well.

If the mother is breast-feeding the child, it is not necessary to discontinue nursing to correct the sleep onset association. It is necessary only to dissociate the act of nursing from falling asleep. Association problems are most likely present when the infant falls asleep during nocturnal breast-feedings after nursing for only a few moments. Instead of nursing at bedtime, it is often better to recommend moving the last

feeding of the evening to a time several hours earlier. If the child tends to fall asleep during breast-feeding, the mother may discontinue the feeding before the child falls asleep and place the child in the crib or bed. The same techniques may be used during daytime naps.

Excessive Nocturnal Fluids

Although this condition is considered under the rubric of behavioral etiologies, excessive nocturnal fluids may have a physiologic basis for causing sleeplessness. In older children and adults, bladder distention typically results in an arousal response (see Chapter 27). In children with primary functional nocturnal enuresis, this arousal response appears to be developmentally delayed. Other evidence that bladder distention has a central arousal effect stems from observations that parasomnias (disorders of sleep stages and partial arousal from sleep) appear to be exacerbated by bladder distention.

Clinical Presentation and Diagnosis

Infants consuming excessively large quantities of fluid during the night typically awaken continuously and frequently. This problem occurs in both breast- and bottle-fed infants. The volume of fluid consumed during the night may range from 8 to 32 ounces, and these children awaken from 3 to 8 times per night.[27] The diapers are usually heavily soaked by morning.

From 7 to 12 months of age, infants no longer have a physiologic need for feeding during the night. Awakening to eat may be secondary to one of three major factors: there may be an association of feeding with sleep onset and returning to sleep; there may be learned hunger during the night; or bladder distention may be present and causing the arousal. Children awakening and feeding due to inappropriate sleep onset associations typically awaken less often than those awakening due to excessive nocturnal fluids. Fluid intake during arousals is also less. The presence of only one or two arousals per night, with a rapid return to sleep after only a brief period at the bottle, breast, or pacifier, suggests that the nipple or parent is more important than the fluid intake. If sleep onset association problems are present, the fluid intake is usually less than 6 ounces per night. More frequent awakenings and the consumption of large volumes of fluid

(8 to 32 ounces) suggest excessive fluid intake as the problem. Breast-feeding more than two times per night and nursing sessions of longer than 2 to 3 minutes suggest excessive fluid intake. Finally, if the child has learned to eat during the night, frequent nocturnal awakening will occur. Habitual nocturnal feedings may distort the circadian hunger rhythm and disrupt the sleep–wake cycle as much as the fluid/food intake.

Treatment

Although nocturnal awakenings are typically frequent and severe in patients ingesting excessive nocturnal fluids, treatment is straightforward and not difficult. The aim of therapy is to *gradually* discontinue the nocturnal fluids. For the bottle-fed infant, gradually decreasing the volume of fluid in each nocturnal bottle over the course of 1 to 2 weeks will usually result in rapid improvement. Often infants will discontinue awakening for feeding when only 1 or 2 ounces are provided. One alternative is to gradually dilute the formula with water before weaning from the bottle. However, it is important in either case that during the treatment phase, the association of sleep onset with suckling not be established. If this is the case, the regimen should be modified to include the principles discussed in the section on the treatment of sleep onset association disorder. Treatment of the breast-fed infant ingesting excessive nocturnal fluids is slightly more problematic. Nursing mothers may experience a letdown on hearing their crying infant. It may be necessary for the nursing mother to manually express her milk (or use a breast pump) and have the father or other caretaker respond. Diluting the mother's milk with water and gradually weaning the child from the bottle are then conducted in the same manner as that for formula-fed infants. Once the infant is sleeping through the night, maternal letdown during sleep will usually resolve.

Colic

Colic is one of the more common disorders affecting sleep in young infants, affecting about one in five.[28] The patient is usually less than 4 months of age, and the typical complaint is one of inconsolable fussiness during late afternoon or evening hours. Symptoms of colic will often

resolve, but disordered sleep remains. The problem does not appear to be biologically based, although it may reflect altered chronophysiologic factors during development. The sleep problem more likely occurs in response to altered sleep–wake schedules and habitual patterns of parental responsiveness persisting into the postcolic period.[1]

Weissbluth has stated that colicky behavior appears to be a reflection of the development of the CNS during the first few months of life.[28] Subsequently, some colicky infants develop irregularity of behavior, heightened activity or arousal, and sensitivity to stimuli that cause, directly or indirectly, difficulty in maintaining regular, prolonged, and consolidated sleep patterns. Mismanagement of the infant's sleep schedule and habits after the colicky period has passed, a result of early difficulties in handling the infant, is thought to be the most common cause of persistence of sleep problems after 4 months of age.

Clinical Presentation and Diagnosis

Patients appear to suffer violent, rhythmic, screaming attacks that are unresponsive to parental intervention and for which no other cause could be found.[29] Wessel and colleagues described colicky infants as those who experience paroxysms of irritability, fussing, or crying lasting for a total of more than 3 hours a day, occurring more than 3 days per week, and continuing or recurring for more than 3 weeks.[30]

The age of onset, time of occurrence, and age at the resolution of symptoms are characteristic. "Attacks" generally do not occur during the first few days of life. Symptoms typically begin during the third (80%) and fourth (100%) weeks of life.[30] An important exception is the premature infant. Three studies have documented the onset of colic in the premature infant within 2 weeks after the infant's expected date of birth (70% between the 39th and 44th gestational weeks) regardless of the gestational age at birth.[31-33] Once the symptoms begin in the preterm infant, the duration of colic appears to be similar to that of term infants. Thus, the ages of the onset and disappearance of colic appear to be locked in time to conceptional age. Episodes of colic tend to start between 5:00 and 8:00 PM and end at about midnight. By 2 months of age almost half of the infants suffering from colic will have a resolution of symptoms, which will subside in 90% of all infants with colic who have no more attacks by 4 months of age.

Another characteristic feature of colic is relatively uninhibited motor activity. During the crying spells, affected infants have been described as hypertonic or neurolabile. This does not occur at other times during the day or night. Physical movements during the colicky spell include tonic stiffening of the entire body with fists tightly clenched; legs flexed rigidly over the abdomen; writhing, twisting, and turning motions; and jerky, uncoordinated movements such as batting or flapping of the arms and kicking of the legs. Facial grimacing suggests severe pain, and affected infants seem unusually sensitive to light.[34]

Daytime sleep periods for colicky infants appear to be extremely irregular and brief. Some infants will temporarily discontinue daytime naps during the period of maximum fussiness (approximately 6 weeks of age). Colicky infants miss periods of quiet sleep during their evening attacks.[28] It is interesting to note that after the cessation of daytime and night-time spells, the infant invariably falls asleep. This may be secondary to exhaustion or the time of day or could represent a period of transient but excessive neurologic arousal, excitation, or lack of inhibition that is terminated by naturally occurring periods of quiet sleep or increased inhibition.[28]

A number of studies have evaluated the sleep patterns of infants in the postcolic period.[35-37] The parents of infants who have had colic report shorter total sleep duration at 4 to 5 months of age. A history of colic appears to be significantly associated with frequent night-time awakenings when compared with infants with no history of colic (a ratio of almost 2.5 to 1). The duration of night-time awakenings is a problem for some infants, as is frequency and duration in others.

Some postcolic infants are exquisitely sensitive to irregularities in their sleep–wake schedules. Disruptions of sleep–wake routines because of illness, holidays, or vacations cause extreme disruptions of settling and night-time awakenings that may last several days. According to Weissbluth, these prolonged recovery periods might reflect easily disorganized, endogenous biologic rhythms caused by enduring congenital imbalances in arousal/inhibition of sleep–wake control mechanisms.[28] This suggests that disordered chronophysiologic mechanisms may be significant in postcolic sleep–wake disturbances, and treatment should focus on mechanisms that may functionally reset and entrain the endogenous circadian pacemaker.

Treatment

The clinical observations of infants who suffer from frequent night-time awakenings and short sleep period times in the postcolic period may be successfully treated only if the parents establish and maintain a regular sleep schedule. It seems that most postcolic sleep problems are the result of the parents' failure to establish regular sleep patterns when the colic dissipates at approximately 4 months of age. Therefore, treatment should focus on the reestablishment of a normal sleep–wake routine. If the parents strictly program their child's sleep schedule, regular daytime and night-time sleep patterns will reemerge. The most powerful point of entrainment is the *morning wake-up time,* which must be fixed and consistent. Nocturnal bedtime and nap times must also be strictly adhered to. *Consistency* and *persistency* are essential in establishing a successful regimen. The maintenance of a sleep diary for 1 to 2 weeks before instituting therapy and during the course of treatment will greatly assist parents in maintaining an appropriate routine and provide accurate feedback for the practitioner regarding the success of the regimen during follow-up visits.

MEDICAL DISORDERS RESULTING IN SLEEPLESSNESS

Cow's Milk Allergy

An allergy to cow's milk protein may result in a severe disturbance of sleep during early infancy. It is often difficult to clinically differentiate cow's milk allergy from colic, since both may begin at similar ages and are associated with sleeplessness, fussiness, intermittent crying episodes, and short sleep period times.

Clinical Presentation and Diagnosis

Frequent night-time awakenings (five or more times per night) and short total sleep times (often as low as 4.5 hours) are the typical sleep complaints.[1,38] Infants with cow's milk allergy often cry frequently during daytime hours and are described by their parents as fussy. The physical exam may be unremarkable; however, anemia and hematochezia may be present in some infants. Polysomnographic analysis reveals a significantly disturbed sleep pattern and is useful in determining the absence of other causes of arousal and short total sleep times. The diagnosis is based on a high clinical index of suspicion of atopy. Allergy testing usually reveals elevated immunoglobulin E levels, and radioallergosorbent testing is often positive for cow's milk protein. Discontinuing a cow's milk–based formula and substituting a hydrolyzed milk protein formula result in the resolution of symptoms.

Treatment

Once the diagnosis is established, treatment consists of the removal of cow's milk protein and the beginning of hydrolyzed milk-protein formula. Within 2 weeks of dietary modifications, sleep patterns will generally normalize. A decrease or complete resolution of daytime symptoms occurs, total sleep time increases to a developmentally normal level, and nocturnal awakenings resolve. Reintroduction of cow's milk protein formula will result in the exacerbation of symptoms. At times, exacerbation is severe and clinical judgment should determine whether reintroduction of the responsible protein is prudent. In general, it should be done under only rare circumstances and only under highly controlled conditions.

Otitis Media

Any condition that results in pain, discomfort, or fever may be associated with sleep disruption and sleeplessness. Otitis media is one of the most common childhood illnesses presenting to the practitioner, and acute middle ear disease rarely goes unrecognized. The cause of the child's sleep complaint is often readily apparent. In contrast, chronic middle ear disease is often present despite a paucity of clinical symptoms. Serous or secretory otitis media associated with persistent middle ear effusions may be clinically asymptomatic except for the presence of disrupted sleep.

Clinical Presentation and Diagnosis

Children with acute suppurative otitis media often present with fever, otalgia, changes in appetite, and vomiting. Frequent and prolonged nocturnal arousals, associated daytime sleepiness, and a significant decrease in daytime activity often occur. The physical exam reveals a bulging tympanic membrane, with the loss of normal landmarks and immobility of the drum on pneumo-otoscopy and/or tympanography.

Chronic serous or secretory otitis media is often associated with only a few symptoms. Hearing may be decreased; however, this may not be clinically apparent. Complaints of otalgia are often absent. The physical exam may reveal a retracted, immobile tympanic membrane. Evidence of eustachian tube dysfunction is often present, and air and/or fluid levels may be visualized. Regardless of the absence of clear clinical complaints during the day, sleep may be significantly disrupted.

Treatment

Treatment of the sleep disturbance associated with acute or chronic middle ear disease first focuses on the adequate management of the underlying pathology. Appropriate courses of antibiotic therapy for acute suppurative otitis media should result in the resolution of sleep complaints. Treatment of chronic serous or secretory otitis media and persistent middle ear effusion has included tympanocentesis, tympanotomy tube placement, chronic antibiotic therapy, and/or a combination of antibiotics and a short course of steroid treatment. Resolution of the effusion will often result in the concomitant resolution of nocturnal symptoms. During the course of medical and/or surgical therapy, appropriate attention must be paid to the principles of sleep hygiene. Sleep schedules must be regularized and parents should adhere to strict patterns of age-appropriate sleep–wake timetables.

Neurologic Disorders

Neurologically impaired children frequently awaken at night and exhibit disordered sleep–wake schedules. It has been thought that this sleep disruption may be due to chronic cerebral irritation; however, sleeplessness and night-time awakening are also reported by the parents of children with significant handicaps that are not associated with cortical irritability. Children with static encephalopathies, noncortical blindness, and deafness may exhibit significant disorders of sleep–wake cycles.

Clinical Presentation and Diagnosis

Sleep problems in children with neurologic disorders may be due to various underlying etiologies. Indeed, a child with obvious neurologic impairment may also exhibit symptoms of sleeplessness secondary to any of the other nonneurologic conditions discussed in this chapter. Therefore, the assessment of the child's sleep problem must include a comprehensive evaluation without prematurely attributing the disorder of sleep to the prominent neurologic condition. All factors that may result in sleeplessness should be considered.

The primary neurologic diagnosis is often clinically obvious. However, the characteristics of the sleep problem may be more obscure, and maintenance of a sleep diary is extremely important in evaluating the sleep–wake cycle of the neurologically impaired child. Reasonable data may be collected to differentiate a primarily behavioral etiology from one secondary to impairment of the neurologic mechanisms responsible for controlling sleep–wake cycles, sleep onset, and/or sleep maintenance. The medications used for the management of the principal neurologic condition may themselves be responsible for disordered sleep. Nocturnal polysomnography is often helpful in determining a central origin of the sleep disorder and will assist in detecting nocturnal seizure activity that may not be apparent during the day. The diagnosis of an organic basis for disordered sleep is exclusionary. Only after the comprehensive evaluation of other possible mechanisms has failed to reveal the etiology should neurologic mechanisms be considered causative.

Treatment

Treatment of sleeplessness in the neurologically impaired child is dependent on the identified underlying cause. Attention should be paid first to all the factors that may influence sleep and the sleep–wake cycle, other than the neurologic disorder. If a behavioral or parent management problem is suspected, it may be handled in the manner previously described. However, it might be necessary to conduct the therapeutic regimen more slowly than it would be in the non-neurologically impaired child. Appropriate attention should be paid to the child's sleep–wake schedule, especially in children with special sensory disorders such as blindness. The correction of these schedule abnormalities is usually not difficult and will result in the rapid improvement of sleep patterns and daytime function.

If the medication used in the treatment of the principal neurologic disorder is considered to be responsible for the sleep problem, attention should be paid to the dosage and timing of administration of the drug. Windows of time exist in which a particular medication may significantly affect circadian timekeeping mechanisms. Administration within the window will result in significant shifts of circadian rhythm, and administration of the same medication and dosage outside of the window will result in little change in pacemaker timing. Therefore, a shift in the time of administration of prescribed medications may greatly change the child's sleep–wake patterns. Under certain circumstances, the dosage of the medication may be modified to improve the child's sleep. In other situations, though less commonly, specific medications may require discontinuation with substitution of an alternative drug for improvement in sleep to occur.

In situations in which the underlying neurologic abnormality is considered the cause of sleeplessness, attention should still be paid to appropriate sleep hygiene. If an improvement in reduced sleeplessness occurs with mild medications, such as diphenhydramine, the child will most often show similar improvement without the use of drugs. Hypnotic or sedative medication is occasionally required. Chloral hydrate is often effective in the treatment of sleeplessness in children with neurologic or special sensory impairment. If medication is necessary, it is usually best to use adequate dosages. It is more appropriate to begin with a dosage schedule that is significant enough to control the symptoms rather than beginning with a small dose and slowly increasing it until a response occurs. However, in the neurologically impaired child, the development of medication resistance occurs less commonly than in children without neurologic disorders. Once medication is instituted, it is important to monitor the child's daytime function to ensure improvement. Periodic withdrawal of medication is also recommended. Once the symptoms of sleeplessness are controlled, it may be possible to discontinue the medication without exacerbation of symptoms.[39]

Attention Deficit Hyperactivity Disorder

The parents of hyperactive children consider their children to have many more sleep problems than the parents of children without hyperactivity do.[40] Most commonly, night-time awakenings and restless sleep are reported. In a study by Salzarulo and Chevalier, the parents of children with attention deficit hyperactivity disorder (ADHD) reported sleep onset problems 16.5% of the time and night-time awakenings 39% of the time.[41] The Diagnostic and Statistical Manual of Mental Disorders (Third Edition) lists motor restlessness during sleep as one of the defining characteristics of hyperactivity,[42] even though support from sleep studies is ambiguous and controversial results do exist.[43,44] It is most likely that hyperactivity and attention deficits are symptoms of a heterogeneous group of disorders with varied etiologies, manifesting increased daytime activity and disordered sleep. For example, children with obstructive sleep apnea syndrome manifest daytime symptoms that are virtually indistinguishable from those with ADHD on clinical grounds alone. Attention span problems may reflect the daytime results of sleep deprivation with the appearance of microsleep episodes. It is obvious that further investigation is necessary to determine whether dysfunctional sleep is a cause or effect of ADHD in some children.

Clinical Presentation and Diagnosis

The diagnosis of ADHD may be difficult. These children tend to be fidgety, have difficulty staying on and completing tasks, often disturb other children in school, are easily distracted, often cry easily, and have rapid mood swings. They may exhibit restlessness and increased activity. They are often easily frustrated in their efforts and

may become destructive. The physical exam is often normal, and the child may not exhibit increased activity during the clinical evaluation. Soft neurologic signs may be present in some children; however, the significance of these findings is questionable. Visual tracking may be poor and speech dysfluency may be present. Letter reversals on writing from dictation, dysdiadochokinesia with significant overflow-associated movements, difficulty hopping and skipping, and right/left confusion have also been reported with increased frequency in children with ADHD.[45,46]

Night-time awakenings and restless sleep are characteristic sleep complaints. However, there does not appear to be a difference in sleep-onset latency or total sleep time between children with ADHD and normal children. Enuresis and night sweats have also been reported more frequently in hyperactive children than in control subjects.[40] Differentiating the sleep disruption of ADHD from that of obstructive sleep apnea may be difficult. The parents of virtually all children with obstructive sleep apnea syndrome will admit that significant snoring is present. Daytime symptoms of hyperactivity may also alternate with periods of somnolence in children with obstructive sleep apnea syndrome. Traditional nocturnal polysomnography may or may not be helpful. If significant sleep-related airway obstruction is present, the polysomnogram may reveal apneas, hypopneas, oxygen desaturation, and arousals. However, in many instances the results of noninvasive sleep studies are inconclusive. Despite increased respiratory resistive load during sleep, clear-cut apneas and hypopneas may be absent. Diagnosis would then require more invasive techniques, such as continuous monitoring of intrathoracic pressure through an indwelling esophageal balloon manometer. Noninvasive techniques for continuous monitoring of intrathoracic pressure during sleep are currently being investigated.

Treatment

The appropriate treatment for ADHD is controversial and beyond the scope of this text. Stimulant medication, counseling, and behavior modification are the most widely accepted methods of therapy. Sleep problems tend to improve along with daytime symptoms despite the use of stimulants that often result in sleeplessness in children without ADHD. At the present time, how the medication functions to improve the daytime and night-time symptoms of ADHD is obscure. It is interesting to speculate on the mechanism of this paradoxical effect. First, stimulant medication may provide enough cortical stimulation to result in an alerting response. Children may then be more capable of focusing attention on the task at hand. On the other hand, if microsleep episodes are present and responsible for attention span deficits and concomitant symptoms, stimulant medication may decrease the frequency or eliminate these microsleep episodes, resulting in better attention and focus. If microsleep episodes are frequent and sleep begins to accumulate during daytime hours, nocturnal sleep may be disrupted. Administration of stimulant medication may then result in the reduction in frequency or elimination of microsleep episodes. Since daytime sleep accumulation does not take place, nocturnal sleep improves. Though engaging, these explanations are highly speculative and await documentation.

Medications

Virtually any medication may cause sleep disruption. Hypnotics are the most commonly prescribed drugs in the United States. It has become apparent that this classification of medication has generally resulted in more significant exacerbation of sleep problems than cures. Hypnotics and sedatives are often inappropriately used in children. Rarely will the use of hypnotics result in long-term improvement of sleep in children who are otherwise normal. If there is improvement initially, a behavioral approach and attention to appropriate sleep hygiene most likely would have resulted in the resolution of symptoms as well without the risk of side effects. The most commonly prescribed medications in childhood are antihistamines (which may themselves cause sleeplessness), major sedatives (such as chloral hydrate and phenobarbital; which may themselves cause paradoxical hyperactivity), and short-acting benzodiazepines. These classes of medication may also adversely affect the child's performance the next day.

Relatively innocuous medications prescribed for acute or chronic illness may also be responsible for sleeplessness. Antibiotics, especially liquid preparations, have been associated with DIMS.[39] It is thought that the vehicle and not the antibiotic itself is responsible for the sleep disruption. Over-the-counter medications, especially combination drugs, may also be implicated. Oral bronchial smooth muscle relaxant medications often cause sleep disruption, although the exact mechanism is unclear.

Clinical Presentation and Diagnosis

A comprehensive medication history should be taken from the parents. It is important to include over-the-counter medication, since the vehicle may be responsible for sleep disruption. If the child is taking medications, it is important to determine their dosage and timing of administration. The history may suggest the onset of the sleep problem commensurate with the institution of medication. Most medications do not result in any typical patterns of sleep disruption. Nocturnal settling and awakening problems may be present. Hypnotics, sedatives, and neuroleptics may cause significant changes in sleep architecture, and nocturnal polysomnography may be useful in assisting in the diagnosis. Depending on the medication, total sleep time may be decreased or shifts in sleep–wake scheduling problems may occur. Maintenance of a sleep diary for a period of two weeks may be of great value in accurately documenting the child's typical circadian sleep–wake rhythm.

Treatment

If possible, the suspected offending medication might be discontinued. If this is not possible, modification of the timing of administration and/or dosage may be attempted. Switching to a similar medication or the same medication prepared differently may be successful (e.g., changing from oral bronchodilators to inhaled preparations). At times, merely changing brands of medication will result in the resolution of the sleep problem.

Chronic Illness

Any chronic condition may contribute to persistent sleep problems. Pain or discomfort from the illness or from treatment regimens may be contributory. Disorders such as migraine cephalgia, asthma, diabetes mellitus, gastroesophageal reflux, and seizures have all been associated with sleep disturbances. The problem of sleeplessness may be directly caused by the underlying disorder or may be an indirect consequence of therapy, medication, or anxiety.

Clinical Presentation and Diagnosis

The underlying disturbance may be readily apparent or may be obscure. For example, a child whose sleep is disrupted because of pruritis associated with chronic eczematous dermatitis will most frequently have easily diagnosable signs. On the other hand, a sleepless child awakening from pain secondary to esophagitis and chronic gastroesophageal reflux may exhibit only a few findings. Likewise, chronic serous or secretory otitis media may present with only a few subjective symptoms.

However, it is often difficult to sort out which factors related to the illness are precipitating the sleep problems. Confusion regarding whether sleep disruption is caused by the primary illness, associated symptoms, the side effects of medication or therapy, or the family's and/or the child's response to the illness is frequently present. Diagnosis rests on a comprehensive history and physical exam.

Treatment

Treatment is based on management of the underlying chronic disorder, control of associated symptoms, and appropriate attention to sleep hygiene. If parental or patient anxiety about the chronic illness is suspected, appropriate supportive interventions should be recommended.

PSYCHOSOCIAL FACTORS RESULTING IN SLEEPLESSNESS

Childhood Affective Disorders

It is extremely difficult to diagnose depression in children because the clinical picture may vary depending on the child's age and developmental level.[47-49] Disrupted sleep has long been noted as part of the symptom complex. The polysomnographic characteristics seen in adult patients with affective disorders have been well defined

and reproducible. Kane and associates[47] have described a patient with childhood depression who manifested polysomnographic variables different from the adult, but similar in characteristics to adult studies when compared with normative data for children of the same age. A significant disturbance in sleep continuity was described. Early morning awakening, problems settling, and intermittent nocturnal arousals were all present. Sleep efficiency was decreased, and a stable but persistently shortened REM latency was also noted. Although the REM latency was at the lower end of normal for the patient's age, it was significantly shorter than the mean value for the patient's age group.

Stress may be associated with sleeplessness in children. Transient DIMS may be precipitated by acute life events, such as the death of a grandparent or parental marital discord. Persistent disorders of sleeplessness in the child is more likely due to parental mismanagement of transient sleeplessness caused by acute stress reactions. Another possibility is that stressful life events do not affect children directly but rather are mediated by parental affect and changes in their responsiveness and caretaking, especially during infancy, when an infant's sleep–wake organization may be affected by responsive caretaking.[50]

Depression is not just another problem but a central link between many kinds of problems, among them those that lead to depression and those that may follow.[51] Psychosocial factors identified as being associated with sleep problems may represent a parent's withdrawal of psychological attention.[52] There is evidence that an association exists between parental depressed feelings and a child's sleep problems. Depressed maternal feelings, rather than other measured psychosocial stresses, such as separation experiences, are associated with the development of sleep problems. Long-term sleep continuity problems and the association of persistent sleep problems with parental difficulty in behavior management have been reported.[14]

To determine whether the sleep problems commonly seen in pediatric practice are associated with more pervasive disturbances in the child or family, Lozoff and coworkers studied two groups of healthy children.[52] Five experiences distinguished children with sleep problems from those without them: an accident or illness in the family, an unaccustomed absence of the mother during the day, maternal depressed mood(s), sleeping in the parental bed, and the maternal attitude of ambivalence toward the child. These findings attest to the importance of sleep problems as an early childhood symptom. Bedtime conflicts and night-time awakening seem to be quantifiable, easily ascertainable behavior patterns that could alert pediatric health professionals to the existence of more pervasive disturbances in the child and family.

Night-time Fears

Childhood fears are normal. Most often they are developmentally related and are manifested in a variety of ways. Children 2 to 3 years old may exhibit aggression directed toward siblings (sibling rivalry), may fear death or the loss of a parent, or may be troubled by separation from parents and emerging socialization. The clinical presentation may vary significantly, and developmentally appropriate fears may be generally obscure. Children may complain of a fear of robbers or monsters. These fears may be manifested as frightening dreams. In general, the etiologies of nocturnal fears and nightmares are similar.[1] If these fears are extreme, excessively strict limit setting by parents will require the child to deal with these fears alone, are usually unsuccessful in resolving the sleep disturbance, and may be detrimental to the emotional health of the child.

To determine the origin of the fears that may be manifested at night and by sleep disturbances, evaluation should occur during waking hours. Evaluation and intervention by a psychologist or psychiatrist should be considered, especially if the problem has persisted for a significant period of time. If fears (and symptoms) have been present for only a short period of time, parental understanding and firm support may be all that is necessary. Positive reinforcement, progressive relaxation techniques, biofeedback, and techniques of self-control may be attempted. A change in the bedtime ritual, with the parent remaining close to the child for support and with gradual withdrawal, may be successful in some children. Others may respond well to modifications in the physical sleeping environment.

Inadequate Limit Setting

Disordered sleep secondary to inadequate limit-setting is most often seen in children during middle childhood and early adolescence. The usual complaint is one of difficulty settling at night and bedtime struggles. The child will often refuse to remain in bed and frequently even in the bedroom. Although the child is physiologically prepared for sleep, the parents give in to the child's protestations easily and are unwilling or unable to enforce night-time rituals and routines consistently. Therefore, the child does not remain in bed long enough for sleep onset to occur. The child repetitively gets out of bed and protests, the parents become disturbed, tension escalates, and the parents ultimately give in and the child's behavior is reinforced. Parents may lack knowledge regarding limit setting or be unaware that they are not appropriately setting limits for the child. Environmental factors, such as sharing a bedroom with a sibling or with parents, and/or marital discord, may contribute to sleep disruption. Parental lack of recognition of the intensity of the child's fears and the inability to provide supportive firmness in the face of the child's protestations may increase anxiety and exacerbate the problem.

Bedtime struggles in children who are not physiologically ready for sleep due to circadian rhythm disturbances or who suffer from inordinate night-time fears may present in a manner similar to that in children who do not have appropriate limits set. Clinical differentiation may be difficult, and evaluation of the family, intrafamilial relationships, and adequacy of parenting is necessary.

If inappropriate limit setting is suggested clinically, treatment should be designed to address the underlying etiology. Psychological causes and parental dysfunction should be addressed first. Parents should be counseled on mechanisms to enforce consistency and to provide *supportive* firmness. A regular bedtime ritual should be implemented and parents must be unwilling to modify the regimen, regardless of protestations by the child. Closing the door or a gate might be used to keep the child in his/her room. However, door closing must be associated with a supportive parental response, and this may be difficult if significant parental dysfunction is concomitantly present. Anger, punishment, and escalation of tension must be eliminated. Children over 3 years of age may respond to specific behavior modification techniques and negotiations using positive reinforcement for appropriate behavior and compliance with objectives of the regimen. The concepts of *persistency*, *consistency*, and *winning* should be stressed. The parents must decide who is going to win, they or the child. Parental patience and persistency are frequently less than those of the child, believing it is easier to give in to the child than to struggle. By letting the child win, the parents reinforce similar behaviors that are often manifested during waking hours as well.

CHRONOPHYSIOLOGIC FACTORS RESULTING IN SLEEPLESSNESS

Advanced Sleep Phase Syndrome

Advanced sleep phase syndrome is a less common chronophysiologic disorder resulting in sleeplessness. Total sleep time is normal; however, sleep occurs at an inappropriate time. When sleep phase is advanced, children retire and settle early and easily. Bedtime struggles are not common, and children may become cranky and disagreeable if kept awake when they are physiologically ready for sleep. Nocturnal awakenings and protestations are infrequent or absent. Parental complaints most often center around early morning awakening. The child is awake, alert, happy, and playful during early morning hours. Children with an advanced sleep phase will often go unrecognized because early bedtime and awakening time may fit well with parental schedules and cause little social interruption. School attendance and performance are rarely affected, and parents may appreciate the free time afforded to them in the evening. Maintenance of a sleep diary will greatly assist in the diagnosis.

Treatment is straightforward and a rapid response should be expected. Delaying the sleep phase is significantly easier than advancing it, since the master circadian pacemaker, under free-running, non-entrained conditions, is spontaneously delayed (usually by 1 hour for each 24-hour period). Bedtime should be gradually delayed by 30 to 60 minutes each night, depending on the developmental level of the child. Morning awakenings should remain spontaneous and will be delayed reflexively once settling is delayed. When the desired bedtime and awakening time have been achieved, they should be fixed and enforced every night (including weekends and holidays). Again, persistency and consistency are imperative for the success of the regimen. A sleep diary should be maintained during the course of treatment to objectively monitor progress.

Delayed Sleep Phase Syndrome

Delayed sleep phase syndrome is the result of a shift from the normal period of sleep to a time later than that expected or desired. The characteristics of sleep are normal, but the children sleep at the wrong times. Children are physiologically ready for sleep late in the evening, and the morning spontaneous awakening time may occur during the late morning or early afternoon hours, depending on the degree of the shift). Nocturnal awakenings do not appear to be a problem. Once the child is asleep, s/he tends to stay asleep. Parental expectations for bedtime may be quite earlier than the time the child is biologically ready for sleep, resulting in the typical complaint of sleep onset difficulties and significant bedtime struggles. Because the normal sleep period has shifted to a time later in the day, parents will usually report profound difficulties in waking up the child in the morning. The child's behavior and activity in the morning hours are quite sluggish. School performance in the morning classes may be poorer than that in the afternoon classes, and the child may fall asleep in school, especially at the beginning of the week. On weekends and holidays, when bedtime tends to be later in the evening, there are fewer struggles and the latency from "lights out" to sleep is shorter. Children suffering from delayed sleep phase syndrome tend to be sleep deprived during the week because of the early morning awakenings but catch up on the weekends. It may be difficult to differentiate delayed sleep phase syndrome from other disorders presenting with sleep onset difficulties, such as disorders of inappropriate and inconsistent limit setting. A comprehensive evaluation and maintenance of a sleep diary for 2 to 3 weeks are of great assistance in evaluating a child for sleep phase delays.

Small phase shifts in younger children are usually best treated with a controlled phase advance. The regimen should begin when the child does not have important daytime social and developmental responsibilities (i.e., school), since some degree of sleep deprivation occurs during the first few days of management. The regimen begins by initially delaying the hour of bedtime for 2 or 3 days until the child is physiologically ready for sleep and sleep onset latency is relatively normal; bedtime struggles will disappear quickly. Also at the beginning of the regimen, the morning wake-up time should be strictly fixed and maintained at an appropriate time, even on weekends and holidays. If it is developmentally appropriate, naps should be continued but prolonged naps avoided. If the child does not normally nap, daytime sleep should not be permitted, since the child may accumulate sleep during these hours at the expense of nocturnal sleep. Once the child is settling easily, the bedtime should be slowly advanced until the desired time is reached. The degree of advance should be determined by the child's tolerance and response to treatment. However, it must be remembered that the total sleep time should be commensurate with the child's age and development. Parents should be counseled regarding appropriate sleep period times at various ages and should expect realistic compliance from their child. Again, maintenance of a sleep diary will greatly assist in the assessment and monitoring of the therapeutic regimen.

Treatment of extensive sleep phase delays in adolescent patients may involve further delay of the sleep phase around the clock (moving in the direction of a free-running pacemaker) until the desired sleep and wake-up times are reached. This should be accomplished only when the youngster has no other social responsibilities, since s/he will be sleeping all day and remaining awake all night for a time. In addition, a parent may have to stay up with the youngster and phase delay with him/her in order for the regimen to succeed. This form of treatment may be extremely difficult and inappropriate for younger adolescents and prelatency children.

Exposure to intense light, especially when it occurs during windows of entrainment, may quickly shift the sleep phase to an appropriate time. This form of therapy appears promising for the adult patient, although it is still experimental. Similar trials have not been performed in children with phase shifts.

Regular but Inappropriate Sleep–Wake Schedule

Children may present with a complaint of napping too late or too early in the day. Naps may be too frequent or prolonged. Daytime sleep may also be too infrequent for the child's developmental level. Occasionally, the child complains of an inappropriately early bedtime or early morning awakenings (which appear similar to a phase advance), but significant daytime sleep also occurs, resulting in appropriate total sleep times. Although any of these symptoms may be present, they tend to be consistent and recur daily. A sleep diary for a period of 2 to 3 weeks will reveal these regularly recurring but inappropriate times of sleep.

Treatment is directed at normalization of the sleep–wake schedule. Once a regular and appropriate sleep–wake schedule is attained, sleep normalizes.

Irregular Sleep Schedule

Entrainment of circadian rhythms occurs only if appropriate zeitgebers are present and sleep–wake schedules remain constant. Inappropriate naps and schedules may result in internal desynchronization of other systems as well. In these patients, not only bedtime is disrupted but also daily living in general is chaotic and lacks formal structure. Social instability is often present. Meal times tend to be irregular from day to day, and meals may be taken by different family members at different times.

Family dysfunction must be addressed first. With little structure in the lives of all members of the household, there is little chance that structuring sleep for the child will be successful unless the entire ecology of the family is treated. Sleep should be charted regularly and appropriate schedules for meals and sleep established. Appropriate time cues must be provided, and structured wake-up times and bedtimes must be maintained in a consistent and persistent manner.

OTHER FACTORS RESULTING IN SLEEPLESSNESS

Childhood Onset of Disorders of Initiating and Maintaining Sleep

One form of primary insomnia in adults has the onset of symptoms before puberty. Some evidence may place the presence of this disorder early in infancy.[53] Sleep onset and/or sleep maintenance complaints may be present. Daytime symptoms of inadequate sleep may occur. It is difficult to differentiate this form of DIMS from others, since it may be finally diagnosed only if the sleep complaint persists through puberty and into adulthood. There seems to be no identifiable precipitating cause. Childhood-onset DIMS may also constitute a shift in the balance of the circadian pacemaker responsible for generation of the sleep–wake rhythm. The patterns of poor sleep are often more difficult to treat than the other forms of insomnia during childhood, and poor sleep tends to continue throughout both the negative and positive periods of emotional and developmental adaptation. This group is also differentiated from short sleepers by the presence of daytime symptoms of fatigue, irritability, tenseness, mild depression, difficulties in waking attention, and at times daytime sleepiness.

Short Sleeper

Although it is not typically discussed in the pediatric literature, the short sleeper is presented here because it may be genetically or congenitally determined. *Short sleeper* is the designation for an individual who consistently sleeps substantially less in a single day than the customary amount of sleep for the patient's age and developmental level.[53] Sleep, though short, is normal. There are typically no specific complaints about the quality of sleep, although the symptoms of bedtime struggles and/or early morning awakenings may occur during childhood. Daytime sleepiness, difficulty with daytime behavior, and poor performance are notably absent. True DIMS does not exist despite the occasional desire and unsuccessful attempts to sleep longer. Short sleep appears to be at one end of the normal individual sleep requirement continuum.

As previously mentioned, short sleep has been linked to reduced life expectancy. This relationship probably has its source mainly in short total sleep time patterns resulting from medical and/or other sleep pathologies and not in short sleep itself, as represented by the short sleeper.[53]

Insomnia is a symptom and not a diagnosis. The causes of insomnia are varied and range from the medical (i.e., drug-related, pain-induced, associated with primary sleep disorders such as obstructive sleep apnea) to the behavioral (i.e., associated with poor sleep hygiene or sleep onset association disorder) and are often a combination of these factors. In adults insomnia is generally defined as difficulty initiating and/or maintaining sleep and/or early morning awakening and/or nonrestorative sleep. However, the definition of insomnia or problematic sleep in children is much more challenging for a number of reasons. Clinically significant sleep problems, like many behavioral problems in childhood, may best be viewed as more loosely occurring along a continuum of severity and chronicity that ranges from a transient and self-limiting disturbance to a disorder that meets specific diagnostic criteria. Unlike strict research definitions of sleep problems, the validity of parental concerns and opinions regarding their child's sleep patterns and behaviors and the resulting stress on the family must be considered in defining sleep disturbances in a clinical context. The relative prevalence and the various types of sleep problems that occur throughout childhood must also be understood in the context of normal physical, cognitive, and emotional phenomena that are occurring at different developmental stages. Parental recognition and reporting of sleep problems in children also vary across childhood, with the parents of infants and toddlers more likely to be aware of sleep concerns than those of school-aged children and adolescents. Thus, the range of sleep behaviors that may be considered "normal" or "pathologic" is broad and the definitions are often highly subjective.

To more clearly define the clinical situations in which the use of pharmacotherapy for pediatric sleep problems might be appropriate, a consensus panel of pediatric sleep medicine specialists agreed that the development of a **consensus definition** of pediatric insomnia was a necessary and important first step. The following key components of the consensus definition were developed by the panel.

1. Pediatric insomnia may be defined as difficulty initiating or maintaining sleep that is viewed as a problem by the child or caregiver.
2. The significance of the sleep problem may be characterized by

   - its severity, chronicity, and frequency *and*
   - associated impairment in daytime function for the child or family.

3. The sleep problem may be due to a primary sleep disorder or occur in association with other sleep, medical, or psychiatric disorders.

Although prevalence rates are only approximations because the definition of difficulty initiating or maintaining sleep in children varies across studies, approximately 25% of all children are reported to experience some type of sleep problem at some point during childhood. Specific studies have reported an overall prevalence of a variety of parent-reported sleep problems ranging from 25% to 50% in pre–school-aged samples[54] to 37% in a community sample of 4 to 10 year olds[55] to up to 40% in adolescents.[56] Furthermore, sleep concerns are one of the most frequent parental complaints in pediatric practices, reported as the fifth leading concern of parents after illness, feeding, behavior problems, and physical abnormalities.[57]

Although these sleep disturbances are transient in many children, there is considerable evidence that sleep problems may persist or recur in a substantial percentage of them.[7,8] In addition to their high prevalence and chronicity, recent evidence also suggests that sleep disorders may have significant short- and long-term consequences on children's academic and social functioning and on their health.[9,10] A wealth of empirical evidence from several lines of research clearly indicates that children and adolescents experience significant daytime sleepiness as a result of inadequate or disturbed sleep and that significant performance impairment and mood dysfunction are associated with daytime sleepiness. Higher-level cognitive functions, such as cognitive flexibility and abstract thinking/reasoning, seem to be particularly sensitive to the effects of disturbed or insufficient sleep. Finally, the health outcomes of inadequate sleep include

an increase in accidental injuries (ranging from minor injuries to drowsy driving–related motor vehicle fatalities) and the potentially deleterious effects on the cardiovascular, immune, and various metabolic systems, such as glucose metabolism and endocrine function. Sleep problems are also a significant source of distress for families and may be one of the primary reasons for caregiver stress in those families with children who have chronic medical illnesses or severe neurodevelopmental delays.

SCREENING FOR SLEEP PROBLEMS

A number of studies have suggested that screening for sleep problems in pediatric practice is inadequate and may result in significant underdiagnosis of sleep disorders. For example, in a recent survey of over 600 community-based pediatricians, over 20% of the respondents did not routinely screen for sleep problems in school-aged children in the context of the well-child visit, and less than 40% questioned adolescents directly about their own sleep habits. Recognizing this gap, the task force recommended that all children be regularly screened for sleep problems in pediatric clinical practice. One simple sleep-screening algorithm is **BEARS** (**B**edtime problems, **E**xcessive daytime sleepiness, **A**wakenings at night, **R**egularity and duration of sleep, **S**noring. The key areas of inquiry that are included in the BEARS screening for sleep problems in children and adolescents are (1) bedtime resistance and delayed sleep onset; (2) frequent and/or prolonged night-time awakenings; (3) regularity, pattern, and duration of sleep; (4) snoring and other symptoms of sleep-disordered breathing; (5) sleep-related anxiety behaviors (e.g., nightmares, night-time fears); and (6) excessive daytime sleepiness (e.g., difficulty awakening in the morning, naps). A number of other brief parent and self-reporting sleep survey tools have also been developed that can facilitate the screening process and yield important information about the nature and severity of any coexisting sleep complaints.

EVALUATION OF SLEEP COMPLAINTS

The clinical evaluation of a child presenting with a sleep problem involves a careful medical history to assess the potential medical causes of sleep disturbances, such as allergies, concomitant medications, and acute or chronic pain conditions. A developmental history is important because of the aforementioned frequent association of sleep problems with severe developmental delay. Assessment of the child's current level of functioning (e.g., school, home) is key in evaluating the possible mood, behavioral, and neurocognitive sequelae of sleep problems. Current sleep patterns, including the usual sleep duration and sleep–wake schedule, are often best assessed with a sleep diary, in which parents record daily sleep behaviors for an extended period. A review of sleep habits, such as bedtime routines, daily caffeine intake, and the sleeping environment (e.g., temperature, noise level) may reveal environmental factors that contribute to the sleep problems. The use of additional diagnostic tools such as polysomnographic evaluation are seldom warranted for the routine evaluation of pediatric insomnia but may be appropriate if organic sleep disorders such as obstructive sleep apnea or periodic limb movements are suspected.

Finally, referral to a sleep specialist for diagnosis and/or treatment should be considered under the following circumstances: children or adolescents with persistent or severe bedtime issues that are not responsive to simple behavioral measures or are extremely disruptive; children or adolescents with parasomnias who also present with symptoms of another underlying sleep disrupter (e.g., sleep disordered breathing) or for whom pharmacologic treatment is being considered; children with associated medical, psychiatric, and/or developmental conditions that create additional management challenges; and children and adolescents with circadian rhythm disorders.

Currently, there are no medications approved by the Food and Drug Administration for the treatment of difficulty initiating and/or maintaining sleep in the pediatric population. Although it is clear that the ideal pediatric hypnotic medication does not exist, the task force members agreed that it was important to consider the characteristics that would be present in the optimum clinical situation to allow the practitioner to compare the pharmacologic options that are currently available. The pharmacokinetic properties of the ideal pediatric hypnotic would include the high oral bioavailability, a property that encompasses solubility, rapid absorption, stability, and invulnerability to extensive first-pass metabolism by the liver and/or the gut to ensure rapid, consistent, and reliable clinical responses and allow appropriate dosages to be accurately predicted. Metabolism should be to inactive products or active metabolites with short half-lives that are no longer than that of the parent compound to minimize the metabolite-associated side effects. Elimination half-life should be short (2 to 3 hours).

Pharmacodynamic properties would include a rapid onset of effect, preferably within 30 minutes, so that it could be administered shortly before bedtime and a duration of action that would be sufficiently long so that only once nightly dosing is necessary but not excessively long so as to avoid residual daytime sedation. There should also be no associated rebound, tolerance, or withdrawal and only a few side effects—preferably the tolerability profile of placebo—with little or no potential for drug–drug interactions. The ideal hypnotic should also not affect sleep architecture because changes in slow-wave sleep, for example, might lead to alterations in hormone levels such as human growth hormone.[35] Finally, the medication should be available in a palatable oral liquid as well as a tablet/capsule formulation.

Disorders of Sleep Onset Associations

Treatment

The discussion of a variety of treatment modalities along with their essential components is provided in the following sections.

DIET AND LIFESTYLE

- Treatment for this disorder and most other disorders associated with the problem of sleeplessness in childhood involves implementation of the principles of sleep hygiene.
- The sleeping environment should be quiet and dark.
- Morning awakening time should be firmly fixed and consistently enforced. It is the most powerful time for the entrainment of the sleep–wake cycle.
- Bedtime should be firmly enforced. However, some flexibility must be allowed for a normal family lifestyle.

- Environmental temperatures should remain at a comfortable level, generally less than 75° F. Excessively hot temperatures can disturb sleep continuity.
- Hunger at bedtime should be avoided by the provision of a small bedtime snack.
- Excessive bedtime and nocturnal fluids should be avoided.
- Children must learn to fall asleep on their own, without parental intervention. Infants and children should be placed in their cribs or beds in a drowsy but awake state at the beginning of their nocturnal sleep period.
- Vigorous activity should be avoided for 1 to 2 hours before bedtime. Baths are stimulating for children and should be moved to the morning hours if there are problems settling at the beginning of the nocturnal sleep period.
- Food or beverages containing caffeine (or other methylxanthines) should be avoided for several hours before bedtime. Common foods and beverages containing caffeine include but are not limited to colas, chocolate, tea, and coffee.
- A variety of medications contain alcohol (elixirs) or caffeine and should be avoided for several hours before bedtime.
- Naps should be developmentally appropriate. Prolonged naps close to the desired bedtime and naps taken too frequently should be avoided.
- A faded-response program is typically the most reliable method to change sleep onset associations and assist the child in learning to fall asleep without the need for parental intervention.[16] Faded response requires work on the parents' part. A resolution tends to occur rapidly if caretakers are persistent and consistent with the intervention.
- Since the sleeping environment must be safe and secure, the youngster needs to be assured that s/he can get his/her parents if needed. But s/he should not need his/her parents in order to fall asleep.
- The youngster should be allowed to protest for a developmentally appropriate period of time before the parents respond. Once the protestation reaches this developmentally determined time limit, the parents respond and calm down the child. Once s/he is calm but awake, they should again leave the room and allow the child to protest slightly longer before they respond. Each intervention should result in the child being calm, in bed, and awake when the parent leaves the sleeping environment.
- This process should be continued until the child is asleep. Several hours of repeated interventions may be required during the initial few nights of treatment. Parents should be prepared for this and understand that if they are consistent and persistent, the problem will be resolved quickly.

PHARMACOLOGIC TREATMENT

- Pharmacologic treatment is not indicated.

INTERVENTIONAL PROCEDURES

- Other interventions, such as environmental manipulation (rearranging the bedroom), night-lights, white noise, and other safe transitional objects, may be used in combination with sleep hygiene and faded response.

ASSISTANCE DEVICES

- White-noise generators, sound machines, and continuous-playing compact disc players may assist in masking environmental noise that may result in nocturnal awakening.

OTHER TREATMENTS

- Other behavior modification techniques have been used. Permitting the child to "cry it out" has been recommended; this can be successful for some children but is often very difficult for the child and the family. As previously noted, security is quite important and permissive for sleep onset to occur. Anxiety related to an inability to alert parents to illness, pain, or other discomfort may create other sleep-related problems and settling difficulties.
- The treatment goal for excessive and repetitive nocturnal fluid intake is to gradually wean the youngster from the fluids at night. Abruptly discontinuing the fluids may be difficult and can create ongoing sleep maintenance problems.
- Weaning from a bottle is often quick and simple. The volume of fluid is decreased by ¼ to ½ oz every night until there is a minimum amount in the bottle. If the child has difficulty with this level of reduction in fluid intake, the decrease may occur more slowly (e.g., every other night, every third night).
- The child should not be permitted to fall asleep with the bottle.

- Once a minimum amount of fluid has been ingested, switching to a pacifier may be attempted.
- Weaning from breast-feeding, when associated with excessive nocturnal fluids, may be somewhat more difficult, but attention to the time spent nursing or switching to nocturnal feeding with a bottle and then weaning (as mentioned above) might be considered. Nurturing may still be provided, but care must be taken not to establish the nursing activity as a sleep onset association. The nursing mother is the best suited to assess this need. If the nursing period at night is considerably different, less vigorous, and shorter than diurnal feedings, the nursing may have developed into a sleep onset association. The child should not be permitted to fall asleep at the breast and should be placed in the desired sleeping environment in a drowsy but awake state.

Neurologic Disorders

Treatment

Treatment of problem sleeplessness in the neurologically challenged child depends on the identified underlying etiology. All of the factors that influence sleeplessness and affect the sleep–wake cycle require attention. If behavioral or parental management of the sleeplessness is suspected, it may be managed by attention to appropriate sleep hygiene. However, it might be necessary to conduct the therapeutic regimen more slowly than it would be in a non-neurologically impaired child. Appropriate attention should be paid to the child's sleep–wake schedule, circadian rhythm, and time cues, which are particularly important for children with impairments of special senses (e.g., blindness). Correction of these schedule abnormalities is usually not difficult and rapidly improves sleep patterns and daytime function.

Pharmacologic Treatment

Pharmacologic treatment is often required in children with neurologic challenges. Treatment may be for the short or long term and may be influenced by significant comorbidity. The most common pharmacologic agents used for problem sleeplessness in children with neurologic challenges are listed below.[17–19]

- Diphenhydramine
  - Standard dosage: 2 to 6 years of age, 12.5 to 25 mg at bedtime; 6 to 12 years of age, 25 mg at bedtime; over 12 years of age, 25 to 50 mg at bedtime.
  - Contraindications: Narrow-angle glaucoma, gastrointestinal or genitourinary obstruction.
  - Main drug interactions: May interact with antihypertensive or antidepressant medications; increased sedation when combined with alcohol.
  - Main side effects: Nervousness, dizziness, hypertension, excitability, and drowsiness.
  - Special points: Over-the-counter preparations are often combined with other medications (e.g., pseudoephedrine) as decongestants. Elixirs contain 5% to 6% alcohol. Multiple preparations are available. Patients' parents should be instructed to read the medication label before purchase and administration.
- Chloral hydrate
  - Standard dosage: Sedation and anxiety, 25 to 50 mg/kg (oral or rectal) every 8 hours, with a maximum of 500 mg; Hypnotic, one dose 50 mg/kg (oral or rectal), with a maximum of 2 g.
  - Contraindications: Hypersensitivity to chloral hydrate; hepatic or renal impairment; gastritis or ulcers; severe cardiac disease.
  - Main drug interactions: May potentiate the effects of warfarin, CNS depressants, and alcohol; concomitant intravenous administration of furosemide may result in flushing, diaphoresis, and blood pressure changes.
  - Main side effects: Disorientation, excitement, dizziness, fever, headache, ataxia, rash, urticaria, gastric irritation with nausea, vomiting, or diarrhea; respiratory depression when combined with other sedatives or narcotics.
  - Special points: Patients develop tolerance to the hypnotic effects, so chloral hydrate is not recommended for use for longer than 2 weeks; taper dosage to avoid withdrawal with prolonged use.
- Imipramine
  - Standard dosage: Imipramine is typically used for the treatment of various forms of depression, often in conjunction with psychotherapy, and enuresis in children and has been used as an analgesic for certain chronic

and neuropathic pain. Hypnotic doses have not been clearly delineated. Depression, 1.5 mg/kg/day, with dosage increments of 1 mg/kg every 3 to 4 days; maximum dose is 5 mg/kg/day in 1 to 4 divided doses. Enuresis, 10 to 25 mg at bedtime.

- Contraindications: Hypersensitivity to imipramine (cross-sensitivity to other tricyclic antidepressants may occur); patients receiving monoamine oxidase inhibitors within the past 14 days; narrow-angle glaucoma.
- Main drug interactions: May decrease or reverse the effects of guanethidine and clonidine; may increase the effects of CNS depressants, adrenergic agents, anticholinergic agents, and alcohol; hyperpyrexia, tachycardia, hypertension, seizures, and death may occur with monoamine oxidase inhibitors; similar interactions with other tricyclic antidepressants may occur.
- Main side effects: Drowsiness, confusion, dizziness, fatigue, anxiety, nervousness, seizures, rash, photosensitivity, nausea, vomiting, constipation, dry mouth, decreased appetite; urinary retention, blood dyscrasia, hepatitis, blurred vision, increased intraocular pressure, weakness, and hypersensitivity reactions.
- Special points: Do not discontinue abruptly in patients receiving long-term, high-dose therapy; use with caution in patients with cardiovascular disease, conduction disturbances, seizure disorders, urinary retention, anorexia, or hyperthyroidism or those receiving thyroid replacement.

- Hydroxyzine
  - Standard dosage: 0.5 mg/kg orally 30 minutes before bedtime.
  - Contraindications: Hypersensitivity to hydroxyzine or any of its components.
  - Main drug interactions: May potentiate other CNS depressants or anticholinergics and can antagonize the vasopressor effects of epinephrine.
  - Main side effects: Hypotension, dizziness, headache, ataxia, dry mouth, urinary retention, and weakness.
  - Special points: Competes with histamine for H1-receptor sites on effector cells in the gastrointestinal tract, blood vessels, and respiratory tract.

- Diazepam
  - Standard dosage: 0.04 to 0.25 mg/kg at bedtime.
  - Contraindications: Hypersensitivity to benzodiazepines; should not be used in patients with preexisting CNS depression, respiratory depression, narrow-angle glaucoma, or severe and uncontrolled pain.
  - Main drug interactions: Inducers of cytochrome P_{450} 2c may increase the metabolism of diazepam. There is increased toxicity in the presence of CNS depressants. Cimetidine may decrease the metabolism of diazepam. Cisapride can significantly increase diazepam levels. Valproic acid may displace diazepam from binding sites, which may result in an increase in sedative effects. Selective serotonin reuptake inhibitors (e.g., fluoxetine, sertraline, paroxetine) have greatly increased diazepam levels by altering clearance.
  - Main side effects: Drowsiness, confusion, dizziness, amnesia, slurred speech, ataxia, paradoxical excitement, blurred vision, decreased respiratory rate, and apnea.
  - Special points: Depresses all levels of the CNS, including the limbic system and reticular formation. Benzodiazepines must be used with caution in the presence of other CNS depressants and also in patients with CNS lesions that affect the brainstem and respiratory centers.

- Clonazepam
  - Standard dosage: Start at 0.01 mg/kg at bedtime. Maximum dose should not exceed 0.025 mg/kg.
  - Contraindications: Hypersensitivity to clonazepam or other benzodiazepines; severe liver disease and acute narrow-angle glaucoma.
  - Main drug interactions: Concomitant use with other CNS depressants will increase sedation; phenytoin and barbiturates increase clearance of clonazepam.
  - Main side effects: Changes in behavior and personality, dizziness, headache, memory impairment, decreased concentration, hangover effect, and paradoxical insomnia.
  - Special points: Clonazepam-induced behavioral problems may be more frequent in children with mental handicaps; when discontinuing treatment, taper slowly.

- Lorazepam
  - Standard dosage: 0.05 mg/kg at bedtime.
  - Contraindications: Hypersensitivity to benzodiazepines; should not be used in patients with preexisting CNS depression, respiratory depression, narrow-angle glaucoma, or severe and uncontrolled pain.
  - Main drug interactions: Other CNS or respiratory center depressants may increase the adverse effects of lorazepam.
  - Main side effects: Drowsiness, lethargy, hangover effect, dizziness, transitory hallucinations, and ataxia.
  - Special points: Use with caution in patients with hepatic or renal impairment. Care should be taken when used in patients with compromised pulmonary function.
- Clonidine
  - Standard dosage: Initial dosage is 2.5 to 5 µg/kg at bedtime.
  - Contraindications: Hypersensitivity to clonidine hydrochloride or any component.
  - Main drug interactions: Tricyclic antidepressants antagonize the hypotensive effects of clonidine. Beta-blocking agents may potentiate bradycardia, and withdrawal may result in rebound hypertension. CNS depressants and alcohol may increase the sedative effects.
  - Main side effects: Palpitations, drowsiness, sedation, headache, insomnia, anxiety, depression, rash, constipation, and fatigue.
  - Special points: Clonidine is a very potent REM sleep suppressant. On abrupt withdrawal, there is considerable REM sleep rebound.
- Melatonin
  - Standard dosage: There are only a few well controlled studies of the use of melatonin in children. Typical doses have ranged from 0.5 mg to 10 mg taken 1 to 5 hours before bedtime.[20]
  - Contraindications: None.
  - Main drug interactions: None.
  - Main side effects: One report has shown an increase in seizure activity in children with significant neurologic conditions and seizures.[21] No other significant side effects have been reported.
  - Special points: Many over-the-counter preparations may contain other ingredients. Since formulations are proprietary, other ingredients may not be known. Pure synthetic melatonin is not soluble in water, and liquid preparations may contain 7% to 13% alcohol.

INTERVENTIONAL PROCEDURES

In some patients with hypertonicity, decreasing muscle tone may result in improved sleep. Medication used to decrease tone and spasticity may result in more consolidated sleep.

Surgical interventions are not specific to the child's sleep-related disorder; they are aimed at improvement of the underlying neurologic condition (e.g., tendon release in spastic quadriplegia, posterior fossa decompression in patients with Chiari II malformations). A beneficial effect on sleep is secondary to improvement in the youngster's underlying condition.

Approaches to the child with underlying neurologic conditions are similar to those used in other youngsters. White-noise devices or sound generators, compact disc players, night-lights, and other assistance devices may be used for problem sleeplessness in children with neurologic disorders.

PHYSICAL/SPEECH THERAPY AND EXERCISE

Physical therapy and functional improvement may also ameliorate problem sleeplessness. Brushing or combing for 15 to 20 minutes before bedtime may be helpful for youngsters with sensory integration problems. A soft brush is rhythmically stroked directly on the skin of the arms, legs, chest, abdomen, and back. Brushing may be done 2 to 3 times per day and should cease before sleep onset so that it will not become a sleep onset association.

Advanced Sleep Phase Syndrome

Treatment

DIET AND LIFESTYLE

- Increase early evening activity and bathe the child before the desired bedtime.
- Increase environmental light exposure during the late afternoon and early evening hours. Decrease environmental light exposure during the early morning hours.
- Bedtime may be delayed from 30 minutes to 2 hours, depending on the child's age and developmental level.
- If it is developmentally appropriate, provide a brief mid-afternoon nap.

PHARMACOLOGIC TREATMENT

In adults, 0.5 to 10 mg of melatonin taken after 4:00 AM or at the time of morning sleep offset has been recommended. Similar data in children are lacking, and it is unclear whether melatonin has a place in the treatment of advanced sleep phase syndrome in children.

Delayed Sleep Phase Syndrome

Treatment

The therapeutic components constituting diet and lifestyle as well as pharmacology in the treatment and management of delayed sleep phase syndrome are discussed below.

Diet and Lifestyle

- Small phase shifts are typically best treated with a controlled phase advance. The regimen should begin when the child does not have important daytime responsibilities, since some degree of sleep deprivation will occur.
- The regimen begins by delaying the hour of bedtime for 2 to 3 days to a point at which the child is physiologically ready for sleep. If there is significant stimulation during the evening before bedtime, this should be minimized and switched to the morning hours.
- Watching television before bedtime should be avoided. Television programming requires the child to delay sleep onset in order to finish watching the show. Videotapes that may be stopped and restarted may help.
- Exposure to bright light in the evening and at around bedtime should be avoided. Bright light and stimulation from computer games and activities may both result in delayed sleep onset.
- Morning awakening time should be firmly fixed. It should not vary by more than 1 to 1.5 hours on school days, weekends, and holidays.
- Exposure to bright light in the morning may assist in the slow advance of the sleep phase. Bright light may be provided through a variety of phototherapy devices or exposure to sunlight. Bright computer screens surrounded by other lamps may also provide the intensity of light required for assisting in the advance of the sleep phase.

- If it is developmentally appropriate, naps should continue but prolonged naps should be avoided.
- If the child does not normally nap, daytime sleep should be avoided.
- Once the youngster is settling easily, the bedtime may be slowly advanced until its desired time is reached. The child's tolerance and response to treatment should determine the degree of advance.
- Total sleep time should remain appropriate to the child's age and development.
- Parental expectations should be realistic.
- Occasionally, large phase delays in adolescents may be managed by a continuous (around-the-clock) phase delay.

PHARMACOLOGIC TREATMENT

- Melatonin has been used for the short term in adults with delayed sleep phase syndrome and has been reported to aid in the achievement of and adherence to a new sleep schedule. In addition, chronic use may assist in maintaining the schedule. Nonetheless, no data are similarly available in children.
- Over-the-counter hypnotics and sedatives as well as prescription medication have not been shown to be effective in the long-term resolution of delayed sleep phase syndrome.

Non–24-Hour Sleep–Wake Schedule

Treatment

This sleep-related disorder is more common in sightless children. It is also common in children with middle fossa tumors both before and after surgical and/or radiologic intervention.

- Begin and maintain a firm sleep–wake schedule.
- Morning awakening time should be firmly fixed.
- Providing sufficient and powerful time cues is essential in assisting entrainment to a 24-hour sleep–wake cycle.
- Caffeine-containing food and beverages should be avoided after 2:00 PM.

PHARMACOLOGIC TREATMENT

- Melatonin 0.5 to 10 mg may be taken 1 to 4 hours before the desired bedtime.
- Vitamin B_{12} has been reported to be helpful in some adult patients. Doses range from 0.5 to 3 mg per day.

Primary Insomnia in Childhood

Treatment

- Treatment is centered on the institution of a comprehensive program of sleep hygiene and appropriate attention to sleep–wake patterns across the 24-hour continuum.
- The sleeping environment should be quiet and dark.
- Morning awakening time should be firmly fixed and consistently enforced.
- Bedtime should be firmly enforced.
- The environmental temperature should remain at a comfortable level.
- Hunger at bedtime should be avoided by the provision of a small bedtime snack.
- Excessive fluids before bedtime should be avoided.
- Children must learn to fall asleep on their own, without parental intervention.
- Vigorous activity should be avoided for 1 to 2 hours before bedtime.
- Food or beverages containing caffeine (or other methylxanthines) should be avoided for several hours before bedtime.
- A variety of medications contain alcohol (elixirs) and should be avoided for several hours before bedtime.
- Naps should be developmentally appropriate.
- Appropriate parental expectations should be established. These expectations should be based on principles related to the ontogeny of the sleep–wake cycle.
- Some children require less sleep than others. The timing of the nocturnal sleep period should be coincident with the youngster's normal sleep requirements.
- Behavioral approaches should be attempted before other interventions.
- When behavioral interventions fail to resolve problem sleeplessness, assessment of the parents' or caretakers' ability to comply with the therapeutic protocol is warranted.
- When compliance fails, more intensive behavioral and family counseling may be indicated.

Pharmacologic Treatment

General recommendations for the use of medications in pediatric insomnia:

- Since the ideal pediatric hypnotic does not currently exist, rational treatment selection should be based on the clinician's judgment of the *best possible match* between the clinical circumstances (e.g., type of sleep problem, patient characteristics) and the individual properties of currently available drugs (e.g., onset and duration of action, safety, tolerability). This principle presumes some degree of clinician familiarity with the pharmacologic profile of the available sedatives/hypnotics currently available for use in the pediatric population.
- Treatment must be *diagnostically driven* and based on a careful clinical evaluation of the symptoms and consideration of all possible differential diagnoses. It is incumbent upon the clinician to choose the most appropriate pharmacologic and/or behavioral therapies based on the actual diagnosis rather than the symptom complex. For example, sleep initiation insomnia may be due to a primarily behavioral sleep disorder (e.g., limit-setting sleep disorder), a physiologically based sleep disorder (e.g., restless legs syndrome, delayed sleep phase syndrome), or a combination of these two disorders (e.g., psychophysiologic insomnia), each necessitating a different treatment approach.
- Sleep problems in infants and very young children are almost always related to developmental asynchrony between the child's sleep development and parental expectations (e.g., the development of nocturnal-diurnal sleep–wake rhythms, "sleeping through the night"). Therefore, medication is rarely if ever indicated in this age group.
- In almost all cases, medication is *not* the first treatment choice nor the sole treatment strategy. Medication use, except for very self-limiting circumstances such as travel, should be viewed only within the context of a more comprehensive treatment plan.
- Medication should always be used *in combination* with nonpharmacologic strategies (e.g., behavioral interventions, parent education). This is analogous to a number of other conditions in children, such as attention deficit hyperactivity disorder (ADHD), in which a combination of pharmacologic and behavioral strategies are often superior to drug treatment alone.
- Before consideration of pharmacologic treatment, *sleep hygiene* should always be optimized. All sleep disorders in children may be

exacerbated by poor sleep habits, such as excessive caffeine use and irregular sleep-wake schedules, which must be addressed before medication is recommended.

- Treatment goals should be realistic, clearly defined, and discussed with and agreed upon by the family before treatment is initiated. In addition, there must be a clear plan for the followup and reassessment of therapeutic goals. In particular, the parental expectations regarding the degree of amelioration of the sleep problem by medication and the anticipated duration of drug treatment should be clearly established.
- Medication should be used only for the short term; no prescription refills should be given without reassessment of the target symptoms and assessment of patient compliance with both pharmacologic and behavioral management.
- Adolescents should be screened for alcohol/drug use and pregnancy before the initiation of therapy. Many recreational substances may have synergistic clinical effects when combined with sedatives/hypnotics. In addition, hypnotics with high toxicity levels in overdose should be used with extreme caution in situations in which there is any risk of nonaccidental overdose.
- Patients should also be screened for the concurrent use of self-initiated nonprescription sleep medications (e.g., Excedrin PM, melatonin, herbals). Some of these medications have similar ingredients (e.g., diphenhydramine is the soporific ingredient in both Benadryl and Tylenol PM); while generally viewed by parents as safe, the potential drug–drug interactions between most herbal preparations and sedatives/hypnotics are largely unknown.
- Medication selection, particularly in terms of duration of action, should be *appropriate to the presenting complaint*—that is, for problems with sleep onset, a shorter-acting medication is generally desirable. For problems with sleep maintenance, longer-acting medications may be considered but are more likely to result in "hangover" effects the following morning.
- All medications should be used with caution and monitored closely for efficacy and side effects. Since there are so few data on the safety and efficacy of these medications in children, a conservative approach similar to that which should be exercised with any pediatric off-label drug use is warranted.

- There are potential indications for hypnotic use in otherwise normal children (generally short-term).
- The safety or welfare of the child is threatened—for example, the parent is overwhelmed and/or unable to implement nonpharmacologic interventions. Because of their rapid onset of action, in this situation medications may assist in "breaking the cycle" and allow for the implementation of effective behavioral strategies.
- There is a failure of, or an inability to comply with, an adequate trial of accepted nonpharmacologic and/or behavioral treatment, for example, the older child or adolescent with psychophysiologic insomnia who fails to respond to standard behavioral management tools such as stimulus control and sleep restriction.
- Medication is used as an adjunct to sleep hygiene and/or chronotherapy in circadian rhythm disturbances, for example, in an otherwise normal adolescent with delayed sleep phase syndrome.
- The insomnia occurs in the setting of medical illness with associated issues, including pain control, concomitant medications, and hospitalization, for example, a child on steroids for chronic illness.
- The insomnia occurs in the context of an acute stressor, for example, a death in the family.
- The insomnia occurs or is anticipated in the context of travel, for example, a prolonged plane ride with an accompanying time change.

Contraindications to hypnotic use in otherwise normal children:

- The insomnia occurs in the presence of untreated sleep-disordered breathing, for example, obstructive sleep apnea. Not only is hypnotic medication often inappropriate for treating the underlying condition but also sedatives with respiratory depressant properties (e.g., chloral hydrate) may be dangerous in the situation of a comorbid sleep-related breathing disorder.
- The insomnia is due to developmentally based normal sleep behavior; for example, there are inappropriate expectations from the parents or practitioner regarding the child's sleep behavior.
- The insomnia is due to a self-limiting condition that temporarily results in night-time awakenings, for example, teething.

- There are potential drug interactions with concurrent medications (e.g., opiates) or unrecognized substance abuse or alcohol use.
- There is a limited ability to follow up with and monitor the patient; for example, the parent frequently misses scheduled appointments.

PHARMACOLOGIC TREATMENT OF PEDIATRIC INSOMNIA IN CHILDREN WITH SPECIAL NEEDS

Sleep disturbances are a prominent part of the morbidity of neurobehavioral, psychiatric, and chronic medical conditions. Whether it is the primary condition or is secondary to the chronic condition, pediatric insomnia may contribute to the exacerbation of these conditions and have an adverse impact on the quality of life for the child and family. Children with chronic medical and developmental conditions are particularly prone to insomnia because of the unique combinations of family stresses, caregiver interactions, social (peer) relationships, medical needs, sedating or activating medications, physical challenges, and psychiatric morbidity. For example, the factors common to many medical conditions that can also create or exacerbate insomnia include pain, pruritis, cough, abnormal movements, and other disturbances. The physician must consider each of these potential factors, realizing that several may coexist and frustrate therapeutic interventions.

Because the neural and cognitive requisites to develop and express most sleep symptoms are basic, children with chronic medical and developmental conditions are susceptible to the same emotional, behavioral, medical, and circadian sleep disorders as normal children. Therefore, these common causes of insomnia should be considered first in children with chronic health conditions and developmental disabilities and treated appropriately. As is the case with normal children, it is preferable to identify and control the underlying process that creates a sleep disturbance instead of simply prescribing symptomatic therapy for insomnia. However, sleeplessness may overshadow other indicators of primary medical and psychiatric disorders and thus appear to arise de novo in an otherwise healthy child. For example, insomnia is often a presenting symptom of many psychiatric disorders, such as depression, post-traumatic stress disorder, and generalized anxiety disorder. If they are not carefully sought, other symptoms of psychi-atric and medical conditions may be missed and an opportunity to eliminate the basis of the insomnia would be lost.

Children with neurologic injury and specific genetic, psychiatric, and behavioral syndromes and conditions are particularly susceptible to specific types of insomnia. Examples include autism and pervasive developmental disorder, blindness (circadian rhythm disorders), Smith-Magenis syndrome (severe insomnia), Williams syndrome (periodic limb movement disorder), Rett syndrome (prolonged sleep onset latency, sleep fragmentation), and Tourette's syndrome (increased nocturnal movements and awakenings). Children with attention deficit hyperactivity disorder are often reported by parents to have sleep onset difficulties and restless sleep and present one of the more common chronic conditions for which sedatives are recommended by pediatric practitioners. Children with asthma and atopy, renal failure, and epilepsy are also highly prone to sleep disruption related to the underlying chronic condition and/or medication. Thus, the physician may be guided by the literature relevant to the specific diagnosis.

The approach to insomnia in children with underlying medical or developmental conditions must take into account the expected efficacy in light of a patient's behavioral strengths and challenges, the capabilities and needs of families and caregivers, health care priorities or urgencies that may temporarily supersede long-term interests, and the impact of insomnia therapy on underlying medical conditions and concurrent medications. For example, a teenager with mild mental retardation might not be able to take a hypnotic in a reliable manner; a family in crisis may need the rapid effect of a hypnotic until behavioral interventions take effect; and melatonin has the potential to lower the seizure threshold in a child with an underlying seizure disorder. In addition, because of frequent concurrent use of other medications and the idiosyncratic response that these children may have to sedatives/hypnotics, extreme caution should be exercised with regard to the choice of medication and monitoring of side effects.

Therefore, the task force recommends that the specific history about the quality of sleep be an integral part of the evaluation and maintenance care of children with chronic medical and/or mental health conditions. Pharmacologic therapy should be considered for sleep problems as a part of the overall management strategy in conjunction with behavioral therapy and sleep hygiene. Sleep problems in these children should be managed aggressively to avoid exacerbation of the underlying condition and improve the overall quality of life; a longer duration of drug therapy is often necessary. Consultation with a pediatric neurologist, developmental/behavioral pediatrician, and/or sleep specialist is often warranted.

- Pharmacologic management of primary insomnia in childhood is rarely indicated. Behavioral management is indicated in almost all cases. Nevertheless, certain situations exist that justify pharmacologic treatment in some cases of primary childhood insomnia. These situations include those children with developmental delays, neurologic problems, and sensory integration issues.
- Pharmacologic management may also be indicated in some situations in which childhood problem sleeplessness is the primary and underlying cause of family dysfunction.
- Once the situation indicates pharmacologic management, treatment should be for the short term (<3 weeks).
- Pharmacologic management must be used in conjunction with other behavioral/family interventions that should continue beyond the limited use of medication.

The most common medications used for this limited purpose are listed below.

- Diphenhydramine
  - Standard dosage: 2 to 6 years of age, 12.5 to 25 mg at bedtime; 6 to 12 years of age, 25 mg at bedtime; over 12 years of age, 25 to 50 mg at bedtime.
  - Contraindications: Narrow-angle glaucoma, gastrointestinal or genitourinary obstruction.
  - Main drug interactions: May interact with antihypertensive or antidepressant medications; increased sedation when combined with alcohol.
  - Main side effects: Nervousness, dizziness, hypertension, excitability, and drowsiness.
  - Special points: Over-the-counter preparations are often combined with other medications (e.g., pseudoephedrine) as decongestants. Elixirs contain 5% to 6% alcohol. Multiple preparations are available. The patients'

parents should be instructed to read the medication label before purchase and administration.
  - Cost-effectiveness: 25 mg capsules, $0.03; 12.5 mg elixir, $0.13 per teaspoon.
- Hydroxyzine
  - Standard dosage: 0.5 mg/kg orally 30 minutes before bedtime.
  - Contraindications: Hypersensitivity to hydroxyzine or any of its components.
  - Main drug interactions: May potentiate other CNS depressants or anticholinergics, and can antagonize the vasopressor effects of epinephrine.
  - Main side effects: Hypotension, dizziness, headache, ataxia, dry mouth, urinary retention, and weakness.
  - Special points: Competes with histamine for H1-receptor sites on effector cells in the gastrointestinal tract, blood vessels, and respiratory tract.
- Lorazepam
  - Standard dosage: 0.05 mg/kg at bedtime.
  - Contraindications: Hypersensitivity to benzodiazepines; should not be used in patients with preexisting CNS depression, respiratory depression, narrow-angle glaucoma, or severe and uncontrolled pain.
  - Main drug interactions: Other CNS or respiratory center depressants may increase the adverse effects of lorazepam.
  - Main side effects: Drowsiness, lethargy, hangover effect, dizziness, transitory hallucinations, and ataxia.
  - Special points: Use with caution in patients with hepatic or renal impairment. Care should be taken when used in patients with compromised pulmonary function.

References

1. Ferber R: Sleeplessness in the child. In Kryger MH, Roth T, Dement WC (eds): Principles and Practice of Sleep Medicine. Philadelphia, WB Saunders, 1989, pp 633-639.
2. Anders TF: Night-waking in infants during the first year of life. Pediatrics 1979;63:860-864.
3. Carey WB: Night waking and temperament in infancy. J Pediatr 1974;84:756-758.
4. Palmer CD, Harrison GA, Hiorns RW: Sleep patterns and life style in Oxfordshire villages. J Biosoc Sci 1980;12:437-467.
5. California Assessment Program: Student Achievement in California Schools: 1979-1980. Annual

report, prepared under the direction of Alexander I. Law, Chief, Office of Program Evaluation and Research, 1980.

6. Hayashi Y: On the sleep hours of school children of 6 to 20 years. Psychological Abstracts 1927; 1:439.

7. Bax MCO: Sleep disturbance in the young child. Br Med J 1980;280:1177-1179.

8. Weissbluth M, Poncher J, Given G, et al: Sleep duration and television viewing. J Pediatr 1981; 99:486-488.

9. Jenkins S, Bax MCO, Hart, H: Behaviour problems in preschool children. J Child Psychol Psychiatry 1980;21:5-17.

10. Richman N, Stevenson JE, Graham PJ: Prevalence of behaviour problems in 3-year-old children: An epidemiological study in a London borough. J Child Psychol Psychiatry 1975;16:277-287.

11. Anders TF: Night-waking in infants during the first year of life. Pediatrics 1979;63:860-864.

12. Metcalf D: The ontogenesis of sleep-awake states from birth to 3 months. Electroencephalogr Clin Neurophysiol 1970;28:421.

13. Moore T, Ucko LE: Night waking in early infancy. Arch Dis Child 1957;32:333-342.

14. Zuckerman B, Stevenson J, Bailey V: Sleep problems in early childhood: Continuities, predictive factors, and behavioral correlates. Pediatrics 1987; 80:664-671.

15. Kataria S, Swanson MS, Trevathan GE: Persistence of sleep disturbances in preschool children. J Pediatr 1987;110:642-646.

16. Jones DPH, Verduyn CM: Behavioural management of sleep problems. Arch Dis Child 1983; 58:442-444.

17. Wilks JM: The sleepless child (letter). Br Med J 1977;2:704-705.

18. Weissbluth M: Sleep duration and infant temperament. J Pediatr 1981;99:817-819.

19. Thomas A, Chess S, Birch HG: Temperament and Behavior Disorders in Children. New York, NYU Press, 1968.

20. Oberklaid F, Prior M, Sanson A, et al: Assessment of temperament in the toddler age group. Pediatrics 1990;85:559-566.

21. Lounsbury ML, Bates JE: The cries of infants of differing levels of perceived temperamental difficulties: Acoustic properties and effects on listeners. Child Dev 1982;53:677-686.

22. Snow ME, Jacklin CN, Maccoby EE: Crying episodes and sleep-wakefulness transitions in the first 26 months of life. Infant Behav Dev 1980; 3:387-394.

23. Lozoff B, Wolf AW, Davis NS: Cosleeping in urban families with young children in the United States. Pediatrics 1984;74:171-182.

24. Monroe LJ: Transient changes in EEG sleep patterns of married good sleepers: The effects of altering sleeping arrangement. Psychophysiology 1969; 6:330-337.

25. Caudill W, Ploth D: Who sleeps by who. Psychiatry 1964;32:12-43.

26. Ferber R: Solve Your Child's Sleep Problems. New York, Simon and Schuster, 1985.

27. Ferber R, Boyle MP: Nocturnal fluid intake: A cause of, not treatment for, sleep disruption in infants and toddlers. Sleep Res 1983;12:243-249.

28. Weissbluth M: Sleep and the colicky infant. In Guilleminault C (ed): Sleep and Its Disorders in Children. New York, Raven Press, 1987, pp 129-141.

29. Illingworth RS: "Three months" colic. Arch Dis Child 1954;29:167-174.

30. Wessel MA, Cobb JC, Jackson EB, et al: Paroxysmal fussing in infancy, sometimes called colic. Pediatrics 1954;14:421-434.

31. Pierce P: Delayed onset of "three months" colic in premature infants. Am J Dis Child 1948; 75:190-192.

32. Breslow L: A clinical approach to infantile colic: A review of 90 cases. J Pediatr 1957;50:196-206.

33. Meyer JE, Thaler MM: Colic in low birth weight infants. Am J Dis Child 1971;122:25-27.

34. Jorup S: Colonic hyperperistalsis in neurolabile infants: Studies in so-called dyspepsia in breast fed infants. Acta Paediatr 1952;85:1-92.

35. Weissbluth M, Christoffel KK, Davis AT: Treatment of infantile colic with dicyclomine hydrochloride. J Pediatr 1984;104:951-955.

36. Weissbluth M, Liu K: Sleep patterns, attention spans, and infant temperament. J Dev Behav Pediatr 1983;4:34-36.

37. Weissbluth M, Davis AT, Poncher J: Night waking in 4- to 8-month-old infants. J Pediatr 1984; 104:477-480.

38. Kahn A, Mozin MJ, Casimir G, et al: Insomnia and cow's milk allergy in infants. Pediatrics 1985; 76:880-884.

39. Ferber R: The sleepless child. In Guilleminault C (ed): Sleep and Its Disorders in Children. New York, Raven Press, 1987, pp 141-163.

40. Kaplan, BJ, McNicol J, Conte RA, Maghadam HK: Sleep disturbance in preschool-aged hyperactive and nonhyperactive children. Pediatrics 1987; 80:839-844.

41. Salzarulo P, Chevalier A: Sleep problems in children and their relationship with early disturbances of the waking-sleeping rhythms. Sleep 1983; 6:47-51.

42. Diagnostic and Statistical Manual of Mental Disorders, 3rd ed. Washington, DC, American Psychiatric Association, 1980.

43. Greenhill L, Puig-Antich J, Goetz R, et al: Sleep architecture and REM sleep measures in pre-pubertal children with attention deficit disorder with hyperactivity. Sleep 1983;6:91-101.

44. Busby K, Firestone P, Pivik RT: Sleep patterns in hyperkinetic and normal children. Sleep 1981; 4:366-383.

45. Peters JE, Romaine JS, Dyckman RA: A special neurological examination of children with learning disabilities. Dev Med Child Neurol 1975; 17:63-78.

46. Touwen BCL, Prechtl HFR: Neurological Examination of the Child with Minor Nervous Dysfunction. London, Spastics International Medical Publications, 1970.

47. Kane J, Coble P, Conners K, Kupfer DJ: EEG sleep in a child with severe depression. Am J Psychiatry 1977;134:813-814.

48. Cytryn L, McKnew D: Proposed classification of childhood depression. Am J Psychiatry 1972; 129:149-155.

49. Poznanski E, Frull JP: Childhood depression: Clinical characteristics of overtly depressed children. Arch Gen Psychiatry 1970;23:8-15.

50. Sander LW, Stechler G, Burns P, et al: Early mother-infant interaction and 24-hour patterns of activity and sleep. J Am Acad Child Psychiatry 1970;9:103-123.

51. Brown GW, Harris T: Social Origins of Depression. London, Tavistock Publications, 1978.

52. Lozoff B, Wolf AW, Davis NS: Sleep problems seen in pediatric practice. Pediatrics 1985;75:477-483.

53. Association of Sleep Disorders Centers: Diagnostic Classification of Sleep and Arousal Disorders, 1st ed. Prepared by the Sleep Disorders Classification Committee, H.P. Roffwarg, Chairman. *Sleep* 1979; 2:1-137.

54. Mindell JA, Carskadon MA, Owens JA: Developmental features of sleep. Child Adolesc Psychiatr Clin N Am 1999;8:695-725.

55. Owens J, Spirito A, McGuinn M, Nobile C: Sleep habits and sleep disturbance in school-aged children. J Dev Behav Pediatr 2000;21:27-36.

56. Gianotti F, Cortesi F: Sleep patterns and daytime functions in adolescents: An epidemiological survey of Italian high school student population. In Carskadon MA (ed): Adolescent Sleep Patterns: Biological, Social, and Psychological Influences. New York, Cambridge University Press, 2002.

57. Mindell J, Owens J: Sleep in the pediatric practice. In Mindell J, Owens J (eds): A Clinical Guide to Pediatric Sleep: Diagnosis and Management of Sleep Problems in Children and Adolescents. Philadelphia, Lippincott-Williams-Wilkins, 2003, pp 1-10.

Attention Deficit, Hyperactivity, and Sleep Disorders

12

Ronald D. Chervin

Pediatric sleep medicine once focused mainly on nocturnal behavior: parasomnias, bedtime rituals, and interactions between children and their parents. More recently, clinicians have realized that intrinsic dyssomnias such as obstructive sleep apnea, upper airway resistance syndrome, restless legs syndrome (RLS), and periodic limb movement disorder (PLMD) also occur in children and may have important effects on *daytime* behavior. Furthermore, these effects differ from those seen in adults with the same disorders. Whereas adults often display overt, excessive daytime sleepiness, children are more likely to present with cognitive and behavioral morbidity. For example, some affected children show inattentive and hyperactive behaviors that lead to a diagnosis of attention deficit hyperactivity disorder (ADHD) and treatment with stimulants before the underlying sleep problem is recognized. This chapter will highlight evidence that abnormal daytime behaviors, many reminiscent of ADHD, are among the most important outcomes of childhood sleep disorders. Data that have challenged or qualified this hypothesis also will be discussed.

SLEEP, ADHD, AND POTENTIAL PATHOPHYSIOLOGIC LINKS

The American Psychiatric Association's Diagnostic and Statistical Manual of Mental Disorders (DSM) once listed disturbed sleep as one of the diagnostic features of ADHD. Although the current edition has dropped this criterion, the parents of children with ADHD commonly note disturbed and restless sleep in their children.[1-4] In practice, sleep disruption is often attributed to stimulant medications or to persistence of daytime hyperactivity into nocturnal hours. Monitoring of movement (actigraphy) during 5-day intervals in children with ADHD did not demonstrate nocturnal over-activity but did show relative instability of sleep onset and total sleep time in comparison with controls.[5] Polysomnographic studies in ADHD children did not identify specific primary sleep disorders.[6-11] A review of polysomnographic studies of ADHD,[12] as well as a subsequent video-polysomnographic study,[13] failed to identify consistent abnormalities except for increased movements during sleep. However, these studies usually were performed with a focus on sleep staging; they did not record breathing or leg movement data later found to be as important in children as they are in adults. Clinicians and researchers without subspecialty interest in sleep medicine often do not consider the possibility that primary sleep disorders could contribute to ADHD or related symptoms.[14-17] However, growing evidence suggests that sleep disorders, because of associated daytime sleepiness or other consequences, could promote inattentive and hyperactive behaviors.

Several types of studies indicate that hyperactive children tend to have deficient levels of arousal. More than 60 years ago, Bradley and Bowen observed that stimulants rather than sedatives provide effective treatment for hyperactivity.[18,19] In contrast, sedatives can worsen the behavior. Early electrophysiologic studies—based on skin conductance, EEG, and auditory and sensory evoked responses—also suggested that children with ADHD show hypoarousal rather than hyperarousal.[20] Recent multiple sleep latency tests among 26 ADHD children and 21 controls showed increased daytime sleepiness in the ADHD subjects,[21] and a survey of the parents of more than 800 children at general pediatrics clinics suggested a substantial association between sleepiness and behavior that characterizes ADHD.[22]

The behaviors that define ADHD may be a product of cognitive changes, particularly deficits in executive functioning,[23] that can result from disordered sleep or daytime sleepiness. In adults, cognitive abilities are sensitive to sleep disorders,[24-26] and executive functioning, which includes working memory, decision making, and the ability to apply old information to new challenges, is especially vulnerable. Research in children has been limited but does include a study of 16 children randomized to either 5 or 11 hours of sleep for one night: On the following day, the sleep-deprived group showed impairment of verbal creativity and abstract thinking.[27] Another study of 82 children randomized to either 4 or 10 hours of sleep for one night showed increased inattentive behaviors after sleep deprivation but not hyperactive-impulsive behavior or impaired performance on tests of response inhibition and sustained attention.[28]

Cognitive deficits after sleep disruption may localize to the prefrontal cortex.[29] Adults with obstructive sleep apnea show neuropsychological deficits, particularly in executive functioning, that can be attributed to the prefrontal cortex and sometimes improved by treatment.[30] Preliminary data from functional magnetic resonance imaging in adults with obstructive sleep apnea show decreased activity of the dorsolateral prefrontal cortex during performance of a working memory task and restoration of normal activity levels after treatment.[31] Prefrontal cortical activity is also affected by experimental sleep deprivation in adults.[32-34] These data combine to suggest a potential mechanism for cognitive and behavioral changes in childhood dyssomnias: Insufficient or inadequate sleep may contribute to prefrontal cortical dysfunction and impair executive functions such as behavioral inhibition, emotional regulation, and working memory and thereby promote inattentive and hyperactive behaviors (Fig. 12–1).[35]

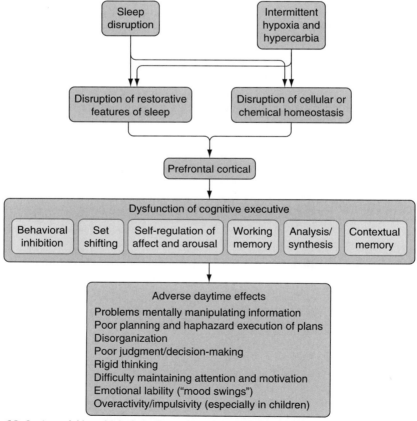

Figure 12–1. A model by which sleep disruption or physiologic effects of sleep apnea could alter daytime behavior in children. (Reprinted with permission from Beebe DW, Gozal D: Obstructive sleep apnea and the prefrontal cortex: Towards a comprehensive model linking nocturnal upper airway obstruction to daytime cognitive and behavioral deficits. J Sleep Res 2002;11:1-16.)

Other pathophysiologic mechanisms may pertain to specific sleep disorders. Obstructive sleep apnea is associated with hypoxemia, which could affect brain development. A model of sleep apnea, produced by subjecting young rats to intermittent hypoxia, has produced evidence of hippocampal and cortical apoptosis.[36] Although the histologic changes are transient, associated deficits in a spatial learning task do not completely resolve 2 weeks after the insult. Furthermore, rats seem to have an age-specific window of vulnerability that may have important analogies in human development: Fifteen- to 20-day-old animals show prominent neuronal apoptosis after intermittent hypoxia, whereas the effect is much less at younger and older ages.[37] Although it is attractive as a potential explanation for the neurobehavioral problems seen in obstructive sleep apnea, hypoxemia cannot explain similar problems seen in children with upper airway resistance syndrome or other sleep disorders.[38]

COGNITIVE AND BEHAVIORAL CHANGES IN CHILDREN WITH SPECIFIC SLEEP DISORDERS

Obstructive Sleep Apnea

In 1976, the first published series of children with obstructive sleep apnea described learning difficulties, inattention, and hyperactivity as prominent daytime symptoms.[39] Subsequent series in the early 1980s re-emphasized the frequency of these behaviors, noted that some of these children had been diagnosed with ADHD before presentation to a sleep center, and found that the symptoms of ADHD improved or disappeared after treatment for sleep-disordered breathing.[38,40] Although no subsequent randomized, placebo-controlled, double-blind studies tested these observations, one study did use a quasiexperimental design: Twelve children with sleep-disordered breathing and scheduled to undergo tonsillectomy were compared with 11 primary snorers also scheduled for tonsillectomy and with 10 control subjects, most of whom had been scheduled for unrelated surgery.[41] Postoperatively, validated parental scales for aggression, inattention, and hyperactivity and a continuous performance test all showed improvement in the group with sleep-disordered breathing but no change in the control group. Children with primary snoring showed improvement in some areas.

Another study used a validated pediatric sleep questionnaire to compare 27 ADHD patients at a child psychiatric clinic, 43 patients with other diagnoses at the same clinic, and 73 children at a general pediatric clinic.[42] The ADHD children were three times as likely as the non-ADHD psychiatric patients and the general pediatric patients to have a history of habitual snoring. Habitual snoring explained 16% of the variance in a DSM-IV–based inattention and hyperactivity scale. In a subsequent study, the parents of 866 children attending two general pediatric clinics completed a validated 22-item pediatric sleep-disordered breathing scale and the hyperactivity index of the Conners' Parent Rating Scale (CPRS).[22] High CPRS scores, defined as greater than 1 standard deviation (SD) above normal, were found in 13% (95% confidence interval [CI], 11, 16) of all subjects, 22% (95% CI, 15, 29) of habitual snorers, and 12% (95% CI, 9, 14) of nonsnorers. High CPRS scores were associated with high overall sleep-disordered breathing scores ($P < .01$). Stratification by age and sex showed that most of the association between hyperactivity and snoring derived from boys less than 8 years old (Table 12–1). These findings suggest that if sleep-disordered breathing does contribute to hyperactive behavior, young boys may be the most vulnerable to this effect.

In an evidence-based review, an American Academy of Pediatrics subcommittee found 12 publications that evaluated the association between sleep-disordered breathing and a range of cognitive and behavioral problems.[43] No report was a randomized trial, and each was a cross-sectional or cohort study or a case series. When the authors pooled the results of six cross-sectional studies, they concluded that the combined odds ratio (OR) for neurobehavioral problems and snoring in children was 2.93 (2.23, 3.83).

Published reports that hyperactivity is particularly common in children with sleep-disordered breathing generally have not prospectively evaluated children using DSM-IV criteria. The preliminary results of one study did include psychiatric evaluations of 5- to 13-year-old children scheduled for adenotonsillectomy (AT) and a control group scheduled for general surgery.[44]

Table 12–1.   Conditional Logistic Regression Coefficients and Odds Ratios for Hyperactive Behavior and Habitual Snoring (Present vs Absent) in a Study of Children Aged 5 to 13 Years*

Age and Gender (N)	Regression Coefficient (SE)	Estimated Odds Ratio (95% CI)	P
All subjects (866)	0.81 (0.25)	2.2 (1.4, 3.6)	.0011
Boys (469)	1.05 (0.31)	2.8 (1.5, 5.2)	.0008
Girls (397)	0.39 (0.43)	1.5 (0.6, 3.3)	.3633
Age < 8 yr (565)	1.02 (0.30)	2.8 (1.5, 4.9)	.0007
Age ≥ 8 yr (301)	0.32 (0.46)	1.4 (0.5, 3.3)	.4831
Boys < 8 yr (295)	1.46 (0.38)	4.3 (2.0, 9.1)	<.0001
Remaining children (571)	0.33 (0.35)	1.4 (0.7, 2.7)	.3500

*Results adjusted for age and sex. Hyperactive behavior defined as Conners' Parent Rating Scale hyperactivity index; T score > 60.
CI, confidence interval; SE, standard error.
Data from Chervin RD, Archbold KH, Dillon JE, et al: Inattention, hyperactivity, and symptoms of sleep-disordered breathing. Pediatrics 2002;109:449-456.

Nearly all of the AT children were suspected by their otolaryngologists of having sleep-disordered breathing, although many also had additional surgical indications. Although the child psychiatrists who evaluated the children were not blinded to surgical group, they did use two well-validated structured interviews, the Diagnostic Interview Schedule for Children and the Children's Psychiatric Ratings Scale. A disruptive behavior disorder—ADHD, oppositional defiant disorder, or conduct disorder—was diagnosed in 20 (44%) of 45 AT children but in 0 (0%) of 8 control subjects (Fisher's exact test; P = .019). Among the AT children, 7 (16%) had the ADHD-inattentive subtype, 2 (4%) had the ADHD-hyperactive subtype, 6 (13%) had the ADHD-combined type, and 9 (20%) had oppositional defiant disorder. The children were also evaluated for several other major DSM-IV diagnoses—social phobia, seasonal affective disorder, generalized anxiety disorder, obsessive-compulsive disorder, post-traumatic stress disorder, enuresis, encopresis, tic disorder, major depressive disorder, dysthymia, mania, hypomania, and pervasive development disorder—but none showed increased frequency in the AT group. These data suggest that DSM-IV–based diagnoses of disruptive behavior disorders are particularly common among children scheduled for AT, most of whom carry a clinical diagnosis of sleep-disordered breathing.

In addition to these behavioral problems, cognitive changes in children with sleep-disordered breathing have been the subject of a small but growing body of literature. One study focused on 16 obese children, among whom 5 had obstructive sleep apnea on polysomnography.[45] The children with sleep apnea demonstrated deficits in learning, memory, and vocabulary, and in the entire sample, apnea severity correlated inversely with memory and learning performance. A second study compared neurocognitive functioning in 16 childhood snorers, who had little or no sleep apnea, to that in 16 nonsnorers.[46] The snorers showed lower attention, memory, and intelligence scores but no differences in social competency and problematic behavior. A third study of 28 children with obstructive sleep apnea and 10 control subjects found preliminary evidence that the former group had significantly more somatic complaints, mood problems, and difficulty relating to peers.[47] However, many measures showed no differences between groups, and children with mild sleep apnea showed more behavioral and emotional problems overall than those with severe sleep apnea. Finally, data from the study of children scheduled for AT or other procedures show that although the two groups did not differ significantly with respect to age, grade, verbal IQ, and performance IQ, the AT children performed more poorly on academic achievement tests, including mathematical reasoning, spelling, and numeric operations.[48] A similar trend emerged for basic reading performance, though not for a measure of reading comprehension. In aggregate, these studies suggest specific academic deficits in children with sleep-disordered breathing that would predict an important practical impact, including poor school performance.

School performance was the main outcome variable in one study that enrolled 297 poorly performing first-grade children and screened them for sleep-disordered breathing by parental questionnaire, home oximetry, and capnography: Fifty-four children (18%) were identified as likely to have sleep-disordered breathing.[49] The parents of these children were advised to seek further evaluation and possible treatment. One year later, 24 (44%) of the 54 children had been diagnosed and treated for obstructive sleep apnea. These children showed significant improvement in their school grades, whereas the 30 children with untreated sleep-disordered breathing and the 243 children without evidence of sleep-disordered breathing showed no improvement. In a subsequent survey of 1,588 seventh and eighth graders, students whose performances ranked them in the bottom quartile of their classes were two to three times as likely as top-quartile students to have had frequent and loud snoring between the ages of 2 and 6 years.[50] Finally, a study performed among 201 medical students found that the failure rate for a year-end examination was 13% for 78 nonsnorers, 22% for 99 occasional snorers, and 42% for 24 frequent snorers (P < .01).[51]

Restless Legs Syndrome and Periodic Limb Movement Disorder

Although the prevalence of RLS in children is not well defined, more than one third of 138 adults with this condition reported that symptoms had begun before the age of 10.[52] Early studies of restless legs in children found that many patients had problems with inattention and hyperactivity.[53,54] One report found that 117 (91%) of 129 children referred to a sleep laboratory and confirmed to have periodic leg movements during sleep (>5 movements per hour) also met the criteria for ADHD.[55] Additional data suggested that children with ADHD may be more likely to have restless legs and related complaints than other children.[56,57] These studies focused on children referred for sleep or behavioral concerns, but subsequent data collected at general pediatric clinics also suggested prominent associations between hyperactive behavior and symptoms that characterize RLS and periodic leg movements during sleep.[58] Hyperactivity was assessed with the CPRS and periodic leg movements, restless legs, and growing pains by a validated subscale of the Pediatric Sleep Questionnaire (Fig. 12–2).[59] High hyperactivity indices (>1 SD elevation) were found in 13% of all 866 subjects, 18% of children who had described "restlessness of the legs when in bed," and 11% of those without restless legs (P < .05). The OR for a high hyperactivity score and a 1 SD increase in the periodic leg movement subscale was 1.6 [1.4, 1.9], and this association retained significance after statistical adjustment for sleepiness, snoring, restless sleep in general, or stimulant use.

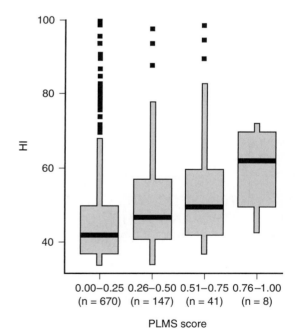

Figure 12–2. Among 866 children aged 5 to 13 years, a validated questionnaire subscale for symptoms of restless legs syndrome and periodic leg movements during sleep (PLMS Score) displayed a dose–response association with the hyperactivity index (HI). Box plots show medians and 10th, 25th, 75th, and 90th percentiles. The horizontal black stripe represents the mean. (Reprinted with permission from Chervin RD, Archbold KH, Dillon JE, et al: Associations between symptoms of inattention, hyperactivity, restless legs, and periodic leg movements. Sleep 2002;25:213-218.)

Further support for the possibility that RLS or periodic leg movements might contribute to ADHD was provided by a report that seven affected children experienced improvement in behavior, as assessed by well validated measures, when their RLS was treated with levodopa or a dopamine agonist.[60] However, as the authors noted, these medications could have improved behavior by a direct effect on brain mechanisms that control behavior rather than through an effect on RLS.

Other Sleep Disorders

Children with sleep disorders other than sleep-disordered breathing or RLS also may suffer from cognitive and behavioral consequences. A case report of a child with delayed sleep phase syndrome carefully documented attention deficit that improved considerably when the circadian rhythm disorder was treated.[61] Children with narcolepsy often have problems with inattention and hyperactivity that may improve upon treatment.[62,63] In the United States, adolescents are often chronically sleep deprived. Those who perform poorly academically tend to obtain less sleep at night than those who receive better grades.[64] Recent efforts to augment high school students' nocturnal sleep and address their tendency to have delayed sleep phases by delaying school start times in some Minnesota school districts have been associated with longer times in bed and slightly higher grades.

DO SLEEP DISORDERS CAUSE COGNITIVE AND BEHAVIORAL MORBIDITY IN CHILDREN?

The evidence presented above suggests that sleep disorders may contribute to cognitive impairment and disruptive behavior in children. However, these studies do not constitute randomized, double-blind, placebo-controlled trials, and proof is still lacking for the hypothesis that substantial minorities of the many children with disruptive behavior disorders have undiagnosed sleep disorders as a contributing factor. In addition, some studies have raised questions or methodological concerns about demonstrated links among sleep, cognition, and behavior.

One study of 113 children, aged 2 to 18 years and referred for suspected sleep-disordered

breathing to a sleep laboratory, found that the 59 children confirmed to have sleep-disordered breathing did show high hyperactivity scores, but these scores were no higher than those of the 54 children without sleep-disordered breathing.[65] Furthermore, hyperactivity levels showed no significant association with the rate of hypopneas and apneas, minimum oxygen saturation, or most negative esophageal pressure (investigated in a subset of 19 children). Instead, the level of hyperactivity was associated with the presence or absence of five or more periodic leg movements per hour of sleep ($P = .02$). The rate of periodic leg movements during sleep showed a linear association with hyperactivity among those subjects with sleep-disordered breathing ($P = .002$) but no association among those without sleep-disordered breathing ($P = .64$). The association between behavior and periodic leg movements rather than apnea, even in a population referred for suspected sleep-disordered breathing, raises some doubt about whether sleep-disordered breathing causes disruptive behavior. Corroborative though preliminary evidence has emerged from a second study.[66] Such data are similar to those obtained from adults with sleep apnea, in whom the major behavioral outcome—sleepiness—shows little correlation with apnea severity.[67,68] One possible explanation for a correlation between periodic leg movements and hyperactive behavior only among children with sleep-disordered breathing is that this disorder acts as an effect modifier. However, the lack of a stronger, direct association between apnea severity and hyperactivity in children raises some doubt about whether sleep apnea directly causes this behavior.

Furthermore, studies that have reported associations between sleep-disordered breathing and either poor school performance or hyperactive behavior have been correlational and could not account for many potential confounding factors.[22,42,49-51] For example, recent data from 146 second and fifth grade students in Ypsilanti, Michigan, showed significant associations between school performance and symptoms of sleep disordered breathing before but not after socioeconomic status was taken into account.[69] These results raise the possibility that previous studies of cognitive and behavioral problems in childhood sleep disorders also would have reached different conclusions if they had accounted for socioeconomic status.

CONCLUSIONS

In short, increasing evidence suggests that a variety of childhood sleep disorders are associated with inattention, hyperactivity, and underlying cognitive impairment that could have significantly adverse effects on such important outcomes as development and school performance. However, proof that sleep disorders cause neurobehavioral deficits in substantial numbers of children is still lacking, and some studies have generated conflicting data. Mechanisms by which sleep disorders may cause cognitive and behavioral changes have been proposed but not yet thoroughly investigated.

If sleep disorders do influence cognition and behavior, then this morbidity may constitute an important public health problem. Problems related to sleep are highly prevalent among children[70] but seldom discussed, recognized, or treated at general pediatric clinics.[71] Furthermore, those children who are suspected of having sleep-disordered breathing usually undergo AT without having any formal polysomnographic, psychiatric, or cognitive testing.[72] Arguments that preoperative evaluation should be more extensive, as now suggested by the American Academy of Pediatrics,[73] will be strengthened if future research more effectively shows cause-and-effect relationships between sleep disorders and neurobehavioral consequences, and if future data more convincingly link specific polysomnographic findings with these important adverse health outcomes.[74]

References

1. Ring A, Stein D, Barak Y, et al: Sleep disturbances in children with attention-deficit/hyperactivity disorder: A comparative study with healthy siblings. J Learn Disabil 1998;31:572-578.
2. Owens JA, Maxim R, Nobile C, et al: Parental and self-report of sleep in children with attention-deficit/hyperactivity disorder. Arch Pediatr Adolesc Med 2000;154:549-555.
3. Marcotte AC, Thacher PV, Butters M, et al: Parental report of sleep problems in children with attentional and learning disorders. J Devel Behav Pediatr 1998;19:178-186.
4. Corkum P, Tannock R, Moldofsky H, et al: Actigraphy and parental ratings of sleep in children with attention-deficit/hyperactivity disorder (ADHD). Sleep 2001;24:303-312.
5. Gruber R, Sadeh A, Raviv A: Instability of sleep patterns in children with attention-deficit/hyperactivity disorder. J Am Acad Child Adolesc Psychiatry 2000;39:495-501.
6. Busby K, Firestone P, Pivik RT: Sleep patterns in hyperkinetic and normal children. Sleep 1981;4:366-383.
7. Greenhill L, Puig-Antich J, Goetz R, et al: Sleep architecture and REM sleep measures in prepubertal children with attention deficit disorder with hyperactivity. Sleep 1983;6:91-101.
8. Haig JR, Schroeder CS, Schroeder SR: Effects of methylphenidate on hyperactive children's sleep. Psychopharmacologia (Berl) 1974;37:185-188.
9. Small A, Hibi S, Feinberg I: Effects of dextroamphetamine sulfate on EEG sleep patterns of hyperactive children. Arch Gen Psychiatry 1971;25:369-380.
10. Palm L, Persson E, Bjerre I, et al: Sleep and wakefulness in preadolescent children with deficits in attention, motor control and perception. Acta Paediatr 1992;81:618-624.
11. Platon MJR, Bueno AV, Sierra JE, Kales S: Hypnopolygraphic alterations in attention deficit disorder (ADD) children. Intern J Neurosci 1990;53:87-101.
12. Corkum P, Tannock R, Moldofsky H: Sleep disturbances in children with attention-deficit/hyperactivity disorder. J Am Acad Child Adolesc Psychiatry 1998;37:637-646.
13. Konofal E, Lecendreux M, Bouvard M, Mouren-Simeoni MC: High levels of nocturnal activity in children with attention-deficit hyperactivity disorder: A video analysis. Psych Clin Neurosci 2001;55:97-103.
14. Zametkin AJ, Ernst M: Problems in the management of attention-deficit-hyperactivity disorder. N Engl J Med 1999;340:40-46.
15. Chervin RD: Attention-deficit-hyperactivity disorder (Letter). N Engl J Med 1999;340:1766-1767.
16. Biederman J: A 55-year-old man with attention-deficit/hyperactivity disorder. JAMA 1998;280:1086-1092.
17. Yuen KM, Pelayo R: Sleep disorders and attention deficit/hyperactivity disorder. JAMA 1999;281:797.
18. Bradley C: The behavior of children receiving Benzedrine. Am J Psychiat 1937;94:577-585.
19. Bradley C, Bowen M: Amphetamine (Benzedrine) therapy of children's behavior disorders. Am J Orthopsychiat 1941;11:92-103.
20. Satterfield JH, Cantwell DP, Satterfield BT: Pathophysiology of the hyperactive child syndrome. Arch Gen Psychiatry 1974;31:839-844.

21. Lecendreux M, Konofal E, Bouvard M, et al: Sleep and alertness in children with ADHD. J Child Psychol Psychiatry 2000;41:803-812.

22. Chervin RD, Archbold KH, Dillon JE, et al: Inattention, hyperactivity, and symptoms of sleep-disordered breathing. Pediatrics 2002;109:449-456.

23. Barkley RA: Genetics of childhood disorders, XVII: ADHD, Part 1: The executive functions and ADHD. J Am Acad Child Adolesc Psychiatry 2000;39:1064-1068.

24. Naegele B, Thouvard V, Pepin JL, et al: Deficits of cognitive executive functions in patients with sleep apnea syndrome. Sleep 1995;18:43-52.

25. Engleman HM, Kingshott RN, Martin SE, Douglas NJ: Cognitive function in the sleep apnea/hypopnea syndrome (SAHS). Sleep 2000;23(Suppl 4):S102-S108.

26. Kim HC, Young T, Matthews CG, et al: Sleep-disordered breathing and neuropsychological deficits: A population-based study. Am J Respir Crit Care Med 1997;156:1813-1819.

27. Randazzo AC, Muehlbach MJ, Schweitzer PK, Walsh JK: Cognitive function following acute sleep restriction in children ages 10-14. Sleep 1998;21:861-868.

28. Fallone G, Acebo C, Arnedt JT, et al: Effects of acute sleep restriction on behavior, sustained attention, and response inhibition in children. Percept Mot Skills 2001;93:213-229.

29. Dahl RE. The impact of inadequate sleep on children's daytime cognitive function. Semin in Pediatr Neurol 1996;3:44-50.

30. Feuerstein C, Naegele B, Pepin JL, Levy P: Frontal lobe-related cognitive functions in patients with sleep apnea syndrome before and after treatment. Acta Neurologica Belgica 1997;97:96-107.

31. Thomas RJ, Rosen BR, Bush G, Kwong KK: Working memory in obstructive sleep apnea: A functional magnetic resonance imaging study. Soc Neurosci Abstr 2001. 27:845-849.

32. Drummond SP, Brown GG, Gillin JC, et al: Altered brain response to verbal learning following sleep deprivation. Nature 2000;403:655-657.

33. Drummond SP, Gillin JC, Brown GG: Increased cerebral response during a divided attention task following sleep deprivation. J Sleep Res 2001;10:85-92.

34. Drummond SP, Brown GG, Stricker JL, et al: Sleep deprivation-induced reduction in cortical functional response to serial subtraction. Neuroreport 1999;10:3745-3748.

35. Beebe DW, Gozal D: Obstructive sleep apnea and the prefrontal cortex: Towards a comprehensive model linking nocturnal upper airway obstruction to daytime cognitive and behavioral deficits. J Sleep Res 2002;11:1-16.

36. Gozal D, Daniel JM, Dohanich GP: Behavioral and anatomical correlates of chronic episodic hypoxia during sleep in the rat. J Neurosci 2001;21:2442-2450.

37. Gozal E, Row BW, Schurr A, Gozal D: Developmental differences in cortical and hippocampal vulnerability to intermittent hypoxia in the rat. Neurosci Lett 2001;305:197-201.

38. Guilleminault C, Winkle R, Korobkin R, Simmons B: Children and nocturnal snoring—evaluation of the effects of sleep related respiratory resistive load and daytime functioning. Eur J Pediatr 1982;139:165-171.

39. Guilleminault C, Eldridge F, Simmons FB: Sleep apnea in eight children. Pediatrics 1976;58:23-30.

40. Guilleminault C, Korobkin R, Winkle R: A review of 50 children with obstructive sleep apnea syndrome. Lung 1981;159:275-287.

41. Ali NJ, Pitson D, Stradling JR: Sleep disordered breathing: Effects of adenotonsillectomy on behaviour and psychological functioning. Eur J Pediatr 1996;155:56-62.

42. Chervin RD, Dillon JE, Bassetti C, et al: Symptoms of sleep disorders, inattention, and hyperactivity in children. Sleep 1997;20:1185-1192.

43. Schechter MS, Section on Pediatric Pulmonology, Subcommittee on Obstructive Sleep Apnea Syndrome. Technical report: Diagnosis and management of childhood obstructive sleep apnea syndrome. Pediatrics 2002;109:e69.

44. Dillon JE, Ruzicka DL, Champine DJ, et al: DSM-IV diagnoses in children scheduled for adenotonsillectomy or hernia repair (Abstract). Sleep 2002; 25:A346-A341.

45. Rhodes SK, Shimoda KC, Wald LR, et al: Neurocognitive deficits in morbidly obese children with obstructive sleep apnea. J Pediatr 1995;127:741-744.

46. Blunden S, Lushington K, Kennedy D, et al: Behavior and neurocognitive performance in children aged 5-10 years who snore compared to controls. J Clin Exp Neuropsychol 2000;22:554-568.

47. Lewin DS, Rosen RC, England SJ, Dahl RE: Preliminary evidence of behavioral and cognitive sequelae of obstructive sleep apnea in children. Sleep Med 2002;3:5-13.

48. Huffman JL, Giordani B, Layne JR, et al: Academic achievement and attention in children scheduled for adenotonsillectomy in comparison to controls (Abstract). Sleep 2002;25:A197-A198.

49. Gozal D: Sleep-disordered breathing and school performance in children. Pediatrics 1998;102: 616-620.

50. Gozal D, Pope DW Jr: Snoring during early childhood and academic performance at ages thirteen to fourteen years. Pediatrics 2001;107:1394-1399.

51. Ficker JH, Wiest GH, Lehnert G, et al: Are snoring medical students at risk of failing their exams? Sleep 1999;22:205-209.

52. Walters AS, Hickey K, Maltzman J, et al: A questionnaire study of 138 patients with restless legs syndrome: The 'Night-Walkers' survey. Neurology 1996;46:92-95.

53. Picchietti DL, Walters AS: Severe periodic limb movement disorder in childhood and adolescence. Sleep Res 1996;25:333.

54. Picchietti DL, Walters AS: Restless legs syndrome and periodic limb movement disorder in children and adolescents: comorbidity with attention-deficit hyperactivity disorder. Child Adolesc Psychiatr Clin North Am 1996;5:729-740.

55. Picchietti DL, Walters AS: Moderate to severe periodic limb movement disorder in childhood and adolescence. Sleep 1999;22:297-300.

56. Picchietti DL, England SJ, Walters AS, et al: Periodic limb movement disorder and restless legs syndrome in children with attention-deficit-hyperactivity disorder. J Child Neurol 1998; 13:588-594.

57. Picchietti DL, Underwood DJ, Farris WA, et al: Further studies on periodic limb movement disorder and restless legs syndrome in children with attention-deficit hyperactivity disorder. Move Disord 1999;14:1000-1007.

58. Chervin RD, Archbold KH, Dillon JE, et al: Associations between symptoms of inattention, hyperactivity, restless legs, and periodic leg movements. Sleep 2002;25:213-218.

59. Chervin RD, Hedger KM: Clinical prediction of periodic leg movements during sleep in children. Sleep Med 2001;2:501-510.

60. Walters AS, Mandelbaum DE, Lewin DS, et al: Dopaminergic therapy in children with restless legs/periodic limb movements in sleep and ADHD. Pediatr Neurol 2000;22:182-186.

61. Dahl RE, Pelham WE, Wierson M: The role of sleep disturbances in attention deficit disorder symptoms: A case study. J Pediatr Psychol 1991;16:229-239.

62. Dahl RE, Holttum J, Trubnick L: A clinical picture of child and adolescent narcolepsy. J Am Acad Child Adolesc Psychiatry 1994;33:834-841.

63. Guilleminault C, Pelayo R: Narcolepsy in prepubertal children. Ann Neurol 1998;43:135-142.

64. Wolfson AR, Carskadon MA: Sleep schedules and daytime functioning in adolescents. Child Dev 1998;69:875-887.

65. Chervin RD, Archbold KH: Hyperactivity and polysomnographic findings in children evaluated for sleep-disordered breathing. Sleep 2001;24: 313-320.

66. Chervin RD, Giordani B, Ruzicka DL, et al: Polysomnographic findings and behavior in children scheduled for adenotonsillectomy or hernia repair (Abstract). Sleep 2002;25:A431.

67. Chervin RD, Aldrich MS: Characteristics of apneas and hypopneas during sleep and relation to excessive daytime sleepiness. Sleep 1998; 21:799-806.

68. Chervin RD, Aldrich MS: The Epworth Sleepiness Scale may not reflect objective measures of sleepiness or sleep apnea. Neurology 1999;52:125-131.

69. Clarke DF, Huffman JL, Szymanski E, et al: School performance, race, and symptoms of sleep-disordered breathing (Abstract). Sleep 2002;25:A83-A84.

70. Archbold KH, Pituch KJ, Panahi P, Chervin RD: Symptoms of sleep disturbances among children at two general pediatric clinics. J Pediatr 2002; 140:97-102.

71. Chervin RD, Hedger KM, Panahi P, Pituch KJ: Sleep problems seldom addressed at two general pediatric clinics. Pediatrics 2001;107:1375-1380.

72. Weatherly RA, Mai EF, Ruzicka DL, Chervin RD: Adenotonsillectomy in children: Indications, practices, and outcomes reported by otolaryngologists (Abstract). Sleep 2000;24(Suppl): A212-A213.

73. Section on Pediatric Pulmonology, Subcommittee on Obstructive Sleep Apnea Syndrome: Clinical practice guideline: Diagnosis and management of childhood obstructive sleep apnea syndrome. Pediatrics 2002;109:704-712.

74. American Thoracic Society: Cardiorespiratory sleep studies in children: Establishment of normative data and polysomnographic predictors of morbidity. Am J Resp Crit Care Med 1999;160:1381-1387.

Narcolepsy in Childhood   13

Suresh Kotagal

In 1880, Gelineau coined the term *narcolepsie* to describe a pathologic condition that was characterized by recurrent, brief attacks of sleepiness.[1] He recognized that the disorder was accompanied by falls, or *astasias,* that were subsequently termed cataplexy. Narcolepsy is a lifelong neurologic disorder of rapid eye movement (REM) sleep in which there are attacks of *irresistible daytime sleepiness, cataplexy* (sudden loss of muscle control in the legs, trunk, or neck in response to emotional stimuli such as laughter, fright, or rage), *hypnagogic hallucinations* (vivid and often terrifying dreams at sleep onset), *sleep paralysis* (momentary inability to move at the time of sleep onset), and fragmented night sleep.[2]

EPIDEMIOLOGY

In a community-based survey in Olmsted County, Minnesota, the incidence of narcolepsy was 1.37 per 100,000 persons per year—1.72 for men and 1.05 for women.[3] It was highest in the 2nd decade of life, followed by a gradual decline. The prevalence was approximately 56 persons per 100,000 persons. In Japan, the prevalence has been estimated at 1 in 600,[4] and in Israel at 1 in 500,000.[5] The exact prevalence of narcolepsy in childhood has been difficult to establish. Nevertheless, between 1957 and 1960, in a series of 400 narcolepsy patients seen at the Mayo Clinic by Yoss and Daly,[6] 15 (4%) were younger than 15 years. These data were, however, gathered prior to the introduction of polysomnography and the establishment of polysomnographic criteria for the diagnosis of narcolepsy. Although the disorder is most often diagnosed in the 3rd and 4th decades, a meta-analysis of 235 subjects derived from three studies by Challamel and coworkers[7] found that 34% of all subjects had onset of symptoms prior to

the age of 15 years, 16% prior to age 10 years, and 4.5 % prior to age 5 years (Fig. 13–1). A lag period of 5 to 10 years between the onset of symptoms and diagnosis has been observed[8] in adult subjects. A similar but shorter lag period perhaps also occurs in childhood narcolepsy. Cataplexy, the most specific clinical feature of narcolepsy, is present in only 50% to 70% of all subjects. Some epidemiologic studies have required the presence of cataplexy as a prerequisite for the diagnosis,[9] whereas others[10] have not made this stipulation. This lack of uniformity in clinical diagnostic criteria may explain variability in estimations of the prevalence of narcolepsy.[11]

CLINICAL FEATURES

Preschool-Aged Children

Narcolepsy is rare in preschool-aged children. Yoss and Daly observed that 11.7% of a group of 85 subjects were below the age of 5 years.[6] In their meta-analysis of 235 children, Challamel and colleagues found that 4.6% were below the age of 5 years at the time of diagnosis.[7] Sharp and D'Cruz have described a 12-month-old with hypersomnia who was subsequently confirmed to have narcolepsy.[12] Nevsimalova and coworkers have described a 2½-year-old who developed hypersomnolence at the age of 6 months, with the presence of as many as 30 cataplectic attacks per day that mimicked atonic seizures, but that subsided after treatment with chlorimipramine.[13] In general, it is difficult to diagnose narcolepsy prior to the age of 4 to 5 years, as even unaffected children of this age tend to take habitual daytime naps and are not able to provide an accurate history of cataplexy, hypnagogic hallucinations, or sleep paralysis. The diagnosis may, however, be facilitated by the documentation

171

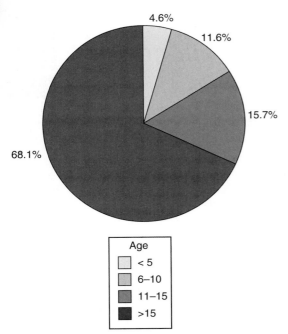

4.6%

11.6%

15.7%

68.1%

Age
☐ < 5
☐ 6–10
☐ 11–15
■ >15

Figure 13–1. The age of onset of narcolepsy. (Adapted from Challamel MJ, Mazzola ME, Nevsimalova S, et al: Narcolepsy in children. Sleep 1994;17S:17-20.)

of cataplectic attacks on video-polysomnography, which shows skeletal muscle atonia and bursts of rapid eye movements coinciding with low-voltage, mixed-frequency activity on the electroencephalogram (EEG).

School-Aged Children

Daytime sleepiness is the most invariant and disabling feature of narcolepsy. It may develop as early as 5 to 6 years of age. There is a background of a constant, foggy feeling from drowsiness, and superimposed on this background are periods of more dramatic sleep attacks. Habitual afternoon napping is uncommon in most 5- to 6-year-olds and should raise suspicion. Lenn reported a 6-year-old who would fall asleep 5 to 10 times a day.[14] Wittig and colleagues described a 7-year, 5-month-old boy with narcolepsy who tended to fall asleep while watching television for longer than a half hour, at the dinner table, and while seated in his mother's lap at a doctor's office.[15] The naps in children with narcolepsy tend to be longer (30 to 90 minutes) than those in adult patients, but they are not consistently followed by a refreshed feel-

ing.[16] These attacks of sleepiness are most likely to occur when the patient is carrying out sedentary activities such as sitting in a classroom or reading a book. The daytime sleepiness frequently leads to automatic behavior of which the subject is unaware, to impaired consolidation of memory, to decreased concentration, to executive dysfunction, and to emotional problems. Mood swings are also common.[17,18] Children with daytime sleepiness may be mistakenly labeled "lazy" and frequently become the target of negative comments from their peers. Excessive sleepiness may also be overlooked by the parents until it starts adversely impacting mood, behavior, or academic performance. Adults who have been diagnosed with narcolepsy frequently give a history of "attention deficit disorder" in childhood.[19] Pollack studied the circadian sleep–wake rhythms in subjects with narcolepsy who were isolated from their environmental cues.[20] He found that the major sleep episode was still about 6 hours long, and it occurred about once every 24 hours, thus indicating that the circadian clock was functioning normally. Pollack confirmed that patients with narcolepsy tended to sleep *more often*, but *not longer* than people without narcolepsy.

Cataplexy, the second most common but most specific feature of narcolepsy, consists of a sudden loss of muscle tone in the extensor muscles of the thighs, back, or neck in response to emotional triggers such as fright, rage, excitement, surprise, or laughter. It is caused by the intrusion of the skeletal muscle atonia of REM sleep into wakefulness.[21,22] It is accompanied by hyperpolarization of spinal alpha motor neurons, with resultant active inhibition of skeletal muscle tone and suppression of the monosynaptic H-reflex and tendon reflexes. A history of cataplexy may be difficult to elicit in young children. I recall a 6-year-old girl with proven narcolepsy who denied any episodic muscle weakness but would repeatedly fall down whenever she jumped on a trampoline. Consciousness remains fully intact during the cataplexy episodes, which can last 1 to 30 minutes. Respiration and cardiovascular functions remain unaffected. Challamel and coworkers[7] found cataplexy in 80.5% of idiopathic narcolepsy and in 95% of symptomatic narcolepsy subjects.

Hallucinations at sleep onset (*hypnagogic*) or upon awakening from sleep (*hypnopompic*) are seen in 50% to 60% of narcolepsy patients and may have an unpleasant, frightening quality to them. They may be auditory or visual in nature. *Sleep paralysis* is a sudden momentary inability to move as one is drifting off to sleep or awakening from sleep. Like cataplexy, both sleep paralysis and hypnagogic hallucinations are caused by the intrusion of fragments of REM sleep into wakefulness.

Night-time sleep is also disturbed, with frequent awakenings. Young and colleagues attributed sleep fragmentation in part to periodic limb movements, which were found in five (63%) of eight children with narcolepsy in their series.[23] Periodic limb movements are rhythmic limb muscle contractions of 0.5 to 5 seconds' duration, with an intermovement interval of 5 to 120 seconds, occurring in series of three or more, usually during stage 1 or 2 of non-REM (NREM) sleep. They may or may not be associated with EEG evidence of cortical arousal. Similarly, they may or may not be accompanied by a feeling of restlessness in the limbs. Sleep fragmentation in narcolepsy may also occur, unrelated to periodic limb movements or restless leg syndrome.

Neuropsychological and behavioral manifestations are common in childhood narcolepsy, but they have not been adequately studied, partly because of difficulties in developing valid and practical batteries of neuropsychological tests for sleepy children. It is not uncommon for children with narcolepsy to present with inattentiveness or mild depression. Adult patients with narcolepsy have demonstrated selective cognitive deficits in response latency, word recall, and estimation of frequency.[24] Rogers and Rosenberg[25] performed a battery of neuropsychological studies on 30 adults with narcolepsy and age-matched controls. The subjects with narcolepsy experienced more difficulty in maintaining attention than controls, as evidenced by more perseveration errors on Strub and Black's List of Letters. It is unclear whether children with narcolepsy exhibit similar deficits.

PATHOPHYSIOLOGY

Narcolepsy in Animals

Over the past 2 decades, the study of narcolepsy in animals has advanced understanding of the various phenomena that are also observed in humans. Narcolepsy has been studied in cats, miniature horses, quarter horses, Brahman bulls, and about 15 breeds of dogs, and it shows a monogenic, autosomal recessive pattern of inheritance.[26-28] Cataplexy can be induced in cats by the injection of carbachol (an acetylcholine-like substance) into the pontine reticular formation.[29] Specifically, muscarinic type-2 receptors of acetylcholine have been implicated.[30,31] The food-elicited cataplexy test, used to study cataplexy in dogs, uses the finding that the time taken for the consumption of food by narcoleptic animals whose eating is interrupted by cataplexy attacks is much longer than in animals without narcolepsy.

In 1999, Lin and coworkers demonstrated that canine narcolepsy is caused by a mutation in the hypocretin receptor-2 (orexin-2) gene.[32] Around the same time, Chemelli and colleagues established that a null mutation for the hypocretin-1 and hypocretin-2 peptides in mice produces aspects reminiscent of human narcolepsy, including cataplexy.[33] The hypocretin-containing neurons are located primarily in the dorsolateral hypothalamus, but they have widespread projections to remote areas such as the basal forebrain, amygdala, medial nuclei of the thalamus, periaqueductal gray matter, reticular formation, pedunculo-pontine nucleus, locus coeruleus, raphe nucleus, pontine tegmentum, and dorsal spinal cord.[32,34] Hypocretins 1 and 2 are peptides that are synthesized from preprohypocretin, and have corresponding receptors. Although the hypocretin type 1 receptor binds only to hypocretin-1, the hypocretin type 2 receptor can bind to both type 1 and type 2 ligands. Hypocretins stimulate food intake, increase the basal metabolic rate, and promote arousal.[34] Decreased activation of the hypocretin system is the underlying theme in canine and murine narcolepsy. This receptor downregulation may occur as a result of either exon-skipping mutations in the hypocretin receptors (Labrador and Doberman models),[33] or after point mutations in the Hcrt2 receptor gene, with an amino acid change from glutamic acid to lysine in the N-terminus portion of the receptor (Dachshund model).[35] Also of significance is the finding that the intravenous administration of hypocretin-1 (orexin A) in narcoleptic Doberman pinschers reduces cataplexy for up to 3 days, increases activity, promotes waking, and reduces sleep fragmentation in a dose-dependent manner.[36]

Histocompatibility Antigens and Human Narcolepsy

In 1984, an association between narcolepsy and histocompatibility leukocyte antigen (HLA) DR2 was reported in Japan by Juji and coworkers.[37] This association was subsequently observed in other geographic regions of the world as well.[38,39] Consequently, an immunologic mechanism was suspected in the pathogenesis of human narcolepsy, but this has not been established. It was then demonstrated that the association with DR2 is only secondary, and that there is a stronger association of narcolepsy with the HLA DQ antigens, specifically DQB1*0602 and DQA1*0102, which are present in 95% to 100% of patients, as compared to a 12% to 38% prevalence in the general population.[40] In a study of 525 healthy subjects, Mignot and colleagues demonstrated that DQB1*0602 positivity was linked to shorter REM latency, increased sleep efficiency, and decreased time spent in stage 1 NREM sleep.[41] Pelin and coworkers have demonstrated that homozygosity for these two haplotypes is associated with a twofold to fourfold increase in the likelihood of developing narcolepsy over heterozygotes, but that the presence of these antigens does not influence the *severity* of the disease.[42]

Hypocretins and Human Narcolepsy

Unlike narcolepsy in dogs and mice, human narcolepsy is generally not associated with abnormalities in hypocretin receptors but rather with low to absent levels of cerebrospinal (CSF) hypocretin-1.[43] In a postmortem study of human narcolepsy, Thannickal and colleagues found an 85% to 95% reduction in the number of hypocretin neurons in the hypothalamic region,[44] whereas melanin-concentrating hormone neurons, which are intermingled with the hypocretin neurons, remained unaffected, thus suggesting a targeted neurodegenerative process. Using a radioimmunoassay, Nishino and coworkers[45] found that the mean CSF level of hypocretin-1 in healthy controls was 280.3 ± 33.0 pg/mL, and in neurologic controls it was 260.5 ± 37.1 pg/mL,

whereas in those with narcolepsy, hypocretin-1 was either undetectable or below 100 pg/mL. The diagnostic sensitivity of low levels (less than 100 pg/mL) was 84.2%. Low to absent levels were found in 32 out of 38 patients, who were all HLA DQB1*0602 positive. HLA-negative narcolepsy patients had normal to high CSF hypocretin-1 levels. In another recent study, 92.3% of patients who were both DQB1*0602 and cataplexy positive had undetectable CSF hypocretin-1 levels, whereas DQB1*0602-negative patients with cataplexy and DQB1*0602-negative patients without cataplexy had normal levels.[46] In a study of narcolepsy with cataplexy, narcolepsy without cataplexy, and idiopathic hypersomnia, Kanbayashi and colleagues[47] found that all nine CSF hypocretin-deficient patients were HLA DR2 positive (including three preadolescents). In contrast, narcolepsy without cataplexy and idiopathic hypersomnia patients had normal CSF hypocretin levels (Fig. 13–2).

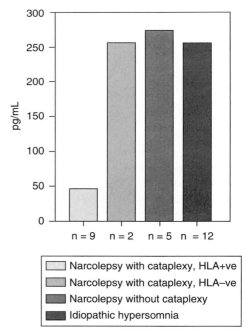

Figure 13–2. Mean cerebrospinal fluid hypocretin-1 levels in various categories of hypersomnia. The narcolepsy-cataplexy group included three prepubertal children of ages 6, 7, and 10. (Adapted from Kanbayashi T, Inoue Y, Chiba S, et al: CSF hypocretin-1 (orexin-A) concentrations in narcolepsy with and without cataplexy and idiopathic hypersomnia. J Sleep Res 2002;11:91-93.)

The routine application of CSF hypocretin-1 assays in the diagnosis of narcolepsy is around the corner. The assay is most useful when an HLA DQB1*0602-positive patient with suspected narcolepsy-cataplexy is receiving CNS stimulants on initial presentation to the sleep specialist, and when discontinuation of medications for the purpose of obtaining a multiple sleep latency test (MSLT) is inconvenient or impractical.

The Two-Hit Hypothesis

The presence of histocompatibility antigen DQB1*0602 or DQA1*0102 is, per se, insufficient to precipitate narcolepsy. This is substantiated by the fact that DQB1*0602-positive monozygotic twins have been incompletely concordant for narcolepsy, with one of the pair developing narcolepsy-cataplexy at age 12 years and the other not until after having suffered emotional stress and sleep deprivation at the age of 45 years.[48] Human narcolepsy is thus best explained on the basis of a *two-threshold hypothesis,* with an interplay between genetic susceptibility and environmental factors—major life events, such as a systemic illness, an injury, or bereavement, have been reported to be present in 82% of narcolepsy patients, compared with a 44% incidence in controls[49] ($P < .001$). The combination of genetic susceptibility and an acquired stress seems to trigger most cases of narcolepsy.

Monoamine Disturbances

Hypocretin deficiency in humans leads to down-regulation of arousal-mediating noradrenergic and dopaminergic pathways in the brainstem, and to upregulation of REM sleep–facilitating cholinergic pathways.[50] Montplaisir and coworkers[51] measured serum and CSF levels of several biogenic amines and their metabolites—dopamine (the metabolite homovanillic acid), norepinephrine (the metabolite 3-methoxy-4-hydroxyphenylethyleneglycol), epinephrine, and serotonin (the metabolite 5-hydroxy indoleacetic acid)—in patients with narcolepsy, in those with idiopathic hypersomnia, and in normal controls. Both narcolepsy and idiopathic hypersomnia patients had significantly decreased concentrations of dopamine and indoleacetic acid, a metabolite of tryptamine. Dopamine and tryptamine are usually present in high concentrations in the basal ganglia. A relative deficiency of these compounds, probably mediated by down-regulation of hypocretin, is involved in the evolution of sleepiness. Stimulants such as dextroamphetamine and methylphenidate, which are used in the treatment of hypersomnolence, are known to enhance dopamine release from presynaptic terminals. Activation of selective dopamine D_2 receptor agonists also suppresses cataplexy.[52] This inhibition is believed to be indirectly mediated via activation of noradrenergic pathways. A reduction in central dopamine activity might also underlie the periodic leg movements that are common in the night sleep of patients with narcolepsy—they are usually relieved by treatment with levodopa or dopamine agonists. A cholinergic disturbance also coexists—physostigmine, a cholinergic agent, leads to a transient increase of cataplexy.

Secondary Narcolepsy

Although the majority of narcolepsy is *idiopathic,* structural lesions of the diencephalon or brainstem may on rare occasion precipitate *secondary narcolepsy* in those who are biologically predisposed, perhaps subsequent to disruption of the hypocretin pathways. Cerebellar hemangioblastomas, temporal lobe B-cell lymphomas, pituitary adenoma, third ventricular gliomas, craniopharyngiomas, head trauma, viral encephalitis, ischemic brainstem disturbances, sarcoidosis, and multiple sclerosis have been associated with narcolepsy.[53-60] In such patients, the finding of cataplexy increases the likelihood that the hypersomnolence is narcolepsy related. Isolated cataplexy has also been observed in Niemann-Pick type C disease,[61] but these patients cannot be labeled as having secondary narcolepsy as they lack other prerequisite clinical and polysomnographic features. Arii and colleagues described a hypothalamic tumor in a 16-year-old girl who manifested hypersomnolence, obesity, and low CSF hypocretin-1 levels, without cataplexy.[62] Although this patient did not meet the criteria for the diagnosis of narcolepsy, the report highlights the importance of hypocretins in the regulation of alertness.

DIAGNOSIS

The diagnosis of narcolepsy is established on the basis of the history, combined with characteristic findings on the nocturnal polysomnogram and a multiple sleep latency test.[63] In preparation for the sleep studies, the patient should be withdrawn from all central nervous stimulants, hypnotics, antidepressants, and any other psychotropic agents for 2 weeks prior to the sleep studies, as these drugs may impact sleep architecture. In the case of drugs with a long half-life, such as fluoxetine, the drug-free interval may need to be 3 to 4 weeks. During this time, the patient should maintain a regular sleep–wake schedule, which can be verified by wrist actigraphy and sleep logs that are maintained by the patient for 1 to 2 weeks prior to the sleep studies.[64] A general physical examination should also be carried out to assess the Tanner stage of sexual development, as normal values for nocturnal total sleep time, daytime sleep latency, and daytime REM sleep latency are closely linked to the Tanner stages.[65]

During the nocturnal polysomnogram, multiple parameters of physiologic activity, such as the EEG (C3-A1, O2-A1 montage), eye movements, chin and leg electromyogram, nasal pressure, thoracic and abdominal respiratory effort, and oxygen saturation, are recorded simultaneously on a computerized sleep monitoring and analysis system.[66] The test helps exclude sleep pathologies such as obstructive sleep apnea, the periodic limb movement disorder,[67,68] and idiopathic hypersomnia[69,70] that can also lead to daytime sleepiness and mimic narcolepsy.

Patients with narcolepsy may exhibit onset of REM sleep within 15 minutes of sleep onset (sleep-onset REM period). Gross sleep efficiency is generally high (greater than 90%), but there may be fragmentation of sleep from an increased number of arousals and periodic limb movements. There is no significant disordered breathing or oxygen desaturation. A useful clue to narcolepsy in adolescents is the presence of decreased nocturnal REM sleep latency (the time between sleep onset and the onset of the first 30-second epoch of REM sleep). For example, in one study,[71] the nocturnal REM sleep latency in narcoleptic subjects was less than 67 minutes (mean, 24.5 minutes; standard deviation, 30; range, 0 to 66.5 minutes; $n = 8$), as compared to a mean nocturnal REM sleep latency of 143.7 minutes in age-matched controls (range, 82.5 to 230.5; SD, 50.9 minutes; $P < .001$). A similar conclusion was reached by Challamel and coworkers in their meta-analysis of 235 subjects,[7] and in the pioneering work of Carskadon and colleagues.[72]

An MSLT should be started at 2 hours after the final morning awakening. It consists of four to five nap opportunities of 20-minute lengths at 2-hour intervals in a darkened, quiet room (e.g., at 1000, 1200, 1400, and 1600 hours).[63] Eye movements, chin electromyogram and electroencephalogram (generally C3-A2, O2-A1) are recorded. The MSLT provides quantitative information about the degree of sleepiness and qualitative information about the nature of the transition from wakefulness into sleep (i.e., wakefulness → NREM sleep, or wakefulness → REM sleep). The time interval between "lights out" and sleep onset is termed the *sleep latency;* a *mean sleep latency* is then derived from all the naps. A urine drug screen is obtained between the naps if the patient appears to be falling asleep very quickly. A concerted effort should be made to ensure that the patient does not accidentally fall asleep between the naps. Typically, the mean sleep latency is markedly shortened to less than 5 minutes in patients with narcolepsy, whereas in controls it is generally 15 to 18 minutes[66] (Table 13–1).

In unaffected children, the initial transition is from wakefulness into NREM sleep. Narcolepsy is, however, associated with a transition from wakefulness directly into REM sleep (*sleep-onset REM period* [SOREMP]). This diagnostic feature of two or more SOREMPs may not be consistently present in the early stages of the disorder in children and young adults, and sometimes serial sleep studies are needed to establish a definitive diagnosis[73] (Fig. 13–3). Opinions differ about normative values for the MSLT-derived mean sleep latency in preadolescents. Although the normative data derived by Carskadon[65] are widely used, it is conceivable that mean sleep latencies may be greater than 20 minutes in preadolescents.[74,75]

Serologic testing for the HLA DQB1*0602 haplotype is an adjunctive test, but it cannot be used alone to diagnose narcolepsy, as this haplotype is also present in 12% to 38% of the general population.[41] CSF hypocretin analysis is useful

Table 13–1.	Normal Values for the Multiple Sleep Latency Test	
Stage of Development	**Mean Sleep Latency (min)**	**Standard Deviation**
Tanner stage I	18.8	1.8
Tanner stage II	18.3	2.1
Tanner stage III	16.5	2.8
Tanner stage IV	15.5	3.3
Tanner stage V	16.2	1.5
Older adolescents	15.8	3.5

Adapted from Carskadon MA: The second decade. In Guilleminault C (ed): Sleeping and Waking Disorders: Indications and Techniques. Menlo Park, Calif, Addison-Wesley, 1982, pp 99-125.

in establishing the diagnosis when psychotropic medications cannot be discontinued for safety reasons. Unfortunately, the testing is not readily available, so nocturnal polysomnography and the MSLT remain the gold standard at this time for making a definitive diagnosis of narcolepsy.

DIFFERENTIAL DIAGNOSIS

By far, the most common disorder leading to excessive daytime sleepiness in an adolescent is

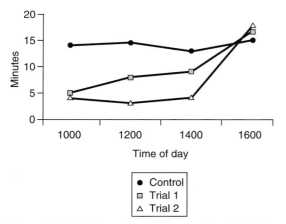

Figure 13–3. Serial multiple sleep latency tests (MSLTs) in a 13-year-old child with evolving narcolepsy. MSLT trials 1 and 2 were carried out 9 months apart. They are compared with the MSLT findings of a healthy control. There is progressive decrease over time in the sleep latencies of the patient at 1000, 1200, and 1400 hours, along with an increase in the number of sleep-onset rapid eye movement periods. Sleep latencies in the final nap (1600 hours) may be physiologically prolonged in children as a result of anticipation about going home—the "last nap" effect. (Reproduced from Kotagal S, Swink TD: Excessive daytime sleepiness in a 13 year old. Semin Pediatr Neurol 1996;3:170-172.)

insufficient nocturnal sleep.[76] To begin with, there is a physiologic shift in the sleep-onset time of most teenagers to between 10:30 and 11:00 PM.[77] Also, the physiologic delay in the onset of dim-light melatonin secretion to a later time at night and the resultant postponement of sleep onset is associated with a corresponding shift to a later morning awakening time in most adolescents. Linked to this phase shift, Carskadon and coworkers have documented SOREMPs during the MSLT of 12 of 25 healthy students.[78] Superimposed on this may be elements of *abnormal sleep hygiene* (e.g., use of stimulants, late-night television viewing/phone calls/computer chats), or circadian rhythm disturbances such as the *delayed sleep phase syndrome*.[79,80] The use of prescription drugs or over-the-counter sedatives such as antihistamines should also be considered as a possible cause of sleepiness. A high index of suspicion should be maintained for illicit drug use.

It is not uncommon for narcolepsy to present with obesity and nocturnal snoring, thus mimicking *obstructive sleep apnea*. The most common causes of childhood obstructive sleep apnea are adenotonsillar hypertrophy, neuromuscular disorders, and craniofacial anomalies such as Crouzon syndrome and Down syndrome.[81-83] The *upper airway resistance syndrome* is another under-recognized disorder leading to chronic daytime sleepiness. It is characterized by habitual snoring, an increased number of breathing-related microarousals, and increased negative intrathoracic pressures on monitoring of esophageal pressures during polysomnography using balloons.[84]

The *Kleine-Levin syndrome*, or *periodic hypersomnia*, is characterized by recurrent periods of sleepiness.[85] The disorder is common in adolescent males, who manifest 1- to 2-week periods of excessive sleep, in association with hyperphagia and hypersexual behavior. There may be a 2- to 10-pound weight gain during the sleepy periods, which then remit spontaneously, only to reappear a few weeks later. No specific etiology has been found. The disorder subsides gradually over time. The nocturnal polysomnogram shows a high sleep efficiency and a decreased percentage of time spent in stages 3 and 4 of NREM sleep.[86] The MSLT shows moderate daytime sleepiness with a shortened mean sleep latency of 5 to 10 minutes, but fewer than two SOREMPs.

Idiopathic hypersomnia should also be considered in the differential diagnosis of narcolepsy. It is defined as a disorder associated with non-imperative sleepiness, long unrefreshing naps, difficulty reaching full awakening after sleep, and sleep drunkenness, as well as absence of SOREMPs during the MSLT.[70,87] Night sleep is quantitatively and qualitatively normal. The MSLT shows a short mean sleep latency, generally in the range of 5 to 10 minutes, but two or more SOREMPs, which would be suggestive of narcolepsy, are not seen. I have studied six children with narcolepsy who underwent serial nocturnal polysomnograms and MSLTs for the assessment of daytime sleepiness.[71] Long, unrefreshing naps were common. Although the initial battery of sleep studies showed shortened mean sleep latencies (less than 10 minutes), suggesting moderate daytime sleepiness, they lacked the necessary (two or more) SOREMPs to diagnose narcolepsy. Initially, therefore, they met the diagnostic criteria for idiopathic hypersomnia. A repeat battery of sleep studies several months later, however, showed the appearance of two or more SOREMPs on the MSLT of each subject, characteristic of narcolepsy. In some children, therefore, idiopathic hypersomnia may be a transitional phase that precedes the development of classic narcolepsy.

MANAGEMENT

Because narcolepsy requires lifelong treatment, the nocturnal polysomnogram and MSLT findings should be unequivocally positive before making the diagnosis. Drugs commonly used for treatment are listed in Table 13–2. *Daytime sleepiness* is countered with stimulants such as methylphenidate (regular or extended-release

Table 13–2.   Drugs Used Commonly in the Treatment of Narcolepsy

Symptom	Drug (Trade Name)	Dosage
Daytime sleepiness	Methylphenidate hydrochloride	5 mg bid to a maximum of 60 mg
	Ritalin	20 mg bid to a maximum of 60 mg
	Ritalin SR	18 mg qid to a maximum of 54 mg/day
	Concerta	10 mg qid to a maximum of 60 mg/day
	Metadate	100-500 mg/day in 1-2 doses
	Modafinil (Provigil)	10-40 mg/day
	Dextroamphetamine (Dexedrine)	20-25 mg/day
	Methamphetamine (Desoxyn)	10-40 mg/day
	Amphetamine/dextroamphetamine mixture (Adderall)	
Cataplexy	Clomipramine (Anafranil)	25-75 mg/day in 1-2 divided doses
	Imipramine	25-100 mg/day
	Protriptyline (Vivactil)	2.5-10 mg/day in 1-2 divided doses
	Sodium oxybate (Xyrem)	3-9 g in two divided doses at night
Emotional problems	Fluoxetine (Prozac)	10-30 mg/day every morning
	Sertraline (Zoloft)	25-100 mg/day every morning
Periodic leg movements	Clonazepam (Klonopin)	0.5-1.0 mg at bedtime
	Levodopa-carbidopa (Sinemet)	25/100 or 50/200 at bedtime
	Pramipexole (Mirapex)	0.125-0.25 mg at bedtime

formulations) or various preparations of amphetamine.[88-91] The side effects of these agents include loss of appetite, nervousness, tics, headache, and insomnia. Modafinil (Provigil), a drug with an unspecified mode of action, has also been reported to be effective in enhancing alertness and improving psychomotor performance in doses of 100 to 400 mg/day in one or two divided doses. The side effects include headache, nervousness, anxiety, and nausea.

Because cataplexy is mediated by cholinergic pathways in the brainstem, drugs with anticholinergic properties such as protriptyline and clomipramine have been used for its control. Sodium oxybate (gamma hydroxybutyrate), an endogenous neurotransmitter/neuromodulator, has recently been found to alleviate cataplexy in a randomized, double-blind, placebo-controlled, multicenter study.[92] It leads to consolidation of sleep and a marked increase in stage 3-4 NREM sleep at night. It is unclear whether the significant improvement in cataplexy and the modest improvement in daytime alertness with sodium oxybate are linked to consolidation in the disrupted night-sleep that is so characteristic of narcolepsy, or to other unknown mechanisms. Because of its positive effects on mood and libido, it has the potential of being abused as a recreational drug.[50] One or two planned naps per day of 25 to 30 minutes also help enhance daytime alertness and improve psychomotor performance.[93] Supportive psychotherapy and fluoxetine or sertraline might also be indicated if patients develop emotional and behavioral problems.

The *Narcolepsy Network* (www.narcolepsynetwork.org) is a private, nonprofit resource for patients, families, and health professionals. Because of the increased risk of accidents from sleepiness, patients should be cautioned against driving long distances and working near sharp, moving machinery. Future treatments might consist of hypocretin analogues.[50]

References

1. Gelineau J: De la narcolepsie. Gaz Hosp (Paris) 1880;53:626-628.
2. American Sleep Disorders Association: The International Classification of Sleep Disorders: Diagnostic and Coding Manual. Rochester, Minn, American Sleep Disorders Association, 1997.
3. Silber M, Krahn L, Olson E, Pankranz V: The epidemiology of narcolepsy in Olmsted County, Minnesota: A population-based study. Sleep 2002;25:197-202.
4. Honda Y: Clinical features of narcolepsy: Japanese experiences. In Honda Y, Juji T (eds): HLA in Narcolepsy. Berlin, Springer-Verlag, 1988, pp 24-57.
5. Lavie P, Peled R: Narcolepsy is a rare disease in Israel. Sleep 1987;10:608-609.
6. Yoss RE, Daly DD: Narcolepsy in children. Pediatrics 1960;25:1025-1033.
7. Challamel MJ, Mazzola ME, Nevsimalova S, et al: Narcolepsy in children. Sleep 1994;17S:17-20.
8. Zarcone V: Narcolepsy. N Engl J Med 1973; 288:1156-1166.
9. Matsuki K, Honda Y, Juji T: Diagnostic criteria for narcolepsy and HLA-DR2 frequencies. Tissue Antigens 1987;30:155-160.
10. Roffwarg HP, Sleep Disorders Classification Committee, Association of Sleep Disorders: Diagnostic classification of sleep and arousal disorders. Sleep 1979;2:1-137.
11. Hublin C, Partinen M, Kaprio J, Kosekenvuo M, et al: Epidemiology of narcolepsy. Sleep 1994;17(Suppl 1):7-12.
12. Sharp SJ, D'Cruz OF: Narcolepsy in a 12-month-old boy. J Child Neurol 2001;16:145-146.
13. Nevsimalova S, Roth B, Zouhar A, Zemanova H: Narkolepsie-kataplexie a periodicka hypersomnie se zacatkem v kojeneckem veku. Cs Pediatr 1986;41:324-327.
14. Lenn NJ: HLA-DR2 in childhood narcolepsy. Pediatr Neurol 1986;2:314-315.
15. Wittig R, Zorick F, Roehrs T, et al: Narcolepsy in a 7-year-old child. J Pediatr 1983;102:725-727.
16. Kotagal S, Hartse KM, Walsh JK: Characteristics of narcolepsy in pre-teen aged children. Pediatrics 1990;85:205-209.
17. Pearl PL, Efron L, Stein MA: Children, sleep, and behavior: A complex association. Minerva Pediatr 2002;54:79-91.
18. Wise MS: Childhood narcolepsy. Neurology 1998;50(Suppl 1):S37-S42.
19. Navalet Y, Anders TF, Guilleminault C: Narcolepsy in children. In Guilleminault C, Dement WC, Passouant P (eds): Narcolepsy. New York, Spectrum, 1976, pp 171-177.
20. Pollack CP: The rhythms of narcolepsy. Narcolepsy Network 1995;8:1-7.
21. Guilleminault C, Wilson RA, Dement WC: A study of cataplexy. Arch Neurol 1974;31:255-261.
22. Guilleminault C, Pelayo R: Narcolepsy in prepubertal children. Ann Neurol 1998;43:135-142.
23. Young D, Zorick F, Wittig R, et al: Narcolepsy in a pediatric population. Am J Dis Child 1988;142:210-214.
24. Henry GK, Satz P, Heilbronner RL: Evidence of a perceptual encoding deficit in narcolepsy. Sleep 1993;16:123-127.

25. Rogers AE, Rosenberg RS: Tests of memory in narcoleptics. Sleep 1990;13:42-52.

26. Foutz AS, Mitler MM, Cavalli-Sforza LL, et al: Genetic factors in canine narcolepsy. Sleep 1979;1:413-421.

27. Knecht CD, Oliver JE, Redding R, et al: Narcolepsy in a dog and a cat. J Am Vet Med Assoc 1984;162:1052-1053.

28. Strain GM, Olcott BM, Archer RM, et al: Narcolepsy in a Brahmin bull. J Am Vet Med Assoc 1984;185:538-541.

29. Mitler MM, Dement WC: Cataplectic-like behavior in cats after microinjection of carbachol in the pontine reticular formation. Brain Res 1974;68:335-343.

30. Nishino S, Reid MS, Dement WC, Mignot E: Neuropharmacology and neurochemistry of narcolepsy. Sleep 1994;17(Suppl 1):S84-92.

31. Reid MS, Tafti M, Geary JN, et al: Cholinergic mechanisms in cataplexy: I. Modulation of cataplexy via local drug administration into the paramedian pontine reticular formation. Neuroscience 1994;59:511-522.

32. Lin L, Faraco J, Li R, et al: The sleep disorder, canine narcolepsy, is caused by a mutation in the hypocretin (orexin) receptor 2 gene. Cell 1999;98:365-376.

33. Chemelli RM, Willie JT, Sinton CM, et al: Narcolepsy in orexin knock-out mice: Molecular genetics of sleep regulation. Cell 1999;98:437-451.

34. Silber MH, Rye DB: Solving the mysteries of narcolepsy: The hypocretin story. Neurology 2001;56:1616-1618.

35. Hungs Fan J, Lin X, Maki RA, Mignot E: Identification and functional analysis of mutations in the hypocretin (orexin) genes of narcoleptic canines. Genome Res 2001;11:531-539.

36. John J, Wu M-F, Siegel JM: Systemic administration of hypocretin-1 reduces cataplexy and normalizes sleep and waking durations in narcoleptic dogs. Sleep Res Online 2000;3:23-28.

37. Juji T, Satake M, Honda Y, Doi Y: HLA antigens in Japanese patients with narcolepsy. Tissue Antigens 1984;24:316-319.

38. Billiard M, Seignalet J, Besset A, Cadilhac J: HLA DR2 and narcolepsy. Sleep 1986;9:149-152.

39. Langdon N, Lock C, Welsh K, et al: Immune factors in narcolepsy. Sleep 1986;9:143-148.

40. Mignot E, Lin L, Rogers W, et al: Complex HLA-DR and -DQ interactions confer risk of narcolepsy-cataplexy in three ethnic groups. Am J Hum Genet 2001;68:686-699.

41. Mignot E, Young T, Lin L, Fin L: Nocturnal sleep and daytime sleepiness in normal subjects with HLA-DQB1*0602. Sleep 1999;22:347-352.

42. Pelin Z, Guilleminault C, Risch N, et al: HLA DQB1*0602 homozygosity increases relative risk for narcolepsy but not disease severity in two ethnic groups. Tissue Antigens 1998;51:96-100.

43. Nishino S, Ripley B, Overeem S, et al: Hypocretin (orexin) deficiency in human narcolepsy. Lancet 2000;355:39-40.

44. Thannickal TC, Moore RY, Nienhuis R, et al: Reduced number of hypocretin neurons in human narcolepsy. Neuron 2000;27:469-474.

45. Nishino S, Ripley B, Overeem S, et al: Low cerebrospinal fluid hypocretin (orexin) and altered energy homeostasis in human narcolepsy. Ann Neurol 2001;50:381-388.

46. Krahn LE, Pankrantz VS, Oliver L, et al: Hypocretin (orexin) levels in cerebrospinal fluid of patients with narcolepsy: Relationship to cataplexy and DQB1*0602. Sleep 2002;25:733-738.

47. Kanbayashi T, Inoue Y, Chiba S, et al: CSF hypocretin-1 (orexin-A) concentrations in narcolepsy with and without cataplexy and idiopathic hypersomnia. J Sleep Res 2002;11:91-93.

48. Honda M, Honda Y, Uchida S, et al: Monozygotic twins incompletely concordant for narcolepsy. Biol Psychiatr 2001;49:943-947.

49. Orellana C, Villemin E, Tafti M, et al: Life events in the year preceding the onset of narcolepsy. Sleep 1994;17(Suppl 1):50-53.

50. Mignot E, Taheri S, Nishino S: Sleeping with the hypothalamus: Emerging therapeutic targets for sleep disorders. Nat Neurosci 2002;5(Suppl): 1071-1075.

51. Montplaisir J, de Champlain J, Young SN, et al: Narcolepsy and idiopathic hypersomnia: Biogenic and related compounds in CSF. Neurology 1982;32:1299-1302.

52. Nishino S, Arrigoni J, Valtier D, et al: Dopamine D2 mechanisms in canine narcolepsy. J Neurosci 1991;11:2666-2671.

53. Autret A, Lucas F, Henry-Lebras F, et al: Symptomatic narcolepsies. Sleep 1994;17S(Suppl 1):21-24.

54. Tridon P, Montaut J, Picard L, et al: Syndrome de Gelineau et hemangioblastome kystique u cervelet. Rev Neurol 1969;121:186-189.

55. Onofrj M, Curatola L, Ferracci F, Fulgente T: Narcolepsy associated with primary temporal lobe B-cell lymphoma in a HLA DR2 negative subject. J Neurol Neurosurg Psychiatry 1992; 55:852-853.

56. Schwartz WJ, Stakes JW, Hobson JA: Transient cataplexy after removal of craniopharyngoma. Neurology 1984;34:1372-1375.

57. Lankford DA, Wellman JJ, Ohara C: Post-traumatic narcolepsy in mild to moderate closed head injury. Sleep 1994;17S(Suppl 1):25-28.

58. Bonduelle C, Degos C: Symptomatic narcolepsies: A critical study. In Guilleminault C, Dement WC, Passouant P (eds): Narcolepsy. New York, Spectrum, 1976, pp 312-332.

59. Rivera VM, Meyer JS, Hata T, et al: Narcolepsy following cerebral ischemia. Ann Neurol 1986;19:505-508.

60. Schrader H, Gotlibsen OB: Multiple sclerosis and narcolepsy-cataplexy in a monozygotic twin. Neurology 1980;30:105-108.

61. Kandt RS, Emerson RG, Singer HS, et al: Cataplexy in variant forms of Niemann-Pick disease. Ann Neurol 1982;12:284-288.

62. Arii J, Kanbayashi T, Tanabe Y, et al: A hypersomnolent girl with decreased CSF hypocretin level after removal of a hypothalamic tumor. Neurology 2001;56:1775-1776.

63. Carskadon MA, Dement WC, Mitler MM, et al: Guidelines for the multiple sleep latency test (MSLT): A standard measure of sleepiness. Sleep 1986;9:519-524.

64. Sadeh A, Hauri PJ, Kripke DF, Lavie P: The role of actigraphy in the evaluation of sleep disorders. Sleep 1995;18:288-302.

65. Carskadon MA: The second decade. In Guilleminault C (ed): Sleeping and Waking Disorders: Indications and Techniques. Menlo Park, Calif, Addison-Wesley, 1982, pp 99-125.

66. Kotagal S, Goulding PM: The laboratory assessment of daytime sleepiness in childhood. J Clin Neurophysiol 1996;13:208-218.

67. American Sleep Disorders Association: Periodic Limb Movement Disorder. In The International Classification of Sleep Disorders: Diagnostic and Coding Manual. Rochester, Minn, American Sleep Disorders Association, 1997, pp 65-68.

68. Chervin RD, Archbold KH, Dillon JE, et al: Association between symptoms of inattention, hyperactivity, restless legs syndrome, and periodic leg movements. Sleep 2002;25:213-218.

69. Roth B: Narcolepsy and hypersomnia: Review and classification of 642 personally observed cases. Scweiz Arch Neurol Neurochir Psychiatr 1976;119:31-41.

70. Basetti C, Aldrich MS: Idiopathic hypersomnia: A series of 42 patients. Brain 1997;120:1423-1435.

71. Kotagal S: A developmental perspective on narcolepsy. In Loughlin GM, Carroll JL, Marcus CL (eds): Sleep and Breathing in Children. New York, Marcel Dekker, 2000, pp 347-362.

72. Carskadon MA, Harvey K, Dement WC: Multiple sleep latency tests during the development of narcolepsy. West J Med 1981;135:414-418.

73. Kotagal S, Swink TD: Excessive daytime sleepiness in a 13-year-old. Semin Pediatr Neurol 1996;3:170-172.

74. Gozal D, Wang M, Pope DW: Objective sleepiness measures in pediatric obstructive sleep apnea. Pediatrics 2001;108:693-697.

75. Palm L, Persson E, Elmquist D, Blennow G: Sleep and wakefulness in normal pre-adolescents. Sleep 1989;12:299-308.

76. Brown LW, Billiard M: Narcolepsy, Kleine-Levin syndrome, and other causes of sleepiness in children. In Ferber R, Kryger M (eds): Principles and Practice of Sleep Medicine in the Child. Philadelphia, WB Saunders, 1995, pp 125-134.

77. Carskadon MA: Factors influencing sleep patterns of adolescents. In Carskadon MA (ed): Adolescent Sleep Patterns: Biological, Social, and Psychological Perspectives. Cambridge, Mass, Cambridge University Press, 2002, pp 18-19.

78. Carskadon MA, Wolfson AR, Acebo C, et al: Adolescent sleep patterns, circadian timing, and sleepiness at a transition to early school days. Sleep 1998;21:871-881.

79. Garcia J, Rosen G, Mahowald M: Circadian rhythms and circadian rhythm disorders in children and adolescents. Semin Pediatr Neurol 2001;8:229-240.

80. Dijk DJ, Bolos Z, Eastman CI, et al: Light treatment of sleep disorders: Consensus report: II. Basic properties of circadian physiology. J Biol Rhythms 1995;10:113-125.

81. Marcus CL: Sleep architecture and respiratory disturbance in children with obstructive sleep apnea. Am J Respir Crit Care Med 2000;162(Part 1): 682-686.

82. Marcus CL: Obstructive sleep apnea symptoms: Difference between children and adults. Sleep 2000;23(Suppl 4):S140-S141.

83. Brooks LJ: Genetic syndromes affecting breathing during sleep. In Loughlin GM, Carroll JL, Marcus CL (eds): Sleep and Breathing in Children. New York, Marcel Dekker, 2000, pp 737-754.

84. Guilleminault C, Pelayo R, Leger D, et al: Recognition of sleep-disordered breathing in children. Pediatrics 1996;98:871-882.

85. Papacostas SS, Hadjivasilis V: Klein Levin syndrome: Report of a case and review of literature. Eur Psychiatr 2000;15:231-235.

86. Gadoth N, Kesler A, Vainstein G, et al: Clinical and polysomnographic characteristics of 34 patients with Klein Levin syndrome. J Sleep Res 2001;10:337-341.

87. Billiard M, Rondouin G, Espa F, et al: Pathophysiology of idiopathic hypersomnia: Current studies and new orientation. Rev Neurol (Paris) 2001;157(Part 2):S101-S106.

88. Stahl SM: Awakening to the psychopharmacology of sleep and arousal: Novel neurotransmitters and wake-promoting drugs. J Clin Psychiatr 2002;63:467-468.

89. Mitler MM: Evaluation of treatment with stimulants in narcolepsy. Sleep 1994;17(Suppl 1): 103-106.

90. Billiard M, Besset A, Montplaisir F, et al: Modafinil: A double blind multicentric study. Sleep 1994;17S:107-112.

91. Littner M, Johnson SF, McCall WV, et al: Practice parameters for treatment of narcolepsy: An update for 2000. Sleep 2001;24:451-466.

92. The U.S. Xyrem Multicenter Study Group: A randomized, double blind, placebo-controlled multicenter trial comparing the effects of three doses of orally administered sodium oxybate with placebo for the treatment of narcolepsy. Sleep 2002;25: 42-49.

93. Garma L, Marchand F: Non-pharmacological approaches to treatment of narcolepsy. Sleep 1994;17S:97-102.

Idiopathic Hypersomnia

Michael H. Kohrman

Excessive daytime sleepiness in the adolescent is epidemic in our society today. In the adolescent population, hypersomnolence is manifested primarily as excessive daytime sleepiness. Symptoms are partially the result of school and lifestyle pressures combined with changes in circadian phase and total sleep time. In contrast, excessive daytime sleepiness being manifested as hypersomnolence is uncommon in young children. The primary manifestation of sleepiness in young children is hyperactivity. Young children respond to the symptoms of sleepiness by increasing their motor activity to maintain alertness. However, even in this group, careful questioning does reveal symptoms of daytime sleepiness. The clinical definition of idiopathic hypersomnolence in childhood must take into account this difference in the clinical response of children to the same "sleep pressure" manifested as excessive daytime sleepiness in adults.

Idiopathic hypersomnia (IH) is characterized by sleepiness and sleep episodes that are usually resistible, long lasting, not refreshing, and not associated with frequent periods of sleep onset with rapid eye movement (REM). In addition, IH is sometimes associated with increased total sleep, difficult awakenings, and sleep drunkenness.[1] Guilleminault and Pelayo have divided IH into three types based on etiology: those patients with a positive family history and positive human leukocyte antigen–Cw2, those with a history of viral infection, and those not included in the first two groups.[2] Bassetti and Aldrich divided their patients into three groups based on clinical symptoms.[1] The "classic IH" group tended to have sleepiness that was not overwhelming, take un-refreshing naps of up to 4 hours, and have prolonged night-time sleep and difficulty awakening. The second group they termed a "narcoleptic" type that presented with overwhelming excessive daytime sleepiness;

took short, refreshing naps; and awakened without sleepiness. The third group was a "mixed" type, with features of both syndromes.

Idiopathic hypersomnolence is by definition a diagnosis of exclusion. A complete evaluation of other causes of hypersomnolence must be undertaken. The differential diagnosis of idiopathic hypersomnolence is quite broad, ranging from mood disorders to narcolepsy to circadian rhythm disturbances. Table 14–1 provides a framework based on etiology for further discussion of the differential diagnosis below.

OBJECTIVE EVALUATION OF SLEEPINESS IN CHILDREN

Objective evaluation of sleepiness begins with a complete sleep history and physical examination to eliminate other causes of excessive daytime sleepiness (Table 14–2) (see Chapter 1). Sleep logs should be obtained to document sleep times, and actigraphy may be utilized to confirm the sleep log data. On the night prior to laboratory testing for daytime sleepiness, a polysomnogram should be obtained to confirm the absence of a primary sleep disorder. Hypersomnolence can be characterized quantitatively via the multiple sleep latency test (MSLT)[3] and maintenance of wakefulness test (MWT).[4] Both tests measure the time to fall asleep during the daytime. The MSLT instructs the patient to fall asleep, while the MWT instructs the patient to stay awake. The mean adult sleep latency is 18.7 minutes. It is generally accepted in the adult population that pathologic average sleep latency is 5 minutes or less as the result of an MSLT with an average sleep latency of 13.4 minutes.[5]

The results of the MSLT and MWT often differ. Bonnet and Arand suggest that the MWT measures sleep propensity and also the arousal system secondary to motivation and posture,

Table 14–1. Differential Diagnosis of Hypersomnolence

Neurologic Disorders

Epilepsy and anticonvulsant therapy
Stroke
Tumor/increased intracranial pressure
Narcolepsy

Primary Sleep Disorders

Insufficient sleep syndrome
Insomnia
Upper airway resistance syndrome
Obstructive sleep apnea syndrome
Restless legs syndrome

Behavioral Disorders

Chronic fatigue syndrome
Kleine-Levin syndrome
Mood disorders

Circadian Disorders

Delayed sleep phase syndrome

Medical Disorders

Infection: acute and chronic
Muscle disease
Metabolic disorders
Prader-Willi syndrome

Table 14–2. Diagnostic Studies to Define Idiopathic Hypersomnia

Sleep log
Polysomnography
Multiple sleep latency test/maintenance
  of wakefulness test
Actigraphy
MRI
EEG
Psychological testing

while the MSLT is done supinely and measures only sleep propensity.[6] Carskadon and Dement have demonstrated that sleep latency in children is age dependent.[7] Using Tanner stages to group children during adolescence, they observed a drop in average sleep latency on the MSLT of 20% between Tanner stages 1 and 3. This decreased sleep latency persisted into later adolescence (Tanner stages 4 and 5). In the same subjects, total sleep time and total REM time remained constant, but total slow-wave sleep (SWS) time decreased by 70%. The mean sleep latency of Tanner stages 1 and 2 children (mean age 12 years, sleeping their habitual average of 9.1 hours) was 18 minutes, compared with the college student (mean age 19 years, habitual sleep 7.1 hours) of less than 5.5 minutes. Thus, the definition of pathologic sleepiness in children must account for this age dependency.

Clinical Presentation

Bassetti and Aldrich reviewed 42 cases of IH.[1] The onset of hypersomnolence began at a mean age of 19 ± 8 years (range 6-43 years). Onset was associated with insomnia in 5, weight gain in 2, viral illness in 4, and minor head trauma in 3. Forty-five percent of the patients snored, and 60% took one or more involuntary naps during the day. These naps lasted 30 minutes or more in over half the subjects in their study, and 77% reported that the naps were un-refreshing. Over 50% of the patients had psychiatric complaints. Polysomnographic recordings demonstrated short sleep latencies of 6.6 ± 5.7 minutes. Mean latency on the MSLT was 4.3 ± 2.1 minutes. In 12 patients who underwent esophageal pressure monitoring, 5 were found to have upper airway resistance syndrome. None of these patients reported improved sleep with continuous positive airway pressure.

Typically, symptoms begin during childhood and include prolonged night-time sleep and awakening difficulties that often proceed to the onset of daytime sleepiness. Roth has reported continuous nonimperative sleepiness; prolonged, un-refreshing naps without dreaming; and difficult arousal.[8]

Polysomnographic studies of the 42 patients of Bassetti and Aldrich[1] demonstrated a sleep efficiency of 93% from a mean of 20 total awakenings of greater than 1 minute, 8% slow-wave sleep, and 18% REM sleep. They also found automatic behaviors in 61% and sleep paralysis in 40%. The amount of sleep per day was 8.4 ± 1.9 hours and arousal time in the morning 42 minutes. Forza and colleagues studied 10 patients with IH.[9] All had onset before the age of 21. There was no statistical difference between IH patients and control subjects for the Tanner stage test or sleep latency. Mean sleep latency was 9.1 minutes. IH patients demonstrated decreased SWS and increased REM sleep percent. Mean sleep latency was 5.7 ± 0.7 minutes.

DIFFERENTIAL DIAGNOSIS OF IDIOPATHIC HYPERSOMNOLENCE

The differential diagnosis of idiopathic hypersomnolence consists of those syndromes that can produce excessive daytime sleepiness. A list based on etiology is seen in Table 14–1. History, physical examination, polysomnography, and assessment of daytime sleep latency can usually exclude most of these diagnoses. Other chapters in this text cover most of these diagnoses, and this chapter will be concerned only with those that are outside the scope of the primary sleep disorders.

Primary Sleep Disorders

While diagnostic criteria are well established for the primary sleep disorders in adults, normative data on which to base clinical decisions have been only recently available for children. Thus, the reader must apply pediatric normative values when diagnosing sleep-disordered breathing[10] or restless legs syndrome/periodic leg movement disorder.[11] Insufficient sleep syndrome is still the primary cause of daytime somnolence in most children. A number of studies have led to conflicting results with regard to school start times and daytime somnolence. Epstein and associates in Israel found decreased total sleep time and increased somnolence in fifth grade pupils who started school at 7:10 AM compared with 8:00 AM.[12] A study in Maryland demonstrated no correlation of total sleep time with academic performance.[13]

Upper airway resistance syndrome remains a diagnosis that must be excluded in this patient population. No consensus has yet been reached on how to best evaluate this syndrome in children. The use of esophageal pressure manometry is controversial, and a consensus on the usefulness of noninvasive measures, nasal pressure, and arterial tonometry has not been established.

Neurologic Disorders

Narcolepsy remains the most difficult clinical syndrome to exclude in this group of disorders.

It can present at as young as 4 years of age, and often cataplexy may not appear until later in life. However, the recent understanding of the absence of Orexin/hypocretin as the pathophysiologic cause of narcolepsy will allow for accurate diagnosis of this patient group as cerebrospinal fluid assay for the absence of Orexin becomes a routine clinical test.[14]

Those central nervous system lesions that produce increased intracranial pressure can be associated with hypersomnia. Subdural hematomas can produce an indolent syndrome of decreasing mental status and lethargy. Associated with increased intracranial pressure are often headache and vomiting. Epilepsy can produce a state in which the patient becomes lethargic and less responsive, the so-called petit mal status or spike-and-wave stupor, because of the atypical continuous spike-and-wave pattern noted on the EEG. This condition is often responsive to valproic acid, with rapid return to a normal state. Anticonvulsants can also produce sedation and excessive daytime sleepiness or paradoxical hyperactivity in children. Sedation appears to be common with carbamazepine, while hyperactivity is more common with phenobarbital.

Behavioral Disorders

Attention deficit hyperactivity disorder is an active area of investigation in terms of its relationship to sleep disruption. Whereas both obstructive sleep apnea syndrome and restless leg syndrome/periodic leg movement disorder are associated with hyperactivity in children, attention deficit hyperactivity disorder is multifactorial in origin and sleep disorders constitute an etiology in only a fraction of children with ADHD.

Chronic fatigue/fibromyalgia syndrome is also a diagnosis of exclusion. While these children often complain of diffuse muscle aches, trigger points may be seen in others. The patients often complain of tiredness rather than true hypersomnia. Polysomnography may demonstrate an alpha–delta pattern on the EEG.[15] Depression and upper airway resistance syndrome must be excluded in chronic fatigue patients as well.

Mood disorders are commonly associated with sleep difficulties in children. They may be manifested as insomnia, early morning awakenings, daytime sleepiness, or hypersomnia. Vgontzas and coworkers found increased sleep latency (54 vs 15 minutes), increased wake time after sleep onset (79 vs 56.8 minutes), and increased total wake time (134 vs 72 minutes) in patients with psychiatric etiologies for their hypersomnia compared with those with IH. In patients with psychiatric disorders REM sleep was decreased, compared with patients with IH.[16] Bipolar disorder may also present with hypersomnia during the depression phase of the illness. At times these children may overlap with Kleine-Levin Syndrome (see Chapter 16).

Circadian Disorders

Delayed sleep phase syndrome may also produce hypersomnolence. However, these children report normal total sleep times in the presence of delayed sleep onset and morning hypersomnia. (see Chapter 9). Non–24-hour sleep–wake cycles as well as advanced sleep phase syndrome may also produce hypersomnolence. Sleep logs and/or actigraphy are often helpful in recognizing these problems.

Medical Disorders

Acute illness often results in hypersomnolence as one attempts to recover from bacterial or viral infections. Hypersomnolence associated with fever and a stiff neck should alert the examiner to possible meningitis. However, a stiff neck and other meningeal signs may be absent in children under 1 year of age. Lumbar puncture should always be performed if any question of meningitis exists. Kubota and colleagues report a case of acute disseminated encephalomyelitis associated with hypersomnolence as the major presenting feature as well as low hypocretin levels in the cerebrospinal fluid.[17] Arii and associates describe hypersomnolence and low hypocretin levels in a child after removal of a hypothalamic tumor.[18]

Metabolic disorders may produce episodic mental status changes which may appear to produce sleepiness and altered mental status. Disorders of ammonia metabolism, lactate and pyruvate metabolism, and mitochondrial metabolism can be associated with episodic hypersomnia. Acute infection or other metabolic stress often precipitates these episodes. Muscle weakness can also be a source of hypersomnolence. Primary muscle disease, comprising the dystrophies, are often associated with decreased respiratory effort secondary to fatigue. Polysomnography demonstrates increasing REM-related central apnea as the first sign of weakness and the need for nocturnal respiratory support.[19]

Prader-Willi syndrome is associated with obesity, craniofacial dysmorphism, hypotonia, hyperphasia, hypersomnia, and hypothalamic dysfunction. Manni et al found sleep-onset REM (SOREM) periods in 5 of 10 children with Prader-Willi syndrome on MSLT.[20] None of the patients were Dr-15 or Dq-6 positive. Hypersomnia and SOREMs could not be accounted for by sleep-disordered breathing alone; however, upper airway resistance syndrome was not excluded in these patients.

TREATMENT

The treatment of IH is focused on symptom control, as the primary etiology remains unknown. The goal of therapy is to allow the patient to enjoy normal, alert functioning and restful nocturnal sleep.

The approach to therapy is sleep hygiene, appropriate use of stimulant medication, and safety for the patient. Sleep hygiene measures should include naps in the afternoon and regular sleep periods of 8 to 10 hours nightly. Drugs, alcohol, or medications that promote sleepiness should be avoided. Stimulant medication should be used at the lowest effective doses tolerated and growth problems secondary to anorexia can be a limiting factor of use in some children. In addition, a balanced plan of stimulant use must be maintained to not interfere with night-time sleep. The newer, longer-acting stimulants (Table 14–3) have been beneficial in management, keeping medicine out of the school setting and decreasing the need for late afternoon dosing. The American Academy of Child and Adolescent Psychiatry has recently produced a practice parameter for stimulant use in children, adolescents, and adults.[21]

SUMMARY

IH remains a diagnosis of exclusion, and at times it can be difficult to differentiate it from the

Table 14–3.   Stimulants Used for Treatment of Idiopathic Hypersomnia

Name	Duration of Action	Contraindications	Special Considerations
Methylphenidate	4-6 hr	Increased risk of	
Time-release preparations	8-12 hr	cardiac arrhythmias	Longer action
Dexmethylphenidate	4-6 hr		Isomer of parent compound
Dextroamphetamine Time spans	4-6hr		
Mixed salts	4-6 hr		
Extended-release preparations	8-12 hr		Longer duration of action
Monafinil	6-8 hr		Non-amphetamine drug
Pemoline	12 hr	High risk of liver disease	

other disorders in Table 14–1. Continued research is necessary to better characterize this disorder in children. Treatment should be symptomatic; naps improve sleep hygiene and stimulants should be used in concert to provide improved quality of life in these children. The role of hypocretin in the etiology of IH in children requires further exploration.

References

1. Bassetti C, Aldrich MS: Idiopathic hypersomnia: A series of 42 patients. Brain 1997;120:1423-1435.
2. Guilleminault C, Pelayo R: Idiopathic Central Nervous System Hypersomnia. In Kryger MH, Roth T, Dement WC: Principles and Practice of Sleep Medicine, 3rd ed. Philadelphia, WB Saunders, 2000, pp 687-692.
3. Carskadon MA, Dement WC, Mitler MM, et al: Guidelines for the multiple sleep latency test (MSLT): A standard measure of sleepiness. Sleep 1986;9:519-524.
4. Mitler MM, Gujavarti KS, Browman CP: Maintenance of wakefulness test: A polysomnographic technique for evaluation of treatment efficacy in patients with excessive somnolence. Electroencephalogr Clin Neurophysiol. 1982;53:658-661.
5. Mitler MM, Carskadon MA, Hirshkowitz M: Evaluating Sleepiness. In Kryger MH, Roth T, Dement WC (eds): Principles and Practice of Sleep Medicine, 3rd ed. Philadelphia, WB Saunders, 2000.
6. Bonnet MH, Arand DL: Arousal components which differentiate the MWT from the MSLT. Sleep 2001;24:441-447.
7. Carskadon MA, Dement WC: Sleepiness in the Normal Adolescent. In Guilleminault C (ed): Sleep and Its Disorders in Children. New York, Raven Press, 1987, pp 53-66.
8. Roth B: Narcolepsy and Hypersomnia. Basel, Karger, 1980.
9. Forza E, Gaudreau H, Petit D, Montplaisir J: Homeostatic sleep regulation in patients with idiopathic hypersomnia. Clin Neurophysiol 2000;111:277-282.
10. Goodwin JL, Enright PL, Morgan WJ, et al: Correlates of obstructive sleep apnea in 6-12 year old children: The Tucson Children Assessment of Sleep Apnea Study (TUCASA) (Abstract). Sleep 2002;25(Suppl):A80.
11. Kohrman MH, Kerr SL, Schumacher S: Effect of sleep disordered breathing on periodic leg movements of sleep in children (Abstract). Sleep 1997;20(Suppl):635.
12. Epstein R, Chillag N, Lavie P: Starting times of school: Effects on daytime functioning of fifth grade children in Israel. Sleep 1998;21:250-256.
13. King J, Gould B, Eliasson A: Association of sleep and academic performance. Sleep Breath 2002;6:45-48.
14. Nishino S, Ripley B, Overeem S, et al: Hypocretin (Orexin) deficiency in human narcolepsy. Lancet 2000;355:39-40.
15. Whelton CL, Salit I, Moldofsky H: Sleep, Epstein-Barr virus infection, musculoskeletal pain and depressive symptoms in chronic fatigue syndrome. J Rheumatol 1992;19:939-943.
16. Vgontzas AN, Bixler EO, Kales A, Criley C, Vela-Bueno A: Differences in nocturnal and daytime sleep between primary and psychiatric hypersomnia: Diagnostic and treatment implications. Psychosomat Med 2000;62:220-226.

17. Kubota H, Kanbayashi T, Tanabe Y, et al: A case of acute disseminated encephalomyelitis presenting hypersomnia with decreased hypocretin level in cerebrospinal fluid. J Child Neurol 2002;17: 537-539.

18. Arii J, Kanbayashi T, Tanabe Y, et al: A hypersomnolent girl with decreased CSF hypocretin level after removal of a hypothalamic tumor. Neurology 2001;56:1775-1776.

19. Kerr SL, Kohrman MH: Polysomnogram in Duchenne muscular dystrophy. J Child Neurol 1994;9:332-334.

20. Manni R, Politini L, Nobili L, Ferrillo F, et al: Hypersomnia in the Prader-Willi syndrome: Clinical- electrophysiological features and underlying factors. Clin Neurophysiol 2001;112: 800-805.

21. Greenhill LL, Plixzka S, Dulcan MK: Work Group on Quality Issues Practice Parameter for the use of stimulant medications in the treatment of children, adolescents, and adults. J Am Acad Child Adolesc Psychiatry 2002;41:26S-49S.

Post-Traumatic Hypersomnia   15

Stephen H. Sheldon

Children who suffer significant head trauma frequently experience significant sleep disturbances after the injury, particularly when the trauma is severe enough to result in major loss of consciousness. Nonetheless, sleep disturbances may also follow minor trauma in which a brief loss of consciousness occurs. In all instances, sleep patterns after the insult vary notably from the pretrauma sleep habits.

Closed-head trauma is the most common event resulting in post-traumatic hypersomnia. Head injury as a result of an automobile accident is the most common cause. Even so, similar symptoms have been reported after neurosurgical procedures and other brain traumas. It appears that the mode of injury is less important than the location. Symptomatically, there is a variable period of initial coma that evolves into a post-traumatic hypersomnolence and excessive daytime sleepiness with or without sleep attacks or unintentional sleep episodes. Nocturnal sleep may or may not be prolonged compared with the preinjury period. When total sleep time within each 24-hour day is increased, the term "post-traumatic hypersomnia" is fitting. Associated symptoms are typically due to daytime sleepiness (e.g., concentration difficulties, amnesia of recent events, fatigue, and occasional visual problems). Chronic headache and minor neurologic signs of traumatic brain injury may also be present.

Less commonly, the initial head injury is followed by problems initiating and maintaining sleep either with or without some degree of subjective daytime sleepiness. Post-traumatic psychogenic insomnia is also seen. Reports of post-traumatic narcolepsy and cataplexy have been described, but as it has been pointed out in some case reports, post-traumatic narcolepsy/cataplexy occurred 5 years after the head injury. Other case reports do not appear to be consistent with the narcolepsy/cataplexy syndrome and more likely represent post-traumatic hypersomnia.[1]

Symptoms resulting from closed-head injury depend on the location of injury within sleep-regulating brain areas. Although data are limited, there appear to be several correlations, with hypersomnolence being the most common feature. Areas of the brain involved are most commonly those related to maintaining wakefulness, including but not limited to the brainstem reticular formation, posterior hypothalamus, and the region of the third ventricle. Shearing forces along the direction of main fiber pathways can lead to microhemorrhages in these areas. High cervical cord trauma has also been known to cause sleepiness and unintentional sleep episodes.[2,3] Whiplash injury may result in hypersomnia, with consequent sleep-disordered breathing. In these cases, the hypersomnolence appears to be secondary to the respiratory abnormality.[4]

Countercoup injuries commonly occur at the base of the skull and may result in organic post-traumatic sleeplessness. These types of injury occur in areas of bony irregularities (especially the sphenoid ridges), with consequent damage to the inferior frontal and anterior temporal regions,[5,6] including the basal forebrain.[7]

Rodrigues and Silva have reported a patient with aggressive body movements during rapid eye movement (REM) sleep and periodic limb movements after a traumatic brain injury—symptoms suggesting REM-sleep behavior disorder.[8] Multiple sleep latency testing revealed extremely short latencies. It was suggested that dopaminergic pathways potentiate hypothalamic hypocretin abnormalities that are involved in the pathophysiology.

Closed-head injury may also involve the suprachiasmatic nucleus within the hypothalamus, resulting in disturbances of circadian rhythmicity. These symptoms then produce a combination of hypersomnia and insomnia. Complete sleep phase reversal has also been reported.[9]

The prevalence of post-traumatic sleep disorders has not been determined. Head injury due to motor vehicle accidents is common and represents over 50% of all reported head injuries in industrialized countries.[10] Unintentional falls, intentional violence, and increased risk-taking behavior also contribute to the frequency of head trauma in children.

Evaluating the underlying cause of hypersomnia in patients who have suffered head trauma involves determining the degree of injury and potential locations within the brain that the trauma may have affected. In patients recovering from coma, the relationship is clear. Nonetheless, a careful history must always be taken, and the presence or absence of prior sleep disturbances of similar types should be determined. Obscure causes of hypersomnolence should also be considered in the evaluation of the patient with suspected post-traumatic hypersomnia. Hydrocephalus, subdural hematoma, meningitis, encephalitis, and seizure disorders should be assessed. The possibility of drug use (pharmacologic and/or recreational) should also be considered. Psychogenic insomnia related to head injury must be assessed. When comprehensive nocturnal polysomnography reveals the presence of sleep-disordered breathing after head trauma, the sleep-related breathing disorders must first be managed before determining the extent to which each comorbid condition contributes to the hypersomnolence. Patients with anatomic risk factors for obstructive sleep disordered breathing may abruptly develop symptoms of head trauma. Similarly, clear-cut narcolepsy with cataplexy has been shown to occur after head trauma in patients who exhibit human leukocyte antigen–DQ B1-0602. The recognition that head trauma can be a precipitating factor to syndromes leading to excessive daytime sleepiness is important, and a comprehensive evaluation of all patients who exhibit excessive sleepiness after head trauma is needed.

Historical information forms the basis for the evaluation of the patient with possible post-traumatic hypersomnia in order to temporally document the association of the hypersomnia with the trauma, determine the presence of preexisting sleep-related pathology, and assess the evolution of symptoms after the head injury. Physical examination can reveal the possibility of minor focal neurologic signs, especially those of brainstem origin.

In the hypersomnolent patient, polysomnography and multiple sleep latency testing should be considered in order to determine the nature of the post-traumatic nocturnal sleep disturbances as well as rule out coexisting pathologies such as obstructive sleep apnea syndrome and periodic limb movement disorder. Polysomnography in patients with post-traumatic hypersomnia generally reveals an increase in sleep duration with or without changes in other aspects of sleep architecture.[11] The findings in patients with post-traumatic insomnia include long sleep latencies, low sleep efficiency, and a decrease in nightly sleep duration, especially in stage 2 sleep.[12]

Continuous polysomnography has confirmed an increase in total sleep per 24 hours in some patients with post-traumatic hypersomnia.[12] It is of interest that polysomnography during the comatose period has prognostic value for the development of full recovery without post-traumatic sleep disturbances. The normal frequency of sleep spindles, K-complexes, and normal non-REM and REM sleep architecture are favorable prognostic signs.[13-16]

If daytime sleepiness is a major complaint, a multiple sleep latency test is of help in determining severity and circadian variation. In post-traumatic hypersomnia with daytime sleepiness, sleep latency may be markedly shortened.[11] Patients with post-traumatic insomnia exhibit prolonged sleep latencies on nocturnal polysomnography, and multiple sleep latency testing may be normal.[12] The presence of obstructive sleep apnea syndrome, other forms of sleep-disordered breathing, and/or sleep onset REM periods (on nocturnal polysomnography and/or multiple sleep latency testing) does not rule out the possibility that head trauma is a precipitating or contributing factor.

Medical evaluation should include assessment of levels of activity and the habitual sleep–wake patterns of the youngster before the head trauma. Assessment should include but not be limited to the following: interviews of parents and teachers, school performance records, prior medical history, and school tardiness and absenteeism.

The exact prognosis of patients with post-traumatic hypersomnia has not yet been elucidated. There are few systematic follow-up studies. Based mostly on anecdotal information, once the hypersomnia has stabilized, sleep disturbances related to the head trauma show little additional change. Patients with post-traumatic hypersomnia generally respond fairly well to treatment, and there are no known specific complications.

Youngsters with post-traumatic hypersomnia may require stimulant medication such as methylphenidate or amphetamines in doses similar to those required for narcolepsy/cataplexy syndrome. In older children the drug of choice may be modafinil, which has fewer side-effects overall than phenylethylamine stimulants. The dosage of modafinil in children has yet to be determined, but a starting dose of 200 mg with gradual titration to 400 mg (if needed) might be attempted. On the other hand, modafinil has no noradrenergic properties, and patients with severe head trauma who have more significant lesions and also complain of intellectual slowness might benefit more from phenylethylamines. These medications will have a general "activating" effect that is not devoted solely to sleepiness.

Any coexisting sleep pathology or neurologic disease requires independent management. Nasal continuous positive airway pressure may be helpful in secondary sleep-disordered breathing. The potential beneficial effects of naps have not been studied; they should probably be restricted to less than 30 minutes to avoid significant sleep inertia after the nap. They should be taken when the patient feels the sleepiest but not within 4 or 5 hours of habitual nocturnal sleep time.

References

1. Bonduelle M, Bouygues P, Faveret C: Narcolepsie post-traumatique. Lille Med 1959;4:719-721.
2. Adey W, Bors E, Porter RW: EEG patterns after high cervical lesions in man. Arch Neurol 1968;19:377-383.
3. Hall CS, Danoff D. Sleep attacks: Apparent relationship to atlantoaxial dislocation. Arch Neurol 1975;32:58-59.
4. Guilleminault C, Yuen KM, Gulevich MG, et al: Hypersomnia after head-neck trauma: A medicolegal dilemma. Neurology 2000;54:653-659.
5. Courville CB: Coup-contrecoup mechanism of cranio-cerebral injuries: Some observations. Arch Surg 1942;55:19-43.
6. Ommaya AK, Grubb RL, Naumann RA: Coup and contre-coup injury: Observations on the mechanics of visible brain injuries in the rhesus monkey. J Neurosurg 1971;35:503-516.
7. Sterman MB, Clemente CD: Forebrain inhibitory mechanisms: Cortical synchronization induced by basal forebrain stimulation. Exp Neurol 1962;6:91-102.
8. Rodrigues RN, Silva AA: Excessive daytime sleepiness after traumatic brain injury: Association with periodic limb movements and REM behavior disorder. Case report. Arquivos de Neuro-Psiquiatria 2002;60:656-660.
9. Billiard M, Negri C, Baldy-Moulignier M, et al: Organisation du sommeil chez les sujets atteints d'inconscience post-traumatique chronique. Rev Electroencephalogr Neurophysiol 1979;9:149-152.
10. Marshall LF, Becker DP, Bowers SA, et al: The National Traumatic Coma Data Bank, Part 1: Design, purpose, goals, and results. J Neurosurg 1983;59:276-284.
11. Guilleminault C, Faull KF, Miles L, van den Hoed J: Posttraumatic excessive daytime sleepiness: A review of 20 patients. Neurology 1983;33:1584-1589.
12. Manseau C, Broughton RJ: Severe head injury: Long term effects on sleep, sleepiness and performance. Sleep Res 1990;19:335.
13. Passouant P, Cadilhac J, Delange M, et al: Different electrical stages and cyclic organization of post-traumatic comas: Polygraphic recordings of long duration. Electroencephalogr Clin Neurophysiol 1965;18:726P.
14. Bergamasco B, Bergamini L, Doriguzzi T: Clinical value of the sleep electroencephalographic patterns in posttraumatic coma. Acta Neurol Scand 1968;44:495-511.
15. Bricolo A, Gentilomo A, Rosadini G, Rossi GF: Long-lasting post-traumatic unconsciousness: A study based on nocturnal EEG and polygraphic recording. Acta Neurol Scand 1968;44:512-532.
16. Lessard CS, Sances A, Larson SJ: Period analysis of EEG signals during sleep and posttraumatic coma. Aerospace Med 1974;45:664-668.

Kleine-Levin Syndrome and Recurrent Hypersomnias

16

Stephen H. Sheldon

Kleine-Levin syndrome is an unusual disorder featuring recurrent episodes of excessive sleepiness and prolonged total sleep time. It is rare, with an onset typically in late adolescence, but cases of younger and older individuals have been reported. It has been suggested that a predisposing event occurs before the onset of symptoms in nearly half of the reported cases. Symptoms that are flulike often precede the onset of episodes of recurrent hypersomnia.

CLINICAL CHARACTERISTICS OF KLEINE-LEVIN SYNDROME

Hypersomnia is the characteristic symptom of Kleine-Levin syndrome. Sleepiness is profound, and during spells patients may sleep continuously for more than 20 hours. This excessive sleepiness and true hypersomnia can develop suddenly. However, symptoms typically have a more gradual onset of 1 to 7 days. During spells of hypersomnia, patients rarely leave their beds and sleep continuously. Sleep may be calm, but at times agitated, restless sleep occurs and vivid dreams are occasionally reported.

In addition to excessively long sleep episodes, abnormal behaviors, including but not limited to compulsive and excessive overeating and sexually acting out behaviors, occur. Other mental disturbances may be present. Compulsive overeating and hypersexuality may not be present with each episode. Excessive caloric intake during spells frequently results in weight gain by the end of the spell.

Overt expression of hypersexuality may include indiscriminate sexual advances, masturbation, and/or public display of sexual fantasies. Sexually acting-out is reported in approximately one third of the males with Kleine-Levin syndrome. Hypersexuality is less often reported in females. The presence of excessive eating and/or hypersexuality is not required for the diagnosis of Kleine-Levin syndrome. In many cases, hypersomnia and its recurrence may be the only symptom.[1] Psychological symptoms vary considerably, and irritability is common. Confusion and visual and auditory hallucinations frequently occur.

Recurrent episodes of hypersomnia may be brief and last less than 1 week or may be prolonged and last up to 30 days. Characteristic of Kleine-Levin syndrome are the *recurrence* of episodes of hypersomnia and abnormal behaviors. Patients are normal between episodes. Nevertheless, neuropsychological sequelae, changes in personality, and a decrease in school performance have been reported after a second hypersomnolent episode. Physical examination is generally normal.

Although Kleine-Levin syndrome is characterized by the triad of recurrent spells of hypersomnolence, hyperphagia, and hypersexuality, it is likely that incomplete manifestation is more common than the complete triad. Isolated, abnormal sleepiness and recurrent periods of hypersomnia without associated symptoms may be a more common manifestation.

Periods of hypersomnia gradually decrease in frequency as the youngster ages. Spells gradually become less severe and eventually resolve.[2] Nonetheless, patients with recurrent episodes of hypersomnia occurring 20 years after the initial onset of symptoms have been reported.[2-4]

The social and professional consequences are not negligible: Students miss classes, and young workers may be fired because of repeated absences.

Menstruation-associated hypersomnia has been reported in female patients. Periods of hypersomnolence recur and are coupled with menses. Occasionally, mental disturbances also occur, frequently during the menstrual cycle.[5]

Several female patients with recurrent hypersomnia had a notable absence of symptoms.[1] The prognosis for menstruation-related hypersomnia is similar to that of Kleine-Levin syndrome.

The cause of recurrent hypersomnia is unknown. A possible viral etiology may be present in some cases, and in others there may be a suggestion of local encephalitis in the region of the diencephalon.[6-8] Recurrent transient episodes of unresponsiveness and clearly identified stage 2 sleep patterns with the presence of sleep spindles due to bilateral paramedian thalamic infarctions have also been reported.[9] Although the exact cause of recurrent hypersomnia and other manifestations is still unclear, the symptoms of hypersomnolence, excessive and compulsive eating, hypersexuality, recurrence, and absence of any identifiable abnormalities between spells are suggestive of a functional abnormality at the level of the diencephalon. The hypothalamus may also be involved. Indeed, identical symptoms have been reported in patients with tumors of the hypothalamus or third ventricle and in patients with epidemic encephalitis. Most of the literature and case reports suggest that this recurrent hypersomnia is caused by dysfunction of the hypothalamus and midbrain limbic system. There also is evidence that brainstem dysfunction may be involved. Recurrent hypersomnia associated with decreased blood flow in the thalamus on single-photon emission computed tomography has also been reported.[10] During the remission period, there were no abnormal data resulting from this testing.

Neuroendocrine function in patients with Kleine-Levin syndrome has been assessed. However, only a limited number of subjects have been investigated, and most of the literature consists of case reports. Investigation is complicated by the inability to predict the timing of episodes, lack of a prodromal period, and relatively rapid recovery once symptoms begin.

Nonetheless, some abnormal laboratory data reported to date include a paradoxical growth hormone response to thyroid-releasing hormone stimulation,[11] a blunted cortisol response to insulin-induced hypoglycemia,[12,13] and an absent thyroid-stimulating hormone response to thyroid-releasing hormone.[13] These findings suggest a possible dysfunction within the hypothalamic–pituitary axis. However, other basal and post-stimulation values of hormones are usually normal, and laboratory values are normal during the asymptomatic periods between spells.

Studies of nocturnal or 24-hour secretory patterns of pituitary hormones have been conducted in a limited number of patients. A normal secretory pattern of growth hormone was reported in one patient, but the sampling at 4-hour intervals was sparse.[14] On the other hand, an elevated growth hormone secretory pattern was reported in two patients.[15] A normal secretory pattern of cortisol and somewhat abnormal patterns of growth hormone have been identified in four other patients.[16] A normal 24-hour pattern of melatonin, prolactin, and cortisol secretion has been reported.[17] Gadoth and colleagues found an increased nocturnal prolactin secretory pattern and an abnormally flat nocturnal luteinizing hormone secretory pattern, whereas follicle-stimulating hormone and thyroid-stimulating hormone secretory patterns were normal.[11] Chesson and Levine compared 24-hour secretions in the symptomatic and asymptomatic periods and found that values obtained during nocturnal sleep showed a significantly decreased growth hormone but increased prolactin and thyroid-stimulating hormone in a direction that supports the hypothesis that dopaminergic tone is reduced during the symptomatic period in Kleine-Levin syndrome.[18] However, Mayer and colleagues found only minor hormonal changes in five patients.[19] Altogether, these data suggest some functional disturbance in the hypothalamic-pituitary axis in Kleine-Levin syndrome, but the disturbance may be in response to the sleep-related and behavioral changes rather than a cause. An observation supporting a diencephalic dysfunction is the occurrence of dysautonomic features in some patients.[20]

Differentiating Kleine-Levin syndrome from organic etiologies is often difficult. Diagnosis is often based on the clinical presentation of recurrence of symptoms with asymptomatic intervals and progressive improvement to resolution. In addition, it is often a diagnosis of exclusion. Hypersomnia may recur with space-occupying lesions of the central nervous system, idiopathic recurring stupor, and certain psychological/psychiatric conditions.

Tumors in the region of the third ventricle, such as cysts, astrocytomas, and/or craniopharyngiomas, may be responsible for intermittent obstruction of the third ventricle, leading to headache, vomiting, sensory disturbances, and intermittent impairment of alertness. Less frequently, tumors in other locations of the central nervous system may result in hypersomnia. Tumors in the middle fossa may disrupt the suprachiasmatic nucleus, and an irregular sleep wake pattern or a free-running state might result. If a free running state occurs, hypersomnia may alternate with sleeplessness at a regular interval as the pacemaker cycles at its inherent rhythm. Recurrent hypersomnia may also develop after encephalitis or head trauma. Periodic hypersomnia has also been reported in a patient with a Rathke cleft cyst.[21]

Major recurrent depression and bipolar affective disorder can be associated with excessive sleepiness.[22] Patients with psychogenic recurrent hypersomnia complain of extreme sleepiness and fatigue and may spend many hours in bed. Continuous night and day polygraphic recording often fails to demonstrate increased total sleep time despite the complaint of sleepiness.[23]

EVALUATION

The diagnosis of Kleine-Levin syndrome is typically based on clinical features. Laboratory evaluations are occasionally useful, since the diagnosis may exclude other similar pathologies. Complete blood cell count, platelet count, electrolytes, renal and liver function tests, calcium, phosphorus, serum protein electrophoresis, immunoglobulin, antinuclear antibodies, rheumatoid factor, and serum titers for herpes simplex, Epstein-Barr virus, cytomegalovirus, varicella zoster, mumps, and measles have all been found to be normal in patients with Kleine-Levin syndrome both during and between episodes. Cerebrospinal fluid evaluation with cultures for bacteria, mycobacterium, virus, and fungi have also been shown to be negative.

Routine EEG obtained during attacks may show generalized slowing of background activity or may be unremarkable. MRI is normal during and between spells of hypersomnia.[19] Prolonged polysomnographic monitoring may reveal the increased total sleep time. During symptomatic periods, the multiple sleep latency test can reveal abnormal sleep latencies and sleep-onset REM periods. Therefore, it has been suggested that the multiple sleep latency test may be useful in diagnosis, especially when polysomnography and multiple sleep latency testing are performed no earlier than the second night after the onset of hypersomnolence.[24] During asymptomatic periods polysomnography and multiple sleep latency testing are both normal.

TREATMENT

Kleine-Levin syndrome is typically treated symptomatically. Interventions are focused on terminating the episode of hypersomnia. Amphetamines, methylphenidate, and modafinil have been used in both treatment and prevention, but no treatment has been consistently successful. Generally, the effectiveness of maintaining wakefulness using this therapeutic approach does not exceed a few hours.

References

1. Kesler A, Gadoth N, Vainstein G, et al: Kleine Levin syndrome (KLS) in young females. Sleep 2000;23:563-567.
2. Critchley M: Periodic hypersomnia and megaphagia in adolescent males. Brain 1962;85:627-656.
3. Gran D, Begemann H: Neue Beobachtungen bei einem Fall von Kleine-Levin Syndrom. Munch Med Wochenschr 1973;115:1098-1102.
4. Bucking PH, Palmer WR: New contribution to the clinical aspects and pathophysiology of the Kleine-Levin syndrome. Munch Med Wochenschr 1978;120:1571-1572.
5. Billiard M, Guilleminault C, Dement WC: A menstruation-linked periodic hypersomnia. Neurology 1975;25:436-443.
6. Takrani LB, Cronin D: Kleine-Levin syndrome in a female patient. Can Psychiatr Assoc J 1976;21:315-318.
7. Carpenter S, Yassa R, Ochs R: A pathological basis for Kleine-Levin syndrome. Arch Neurol 1982;39:25-28.
8. Fenzi F, Simonati A, Crosato F, et al: Clinical features of Kleine-Levin syndrome with localized encephalitis. Neuropediatrics 1993;24:292-295.
9. Bjornstad B, Goodman SH, Sirven JI, Dodick DW: Paroxysmal sleep as presenting symptom of bilateral paramedian thalamic infarction. Mayo Clin Proc 2003;78:347-349.
10. Nose I, Ookawa T, Tanaka J, et al: Decreased blood flow of the left thalamus during somnolent

episodes in a case of recurrent hypersomnia. Psych Clin Neurosci 2002;56:277-278.

11. Gadoth N, Dickerman Z, Bechar M, et al: Episodic hormone secretion during sleep in Kleine-Levin syndrome: Evidence for hypothalamic dysfunction. Brain Dev 1987;9:309-315.

12. Koerber RK, Torkelson R, Haven G, et al: Increased cerebrospinal fluid 5-hydroxytryptamine and 5-hydroxyindoleacetic acid in Kleine-Levin syndrome. Neurology 1984;34:1597-1600.

13. Fernandez JM, Lara I, Gila L, et al: Disturbed hypothalamic-pituitary axis in idiopathic recurring hypersomnia syndrome. Acta Neurol Scand 1990;82:361-363.

14. Gilligan BS: Periodic megaphagia and hypersomnia—an example of the Kleine-Levine syndrome in an adolescent girl. Proc Aust Assoc Neurol 1973;9:67-72.

15. Kaneda H, Sugita Y, Masoaka S, et al: Red blood cell concentration and growth hormone release in periodic hypersomnia. Wak Sleep 1977;1: 369-374.

16. Hishikawa Y, Iijima S, Tashiro T, et al: Polysomnographic Findings and Growth Hormone Secretion in Patients with Periodic Hypersomnia. In Koella WP (ed): Sleep 1980. Basel, S Karger, 1981, pp 128-133.

17. Thompson C, Obrecht R, Franey C, et al: Neuroendocrine rhythms in a patient with the Kleine-Levin syndrome. Br J Psychiatry 1985;147: 440-443.

18. Chesson AL, Levine SN: Neuroendocrine evaluation in Kleine-Levin syndrome: Evidence of reduced dopaminergic tone during periods of hypersomnolence. Sleep 1991;14:226-232.

19. Mayer G, Leonhard E, Krieg J, Meier-Ewert K: Endocrinological and polysomnographic findings in Kleine-Levin syndrome: No evidence for hypothalamic and circadian dysfunction. Sleep 1998;21:278-284.

20. Hegarty A, Merriam AE: Autonomic events in Kleine-Levin syndrome. Am J Psychiatry 1990; 147:951-952.

21. Autret A, Lucas B, Mondon K, et al: Sleep and brain lesions: A critical review of the literature and additional new cases. Neurophysiol Clin 2001;31:356-375.

22. Jeffries JJ, Lefebvre A: Depression and mania associated with Kleine-Levin-Critchley syndrome. Can Psychiatr Assoc J 1973;18:439-444.

23. Billiard M, Cadilhac J: Les hypersomnies recurrentes. Rev Neurol (Paris) 1988;144:249-258.

24. Rosenow F, Kotagal P, Cohen BH, et al: Multiple sleep latency test and polysomnography in diagnosing Kleine-Levin syndrome and periodic hypersomnia. J Clin Neurophysiol 2000;17: 519-522.

Diagnosis of Obstructive Sleep Apnea Syndrome in Infants and Children

17

Eliot S. Katz

Carole L. Marcus

Sleep-disordered breathing (SDB) is a common and serious cause of morbidity during childhood. This chapter is concerned with diagnosing the spectrum of obstructive SDB, ranging from the frank, intermittent occlusion seen in obstructive sleep apnea syndrome (OSAS), to persistent, primary snoring (Fig. 17–1). OSAS is characterized by recurrent episodes of partial or complete airway obstruction resulting in hypoxemia, hypercapnia, and/or respiratory arousal. The sleep fragmentation and gas exchange abnormalities observed with OSAS may produce serious cardiovascular and neurobehavioral impairment. The upper airway resistance syndrome (UARS) is characterized by brief, repetitive respiratory effort–related arousals during sleep in the absence of overt apnea, hypopnea, or gas exchange abnormalities[1] (Fig. 17–2). It has been linked to significant cognitive and behavioral sequelae in children, including learning disabilities, attention deficit, hyperactivity, and aggressive behavior.[2] Obstructive hypoventilation features prolonged increased upper airway resistance accompanied by gas exchange abnormalities, but not frank apnea or hypopnea.[3] Children with primary snoring may have increased respiratory effort, but they lack identifiable arousals, including respiratory effort–related, electroencephalographic (EEG), and subcortical arousals.[4] Although primary snoring has been traditionally defined as a benign condition without polysomnographic abnormalities,[5] recent evidence suggests that the increased respiratory effort in primary snoring per se may be associated with untoward neurobehavioral consequences.[6,7]

Habitual snoring has been reported in 3% to 12% of the general pediatric population, although only 1% to 3% have OSAS.[8-10] It is thus important to distinguish primary snoring from more serious forms of obstruction. Early recognition of SDB is important for effective treatment with adenotonsillectomy or continuous positive airway pressure. Establishing strict criteria for OSAS diagnosis and severity is the basis for optimizing the surgical and medical management of this condition.[11] The diagnosis and management of pediatric OSAS continues to evolve as more precise measures of flow limitation and sleep fragmentation are introduced. Both the intermittent hypoxemia and the sleep fragmentation characteristic of OSAS pose a risk to the vulnerable developing brain. The increased recognition of subtle neurocognitive impairments in children with SDB has forced clinicians to rethink the threshold of disease requiring intervention.

HISTORY AND PHYSICAL EXAMINATION

The high incidence of OSAS in children mandates that screening inquiries about sleep disturbances should be a routine part of the primary care interview[12] (Table 17–1). Particular attention should be given to conditions known to exacerbate SDB, such as craniofacial abnormalities, neuromuscular weakness, and genetic conditions. Parents typically provide the clinical history, as the patients are usually oblivious to their condition. Loud snoring, on a nightly basis, is nearly universal in pediatric OSAS. A parental report of a snoring child is an accurate predictor of polysomnographic snoring, but not of OSAS.[13] The snoring is often accompanied by labored breathing, hyperextension of the neck, and witnessed apneic pauses. Subjective reports of excessive daytime sleepiness are infrequently present in children with OSAS. A recent study reported that only 7.5% of the children with polysomnographically proven OSAS had a history of daytime sleepiness.[14] Using an objective measure of sleepiness, such as a multiple sleep latency

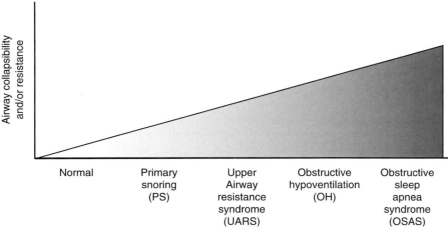

Figure 17–1. Spectrum of obstructive sleep-disordered breathing in children. (Adapted with permission from Loughlin GM: Obstructive sleep apnea syndrome in children: Diagnosis and management. In Loughlin GM, Carroll JL, Marcus CL (eds): Sleep and Breathing in Children: A Developmental Approach. New York, Marcel Dekker, 2000, pp 625-650.)

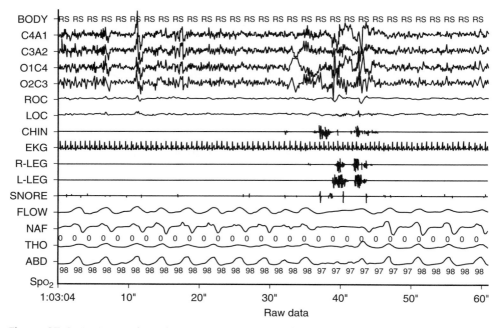

Figure 17–2. A 60-second epoch from a 16 year old with snoring and excessive daytime sleepiness. Note flow limitation in the nasal pressure tracing leading to an EEG arousal. Inspiration is upward. Abd, abdomen; Body, body position; Flow, thermistor; NAF, nasal pressure; RS, right side; Spo₂, pulse oximetry; Tho, thorax.

test, reveals that only 13% of children with OSAS have a sleep latency of less than 10 minutes.[14] Although not considered sleepy by adult standards, children with SDB are sleepier than unaffected children.[15] Increasing body mass index and apnea index (usually greater than 15 to 20 events per hour) were independently correlated with shorter sleep latencies.[14]

The use of standardized screening questionnaires for OSAS has been disappointing. Brouillette and coworkers presented a questionnaire suitable for distinguishing children with

Table 17–1. Clinical History of Obstructive Sleep Apnea Syndrome	
Sleep	**Wakefulness**
Snoring	Poor school performance
Witnessed apnea	Aggressive behavior
Choking noises	Hyperactivity
Increased work of breathing	Attention deficit disorder
Paradoxical breathing	Excessive daytime sleepiness
Enuresis	Morning headaches
Restless sleep	
Diaphoresis	
Hyperextended neck	
Frequent awakenings	
Dry mouth	

OSAS from normal controls.[16] However, subsequent application of this questionnaire to a population of snoring children demonstrated wide-ranging positive predictive values (48.3% to 76.9%) and negative predictive values (26.9%

Table 17–2.   Physical Examination in Obstructive Sleep Apnea Syndrome
General
Sleepiness
Obesity
Failure to thrive
Head
Swollen mucous membranes
Deviated septum
Adenoidal facies
Infraorbital darkening
Elongated face
Mouth breathing
Tonsillar hypertrophy
High arched palate
Overbite
Crowded oropharynx
Macroglossia
Glossoptosis
Midfacial hypoplasia
Micrognathia/retrognathia
Cardiovascular
Hypertension
Loud P2 (heart sound)
Extremities
Edema
Clubbing (rare)

to 83.3%).[16-18] Other questionnaires were also unsuccessful[19,20] or were not validated with polysomnography.[21,22] Although children with OSAS are statistically more likely to have reported symptoms (e.g., witnessed apnea, cyanosis, or labored breathing), the sensitivity and specificity of such observations are low. Thus, the clinical history alone is insufficient to diagnose OSAS in a population of snoring children.[12]

Physical examination of children with OSAS is most often normal, with the exception of adenotonsillar hypertrophy or craniofacial abnormalities (Table 17–2). The majority of OSAS children are of normal height and weight, although both obesity and failure to thrive may occur. Cardiovascular sequelae of SDB such as cor pulmonale and congestive heart failure are infrequently observed in current clinical practice, as heightened awareness has facilitated earlier diagnosis. Although blood pressure is statistically elevated in children with OSAS, the wide range of normal makes this measurement a poor screening tool.[23] The neurocognitive consequences of OSAS, such as poor school performance,[24] aggressive behavior, and hyperactivity,[2,25] are nonspecific.

IMAGING AND LABORATORY EVALUATION

The diagnosis of SDB is firmly established using polysomnography, and ancillary testing is rarely indicated. Further screening may be useful to facilitate perioperative care and to exclude underlying conditions (Table 17–3). For example, concern regarding right ventricular dysfunc-

Table 17–3. **Ancillary Diagnostic Studies in Obstructive Sleep Apnea Syndrome**

Serum Markers

Hematocrit
Serum bicarbonate

Imaging

Brain magnetic resonance imaging (MRI)
Anteroposterior and lateral neck radiograph
Upper airway computer tomography/MRI (complex craniofacial issues)
Dynamic fluoroscopy

Sleep Monitoring

Multiple sleep latency test

Miscellaneous

Echocardiogram
Neurocognitive testing
Electrocardiogram
Flow-volume loop

tion may necessitate an electrocardiogram or an echocardiogram. Occasionally, chronic intermittent hypoxemia may induce polycythemia, and persistent hypercarbia can elevate serum bicarbonate. Routine pulmonary function testing is not indicated in children suspected of having OSAS unless restrictive or obstructive lung disease is suspected. A fluttering pattern in the flow volume loop has been described in adults with OSAS.[26] Magnetic resonance imaging (MRI) of the upper airway in children with OSAS compared to unaffected controls reveals a statistically smaller upper airway luminal volume and elongation of the soft palate, as well as enlarged tonsils and adenoids.[27] However, there is considerable overlap between the groups, rendering MRI a poor screening tool. The measurement of the ratio of the width of the tonsil to the depth of the pharyngeal space on a lateral neck radiograph was reported to have good sensitivity and specificity for distinguishing mild from moderate/severe OSAS in a small number of patients.[28] Dynamic fluoroscopy under sedation may demonstrate glossoptosis, particularly in children with macroglossia, micrognathia, or neuromuscular weakness.[29] Anatomic localization of the site of obstruction may alter the therapeutic approach in some children with craniofacial anomalies. Neck radiographs may be suggestive of adenoidal hypertrophy, but direct or indirect visualization of the adenoids remains the diagnostic standard.

Video/Audio Recordings

Diagnosing OSAS using home audio recordings, in addition to a standard clinical history and physical examination, revealed a sensitivity of 92% but a specificity of only 29%.[30] Subtle forms of SDB are particularly difficult to evaluate using this technique. However, computer-aided processing of audio signals for regularity may improve predictive value.[31] Frequency domain analysis of the snoring signal has also shown promise in distinguishing OSAS from primary snoring.[32] Video recordings yield a noninvasive measure of movement and therefore arousal.[33-35] Video is also a useful adjunct to a comprehensive polysomnogram to evaluate body and head positioning, paradoxical breathing, snoring, and mouth breathing. Studies correlating video scoring systems to standard polysomnography have been encouraging.[34] Future research will be necessary to validate the utility of a particular domiciliary video or audio study in a population with a well-characterized symptomatology.

Overnight Polysomnography

Polysomnography is the gold standard for establishing the presence and severity of SDB in children, and it can be performed in children of all ages. An expert consensus panel has recommended that overnight polysomnography is the diagnostic test of choice in evaluating children with suspected SBD.[12] Guidelines for performing laboratory-based polysomnography in children have been established.[36] The sleep laboratory should be a nonthreatening environment that comfortably accommodates a parent during the study. Personnel with pediatric training should record, score, and interpret the study. The use of sedatives[37] and sleep deprivation[38] may worsen SBD and are therefore not recommended. To the extent possible, sleep studies should conform to the child's usual sleep period. Infants may reasonably be studied during the day, whereas adolescent studies should generally start later at night. The polysomnographic montage will vary with the patient's age and suspected disorder (Table 17–4).

Electroencephalogram

Consensus guidelines for analyzing sleep architecture have been established in infants[39] and adults.[40] Standard practice is to apply adult EEG criteria to children older than 6 months. Sleep staging establishes that an adequate amount of total sleep time and sufficient rapid eye movement (REM) sleep were obtained on the night of the study. In addition to sleep staging, the EEG tracing is useful for scoring cortical arousals and detecting epileptiform discharges. By consensus, an electrocortical (EEG) arousal is defined in adults as an abrupt 3-second shift in EEG frequency.[41] This criterion appears to be appropriate for use in children as well.[42] However, visible EEG arousals are present in only 51% of obstructive events in children,[43] complicating the diagnosis of UARS in children. Frequency domain analysis of

the EEG tracing may further enhance the sensitivity of detecting respiratory events or arousal.[44,45] Initial reports indicated that children with snoring[46] or even severe OSAS may have normal sleep state distribution.[47] However, a large cohort (N = 559) comparing unaffected children to those with OSAS revealed that the latter have increases in slow-wave sleep (23.5% versus 28.8% of total sleep time) and decreases in REM sleep (22.3% versus 17.3% of total sleep time).[48] Furthermore, these authors observed a decline in the spontaneous arousal index in patients with OSAS compared with controls (8.4 versus 5.3), suggesting a homeostatic elevation in the arousal threshold.[48]

Arousal

Arousal from sleep is a protective reflex mechanism that restores airway patency through dilator muscle activation. Both mechanoreceptors and chemoreceptors have a role in initiating the arousal response. Although arousals reverse the airway obstruction, they result in the untoward consequences of sleep fragmentation and sympathetic activation.[49] Polysomnographically, arousal may be associated with EEG changes,[41,45] increased airflow, elimination of airflow limitation, cessation of paradoxical breathing, tachycardia, movement,[35] blood pressure elevation,[50] and autonomic activation. In children, however, approximately 50% of obstructive events do not result in an EEG arousal.[43] In infants, EEG arousals are even less common.[43] Thus, the EEG arousal index is unreliable for the diagnosis of UARS. Frequency domain analysis may reveal evidence of EEG arousal not readily visible, and it may be a clinically useful tool in the future.[44,45]

Obstructive events that terminate with autonomic activation are termed subcortical arousals. Autonomic measures include heart rate variability,[51] blood pressure elevations,[50] pulse transit time,[4] and peripheral arterial tonometry.[52] The pulse transit time was reported to be a more sensitive measure of respiratory arousal than the 3-second EEG arousal.[4] Subcortical arousals alone have been demonstrated to result in neurocognitive impairment in adults.[53]

Measures of Respiratory Effort

A variety of methods to categorize central and obstructive respiratory events are amenable to

Table 17–4.	Example of a Polysomnogram Montage

Electroencephalography (C3/A2, O1/A2)
Electrooculogram (right/left)
Electrocardiogram
Abdominal and thoracic excursion
Oximetry (3-sec averaging value), waveform
End-tidal Pco_2 (peak value, waveform)
Flow: nasal pressure, oronasal thermistor
Snore volume
Body position sensor
pH (in special circumstances)
Esophageal pressure (in special circumstances)
Video/audio taping

overnight polysomnography. Measures of thoracic and abdominal excursion include piezoelectric belts and respiratory inductive plethysmography (RIP). The classification of central and obstructive apneas is achieved by determining if respiratory efforts are present during intervals of reduced flow. Uncalibrated RIP tracings may also be used as an index of thoracoabdominal asynchrony. The highly compliant chest wall in children results in asynchronous motion between the thoracic and abdominal tracings, termed paradoxical breathing. This disparity may be quantified using phase angle analysis that is independent of the relative contributions of the two compartments.[54] Thoracoabdominal asynchrony has been demonstrated in children with increased respiratory effort due to upper airway obstruction and OSAS.[54,55] Paradoxical breathing is normally seen in infants because of the high compliance of their chest wall, particularly during REM sleep, but it is rare after 3 years of age.[56]

Esophageal manometry (P_{es}), the gold standard for quantifying respiratory effort, permits the detection of subtle, partially obstructive events that may produce sleep fragmentation.[57] However, P_{es} monitoring is uncomfortable and may itself alter the frequency of respiratory events.[58] The introduction of noninvasive, nasal pressure measurements has largely supplanted P_{es} for establishing the diagnosis of UARS (see Fig. 17–2). Our current practice is to reserve P_{es} monitoring for children with diagnostic uncertainty even after standard overnight polysomnography.

Measures of Airflow

Airflow can be quantitatively measured using an oronasal mask and a pneumotachograph. However, mask breathing is uncomfortable and has been shown to alter respiratory mechanics. Practically speaking, this methodology is restricted to research settings. Thermistors provide qualitative measures of oronasal airflow by measuring the temperature of expired air. Although thermistors accurately indicate complete cessation of flow, they are not an accurate measure of tidal volume or therefore of hypopnea.[59] As a result, many laboratories have adopted a definition of hypopnea that requires an arterial oxygen desaturation of 3% and/or an

arousal in addition to a reduction in the thermistor signal. Another drawback of the thermistor is its long time constant that obscures the nuance of the flow profile, making the evaluation of flow limitation impossible.[59]

Nasal cannula pressure recordings provide a minimally invasive, semiquantitative measure of airflow.[60,61] The resulting signal has been shown to be proportional to flow squared. Because nasal pressure measurements have a fast time constant, it is possible to detect flattening of the inspiratory nasal pressure signal, termed flow limitation, which occurs in a collapsible tube when flow becomes independent of driving pressure (Fig. 17–3). Limitations of the nasal cannula pressure recordings include obstruction of the tubing with secretions, mouth breathing (especially in children with adenoidal hypertrophy), and the possible increase in nasal resistance caused by obstruction of the nares. In children, the reported signal quality has varied in laboratory-based studies. Trang and coworkers[62] reported an uninterpretable nasal cannula signal during only 4% of total sleep time. However, 17% of subjects had uninterpretable signals for more than 20% of total sleep time. In contrast, Serebrisky and colleagues[63] reported adequate nasal cannula flow signals (in greater than 50% of total sleep time) during sleep in only 71.8% of patients. In a domiciliary study, the nasal cannula channel was not available, overall, for more than 50% of the night.[64]

Airflow may be approximated using RIP by considering that lung volume can be approximated by a two-compartment model (thoracic and abdominal excursion). RIP may be calibrated using an isovolume maneuver or a statistical technique and used to derive a sum channel proportional to tidal volume.[65,66] Thus, the time derivative of the sum channel is proportional to flow. The RIP signal may therefore be analyzed for apnea, hypopnea, and flow limitation. Our current practice is to combine RIP, nasal cannula pressure, and oronasal thermistor in our laboratory-based studies to ensure that a flow signal is likely to be available throughout the night.

Gas Exchange

Pulse oximetry, which is based on the absorption spectra of hemoglobin, is the standard polysomno-

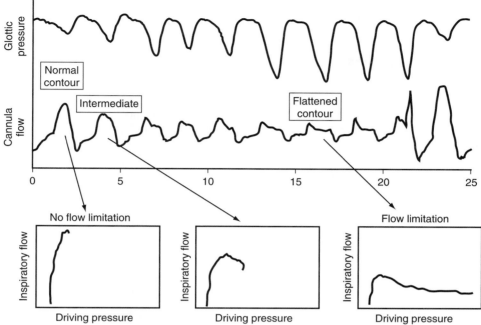

Figure 17–3. Nasal cannula pressure tracing demonstrating that flow becomes independent of driving pressure during flow-limited breaths. (Reproduced with permission from Hosselet J, Norman RG, Ayappa I, Rapoport DM: Detection of flow limitation with a nasal cannula/pressure transducer system. Am J Respir Crit Care Med 1998;157:1461- 1467.)

graphic measure of hypoxemia. The relationship between the arterial oxygen tension (PaO_2) and the oxygen saturation (SpO_2), the oxyhemoglobin curve, is sigmoidal. Patients with normal pulmonary function, whose baseline SpO_2 is on the flat portion of the curve, require large changes in PaO_2 to affect their SpO_2. In contrast, patients with parenchymal lung disease may be operating on the steep portion of the oxyhemoglobin curve, thereby experiencing a profound decline in SpO_2 with small decrements in PaO_2. In sickle cell disease, the oxyhemoglobin curve is variably shifted to the right, thus limiting the utility of SpO_2 measurements.[67]

The adequacy of ventilation can be assessed noninvasively during sleep by sampling CO_2 tension in respired air, termed capnography. Expired gas initially consists of dead space ventilation in the measuring apparatus as well as the physiologic dead space. The terminal expired concentration of CO_2 reaches a plateau and reflects alveolar gas. The concentration of CO_2 in a given alveolus is predicated on the ventilation–perfusion relationship. In subjects with normal lung mechanics, end-tidal $PaCO_2$ ($P_{ET}CO_2$) is approximately 2 to 5 mm Hg below the arterial $PaCO_2$ level.[68] However, in diseases with uneven ventilation–perfusion or altered alveolar time constants, such as cystic fibrosis, the $P_{ET}CO_2$ is not an accurate measure of $PaCO_2$. Also, the rapid respiratory rates characteristic of infants may not permit the alveolar CO_2 to plateau and therefore may underestimate the true CO_2 value.[69] In OSAS, the shape of the capnogram waveform qualitatively reflects flow, whereas the plateau level indicates the overall adequacy of ventilation. Normative data for $P_{ET}CO_2$ during sleep are presented later in Table 17–5. The capnometry signal is prone to artifact because of nasal secretions that obstruct the sampling cannula. Morielli and colleagues[69] reported that 27% of polysomnographic epochs in their laboratory had a poor $P_{ET}CO_2$ waveform, stressing the importance of careful attention to technique. Transcutaneous CO_2 ($TcCO_2$) monitors may be valuable in patients in whom $P_{ET}CO_2$ is not accurate, such as infants or patients with parenchymal lung disease.[69] Although absolute values of $TcCO_2$ are variable, the trend is proportional to the $PaCO_2$, with a lag of several minutes. Sleep is normally associated with a 4- to 6-mm Hg increase in $TcCO_2$.

Normative Polysomnographic Data

Normative data for the EEG and respiratory parameters of sleeping children are shown in Table 17–5.[47,48,70-72] In infants, longitudinal arterial oxygen saturation monitoring revealed a median SpO_2 baseline of 98%, but the SpO_2 was less than 90% during 0.51% of epochs.[73] Marcus and coworkers[72] presented the respiratory data of 50 normal, nonobese children between 1 and 18 years of age (mean, 9.7 ± 4.6), using a thermistor and $P_{ET}CO_2$ monitoring. Nine subjects had at least one obstructive apneic event. One "normal" child had an apnea index of 3.1/hour, although he had a sibling with OSAS. Including this outlier, an apnea index of greater than 1/hour was determined to be statistically abnormal. However, the threshold level at which the apnea index becomes clinically significant has not been established. Only 15% of unaffected children had any hypopneas, with the mean hypopnea index being 0.1 ± 0.1 (range, 0.1 to 0.7).[74] Acebo and colleagues[71] also reported that hypopneas were rare in older children and adolescents. Normative data using nasal pressure during sleep have not been presented in children. Experience from our laboratory indicates that hypopneas and respiratory effort–related arousals do not occur in normal young children.

Normative data for esophageal manometry (ΔP_{es}) from 10 normal subjects in our laboratory, aged 2 to 11 years, showed that control subjects had a mean ΔP_{es} of −8 ± 2 cm H_2O (range, − 6 to −12), a peak ΔP_{es} of −12 ± 3 cm H_2O (range − 9 to −19 cm H_2O), and a ΔP_{es} of less than or equal to −10 cm H_2O for 8% ± 12% of breaths (range, 3% to 61%).[4] Other investigators have considered ΔP_{es} swings of −8 to −14 cm H_2O as normal[75] and have suggested that normal children spend 10% or less of the night with inspiratory esophageal pressure swings of −10 cm H_2O or less.[57] However, our data showed that two control patients spent 21% and 61% of the night with a ΔP_{es} of −10 cm H_2O or less. Thus, normative data from nonsnoring controls reveal considerable variability in respiratory effort. The ΔP_{es} is lower in normal infants (5 to 6 cm H_2O).[76]

Domiciliary and Nap Studies

Attended overnight polysomnography in a designated pediatric sleep laboratory is the gold standard for the diagnosis of SDB children.[36] However, such comprehensive testing is expensive, labor intensive, and not widely available. Recognizing that 10% to 12% of children snore but that only 1% to 3% have OSAS[8,9] has prompted considerable interest in limited, nap, or unattended domiciliary studies. Choosing the most appropriate evaluation is predicated on understanding the relative risks of OSAS and its

Table 17–5. Polysomnographic Data in Unaffected Children

Sleep Parameters		Respiratory Parameters	
EEG arousal index, n/hr	7 ± 2	Obstructive apnea index, n/hr TST	0.0 ± 0.1
Sleep efficiency, %	84 ± 13	Obstructive hypopnea index, n/hr TST	0.1 ± 0.1
Stage 1, % TST	5 ± 3	Central apneas with desaturation, n/hr TST	0.0 ± 0.1
Stage 2, % TST	51 ± 9	Duration of hypoventilation ($P_{ET}CO_2 \geq 45$ mm Hg), % TST	1.6 ± 0.8
Slow-wave sleep, % TST	26 ± 8	Peak $P_{ET}CO_2$, mm Hg	46 ± 3
REM sleep, % TST	19 ± 6	SpO_2 nadir, %	95 ± 1
REM cycles, n	4 ± 1		

Data presented as mean ± 2 SD.
EEG, electroencephalography; $P_{ET}CO_2$, end-tidal arterial carbon dioxide partial pressure; REM, rapid eye movement; SpO_2, oxygen saturation.
See references 47, 48, 70, and 72.

treatments. Testing is indicated to determine the presence and severity of SDB, the type of treatment, the preoperative care, and necessary follow-up.

Polysomnography during a daytime nap may underestimate the degree of SDB.[77,78] REM sleep often does not occur during naps. Furthermore, obstructive respiratory events worsen as sleep progresses.[47] Thus, although the positive predictive value of an abnormal nap study is 100%, the negative predictive value is only 20%.[77,78] Home study devices range in complexity from oximetry alone[79,80] to multichannel recordings.[81] Ambulatory studies may be used to evaluate oxygenation in infants with chronic lung disease, cystic fibrosis, restrictive lung diseases, and neuromuscular conditions. Jacob and colleagues[82] compared laboratory and domiciliary studies in a population of symptomatic children with adenotonsillar hypertrophy. Their multichannel monitor included oxygen saturation, waveform, electrocardiogram, RIP, and video recording, and therefore it cannot be compared to commercially available ambulatory systems.[82] Similar indices of apnea/hypopnea, desaturation, and arousal were observed during attended laboratory-based polysomnograms and domiciliary studies.[82]

Documenting oximeters should include an algorithm for artifact reduction such as a plethysmograph waveform or heart rate detected by the oximeter. The oximetry channel alone has been compared to full polysomnography in a population of snoring children suspected to have SDB with adenotonsillar hypertrophy.[83] Oximetry demonstrated an excellent positive predictive value (97%) but a poor negative predictive ability (53%).[83] Many children with SDB and clinically significant respiratory–effort related arousals do not demonstrate oxygen desaturation.[1,57] Similar observations have been made regarding the limitations of using oximetry as a screening tool for adult OSAS.[79,80] Oximetry is inadequate to diagnose a considerable percentage of pediatric SDB in which arousal and hypoventilation, rather than hypoxemia, predominate.[84]

Night-to-Night Polysomnographic Variability

A single overnight polysomnogram is a well-recognized diagnostic tool for determining the presence and severity of OSAS in symptomatic children.[36] However, few data exist regarding the variability of polysomnographic findings in children. That is, it is unknown whether the frequency and severity of sleep apnea syndrome among snoring children is sufficiently consistent from night to night to be accurately assessed by one polysomnogram. The misclassification of OSAS as primary snoring after a single night of polysomnography has been observed in adults,[85,86] and it may also occur in children. An adaptation effect of the sleep laboratory environment, termed the first-night effect, has been reported to disrupt sleep architecture[87-90] and perhaps to underestimate respiratory disturbance.[88,91]

In children, the clinical diagnosis of either OSAS or primary snoring remained the same in two polysomnographic studies 1 to 4 weeks apart.[92] Although the overall classification of subjects was unchanged, there were minimal changes in OSAS severity between nights. This supports the view that a single polysomnographic night is sufficient for the diagnosis of OSAS in otherwise normal, snoring children with adenotonsillar hypertrophy. No night-to-night systematic bias was observed in any of the mean intersubject respiratory parameters.[90,92] The intrasubject respiratory parameters, however, demonstrated considerable variability, particularly in children with severe disease. The variability in respiratory parameters could not be accounted for by changes in body position or percent REM time. Among the sleep variables, a first-night effect, including increased wakefulness and a reduction of REM sleep, was observed as the result of adaptation to the sleep laboratory environment.[90] Circumstances in which a single study night may not be sufficient include inadequate REM time, technical limitations in acquiring key channels, or when the parents report that the particular study night did not reflect a typical night's sleep.

DIAGNOSTIC AND EVENT CLASSIFICATION

The optimal definition for respiratory events and clinical classification has not been established in children. There are no clinical studies evaluating the relative merit of specific event definitions in relation to clinical outcomes.[93] The poly-somnographic criteria for event scoring and clinical diagnosis, based on our experience, are summarized in Tables 17–6 and 17–7. However, well-designed outcome studies are desperately needed to validate these criteria. Additional abnormal breathing patterns, including tachypnea and increased respiratory effort, have been described in children with OSAS.[94] Normative data for respiratory effort–related arousals and flow limitation are scant in children, and these events appear to be rare. Nevertheless, the clinical classification of symptomatic children cannot be exclusively based on the apnea index alone. Consideration of the apnea-hypopnea index, flow limitation, SpO_2, $P_{ET}CO_2$, and arousal indices also contribute to the diagnosis of OSAS. Thus, diagnostic interpretation of pediatric polysomnography will continue to require consideration of all respiratory parameters.

Table 17–6. Respiratory Pattern Scoring

Obstructive	
Apnea	Absence of oronasal airflow for any duration, with persistent respiratory effort
Hypopnea	*Thermistor:* Reduction of oronasal flow >50% for a 2-breath duration or longer, with persistent respiratory effort accompanied by a desaturation of 3% or greater, or by an arousal
	Nasal pressure: Discernible change in flow shape or amplitude for a 2-breath duration or longer, with persistent respiratory effort accompanied by a desaturation of 3% or greater, or by an arousal
Respiratory effort–related arousal	Evidence of increased respiratory effort or flow limitation leading to an arousal, followed by normalization of effort and flow
Flow limitation	Flattening of the inspiratory limb of the nasal pressure channel
Snoring	Coarse, low-pitched inspiratory sound
Hypoventilation	$P_{ET}CO_2$ > 50 mm Hg for >10% TST, or $P_{ET}CO_2$ peak > 53 mm Hg
	Accompanied by paradoxical breathing or obstructive events
Central	
Apnea	Absence of oronasal airflow for 20 sec or longer without respiratory effort
	Shorter events are scored if associated with arousal, desaturation, or bradycardia.
Hypoventilation	$P_{ET}CO_2$ > 50 mm Hg for >10% TST, or $P_{ET}CO_2$ peak > 53 mm Hg
	Accompanied by decreased respiratory effort
Periodic breathing	Succession of 3 or more central apneas of 3-sec duration, separated by < 20 sec of normal breathing
Miscellaneous	
Mixed apneas	Cessation of flow with a central and obstructive component
Rebreathing	Evidence of increased CO_2 in inspired air

$P_{ET}CO_2$, end-tidal arterial carbon dioxide partial pressure; TST, total sleep time.

Table 17–7. Diagnostic Classification of Sleep-Disordered Breathing

Diagnosis*	Apnea Index (Events/hr)	Spo$_2$ Nadir (%)	P$_{ET}$co$_2$ Peak (torr)	P$_{ET}$co$_2$ > 50 torr (% TST)	Arousals (Events/hr)
Primary snoring	≤1	>92	≤53	<10	EEG < 11
Upper airway resistance syndrome	≤1r	>92	≤53	<10	RERA > 1 EEG > 11
Mild OSAS	1-4	86-91	>53	10- 24	EEG > 11
Moderate OSAS	5-10	76-85	>60	25-49	EEG > 11
Severe OSAS	>10	≤75	>65	≥50	EEG > 11

*Each diagnosis requires one or more of the measures to its right.
EEG, electroencephalographic arousal; OSAS, obstructive sleep apnea syndrome; P$_{ET}$co$_2$, end tidal Pco$_2$; RERA, respiratory-related arousal; Spo2, arterial oxygen saturation; TST, total sleep time.

References

1. Guilleminault C, Stoohs R, Clerk A, et al: A cause of excessive daytime sleepiness: The upper airway resistance syndrome. Chest 1993;104:781-787.
2. Guilleminault C, Korobkin R, Winkel R: A review of 50 children with obstructive sleep apnea syndrome. Lung 1981;159:275-287.
3. Rosen C, D'Andrea L, Haddad G: Adult criteria for obstructive sleep apnea do not identify children with serious obstruction. Am Rev Respir Dis 1992;146:1231-1234.
4. Katz ES, Lutz J, Black C, Marcus CL: Pulse transit time as a measure of arousal and respiratory effort in children with sleep-disordered breathing. Pediatr Res 2003;53:580-588.
5. American Sleep Disorders Association: The international classification of sleep disorders. Diagnostic and coding manual (revised edition). Rochester, Minn, American Sleep Disorders Association, 1997.
6. Urschitz MS, Guenther A, Eggebrecht E, et al: Snoring, intermittent hypoxia and academic performance in primary school children. Am J Respir Crit Care Med 2003;168:464-468.
7. O'Brien LM, Mervis CB, Holbrook CR, et al: Neurobehavioral implications of habitual snoring in children. Pediatrics 2004;114:44-49.
8. Ali NJ, Pitson DJ, Stradling JR: Snoring, sleep disturbance and behaviour in 4-5 year olds. Arch Dis Child 1993;68:360-366.
9. Gislason T, Benediktsdottir B: Snoring, apneic episodes, and nocturnal hypoxemia among children 6 months to 6 years old. Chest 1995;107:963-966.
10. Redline S, Tishler PV, Schluchter M, et al: Risk factors for sleep-disordered breathing in children: Associations with obesity, race, and respiratory problems. Am J Respir Crit Care Med 1999;159:1527-1532.
11. Wilson K, Lakheeram I, Morielli A, et al: Can assessment for obstructive sleep apnea help predict postadenotonsillectomy respiratory complications? Anesthesiology 2002;96:313-322.
12. American Academy of Pediatrics, Section on Pediatric Pulmonology, Subcommittee on Obstructive Sleep Apnea: Clinical practice guideline: Diagnosis and management of childhood obstructive sleep apnea syndrome. Pediatrics 2002;109:704-712.
13. Preutthipan A, Chantarojanasiri T, Suwanjutha 5, Udomsubpayakul U: Can parents predict the severity of childhood obstructive sleep apnoea? Acta Paediatr 2000;89:708-712.
14. Gozal D, Wang M, Pope DW: Objective sleepiness measures in pediatric obstructive sleep apnea. Pediatrics 2001;108:693-697.
15. Melendres MCS, Lutz J, Rubin ED, Marcus CL: Daytime sleepiness and hyperactivity in children with suspected sleep-disordered breathing. Pediatrics 2004;114:768-775.
16. Brouillette R, Hanson D, David R, et al: A diagnostic approach to suspected obstructive sleep apnea in children. J Pediatr 1984;105:10-14.
17. Carroll J, McColley S, Marcus C, et al: Inability of clinical history to distinguish primary snoring from obstructive sleep apnea syndrome in children. Chest 1995;108:610-618.
18. Rosen CL: Clinical features of obstructive sleep apnea hypoventilation syndrome in otherwise healthy children. Pediatr Pulmonol 1999;27:403-409.
19. Croft CB, Brockbank MJ, Wright A, Swanston AR: Obstructive sleep apnoea in children undergoing routine tonsillectomy and adenoidectomy. Clin Otolaryngol 1990;15:307-314.

20. Suen JS, Arnold JE, Brooks U: Adenotonsillectomy for treatment of obstructive sleep apnea in children. Arch Otolaryngol Head Neck Surg 1995;121:525-530.

21. Van Someren VH, Hibbert J, Stothers JK, et al: Identification of hypoxaemia in children having tonsillectomy and adenoidectomy. Clin Otolaryngol 1990;15:263-271.

22. Van Someren VH, Burmester M, Alusi G, Lane R: Are sleep studies worth doing? Arch Dis Child 2000;83:76-81.

23. Marcus CL, Greene MG, Carroll JL: Blood pressure in children with obstructive sleep apnea. Am J Respir Crit Care Med 1998;157:1098-1103.

24. Gozal D: Sleep-disordered breathing and school performance in children. Pediatrics 1998;102: 616-620.

25. Guillemmault C, Winkel R, Korobkin R, Simmons B: Children and nocturnal snoring: Evaluation of the effects of sleep related respiratory resistive load and daytime functioning. Eur Respir J 1982;139:165-171.

26. Haponik EF, Smith PL, Kaplan J, Bleeker ER: Flow-volume curves and sleep-disordered breathing: Therapeutic implications. Thorax 1983;38: 609-615.

27. Arens R, McDonough JM, Costarino AT, et al: Magnetic resonance imaging of the upper airway structure of children with obstructive sleep apnea syndrome. Am J Respir Crit Care Med 2001;164: 698-703.

28. Li AM, Wong E, Kew J, et al: Use of tonsil size in the evaluation of obstructive sleep apnoea. Arch Dis Child 2002;87:156-159.

29. Donnelly LF, Strife JL, Myer CM: Glossoptosis (posterior displacement of the tongue) during sleep: A frequent cause of sleep apnea in pediatric patients referred for dynamic sleep fluoroscopy. AJR Am J Roentgenol 2000;175:1557-1559.

30. Goldstein NA, Sculerati N, Waisleben JA, et al: Clinical diagnosis of pediatric obstructive sleep apnea validated by polysomnography. Otolaryngol Head Neck Surg 1994;111:611-617.

31. Potsic WP: Comparison of polysomnography and sonography for assessing regularity of respiration during sleep in adenotonsillar hypertrophy. Laryngoscope 1987;97:1430-1437.

32. McCombe AW, Kwok VK, Hawke WM: An acoustic screening test for obstructive sleep apnoea. Clin Otolaryngol 1995;20:348-351.

33. Morielli A, Laden S, Ducharme FM, Brouillette RT: Can sleep and wakefulness be distinguished in children by cardiorespiratory and videotape recordings? Chest 1996;109:680-687.

34. Sivan Y, Kornecki A, Schonfeld T: Screening obstructive sleep apnoea syndrome by home videotape recording in children. Eur Respir J 1996;9:2127-2131.

35. Mograss M, Ducharme F, Brouillette R: Movement/arousals. Description, classification and relationship to sleep apnea in children. Am J Respir Crit Care Med 1994;150:1690-1696.

36. American Thoracic Society: Standards and indications for cardiopulmonary sleep studies in children. Am J Respir Crit Care Med 1996;153: 866-878.

37. Hershenson M, Brouillette RT, Olsen E, Hunt CE: The effect of chloral hydrate on genioglossus and diaphragmatic activity. Pediatr Res 1984;18: 516-519.

38. Canet E, Gaultier C, D'Allest AM, Dehan M: Effects of sleep deprivation on respiratory events during sleep in healthy infants. J Appl Phys 1989;66:1158-1163.

39. Anders T, Ende R, Parmelee A: A manual of standardized terminology, technique, and criteria for scoring of states of sleep and wakefulness in newborn infants. Los Angeles, UCLA Brain Information Service, 1971.

40. Rechtschaffen A, Kales A: A manual of standardized terminology: Techniques and scoring systems for sleep stages of human subjects. Los Angeles, UCLA Brain Information Service/Brain Research Institute, 1968.

41. Sleep Disorders Atlas Task Force of the American Sleep Disorders Association: EEG arousals: Scoring rules and examples—A preliminary report. Sleep 1992;15:173-184.

42. Wong TK, Gaister P, Lau TS, et al: Reliability of scoring arousals in normal children and children with obstructive sleep apnea syndrome. Sleep 2004; 27:1139–1145.

43. McNamara F, Issa F, Sullivan C: Arousal pattern following central and obstructive breathing abnormalities in infants and children. J Appl Physiol 1996;81:2651-2657.

44. Bandla HP, Gozal D: Dynamic changes in EEG spectra during obstructive apnea in children. Pediatr Pulmonol 2000;29:359-365.

45. Black JE, Guilleminault C, Colrain IM, Carrillo O: Upper airway resistance syndrome: Central electroencephalographic power and changes in breathing effort. Am J Respir Crit Care Med 2000;162:406-411.

46. Fuentes-Pradera MA, Botebol G, Sanchez-Armengol A, et al: Effect of snoring and obstructive respiratory events on sleep architecture in adolescents. Arch Pediatr Adolesc Med 2003;157: 649-654.

47. Goh DY, Galster P, Marcus CL: Sleep architecture and respiratory disturbances in children with obstructive sleep apnea. Am J Respir Crit Care Med 2000;162:682-686.

48. Tauman R, O'Brien LM, Holbrook CR, Gozal D: Sleep pressure score: A new index of sleep dis-

ruption in snoring children. Sleep 2004;27: 274-278.

49. Somers VK, Dyken ME, Clary MP, Abboud FM: Sympathetic neural mechanisms in obstructive sleep apnea. J Clin Invest 1995;96:1897-1904.

50. Davies RJO, Vardi-Visi K, Clarke M, Stradling JR: Identification of sleep disruption and sleep disordered breathing from the systolic blood pressure profile. Thorax 1993;48:1242-1247.

51. Aljadeff G, Gozal D, Schechtman VL, et al: Heart rate variability in children with obstructive sleep apnea. Sleep 1997;20:151-157.

52. Schnall RP, Shlitner A, Sheffy J, et al: Periodic, profound peripheral vasoconstriction: A new marker of obstructive sleep apnea. Sleep 1999;22:939-946.

53. Martin SE, Wraith PK, Deary IJ, Douglas NJ: The effect of nonvisible sleep fragmentation on daytime function. Am J Respir Crit Care Med 1997;155:1596-1601.

54. Sivan Y, Ward SD, Deakers T, et al: Rib cage to abdominal asynchrony in children undergoing polygraphic sleep studies. Pediatr Pulmonol 1991;11:141-146.

55. Kohyama J, Shiiki T, Shimohira M, Hasegawa T: Asynchronous breathing during sleep. Arch Dis Child 2001;84:174-177.

56. Gaultier C, Praud JP, Canet E, et al: Paradoxical inward ribcage motion during rapid-eye movement sleep in infants and young children. J Dev Physiol 1987;9:391-397.

57. Guilleminault C, Pelayo R, Leger D, et al: Recognition of sleep-disordered breathing in children. Pediatrics 1996;98:871-882.

58. Groswasser J, Scaillon M, Rebuffat E, et al: Naso-oesophageal probes decrease the frequency of sleep apnoeas in infants. J Sleep Res 2000;9: 193-196.

59. Farre R, Montserrat JM, Rotger M, et al: Accuracy of thermistors and thermocouples as flow-measuring devices for detecting hypopneas. Eur Respir J 1998;11:179-182.

60. Norman RG, Ahmed MM, Walsleben JA, Rapoport DM: Detection of respiratory events during NPSG: Nasal cannula/pressure sensor versus thermistor. Sleep 1997;20:1175-1184.

61. Hosselet J, Norman RG, Ayappa I, Rapoport DM: Detection of flow limitation with a nasal cannula/pressure transducer system. Am J Respir Crit Care Med 1998;157:1461-1467.

62. Trang H, Leske V, Gaultier C: Use of nasal cannula for detecting sleep apneas and hypopneas in infants and children. Am J Respir Crit Care Med 2002;166:464-468.

63. Serebrisky D, Cordero R, Mandeli J, et al: Assessment of inspiratory flow limitation in children with sleep-disordered breathing by a nasal

cannula pressure transducer system. Pediatr Pulmonol 2002;33:380-387.

64. Poels PJP, Schilder AGM, van de Berg S, et al: Evaluation of a new device for home cardiorespiratory recording in children. Arch Otolaryngol Head Neck Surg 2003;129:1281-1284.

65. Sackner MA, Watson H, Belsito AS, et al: Calibration of respiratory inductive plethysmograph during natural breathing. J Appl Phys 1989;66:410-420.

66. Adams JA, Zabaleta IA, Stroh D, Sackner MA: Measurement of breath amplitudes: Comparison of three noninvasive respiratory monitors to integrated pneumotachograph. Pediatr Pulmonol 1993;16:254-258.

67. Seakins M, Gibbs WN, Milner PF, Bertles JF: Erythrocyte Hb-S concentration: An important factor in the oxygen affinity of blood in sickle cell anemia. J Clin Invest 1973;52:422-432.

68. Bhavani-Shankar K, Moseley H, Kumar AY, Deiph Y: Capnometry and anesthesia. Can J Anaesth 1992; 39:617-632.

69. Morielli A, Desjardins D, Brouillette RT: Transcutaneous and end-tidal carbon dioxide pressures should be measured during pediatric polysomnography. Am Rev Respir Dis 1993;148: 1599-1604.

70. Uliel S, Tauman R, Greenfeld M, Sivan Y: Normal polysomnographic respiratory values in children and adolescents. Chest 2004;125:872-878.

71. Acebo C, Millman RP, Rosenberg C, et al: Sleep, breathing, and cephalometrics in older children and young adults: Part 1. Normative values. Chest 1996;109:664-672.

72. Marcus CL, Omlin KJ, Basinski DJ, et al: Normal polysomnographic values for children and adolescents. Am Rev Respir Dis 1992;146:1235-1239.

73. Hunt CE, Corwin MJ, Lister G, et al: Longitudinal assessment of hemoglobin oxygen saturation in healthy infants during the first 6 months of age. J Pediatr 1999;134:580-586.

74. Witmans MB, Keens TG, Ward SLD, Marcus CL: Obstructive hypopneas in children and adolescents: Normal values. Am J Respir Crit Care Med 2003;168:1540.

75. Miyazaki S, Itasaka Y, Yamakawa K, et al: Respiratory disturbance during sleep due to adenoid-tonsillar hypertrophy. Am J Otolaryngol 1988;10:143-149.

76. Skatvedt O, Grogaard J: Infant sleeping position and inspiratory pressures in the upper airways and oesophagus. Arch Dis Child 1994;71:138-140.

77. Marcus CL, Keens TG, Ward SL: Comparison of nap and overnight polysomnography in children. Pediatr Pulmonol 1992;13:16-21.

78. Saeed MM, Keens TG, Stabile MW, et al: Should children with suspected obstructive sleep apnea

syndrome and normal nap studies have overnight sleep studies? Chest 2000;118:360-365.

79. Cooper BG, Veale D, Griffiths CJ, Gibson GJ: Value of nocturnal oxygen saturation as a screening test for sleep apnoea. Thorax 1991;46: 586-588.

80. Ryan PJ, Hilton MF, Boldy DAR, et al: Validation of British Thoracic Society guidelines for the diagnosis of the sleep apnoea/hypopoea syndrome: Can polysomnography be avoided? Thorax 1995;50:972-975.

81. Redline S, Tosteson T, Boucher MA, Millman RP: Measurement of sleep-related breathing disturbances in epidemiologic studies: Assessment of the validity and reproducibility of a portable monitoring device. Chest 1991;100: 1281-1286.

82. Jacob SV, Morielli A, Mograss MA, et al: Home testing for pediatric obstructive sleep apnea syndrome secondary to adenotonsillar hypertrophy. Pediatr Pulmonol 1995;20:241-252.

83. Brouillette RT, Morielli A, Leimanis A, et al: Nocturnal pulse oximetry as an abbreviated testing modality for pediatric obstructive sleep apnea. Pediatrics 2000;105:405-412.

84. Kirk VG, Boim SG, Flemons WW, Remmers JE: Comparison of home oximetry monitoring with laboratory polysomnography in children. Chest 2003;124:1702-1708.

85. Mosko S, Dickel M, Ashurst J: Night-to-night variability in sleep apnea and sleep-related periodic leg movements in the elderly. Sleep 1988;11:340-348.

86. Bliwise D, Benkert R, Ingham R: Factors associated with nightly variability in sleep-disordered breathing in the elderly. Chest 1991;100:973-976.

87. Aber W, Block A, Hellard D, Webb W: Consistency of respiratory measurements from night to night during the sleep of elderly men. Chest 1989; 96:747-751.

88. Le Bon O, Hoffman G, Tecco J, et al: Mild to moderate sleep respiratory events: One negative night may not be enough. Chest 2000;118:353-359.

89. Agnew H, Webb W, Williams R: The first night effect: An EEG study of sleep. Psychophysiology 1966;2:263-266.

90. Scholle S, Scholle HC, Kemper A, et al: First night effect in children and adolescents undergoing polysomnography for sleep-disordered breathing. Clin Neurophys 2003;14:2138-2145.

91. Bliwise D, Carey B, Dement W: Nightly variation in sleep-related respiratory disturbance in older adults. Exp Aging Res 1983;9:77-81.

92. Katz ES, Greene MG, Carson KA, et al: Night-to-night variability of polysomnography in children with symptoms of sleep-disordered breathing. J Pediatr 2002;140:589-594.

93. Marcus CL, England S, Annett RD, et al: Cardiorespiratory sleep studies in children: Establishment of normative data and polysomnographic predictors of morbidity. Am J Respir Crit Care Med 1999;160:1381-1387.

94. Guilleminault C, Li KK, Khramstov A, et al: Breathing patterns in prepubertal children with sleep-related breathing disorders. Arch Pediatr Adolesc Med 2004;158:153-161.

Consequences of Obstructive Sleep Apnea Syndrome

18

Louise Margaret O'Brien
David Gozal

Obstructive sleep apnea (OSA) is a frequent condition and is currently estimated to affect between 1% and 3% of 2- to 8-year-old children.[1-3] OSA is characterized by repeated events of partial or complete upper airway obstruction during sleep, resulting in disruption of normal ventilation, hypoxemia, and fragmentation of sleep (Fig. 18–1).[4] However, habitual snoring during sleep is a much more frequent occurrence and affects up to 27% of children,[2,3,5-9] with a decrease in frequency in 9 to 14 year olds.[10]

OSA was first described by McKenzie over a century ago,[11] yet it was not until the mid-1970s that it was recognized in children.[12] Using polysomnography in eight children aged 5 to 14 years, Guilleminault and colleagues published the first detailed report of children with adenotonsillar hypertrophy and OSA and suggested that surgery may eliminate their clinical symptoms. Since this initial report there have been multiple publications on OSA in children, and it is clear that the classic OSA in children is a disorder distinct from the OSA that occurs in adults, in particular with respect to gender distribution, clinical manifestations, polysomnographic findings, and treatment.[13,14] OSA is frequently diagnosed in association with adenotonsillar hypertrophy and is also common in children with craniofacial abnormalities and neurologic disorders affecting upper airway patency.

The primary symptom of OSA is snoring. While snoring is not normal and essentially indicates the presence of heightened upper airway resistance, many snoring children may have primary snoring, that is, habitual snoring without alterations in sleep architecture, alveolar ventilation, and oxygenation. However, the acquisition of definitive criteria allowing for a reliable distinction between primary snoring and OSA will have to wait several years as the consequences of OSA in children become better recognized and

understood and the threshold at which morbidity occurs becomes known. Despite such limitations, it is clear that polysomnographic assessment is currently required for the definitive diagnosis of OSA in children, since a clinical history and physical examination are insufficient to confirm its presence or severity.[15] Nevertheless, it should be emphasized that alternative screening methods have been recently explored[16-19] and that novel technologic advances may allow for improved diagnostic accuracy in the future.[20,21]

The implications of OSA in children are multifaceted and potentially complex. If left untreated or, alternatively, if treated late, pediatric OSA may lead to substantial morbidity that affects multiple target organs and systems and that may not be completely reversed with appropriate treatment. The potential consequences of OSA in children include behavioral disturbances and learning deficits,[2,22-25] pulmonary hypertension,[26] and systemic hypertension[27] as well as compromised somatic growth.[28]

The pathophysiology of OSA in children has been recently reviewed[29] and is discussed in detail in the previous chapter. It is clear that children with OSA have increased upper airway collapsibility[30] and that enlarged tonsils and adenoids are a major contributor to this disorder.[31] However, adenotonsillar hypertrophy alone is not sufficient to cause OSA because some children with "kissing tonsils" do not have OSA, whereas others are not cured after adenotonsillectomy.[32]

As with any other disorder in medicine, morbidity and mortality are the major incentives to intervene and treat it. In subsequent sections of this chapter, we will critically review the various consequences of pediatric OSA. For the purpose of clarity, the spectrum of morbidities associated with OSA can be examined as representing four

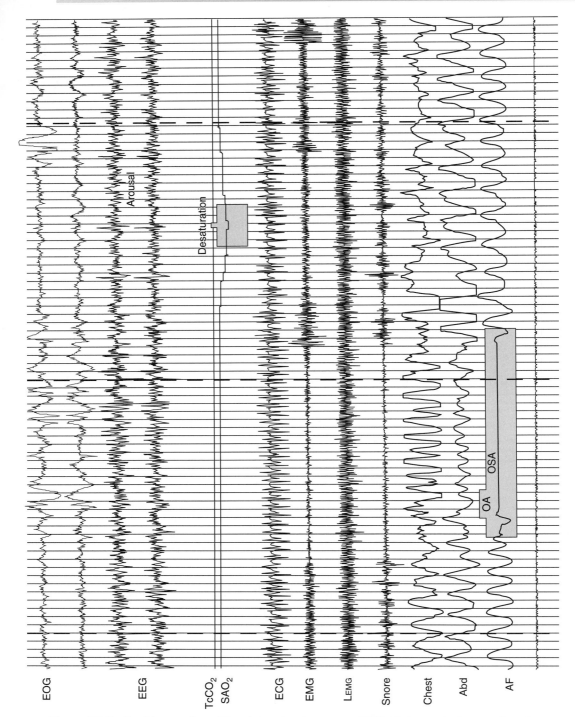

Figure 18–1. Graphic recording of the obstructive sleep apnea (OSA) triad, namely the cessation of airflow in the presence of respiratory effort, oxyhemoglobin desaturation, and sleep arousal. AF, airflow; Abd, abdominal excursion; Chest, chest wall excursion; ECG, electrocardiogram; EEG, electroencephalogram; EMG, chin electromyogram; EOG, electro-oculogram; LEMG, left anterior tibial EMG; OA, obstructive apnea; SaO$_2$, oxyhemoglobin saturation; Snore, sound channel; TccO$_2$, transcutaneous PcO$_2$.

immediate consequences of upper airway obstruction during sleep, namely, increased work of breathing, intermittent hypoxemia, sleep fragmentation, and alveolar hypoventilation. Obviously, the separation of these elements as individual contributors is artificial due to their anticipated interaction in end-organ effects. Nevertheless, this categoric classification permits more accurate representation of the relative contributions of each of these alterations induced by OSA and provides a useful methodological approach to their investigation.

INCREASED WORK OF BREATHING

A logical and potential consequence of increased work of breathing during sleep in children with OSA is the development of failure to thrive (FTT). Although in early reports of children with severe OSA FTT was often present,[28,33,34] it is currently estimated that only a minority of children with OSA will present with this problem, most probably because of earlier recognition and referral. Adenotonsillectomy and complete resolution of OSA will induce significant growth improvements in those children who present with FTT. In a small study of children with OSA and FTT, Brouillette and associates[35] found that adenotonsillectomy resulted in catch-up growth in all six children. In fact, adenotonsillectomy has been shown to increase the height and weight velocities of children with normal growth and OSA.[36] Interestingly, even obese children with OSA will demonstrate weight gain after surgical removal of their enlarged tonsils and adenoids for the resolution of OSA.[37]

Mechanisms for growth deceleration in OSA may be varied. These mechanisms may include, but are not limited to, decreased appetite that is possibly associated with reduced olfaction in children with adenoidal hypertrophy, dysphagia from tonsillar hypertrophy,[38] decreased levels of insulin-like growth factor-1 (IGF-1), IGF binding protein and possibly growth hormone release,[39-42] hypoxemia, acidosis, and the increased metabolic cost of breathing during sleep. While the mechanisms underlying decreased circulating levels of IGF-1 in children with OSA remain unclear, IGF-1 will recover after tonsillectomy and adenoidectomy and parallel the rebound growth that characterizes the responses of these patients.[41] It is possible that disruption of non–rapid eye movement (NREM) sleep that

is not immediately recognizable when using visual inspection of the sleep records may play a role, since growth hormone release and its downstream signaling through IGF-1 occur during NREM sleep in general and more specifically during delta sleep.[43,44] This is particularly applicable to pediatric OSA because even in snorers who do not fulfill the current criteria for OSA, there is evidence of stunted growth and disruption of IGF binding protein–3 circulating levels, suggesting that some of these children may suffer from disrupted sleep that in turn would affect growth hormone release.[42]

Alternatively, changes in energy expenditure during sleep could account for a reduction in the linear growth of children with OSA. Indeed, Marcus and coworkers[45] studied 14 children with moderate OSA (mean age 4 ± 1 years) and demonstrated that increased metabolic requirements were present during sleep and normalized after adenotonsillectomy, with a concomitant gain in body weight. In this study no evidence for decreased appetite was apparent, since caloric intake was similar both before and after surgery in all children. These findings suggest that poor growth in some children with OSA may be secondary to the increased energy expenditure that directly results from the increase in work of breathing during sleep rather than be associated with decreased caloric intake.[1] However, this a priori logical mechanism has been recently challenged by Bland and colleagues[46] in a study of 11 children (mean age 6 ± 2 years) with a polysomnographically confirmed diagnosis of OSA. These investigators found no evidence of increased energy requirements either before or after adenotonsillectomy in these patients; in fact, their total daily energy expenditures were similar to those of healthy age- and gender-matched control subjects.

Thus, the FTT in pediatric OSA does not appear to be associated with increased daily energy requirements but involves a combination of increased night-time energy expenditure caused by increased respiratory effort and, more importantly, disruption of the growth hormone-IGF-1 pathway. In general, complete recovery of growth and resumption of its normal patterns will occur after adenotonsillectomy.[28,34,37] Furthermore, we are unaware of any persistent, residual somatic deficits after the resolution of OSA.

INTERMITTENT HYPOXEMIA

Frequent oxygen desaturations during sleep are common in children with OSA. In a study of 11 children, Gislason and Benediktsdottir[3] found that 73% had three or more respiratory events per hour that were associated with desaturations of >4%. Similarly, Stradling and associates[38] found that 61% of the 61 children selected for adenotonsillectomy because of recurrent tonsillitis had hypoxemia during sleep. Elevation of pulmonary artery pressure due to hypoxia-induced pulmonary vasoconstriction is a serious consequence of OSA in children and can lead to persistent pulmonary hypertension and cor pulmonale.[26] The overall magnitude of pressure increases in the pulmonary circulation is probably smaller than that occurring during the sustained, chronic hypoxemia observed at high altitudes. Indeed, direct measurements of pulmonary artery pressures in rats and mice exposed to hypoxia revealed that the increase in pulmonary artery pressure was greater when continuous hypoxia was applied than it was with episodic hypoxia.[47] In 27 pediatric patients with moderate to severe OSA, radionuclide assessment of right ventricular function revealed reduced ejection fraction in 37% and wall motion abnormality in 45% of children with OSA.[48] These abnormalities were reversible after surgery. However, there is no prospective study assessing the overall prevalence and severity of pulmonary hypertension in a large cohort of children with sleep-disordered breathing (SDB). It also remains unclear whether untreated or long-lasting OSA will be associated with vascular remodeling of the pulmonary circulation in these children. Furthermore, evidence from animal models exposed to hypoxia for a short period of time during early postnatal life reveals that pulmonary hypertension is increased when exposed to hypoxia later in infancy.[49] These authors speculated that the disrupted alveolarization and vascular growth after the brief hypoxic insult may increase the risk of severe pulmonary hypertension later in life.

Normally, the cardiovascular effects of breathing are recognizable in the systemic circulation but are of small magnitude, as revealed by respiratory sinus arrhythmia and minor fluctuations in blood pressure that are synchronous with respiratory periodicity. In the context of OSA, systemic hypertension has emerged as a major cardiovascular consequence in adult patients. Indeed, elevated blood pressures are present during wakefulness in approximately 50% of adult patients with OSA.[50] Although the pathophysiologic mechanisms of such elevation in arterial tension are still under intense investigation, it appears that intermittent hypoxemia is the major contributor to this serious consequence of OSA, with less significant roles being played by sleep fragmentation and episodic hypercapnia. Notwithstanding such considerations, enhanced sympathoadrenal discharge, altered homeostasis of the renin-angiotensin pathway, and heightened sympathetic autonomic nervous system tone will develop along with increases in small arteriolar vasomotor contractility suggestive of endothelial dysfunction.[51-62]

The evidence for alterations in autonomic nervous system tone is clearly not as extensive when addressing the pediatric OSA population. In an earlier study, Aljadeff and coworkers examined heart rate variability (a noninvasive probe of autonomic nervous system tone) in children with moderate to severe OSA and matched control subjects.[63] Inspection of moment-to-moment changes in RR intervals revealed sustained increases in sympathetic activity as well as increased vagal discharge during respiratory events. Similarly, Baharav and colleagues found evidence of increased sympathetic tone as derived from spectral analysis of cardiac periodicities in children with OSA.[64] The marked sensitivity of the sympathetic system to the increased respiratory effort that occurs throughout the night in OSA patients, with the subsequent hypoxia and arousal, will be manifested as changes in vascular hemodynamics that can be derived from the time differential between the R wave (electrical cardiac contraction) and the peripheral pulse waveform, (i.e., pulse transit time). This relatively easy-to-obtain measure may in fact be used as a circulatory corollary of respiratory and arousal events in children[65] and may ultimately become one of the useful parameters for the OSA screening of snoring children.

Because children have greater vascular compliance than adults, the magnitude and severity of blood pressure elevation in pediatric patients with OSA are not as prominent as those described for older patients. Nevertheless, they do occur and are manifested primarily as diurnal elevations of diastolic blood pressure.[27] These autonomic alterations are mediated by both the episodic hypoxia that characteristically accompanies the OSA syndrome and by the repeated arousals and carbon dioxide elevations of this condition. The long-term implications of such effects on cardiovascular morbidity during the later stages of childhood or even adulthood have yet to be explored. However, in preliminary animal experiments, when rodents were exposed to a model of OSA[66] at an age corresponding to that for the peak prevalence of pediatric OSA in childhood, marked attenuation of their baroreceptor function lasting into late adulthood was found.[67] As a result, early childhood perturbations may lead to lifelong consequences; in other words, certain types of adult cardiovascular disease may represent, at least in part, sequelae from a priori "unrelated events" during childhood. Therefore, early identification of children with alterations in baroreceptor and autonomic nervous system functions in the context of pediatric OSA may lead to detection of a population potentially at risk for ulterior development of hypertension and its cardiovascular-associated morbidity.

Evidence for an Effect of OSA on Learning and Behavior

Another potentially very serious consequence of intermittent hypoxia may involve its long-term deleterious effects on neuronal and intellectual functions. Reports of decreased intellectual function in children with tonsillar and adenoidal hypertrophy date back to 1889, when Hill reported on "some causes of backwardness and stupidity in children."[68] School problems have been repeatedly reported in case-series of children with OSA and in fact may underlie more extensive behavioral disturbances such as restlessness, aggressive behavior, excessive daytime sleepiness. and poor test performance.[2,22,24,31,69,70,74] Table 18–1 summarizes the evidence for OSA and neurocognitive and behavioral functions.

The neurocognitive and behavioral consequences of disrupted sleep architecture and intermittent hypoxemia in children with SDB are only now being defined by appropriate scientific methodology. There is increasing evidence to support an association between OSA and attention deficit hyperactivity disorder (ADHD) in children.[77,80,85-88] Several studies have documented that children with SDB often have problems with attention and behavior similar to those observed in children with ADHD.[2,22-24,31] In addition, three separate survey studies encompassing almost 3300 children have documented daytime sleepiness, hyperactivity, and aggressive behavior in children who snored.[2,8,81] It has been further suggested that up to one third of all children with frequent, loud snoring will display significant hyperactivity and inattention,[2] while a reciprocal relation also appears to be true, that is, children with ADHD exhibit more sleep disturbances more frequently than normal children.[81,85]

However, most of these studies of ADHD children have relied on parental reporting rather

Table 18–1.	Brief Summary of Evidence for Obstructive Sleep Apnea and Neurocognitive/Behavioral Function	
Symptom	**Reference(s)**
Based on Parental Report	
Daytime sleepiness	12, 38, 75, 76
Behavior (including hyperactivity, inattention, and aggression)	2, 12, 22-24, 31, 74, 75, 77-81
Depression	82
Enuresis	12, 76
Impaired school performance	12, 71
Objectively Measured	
Behavior	9, 73, 82
Depression	83
Impaired school performance	25, 72, 84

than on objectively collected data (see Table 18–1). In the few instances in which sleep studies were conducted in patients with ADHD, attention was given to sleep architecture alone and did not include cardiorespiratory data.[89,90] In a recent study from our laboratory, both subjective and objective sleep measures were obtained and showed that objectively measured sleep and respiratory disturbances are relatively frequent among children with ADHD, albeit not as frequent as those anticipated from parental reports.[9] In this study we also found that the prevalence of OSA in a cohort of children with ADHD, verified by neuropsychological testing, does not appear to differ from that found in the general population.[2,3,91] However, an unusually high frequency of OSA was found among children with mild to moderate increases in hyperactivity as measured by the Conner Parent Rating Scale,[92] a well validated method for discriminating between children with ADHD and normal control subjects (i.e., without true ADHD). This suggests that while OSA can induce significant behavioral effects being manifested as increased hyperactivity and inattention, it will not overlap with true clinical ADHD when the latter is assessed by more objective tools than just parental perception. Therefore, in a child presenting with parental complaints of hyperactivity and who does not meet the diagnostic criteria of ADHD after undergoing a thorough evaluation, as recently recommended by the American Academy of Pediatrics,[93] a careful sleep history should be taken, and if snoring is present, an overnight polysomnographic evaluation should be performed.

The mechanism or mechanisms by which OSA may contribute to hyperactivity remain unknown. It is possible that both the sleep fragmentation (see below) and episodic hypoxia that characterize OSA will lead to alterations within the neurochemical substrate of the prefrontal cortex, with resulting executive dysfunction.[94] Notwithstanding these considerations, sleep disturbances are frequently reported by the parents of ADHD children even when snoring is excluded.[88] Based on the available literature, the comorbidity of OSA and ADHD could be shared by a substantial number of hyperactive children. In fact, it has been suggested that up to 25% of children with a diagnosis of ADHD may actually have OSA.[24] However, such rather extensive overlap may be less prominent than that previously estimated if medication status and psychiatric comorbidity are accounted for in the analysis.[95]

Inverse relationships among memory, learning, and OSA have been documented.[72,73] In addition, improvements in learning and behavior have been reported after treatment for OSA in children,[25,38,73] suggesting that the neurocognitive deficits are at least partially reversible. In a large cohort of first graders whose academic performance was in the lowest 10th percentile of their class, we found not only a six- to ninefold increase in the expected incidence of OSA but also a significant improvement in school grades after adenotonsillectomy and resolution of OSA. However, since we did not know what the optimal learning potential was for these children, it is possible that long-term residual deficits may occur even after treatment. To further explore this possibility, we examined the history of snoring during early childhood in two groups of 13- to 14-year-old children who were matched for age, gender, race, school attending, and socioeconomic status but whose performances were either in the upper or lower quartile of their class. We found that children who snored frequently and loudly during their early childhood were at greater risk for poor academic performance in later years, well after snoring had resolved.[84] Therefore, these findings suggest that even if a component of the OSA-induced learning deficits is reversible, there may be a long-lasting residual deficit in learning capability and that the latter may represent a "learning debt"; that is, the decreased learning capacity during OSA may have led to such a delay in learned skills that recuperation is possible only with additional teaching assistance. Alternatively, the processes underlying the learning deficit during OSA may have irreversibly altered the performance characteristics of the neuronal circuitry responsible for learning particular skills (Fig. 18–2; see below). More recent work further suggests that snoring children perform poorly on measures of "executive functioning,"[96] that is, the ability to develop and sustain an organized, future-oriented, and flexible approach to problem solving. Executive dysfunction appears to be the most prominent area of cognitive impairment with untreated SDB in adults,[97,98] and our work now extends such observations to the pediatric age range.[9,96]

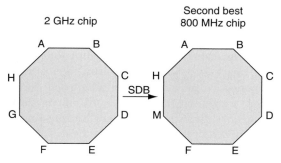

Simple computation: 32 ms versus 44 ms
Complex computation: 2.23 ms versus "freeze"

Figure 18–2. Schematic model illustrating how the loss of a given neuron within a neural circuit to sleep-disordered breathing (SDB) (in this case the neuron labeled "G") leads to its replacement by the next best (2ⁿᵈ Best) option available (in this case the neuron labeled "M"). Such cellular changes, which underlie the fundamental mechanisms of brain plasticity, are accompanied by changes in the intrinsic properties of the neural circuit. Analogous to a computer chip, the performance of the circuit is reduced from 2 GHz to 800 MHz. As such, simple computations such as those required from early-school children would not obligatorily translate into visible learning/performance deficits. However, as the intellectual requirements increase over time, the decrements in performance associated with SDB could translate into "FREEZE," that is, the inability to learn or perform the computational task being requested. Thus, the deficits associated with pediatric OSA may not manifest themselves until later in life.

SLEEP FRAGMENTATION

The physiologic and behavioral effects of sleep loss have been extensively investigated in adults, although the effects of OSA on sleep in children remain poorly understood. In adults OSA is known to cause sleep fragmentation due to multiple arousals. Sleep fragmentation may be achieved by auditory stimuli inducing arousals throughout the night and has been shown to result in performance decrements the following day.[99-101] Functions requiring concentration and dexterity are significantly affected by the excessive daytime sleepiness (EDS) resulting from sleep fragmentation, and subjects are often confused and disoriented. Aggressive outbursts, irritability, anxiety, and depression are all known manifestations of EDS in adults and appear to be fully reversible once sleep recovery is allowed. However, in contrast to adults with OSA, EDS does not appear to be a major feature of childhood OSA when assessed by either parental

reports[15,102] or more objective tools such as the multiple sleep latency test.[103] In fact, EDS occurred in only 13% of the children with OSA and was linearly correlated with the severity of respiratory disturbance such that a multiple sleep latency test of <10 minutes, which is indicative of EDS, was extremely unlikely when the apnea-hypopnea index was <15 events/hr. However, evidence of increased sleepiness, measured by multiple sleep latency testing, was reported by Lecendreux and colleagues in 30 children with ADHD who otherwise had no significant polysomnographic alterations,[104] raising the possibility that a subset of children with hyperactivity may in fact have an arousal disorder .

However, there is no reason to believe that sleep fragmentation affects children differently from adults. If this assumption is true, we would anticipate that sleep fragmentation–related morbidity would be reduced in children, since disruption of sleep architecture appears to be unusual in this population.[105] Indeed, when arousals are scored using criteria developed for adults,[106] children with OSA have fewer EEG arousals than adults with OSA and thus are better able to preserve sleep architecture.[45,102] The lack of arousals may account for the increased frequency of nocturnal enuresis seen in this population. Indeed, in a report by Guilleminault and associates,[22] 18% of children presented with secondary enuresis, while Weider and coworkers[107] reported a 76% improvement in nocturnal enuresis after tonsillectomy and adenoidectomy. Nonetheless, EDS-like morbidity is in fact present in children with OSA, suggesting either that current techniques to define arousal are not sensitive enough to detect sleep fragmentation in children[108] or that functional susceptibility to sleep fragmentation is higher in children. Alternatively, intermittent hypoxia rather than sleep fragmentation may be the major determinant of neurocognitive morbidity in children. As mentioned above, separation of the effects of sleep fragmentation and intermittent hypoxia on behavior and cognition is not possible in children. Thus, the individual role played by each of these factors in relation to neurobehavioral morbidity will be impossible to determine in the context of human studies.

To overcome such constraints, we recently developed a rodent model that allows for separation of the roles played by intermittent hypoxia and sleep fragmentation.[66] We found that intermittent hypoxia during sleep is associated with significant increases in neuronal cell loss and adverse effects on spatial memory tasks in the absence of significant sleep fragmentation or deprivation. Furthermore, when this model was applied to developing rodents, a unique period of neuronal susceptibility to episodic hypoxia during sleep emerged and coincides with ages at which OSA prevalence peaks in children.[109] Since this age coincides with that of the critical period for brain development, it is possible that during this period the delayed diagnosis and treatment of OSA will impose a greater burden on vulnerable brain structures and ultimately hamper the overall neurocognitive potential of children with SDB. This issue has been recently investigated, and indeed, developing rats exhibit greater decreases in the acquisition and retention of spatial tasks.[110] Interestingly, male rats exposed to intermittent hypoxia during sleep also exhibit increased locomotor activity, uniquely reminiscent of the hyperactivity of children with SDB, in whom a male predominance is well established.

ALVEOLAR HYPOVENTILATION

Snoring children with and without OSA represent a classic example of intermittent alveolar hypoventilation resulting from increased upper airway resistance associated with insufficient compensatory respiratory drive mechanisms during sleep. Since children are less prone to collapse their upper airways during sleep,[29] long periods of increased upper airway resistance and hypercapnia with and without hypoxemia will develop during the night rather than more frequent, discrete, obstructive apneic events, leading to the term "obstructive hypoventilation."[13] This feature of OSA in children has led to the recommendation to monitor carbon dioxide levels using both end-tidal and transcutaneous approaches, if possible.[111]

In adults with OSA, a blunted ventilatory drive to hypercapnia during wakefulness may develop and may contribute to the pathophysiology of upper airway obstruction. In addition, daytime hypercapnia may occur in adult patients with OSA and is probably the end result of multifactorial interactions involving respiratory dynamics, obesity, and leptin and other endocrine abnormal-

ities.[112] While intermittent hypercapnia is frequent in pediatric OSA during sleep, it will almost always disappear during wakefulness, indicating that hypercapnic and hypoxic ventilatory drives are intact in children.[27,45] However, arousal responses to hypercapnia are attenuated during sleep, suggesting that interactions among sleep, ventilatory drive, and neural mechanisms underlying upper airway patency affect the recruitment of arousal centers in OSA.[27]

Intermittent elevations in $Paco_2$ not only can exacerbate the effects of intermittent hypoxemia on neural tissue but also can affect cerebral circulation and vasomotor activity.[113] Furthermore, hypercapnia can directly suppress neural function,[114] and it is well established that CO_2 elevations will increase pulmonary artery pressure, possibly through increases in sympathetic tone.[115] Therefore, the typical intermittent hypercapnia that occurs in children with OSA may either directly or, through interactions with episodic hypoxia and arousal, exacerbate end-organ injury in this condition.

CONCLUSIONS

It is becoming increasingly clear that OSA in children can have adverse effects on somatic growth, induce cardiovascular alterations such as pulmonary and systemic hypertension, and lead to substantial neurobehavioral deficits, some of which may not be reversible if treatment is delayed. Based on our current understanding of the morbidity affecting pediatric OSA, it is imperative to direct future efforts toward an improved definition of the spectrum of the OSA-induced syndrome, such as providing more accurate guidelines for treatment.

References

1. Brouillette R, Hanson D, David R, et al: A diagnostic approach to suspected obstructive sleep apnea in children. J Pediatr 1984;105:10-14.
2. Ali NJ, Pitson D, Stradling JR: Snoring, sleep disturbance and behaviour in 4-5 year olds. Arch Dis Child 1993;68:360-366.
3. Gislason, T, Benediktsdottir B: Snoring, apneic episodes, and nocturnal hypoxemia among children 6 months to 6-years-old. Chest 1995;107:963-966.
4. American Thoracic Society: Standards and indications for cardiopulmonary sleep studies in children. Am J Respir Crit Care Med 1995;153:866-878.

5. Teculescu DB, Caillier I, Perrin P, et al: Snoring in French preschool children. Pediatr Pulmonol 1992;13:239-244.

6. Hulcrantz E, Lofstarnd TB, Ahlquist RJ: The epidemiology of sleep related breathing disorders in children. Int J Pediatr Otorhinolaryngol 1995;6 (suppl):S63-S66.

7. Owen GO, Canter RJ, Robinson A: Snoring, apnea and ENT symptoms in the paediatric community. Clin Otolaryngol Allied Sci 1996;21:130-134.

8. Ferreira AM, Clemente V, Gozal D, et al: Snoring in Portuguese primary school children. Pediatrics 2000;106:E64.

9. O'Brien LM, Holbrook CR, Mervis CB, et al: Sleep and neurobehavioral characteristics in 5-7 year old children with parentally reported symptoms of ADHD. Pediatrics 2003;111:554-563.

10. Corbo GM, Forastiere F, Agabiti N, et al: Snoring in 9- to 15-year-old children: Risk factors and clinical relevance. Pediatrics 2001;180:1149-1154.

11. McKenzie M: A Manual of Diseases of the Throat and Nose, Including the Pharynx, Larynx, Trachea, Oesophagus, Nasal Cavities, and Neck. London, Churchill, 1880.

12. Guilleminault C, Eldridge F, Simmons FB, Dement WC: Sleep apnea in eight children. Pediatrics 1976;58:28-31.

13. Rosen CL, D'Andrea L, Haddad GG: Adult criteria for obstructive sleep apnea do not identify children with serious obstruction. Am Rev Respir Dis 1992;146:1231-1234.

14. Carroll JL, McLoughlin GM: Diagnostic criteria for obstructive sleep apnea in children. Pediatr Pulmonol 1992;14:71-74.

15. Carroll JL, McColley SA, Marcus CL, Curtis S, Loughlin GM: Inability of clinical history to distinguish primary snoring from obstructive sleep apnea syndrome in children. Chest 1995;108:610-618.

16. Sivan Y, Kornecki A, Schonfeld T: Screening obstructive sleep apnoea syndrome by home videotape recording in children. Eur Respir J 1996;9:2127-2131.

17. Lamm C, Mandeli J, Kattan M: Evaluation of home audiotapes as an abbreviated test for obstructive sleep apnea syndrome (OSAS) in children. Pediatr Pulmonol 1999;27:267-272.

18. Brouillette RT, Morielli A, Leimanis A, et al: Nocturnal pulse oximetry as an abbreviated testing modality for pediatric obstructive sleep apnea. Pediatrics 2000;105:405-412.

19. Brouillette RT, Lavergne J, Leimanis A, et al: Differences in pulse oximetry technology can affect detection of sleep-disordered breathing in children. Anesth Analg 2002;94:S47-S53.

20. Schnall RP, Shlitner A, Sheffy J, et al: Periodic, profound peripheral vasoconstriction—a new marker of obstructive sleep apnea. Sleep 1999;22:939-946.

21. Lavie P, Shlitner A, Sheffy J, Schnall RP: Peripheral arterial tonometry: A novel and sensitive non-invasive monitor of brief arousals during sleep. Isr Med Assoc J 2000;2:246-247.

22. Guilleminault C, Korobkin R, Winkle R: A review of 50 children with obstructive sleep apnea syndrome. Lung 1981;159:275-287.

23. Guilleminault C, Winkle R, Korobkin R, Simmons B: Children and nocturnal snoring—evaluation of the effects of sleep related respiratory resistive load and daytime functioning. Eur J Pediatr 1982;139:165-171.

24. Chervin R, Dillon J, Bassetti C, et al: Symptoms of sleep disorders, inattention, and hyperactivity in children. Sleep 1997;20:1185-1192.

25. Gozal D: Sleep-disordered breathing and school performance in children. Pediatrics 1998;102:616-620.

26. Shiomi T, Guilleminault C, Stoohs R, Schnittger I: Obstructed breathing in children during sleep monitored by echocardiography. Acta Paediatr 1993;82:863-871.

27. Marcus CL, Greene MG, Carroll JL: Blood pressure in children with obstructive sleep apnea. Am J Respir Crit Care Med 1998;157:1098-1103.

28. Everett AD, Koch WC, Saulsbury FT: Failure to thrive due to obstructive sleep apnea. Clin Pediatr 1987;26:90-92.

29. Marcus CL: Pathophysiology of childhood obstructive sleep apnea: Current concepts. Respir Physiol 2000;119:143-154.

30. Isono S, Shimada A, Utsugi M, et al: Comparison of static mechanical properties of the passive pharynx between normal children and children with sleep-disordered breathing. Am J Respir Crit Care Med 1998;157:1201-1212.

31. Owens J, Opipari L, Nobile C, Spirito A: Sleep and daytime behavior in children with obstructive sleep apnea and behavioral sleep disorders. Pediatrics 1998;102:1178-1184.

32. Suen JS, Arnold JE, Brooks LJ: Adenotonsillectomy for treatment of obstructive sleep apnea in children. Arch Otolaryngol Head Neck Surg 1995;121:525-530.

33. Ahlqvist-Rastad J, Hutcrantz E, Melander H: Body growth in relation to tonsillar enlargement and tonsillectomy. Int J Pediatr Otorhinolaryngol 1992;24:55-61.

34. Freezer NJ, Bucens IK, Robertson CF: Obstructive sleep apnoea presenting as failure to thrive in infancy. J Paediatr Child Health 1995;31:172-175.

35. Brouillette RT, Fernbach SK, Hunt CE: Obstructive sleep apnea in infants and children. J Pediatr 1982;100:31-40.

36. Lind MG, Lundell BP: Tonsillar hyperplasia in children: A cause of obstructive sleep apneas, CO_2 retention, and retarded growth. Arch Otolaryngol 1982;108:650-654.

37. Soultan Z, Wadowski S, Rao M, Kravath RE: Effect of treating obstructive sleep apnea by tonsillectomy and/or adeniodectomy on obesity in children. Arch Pediatr Adolesc Med 1999;153:33-37.

38. Stradling JR, Thomas G, Warley ARH, et al: Effect of adenotonsillectomy on nocturnal hypoxaemia, sleep disturbance, and symptoms in snoring children. Lancet 1990;335:249-253.

39. Waters KA, Kirjavainen T, Jimenez M, et al: Overnight growth hormone secretion in achondroplasia: Deconvolution analysis, correlation with sleep state, and changes after treatment of obstructive sleep apnea. Pediatr Res 1996;39:547-553.

40. Chiba S, Ashikawa T, Moriwaki H, et al: The influence of sleep breathing disorder on growth hormone secretion in children with tonsil hypertrophy (in Japanese). Nippon Jibiinkoka Gakkai Kaiho 1998;101:873-878.

41. Bar A, Tarasiuk A, Segev Y, Phillip M, Tal A: The effect of adenotonsillectomy on serum insulin-like growth factor-I and growth in children with obstructive sleep apnea syndrome. J Pediatr 1999;135:76-80.

42. Nieminen P, Lopponen T, Tolonen U, et al: Growth and biochemical markers of growth in children with snoring and obstructive sleep apnea. Pediatrics 2002;109:e55.

43. Van Cauter E, Copinschi G: Interrelationships between growth hormone and sleep. Growth Horm IGF Res 2000;10(Suppl B):S57-S62.

44. Obal F Jr, Krueger JM: The somatotropic axis and sleep. Rev Neurol (Paris) 2001;157:S12-S15.

45. Marcus CL, Carroll JL, Koerner CB, et al: Determinants of growth in children with the obstructive sleep apnea syndrome. J Pediatr 1994;125:556-562.

46. Bland RM, Bulgarelli S, Ventham JC, et al: Total energy expenditure in children with obstructive sleep apnoea syndrome. Eur Respir J 2001;18:164-169.

47. Fagan KA: Selected contribution: Pulmonary hypertension in mice following intermittent hypoxia. J Appl Physiol 2001;90:2502-2507.

48. Tal A, Leiberman A, Margulis G, Sofer S: Ventricular dysfunction in children with obstructive sleep apnea: Radionuclide assessment. Pediatr Pulmonol 1988;4:139-143.

49. Tang J-R, Le Cras TD, Morris KG Jr, Abman SH: Brief perinatal hypoxia increases severity of pulmonary hypertension after reexposure to hypoxia in infant rats. Am J Physiol. Lung Cell Mol Physiol 2000;278:L356-L364.

50. Shepard JW Jr: Hypertension, cardiac arrhythmias, myocardial infarction, and stroke in relation to obstructive sleep apnea. Clin Chest Med 1992;13:437-458.

51. Fletcher EC, Bao G: Effect of episodic eucapnic and hypocapnic hypoxia on systemic blood pressure in hypertension-prone rats. J Appl Physiol 1996;81:2088-2094.

52. Peled N, Greenberg A, Pillar G, et al: Contributions of hypoxia and respiratory disturbance index to sympathetic activation and blood pressure in obstructive sleep apnea syndrome. Am J Hypertens 1998;11:1284-1289.

53. Brooks D, Horner RL, Floras JS, et al: Baroreflex control of heart rate in a canine model of obstructive sleep apnea. Am J Respir Crit Care Med 1999;159:1293-1297.

54. Fletcher EC, Bao G, Li R: Renin activity and blood pressure in response to chronic episodic hypoxia. Hypertension 1999;34:309-314.

55. Khoo MC, Kim TS, Berry RB: Spectral indices of cardiac autonomic function in obstructive sleep apnea. Sleep 1999;22:443-451.

56. Loredo JS, Ziegler MG, Ancoli-Israel S, et al: Relationship of arousals from sleep to sympathetic nervous system activity and BP in obstructive sleep apnea. Chest 1999;116:655-659.

57. Duchna HW, Guilleminault C, Stoohs RA, et al: Vascular reactivity in obstructive sleep apnea syndrome. Am J Respir Crit Care Med 2000;161:187-191.

58. Fletcher EC: Effect of episodic hypoxia on sympathetic activity and blood pressure. Respir Physiol 2000;119:189-197.

59. Kraiczi H, Hedner J, Peker Y, Carlson J: Increased vasoconstrictor sensitivity in obstructive sleep apnea. J Appl Physiol 2000;89:493-498.

60. Phillips BG, Somers VK: Neural and humoral mechanisms mediating cardiovascular responses to obstructive sleep apnea. Respir Physiol 2000;119:181-187.

61. Fletcher EC: Invited review: Physiological consequences of intermittent hypoxia: Systemic blood pressure. J Appl Physiol 2001;90:1600-1605.

62. Elmasry A, Lindberg E, Hedner J, et al: Obstructive sleep apnoea and urine catecholamines in hypertensive males: A population-based study. Eur Respir J 2002;19:511-517.

63. Aljadeff G, Gozal D, Schechtman VL, et al: Heart rate variability in children with obstructive sleep apnea. Sleep 1997;20:151-157.

64. Baharav A, Kotagal S, Rubin BK, et al: Autonomic cardiovascular control in children with obstructive sleep apnea. Clin Auton Res 1999;9:345-351.

65. Katz ES, Marcus CL: The pulse transit time as a measure of respiratory arousal in children with sleep-disordered breathing. Sleep 2001;24:A207.

66. Gozal D, Daniel JM, Dohanich GP: Behavioral and anatomical correlates of chronic episodic hypoxia during sleep in the rat. J Neurosci 2001;21:2442-2450.

67. Soukhova GK, Roberts AM, Lipton AJ, et al: Early postnatal exposure to intermittent hypoxia attenuates baroreflex sensitivity in adult rats (abstract). Sleep 2002;25:A335-336.

68. Hill W: On some causes of backwardness and stupidity in children and the relief of the symptoms in some instances by nasopharyngeal scarifications. BMJ 1889;II:711-712.

69. Weissbluth M, Davis A, Poncher J, Reiff J: Signs of airway obstruction during sleep and behavioral, developmental and academic problems. Dev Behav Pediatr 1983;4:119-121.

70. Singer LP, Saenger P: Complications of pediatric obstructive sleep apnea. Otolaryngol Clin North Am 1990;23:665-676.

71. Leach J, Olson J, Hermann J, Manning S: Polysomnographic and clinical findings in children with obstructive sleep apnea. Arch Otolaryngol Head Neck Surg 1992;118:741-744.

72. Rhodes SK, Shimoda KC, Wald LR, et al: Neurocognitive deficits in morbidly obese children with obstructive sleep apnea. J Pediatr 1995;127:741-744.

73. Ali NJ, Pitson D, Stradling JR: Sleep disordered breathing: Effects of adenotonsillectomy on behaviour and psychological functioning. Eur J Pediatr 1996;155:56-62.

74. Chervin RD, Archbold KH: Hyperactivity and polysomnographic findings in children evaluated for sleep-disordered breathing. Sleep 2001;24:313-320.

75. Ali NJ, Pitson D, Stradling JR: Natural history of snoring and related behaviour problems between the ages of 4 and 7 years. Arch Dis Child 1994;71:74-76.

76. Stein MA, Mendelsohn J, Obermeyer WH, et al: Sleep and behavior problems in school-aged children. Pediatrics 2001;107:E60.

77. Kaplan BJ, McNichol J, Conte RA, Moghadam HK: Sleep disturbance in preschool-aged and hyperactive and nonhyperactive children. Pediatrics 1987;80:839-844.

78. Hansen DE, Vandenberg B: Neuropsychological features and differential diagnosis of sleep apnea syndrome in children. J Clin Child Psychol 1997;26:304-310.

79. Corkum P, Tannock R, Moldofsky H: Sleep disturbance in children with attention-deficit hyperactivity disorder. J Am Acad Child Adolesc Psychiatry 1998;37:637-646.

80. Corkum P, Tannock R, Moldofsky H, et al: Actigraphy and parental ratings of sleep in children with attention deficit/hyperactivity disorder (ADHD). Sleep 2001;24:303-312.

81. Chervin RD, Archbold KH, Dillon JE, et al: Inattention, hyperactivity, and symptoms of sleep disordered breathing. Pediatrics 2002;109:449-456.

82. Sadeh A, McGuire JP, Sachs H, et al: Sleep and psychological characteristics of children on a psychiatric inpatient unit. J Am Acad Child Adolesc Psychiatry 1995;34:813-819.

83. Benca RM, Obermeyer WH, Thisted RA, Gillin JC: Sleep and psychiatric disorders: A meta-analysis. Arch Gen Psychiatry 1992;49:651-668.

84. Gozal D, Pope DW Jr: Snoring during early childhood and academic performance at ages 13-14 years. Pediatrics 2001;107:1394-1399.

85. Ball JD, Tiernan M, Janusz J, Furr A: Sleep patterns among children with attention-deficit hyperactivity disorder: A re-examination of parental perceptions. J Pediatr Psychol. 1997;22:389-398.

86. Ring A, Stein D, Barak Y, et al: Sleep disturbances in children with attention-deficit/hyperactivity disorder: A comparative study with healthy siblings. J Learn Disabil 1998;31:572-578.

87. Stein MA: Unraveling sleep problems in treated and untreated children with ADHD. J Child Adolesc Psychopharmacol 1999;9:157-168.

88. Owens J, Maxim R, Nobile C, McGuinn M, Msall M: Parental and self-report of sleep in children with attention deficit/hyperactivity disorder. Arch Pediatr Adolesc Med 2000;154:549-555.

89. Busby K, Firestone P, Pivik RT: Sleep patterns in hyperkinetic and normal children. Sleep 1981;4:366-383.

90. Greenhill L, Puig-Antich J, Goetz R, et al: Sleep architecture and REM sleep measures in prepubertal children with attention deficit disorder with hyperactivity. Sleep 1983;6:91-101.

91. Redline S, Tishler PV, Schluchter M, et al: Risk factors for sleep-disordered breathing in children: Associations with obesity, race, and respiratory problems. Am J Respir Crit Care Med 1999;159:1527-1532.

92. Conners CK: Conners' Parent Rating Scales. New York, MHS Publishing, 1989.

93. American Academy of Pediatrics: Clinical Practice Guideline: Diagnosis and Evaluation of the Child with Attention-Deficit/Hyperactivity Disorder. Pediatrics 2000;105:1158-1170.

94. Beebe DW, Gozal D: Obstructive sleep apnea and the prefrontal cortex: Towards a comprehensive model linking nocturnal upper airway dysfunction to daytime cognitive and behavioral deficits. J Sleep Res 2002;11:1-16.

95. Corkum P, Moldofsky H, Hogg-Johnson S, et al: Sleep problems in children with attention-deficit/hyperactivity disorder: Impact of subtype, comorbidity, and stimulant medication. J Am Acad Child Adolesc Psychiatry 1999;38:1285-1293.

96. Gozal D, Holbrook CR, Mehl RC, et al: Correlation analysis between NEPSY battery scores and respiratory disturbance index in snoring 6-year old children: A preliminary report. Sleep 2001;24:A126.

97. Greenberg GD, Watson RK, Deptula D: Neuropsychological dysfunction in sleep apnea. Sleep 1987;10:254-262.

98. Naegele B, Thouvard V, Pepin JL, et al: Deficits of cognitive executive functions in patients with sleep apnea syndrome. Sleep 1995;18:43-52.

99. Stepansky EJ, Lamphere P, Badia P: Sleep fragmentation and daytime sleepiness. Sleep 1984;7:18-26.

100. Stepansky EJ, Lamphere J, Roehrs T: Experimental sleep fragmentation in normal subjects. Int J Neurosci 1987;33:207-214.

101. Chugh DK, Weaver TE, Dinges DF: Neurobehavioral consequences of arousals. Sleep 1996;19:S198-S201.

102. Frank Y, Kravath RE, Pollak CP, Weitzman ED: Obstructive sleep apnea and its therapy: Clinical and polysomnographic manifestations. Pediatrics 1983;71:737-742.

103. Gozal D, Wang M, Pope DW: Objective sleepiness measures in pediatric obstructive sleep apnea. Pediatrics 2001;108:693-697.

104. Lecendreux M, Konofal E, Bouvard M, et al: Sleep and alertness in children with ADHD. J Child Psychol Psychiatry 2000;41:803-812.

105. Goh DY, Galster P, Marcus CL: Sleep architecture and respiratory disturbances in children with obstructive sleep apnea. Am J Respir Crit Care Med 2000;162:682-686.

106. Sleep Disorders Atlas Task Force, Guilleminault C (ed). EEG arousals: Scoring and rules and examples. Sleep 1992;15:173-184.

107. Weider DJ, Sateia MJ, West RP: Nocturnal enuresis in children with upper airway obstruction. Otolaryngol Head Neck Surg 1991;105:427-432.

108. Bandla HPR, Gozal D: Dynamic changes in EEG spectra during obstructive apnea in children. Pediatr Pulmonol 2000;29:359-365.

109. Gozal E, Row BW, Schurr A, Gozal D: Developmental differences in cortical and hippocampal vulnerability to intermittent hypoxia in the rat. Neurosci Lett 2001;305:197-201.

110. Row BW, Kheirandish L, Neville JJ, Gozal D: Impaired spatial learning and hyperactivity in developing rats exposed to intermittent hypoxia. Pediatr Res 2002; 52:449-453.

111. Morielli A, Desjardins D, Brouillette RT: Transcutaneous and end-tidal carbon dioxide pressures should be measured during pediatric polysomnography. Am Rev Respir Dis 1993;148:1599-1604.

112. Gozal D: Determinants of daytime hypercapnia in obstructive sleep apnea: Is obesity the only one to blame? Chest 2002;121:320-321.

113. Loeppky JA, Miranda FG, Eldridge MW: Abnormal cerebrovascular responses to CO_2 in sleep apnea patients. Sleep 1984;7:97-109.

114. Itoh Y, Yoshioka M, Kemmotsu O: Effects of experimental hypercapnia on hippocampal long-term potentiation in anesthetized rats. Neurosci Lett 1999;260:201-220.

115. Myers JL, Domkowski PW, Wang Y, Hopkins RA: Sympathetic blockade blunts hypercapnic pulmonary arterial vasoconstriction in newborn piglets. Eur J Cardiothorac Surg 1998;3:298-305.

Obstructive Sleep Apnea Syndrome in Infants and Children: Clinical Features and Pathophysiology

19

Lee J. Brooks

PATHOPHYSIOLOGY

The anatomy and neural control of the pharynx have evolved to serve its multiple functions as a conduit for air, liquids, and solids. The pharynx must be collapsible to facilitate swallowing and speech. Coordinated neuromuscular action is required to propel food into the esophagus but not the nose or trachea, as well as for speech. However, the collapsibility required for speech and swallowing can be an impediment to respiration, when the patency of the pharynx is required to conduct air from the nose to the larynx. In conscious individuals, the pharynx must remain open at all times except during momentary closure associated with swallowing, speech, regurgitation, and eructation.

The patency of the pharynx is determined by both anatomic and physiologic factors. During inspiration, intraluminal pressure is negative (subatmospheric) and tends to produce pharyngeal collapse. Assuming constant flow, Bernoulli's principle dictates that a smaller airway would result in even more negative intraluminal pressure, with a greater tendency to collapse. Thus, one would expect that individuals with a small pharynx would be at a greater risk for airway collapse during sleep, but this is not necessarily the case. The airway of a child is inherently smaller than that of an adult, yet the prevalence of obstructive sleep apnea (OSA) is about 1% in school-aged children,[1-3] compared with a prevalence of 4% in middle-aged men.[4] Similarly, the prevalence of OSA is higher in men than women,[4] even though women have a smaller pharynx.[5] Thus, the anatomic size of the pharynx cannot be the only factor predisposing an individual to OSA.

Modeling the pharynx as a Starling resistor has been useful in understanding its mechanical properties as a collapsible tube (Fig. 19–1). On inspiration, pressure at the airway opening (nares) is atmospheric, and downstream pressure is equal to tracheal pressure. Therefore, pressure within the pharyngeal lumen is negative with respect to the atmosphere. Collapse occurs when this negative pressure is lower than that surrounding the segment (P_{crit}). In adults P_{crit} is the lowest in nonsnorers, increasing progressively in subjects who snore and those with hypopnea and obstructive apnea. The results of one study showed that subjects with OSA had a positive P_{crit}, indicating that the airway would collapse during sleep.[6] Similar results have been found in children, in whom P_{crit} correlated with the severity of sleep-disordered breathing (Fig. 19–2).[7]

In awake adults, a small pharynx can be overcome by stiffening of the pharynx,[8] probably by augmenting upper airway tone.[9] During sleep this compensatory mechanism can be lost, resulting in airway closure despite (and partially because of) continuing respiratory effort.[10] Hypoxemia and hypercapnia ensue, with the apnea terminating on arousal. Frequent arousal results in sleep fragmentation and daytime sleepiness. Therefore, any factors that decrease pharyngeal size or increase pharyngeal compliance might be expected to predispose an individual to OSA syndrome (OSAS) (Fig. 19–3). In one early description of OSAS in children, 32% had facial dysmorphism, presumably contributing to an anatomically small pharynx, and an additional 12% had underlying neuromuscular disorders, probably causing OSA from pharyngeal hypotonia.[11]

Factors Affecting Pharyngeal Size

The anatomic size of the pharynx stems from a combination of the underlying bony structure and soft tissue, including the tonsils and adenoids. It may also be affected by dynamic factors such as obesity.

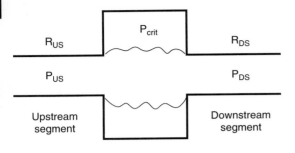

Collapsible segment

Figure 19–1. The Starling resistor model of the upper airway. The upper airway is represented as a tube with a collapsible segment. The upstream (nasal) and downstream (tracheal) segments have fixed diameters and resistances (R_{US}, R_{DS}) and pressures (P_{US}, P_{DS}). Collapse occurs when the pressure surrounding the airway (P_{crit}) is greater than that within the airway. (Redrawn with permission from Marcus et al: Upper airway collapsibility in children with obstructive sleep apnea syndrome. J Appl Physiol 1994;77:918-924.)

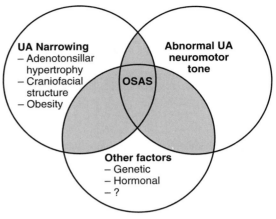

Figure 19–3. Obstructive sleep apnea syndrome (OSAS) in children may result from a combination of factors. Structural anomalies may result in a narrow upper airway (UA), and decreased neuromuscular tone may result in a floppy UA. Genetic, hormonal, or other factors may also have an impact on these conditions.

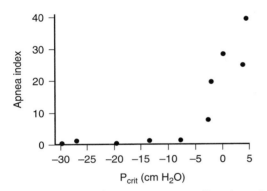

Figure 19–2. P_{crit} (the pressure surrounding the collapsible pharyngeal segment) vs. apnea index (number of obstructive apnea events per hour of sleep). There is a significant correlation between P_{crit} and the severity of obstructive sleep apnea ($r = .80$, $P < .02$). (Redrawn with permission from Marcus et al: Upper airway collapsibility in children with obstructive sleep apnea syndrome. J Appl Physiol 1994;77:918-924.)

The underlying bony structure of the face clearly contributes to the risk for OSAS. Children who snore have a narrower anterior-posterior dimension of the pharynx.[12] Several studies have documented familial aggregation of OSAS[13] independent of weight, body mass index, or neck circumference.[14,15] Family members tended to share a small pharyngeal volume, retroposed maxillae with shorter mandibles,[16] and/or other craniofacial features, such as a high, narrow hard palate.[17] Thus, genetic factors, particularly those controlling pharyngeal structure, can place even normal individuals at a risk for OSAS.

Children with craniofacial abnormalities may be at a particularly high risk for OSAS.[18] Micrognathia is a hallmark of Treacher Collins syndrome and the Robin sequence. Mutations in the fibroblast growth factor receptor genes result in midfacial hypoplasia of children with such disorders as Apert-Crouzon syndrome and achondroplasia. These disorders are discussed in detail elsewhere.

Soft tissues can also narrow the pharynx, particularly in cases of adenotonsillar hypertrophy. The tonsils and adenoids are at their largest, with respect to the underlying bony structures, between 3 and 6 years of age,[19] coinciding with the peak incidence of childhood OSAS. The severity of obstructive events is related to the size of the adenoids[20] and most otherwise normal children with OSAS respond well to adenotonsillectomy.[21] However, OSAS is not caused by adenotonsillar hypertrophy alone. Several studies have been unable to show a correlation between upper airway or adenotonsillar size and the number of respiratory events that occur during sleep.[20,22-24] In addition, some children with adenotonsillar hypertrophy but no other known risk factors for OSAS are not cured by adenotonsillectomy.[21] Finally, Guilleminault and colleagues described a cohort of children who were cured of OSAS by adenotonsillectomy but developed a recurrence during adolescence.[25] Thus, it appears that childhood OSAS is a dynamic process resulting from a combination of structural and neuromotor abnormalities rather than from structural abnormalities alone.

Obesity may narrow the pharynx due to the deposition of adipose tissue within the muscles and soft tissue surrounding the airway.[26] Although most adults with OSAS are obese, children with OSAS are often of normal weight or even fail to thrive.[27] However, obesity does increase the child's risk for OSAS.[20,28-31]

Factors Affecting Pharyngeal Compliance

Women and children have a smaller pharynx than men yet are at a lower statistical risk for OSA. Acoustic studies of the upper airway demonstrate that women have a relatively stiff pharynx compared with men.[5] Children also have different pharyngeal pressure–flow characteristics, suggesting a stiffer upper airway than that in adults.[32] These findings suggest that both genetic and hormonal factors likely affect pharyngeal compliance and hence the risk for OSA. This can be modified by many disease states, particularly those affecting neuromuscular tone. Children with cerebral palsy and other neurologic disorders are at an increased risk for OSA. Children with Down syndrome and Prader-Willi syndrome are at an increased risk for OSA because of decreased neuromuscular tone as well as anatomic factors. Obesity may make the pharynx more compliant and may also increase the risk for sleep-disordered breathing by decreasing oxyhemoglobin saturation because of reduced functional residual capacity and/or blunting of central respiratory drive.

CLINICAL FEATURES

The clinical appearance of children with OSAS is often different from that of adults. However, in both groups the problem is usually first recognized by the female caregiver (wife or mother), and there is often some denial and reluctance on the part of the patient to seek medical care. Unlike adults, gender distribution in children, at

least during the prepubertal years, is approximately equal.[31]

Snoring

Clinical findings may occur during both sleep and wakefulness (Table 19–1). It is important to obtain the clinical history from a parent or even a sibling who shares a room and might have observed the patient while s/he was sleeping; few of us are aware of (and admit to) snoring and other nocturnal symptoms. Snoring is usually the presenting complaint of patients with OSAS. Up to 20% of children snore intermittently, and 7% to 10% of them are habitual or regular snorers.[1,2] From 1% to 3% of school-aged children have significant disease.[1,2] Respiratory pauses, often ending with a snort or gasp, are also often described. The snoring may be cyclical, worsening with a decrease in motor tone associated with rapid eye movement sleep. These symptoms are often the worst when the patient is in the supine position, where gravity pulls the genioglossus to occlude the airway. However, non-obese prepubertal children may breathe better in the supine position,[33] suggesting a different pathophysiology from that in older children and adults.

Not all children who snore have OSAS. No combination of historical or physical factors has been useful in distinguishing OSAS from primary snoring. Several studies have attempted to predict the presence of OSAS in children with a suggestive clinical presentation, including

Table 19–1. Symptoms of Obstructive Sleep Apnea in Children
Nocturnal
Snoring
Respiratory pauses
Restless sleep
Diaphoresis
Paradoxical respiratory movements
Enuresis
Diurnal
Sleepiness
Behavior problems
Poor school performance
Morning headaches

snoring, witnessed apneas, and/or daytime somnolence. However, only one third to one half of
the children suspected of having OSAS satisfied
polysomnographic criteria.[21,34-36] Therefore, laboratory confirmation is essential to confirm the
diagnosis and establish the severity of the disorder so that the appropriate therapy may be
instituted. These studies are best performed in a
laboratory where the staff members are experienced with children; preparation of the child for
study and scoring and interpretation of the study
may be different from that for adults. In general,
children have fewer clear obstructive events than
adults, and close attention must be paid to the
identification of partial obstructive events, or
obstructive hypopneas, in children.[37] An apnea/
hypopnea index of 5 or greater is considered
abnormal in young adults, whereas normal children usually do not have more than one event of
obstructive apnea per hour of sleep.[38] However,
the clinical significance of a small number of respiratory events, even if statistically abnormal, is
not known. Children are also more likely than
adults to have significant oxyhemoglobin desaturation with shorter obstructive events, probably due to lower functional residual capacity and
smaller oxygen stores.

Restless Sleep

Restless sleep may be a sign of frequent arousal
secondary to respiratory pauses. It is often helpful to inquire about the condition of the bedclothes in the morning; the only clue to the
extent of restless sleep may be disheveled sheets
and blankets. The child may prefer to sleep in
the upright position or with his or her neck hyper-
extended to maximize the patency of the upper
airway.

Enuresis

Nocturnal enuresis can occur during any stage of
sleep.[39] Several anecdotal reports describe a relationship between OSAS and enuresis in children.[40,41] In one study, 47% of children with
more than one respiratory event per hour of
sleep had nocturnal enuresis, compared with
17% of children with no or one respiratory event
per hour ($P < .05$).[42] Enuresis was more prevalent among boys than girls but was not related to
obesity. This may be a function of an insufficient

arousal response,[43] impaired urodynamics,[44]
and/or insufficient vasopressin production during sleep.[45]

Obesity or Failure to Thrive

As in adults, obesity may predispose the child to
OSAS.[20,28-31] However, in contrast to adults, children with OSAS may fail to thrive. In one report,
27% of the children with OSAS were failing to
thrive,[46] perhaps due to the increased work of
breathing during sleep.[27] After treatment for
their OSAS, a group of 14 children demonstrated
an increase in weight percentile, accompanied by
a decrease in sleeping energy expenditure.[27]
Endocrine factors such as insulin-like growth
factor–1 (IGF-1) may also play a role. Thirteen
children with OSA showed an improvement in
weight and IGF-1 after adenotonsillectomy.[47]

Conversely, OSA may itself be a risk factor for
the metabolic syndrome, a complex of hyperin-
sulinemia/fasting hyperglycemia, abdominal
obesity, and dyslipidemia. The severity of OSA
correlated with fasting insulin levels in a group
of obese children independent of the degree of
obesity.[48] Treatment of OSA by continuous positive airway pressure in adults with type 2 diabetes resulted in a significant improvement in
their insulin responsiveness.[49] This may be the
result of catecholamine and/or cortisol release
associated with arousal and/or hypoxemia.

Daytime Functioning

Frequent arousal and poor quality of sleep may
result in daytime sleepiness. Sometimes this is
obvious, as in the child who falls asleep in school
or at the dinner table. It is frequently more subtle, being manifested as a short temper, behavior
problems, or academic difficulties. Children
whose parents report snoring and sleep disturbances were believed by their teachers to be more
hyperactive and less attentive than control subjects.[1] These children may be misdiagnosed as
those with attention deficit hyperactivity disorder.
These episodes of daydreaming or inattentiveness may represent brief "microsleeps" as the
child attempts to repay his or her sleep debt.
Children with a lower academic performance in
middle school are more likely to have snored
during early childhood than their better performing schoolmates.[50] Children with sleep-associated

gas exchange abnormalities who were performing poorly in school showed an increase in their grades after adenotonsillectomy.[51] Deficiencies in cognitive function, when they occur, may be the result of intermittent hypoxemia[52] and/or frequent arousal, preventing good-quality nocturnal sleep. Sleepiness in the absence of snoring may suggest narcolepsy or simply inadequate sleep due to insomnia or schedule problems. Nocturnal asthma and gastroesophageal reflux may also disturb nocturnal sleep and result in excessive daytime somnolence.

Mortality

There appears to be an excess mortality in adults with OSAS. Adults with more than twenty apneic events per hour had a significant increase in mortality over those with fewer than twenty such events per hour.[53] The increased mortality may result indirectly from medical risk factors such as hypertension[54] or an increased risk of motor vehicle accidents.[55] Comparable data are not available for children, but pediatric OSAS can be associated with systemic hypertension,[56] ventricular dysfunction, and/or cor pulmonale.[57,58] In one early report 12 of 22 children had cor pulmonale,[46] but this is probably less common now, with greater awareness of the problem resulting in earlier diagnosis and treatment.

SUMMARY

OSA is common in children, resulting from a combination of factors influencing the size and collapsibility of the pharynx. Children with OSAS may present with nocturnal complaints including snoring, restless sleep, and enuresis. In the daytime they may exhibit sleepiness, behavior problems, and/or poor school performance. They may be obese or fail to thrive. OSAS may result in considerable morbidity and perhaps mortality if left untreated.

References

1. Ali NJ, Pitston DJ, Stradling JR: Snoring, sleep disturbance, and behaviour in 4-5 year olds. Arch Dis Child 1993;68:360-366.
2. Gisalson T, Benediktsdottir B: Snoring, apneic episodes, and nocturnal hypoxemia among children 6 months to 6 years old. Chest 1995;107: 963-966.
3. Anuntaseree W, Rookkapan K, Kuasirikul S, Thongsuksai P: Snoring and obstructive sleep apnea in Thai school-age children. Pediatr Pulmonol 2001;32:222-227.
4. Young T, Palta M, Dempsey J, et al: The occurrence of sleep-disordered breathing among middle-aged adults. N Engl J Med 1993;328: 1230-1235.
5. Brooks LJ, Strohl KP: Size and mechanical properties of the pharynx in healthy men and women. Am Rev Respir Dis 1992;146:1394-1397.
6. Gleadhill IC, Schwartz AR, Schubert N, et al: Upper airway collapsibility in snorers and patients with obstructive hypopnea and apnea. Am Rev Respir Dis 1991;144:1300-1303.
7. Marcus CL, McColley SA, Carroll JL, et al: Upper airway collapsibility in children with obstructive sleep apnea syndrome. J Appl Physiol 1994;77: 918-924.
8. Hudgel DW, Brooks LJ, Harasick TM: Measurements of awake upper airway caliber do not predict upper airway resistance during sleep. Am Rev Respir Dis 1989;139:A374.
9. Mezzanotte WS, Tangel DJ, White DP: Waking genioglossal electromyogram in sleep apnea patients versus normal controls (a neuromuscular compensatory mechanism). J Clin Invest 1992;89: 1571-1579.
10. Mezzanotte WS, Tangel DJ, White DP: Influence of sleep onset on upper airway muscle activity in apnea patients versus normal controls. Am J Respir Crit Care Med 1996;153:1880-1887.
11. Guilleminault C, Korobkin R, Winkle R: A review of 50 children with obstructive sleep apnea syndrome. Lung 1981;159:275-287.
12. Kulnis R, Nelson S, Strohl K, Hans M: Cephalometric assessment of snoring and nonsnoring children. Chest 2000;118:596-603.
13. Pillar G, Lavie P: Assessment of the role of inheritance in sleep apnea syndrome. Am J Respir Crit Care Med 1995;151:688-691.
14. Redline S, Tosteson T, Tishler PV, et al: Studies in the genetics of obstructive sleep apnea. Am Rev Respir Dis 1992;145:440-444.
15. Redline S, Tishler PV, Tosteson TD, et al: The familial aggregation of obstructive sleep apnea. Am J Respir Crit Care Med 1995;151:682-687.
16. Mathur R, Douglas NJ: Family studies in patients with the sleep apnea-hypopnea syndrome. Ann Intern Med 1995;122:174-178.
17. Guilleminault C, Partinen M, Hollman K, et al: Familial aggregates in obstructive sleep apnea syndrome. Chest 1995;107:1545-1551.
18. Brooks LJ: Genetic syndromes affecting breathing during sleep in children. In Lee-Chiong TL, Sateia MJ, Carskadon MA (eds): Sleep Medicine. Philadelphia, Hanley & Belfus, 2002, pp 305-314.

19. Jeans WD, Fernando DCJ, Maw AR, Leighton BC: A longitudinal study of the growth of the nasopharynx and its contents in normal children. Br J Radiol 1981;54:117-121.

20. Brooks LJ, Stephens B, Bacevice AM: Adenoid size is related to severity but not the number of episodes of obstructive apnea in children. J Pediatr 1998;132:682-686.

21. Suen JS, Arnold JE, Brooks LJ: Adenotonsillectomy for treatment of obstructive sleep apnea in children. Arch Otolaryngol Head Neck Surg 1995;121:523-530.

22. Fernbach SK, Brouillette RT, Riggs TW, Hunt CE: Radiologic evaluation of adenoids and tonsils in children with obstructive apnea: Plain films and fluoroscopy. Pediatr Radiol 1983;13:258-265.

23. Mahboubi S, Marsh RR, Potsic WP, Pasquariello PS: The lateral neck radiograph in adenotonsillar hyperplasia. Int J Pediatr Otorhinolaryngol 1985;10:67-73.

24. Laurikainen E, Erkinjuntti M, Alihanka J, et al: Radiological parameters of the bony nasopharynx and the adenotonsillar size compared with sleep apnea episodes in children. Int J Pediatr Otorhinolaryngol 1987;12:303-310.

25. Gulleminault C, Partinen M, Praud JP, et al: Morphometric facial changes and obstructive sleep apnea in adolescents. J Pediatr 1989;114: 997-999.

26. Horner RL, Mohiaddin RH, Lowell DG, et al: Sites and sizes of fat deposits around the pharynx in obese patients with obstructive sleep apnoea and weight matched controls. Eur Respir J 1989;2:613-622.

27. Marcus CL, Carroll JL, Koerner CB, et al: Determinants of growth in children with the obstructive sleep apnea syndrome. J Pediatr 1994;125:556-562.

28. Mallory GB, Fiser DH, Jackson R: Sleep-associated breathing disorders in morbidly obese children and adolescents. J Pediatr 1989;115: 892-897.

29. Silvestri JM, Weese-Mayer DE, Bass MT, et al: Polysomnography in obese children with a history of sleep-associated breathing disorders. Pediatr Pulmonol 1993;16:124-129.

30. Marcus CL, Curtis S, Koerner CB, et al: Evaluation of pulmonary function and polysomnography in obese children and adolescents. Pediatr Pulmonol 1996;21:176-183.

31. Redline S, Tishler PV, Schluchter M, et al: Risk factors for sleep disordered breathing in children. Am J Respir Crit Care Med 1999;159:1527-1532.

32. Marcus CL, Lutz J, Hamer A, et al: Developmental changes in response to subatmospheric pressure loading of the upper airway. J Appl Physiol 1999;87:626-633.

33. Fernandes do Prado LB, Li X, Thompson R, Marcus CL: Body position and obstructive sleep apnea in children. Sleep. 2002;25:66-71.

34. Wang RC, Elkins TP, Keech D, et al: Accuracy of clinical evaluation in pediatric obstructive sleep apnea. Otolaryngol Head Neck Surg 1998;118: 69-73.

35. Carroll JL, McColley SA, Marcus CL, et al: Inability of clinical history to distinguish primary snoring from obstructive sleep apnea syndrome in children. Chest 1995;108:610-618.

36. Leach J, Olson J, Herman J, Manning S: Polysomnographic and clinical findings in children with obstructive sleep apnea. Arch Otolaryngol Head Neck Surg 1992;118:741-744.

37. Rosen CL, D'Andrea L, Haddad GG: Adult criteria for obstructive sleep apnea do not identify children with serious obstruction. Am Rev Respir Dis 1992;146:1231-1234.

38. Marcus CL, Omlin KJ, Basinki DJ, et al: Normal polysomnographic values for children and adolescents. Am Rev Respir Dis 1992;146:1235-1239.

39. Bader G, Neveus T, Kruse S, Sillen U: Sleep of primary enuretic children and controls. Sleep 2002;25:579-583.

40. Sakai J, Herbert F: Secondary enuresis associated with obstructive sleep apnea (letter). J Am Acad Child Adolesc Psychiatry 2000;39:140-141.

41. Timms DJ: Rapid maxillary expansion in the treatment of nocturnal enuresis. Angle Orthod 1990;60:229-233.

42. Brooks LJ, Topol HI: Enuresis in children with sleep apnea. J Pediatr 2003;142:515-518.

43. Berry RB, Kouchi KG, Der DE, et al: Sleep apnea impairs the arousal response to airway occlusion. Chest 1996;109:1490-1496.

44. Yokoyama O, Amano T, Lee S, et al: Enuresis in an adult female with obstructive sleep apnea. Urology 1995;45:150-154.

45. Lin C, Tsan K, Lin C: Plasma levels of atrial natriuretic factor in moderate to severe obstructive sleep apnea syndrome. Sleep 1993;16:37-39.

46. Brouillette RT, Fernbach SK, Hunt CE: Obstructive sleep apnea in infants and children. J Pediatr 1982;100:31-40.

47. Bar A, Tarasiuk A, Segev Y, et al: The effect of adenotonsillectomy on serum insulin-like growth factor-1 and growth in children with obstructive sleep apnea syndrome. J Pediatr 1999;135:76-80.

48. de la Eva RC, Baur LA, Donaghue KC, Waters KA: Metabolic correlates with obstructive sleep apnea in obese subjects. J Pediatr 2002;140:654-659.

49. Brooks B, Cistulli PA, Borkman M, et al: Obstructive sleep apnea in obese noninsulin-dependent diabetic patients: Effect of continuous positive airway pressure on insulin responsiveness. J Clin Endocrinol Metab 1994;79:1681-1685.

50. Gozal D, Pope DW: Snoring during early childhood and academic performance at ages thirteen to fourteen years. Pediatrics 2001;107:1394-1399.

51. Gozal D: Sleep-disordered breathing and school performance in children. Pediatrics 1998;102:616-620.

52. Findley LJ, Barth JT, Powers DC, et al: Cognitive impairment in patients with obstructive sleep apnea and associated hypoxemia. Chest 1986;90:686-690.

53. He J, Kryger MH, Zorick FJ, et al: Mortality and apnea index in obstructive sleep apnea: Experience in 385 male patients. Chest 1988;94:9-14.

54. Lavie P, Herer P, Peled R, et al: Mortality in sleep apnea patients: A multivariate analysis of risk factors. Sleep 1995;18:149-157.

55. Teran-Santos J, Jimenez-Gomez A, Cordera-Guevara J: The association between sleep apnea and the risk of traffic accidents. N Engl J Med 1999;340:847-851.

56. Marcus CL, Greene MG, Carroll JL: Blood pressure in children with obstructive sleep apnea. Am J Respir Crit Care Med 1998;157:1098-1103.

57. Tal A, Lieberman A, Margulis G, Sofer S: Ventricular dysfunction in children with obstructive sleep apnea: Radionuclide assessment. Pediatr Pulmonol 1988;4:139-143.

58. Sofer S, Weinhouse E, Tal A, et al: Cor pulmonale due to adenoidal or tonsillar hypertrophy or both in children. Chest 1988;93:119-122.

Enuresis in Children with Sleep Apnea

20

Lee J. Brooks

Several anecdotal reports suggest the likelihood of a relationship between nocturnal enuresis and obstructive sleep apnea (OSA) in both adults[1-6] and children.[7-10] This is further elucidated in case series. A questionnaire study of children in Istanbul showed an increased prevalence of nocturnal enuresis in habitual snorers compared with occasional snorers and nonsnorers.[11] Cinar and colleagues[12] noted that 35% of children operated on for upper airway obstruction reported nocturnal enuresis, and two thirds of those who responded reported complete or partial relief of enuresis 3 months after surgery. Weider and coworkers[13] described a series of 115 children with upper airway obstruction and enuresis. Six months after "some type of surgery to eliminate upper airway obstruction," the group reported a 77% reduction in the number of enuretic nights. However, neither of these reports included a control group and very few of the patients had polysomnography to define and quantify their obstructive sleep apnea. A large population study of home polysomnograms in Hispanic and Caucasian children aged 6 to 11 years found a prevalence of enuresis of 11.3% in children with a respiratory disturbance index (RDI; apneas plus hypopneas per hour of sleep) of greater than 1 compared with a prevalence of 6.3% in children with an RDI of less than 1 ($P < .08$). Enuresis was strongly associated with loud snoring ($P < .007$), a known correlate of sleep-disordered breathing (SDB) in children.[14]

We described 160 pediatric patients (90 boys and 70 girls) who were referred to our sleep center with signs and symptoms suggestive of OSA[15] (Table 20–1). The mean age of the children was 9.6 ± 3.58 years (range, 4.2 to 17.9). There was no relationship between RDI and age ($r_S = -.15$, $P > .20$). A total of 66 children (41%) currently described enuresis, a percentage similar to that found in the data of Cinar et al.[12] Forty-nine per-

cent of the boys were enuretic compared with 31% of the girls ($P < .05$). There was no difference in RDI between the boys and girls ($P = .91$). The mean body mass index (BMI; kg/m^2) was 22.6 ± 8.71 (range, 12.9 to 64.2). There was no relationship between BMI and RDI ($r_S = .09$, $P > .5$) or the presence of enuresis ($X^2 = 3.08$, $P = 0.55$).

Enuresis was more prevalent in the younger children, but at all ages enuresis was more prevalent than in literature controls.[16,17] Of the children who wet the bed, 64% had primary enuresis and 36% had secondary enuresis. Children with an RDI of less than 1 had a significantly lower prevalence of nocturnal enuresis (27%) than did children with an RDI of greater than 1 (47%) ($X^2 = 4.13$, $P < .05$). Of children with an RDI of less than 1, 14% had enuresis frequently, compared with 32% of children with an RDI of greater than 1 ($X^2 = 4.52$, $P < .05$). There was no significant difference in the prevalence of enuresis between children with an RDI between 1 and 5, those with an RDI between 5 and 15, and those with an RDI greater than 15 ($X^2 = .18$, $P = .92$) (Figure 20–1).

These data demonstrate a high prevalence of nocturnal enuresis in children with suspected SDB. Children with more than one respiratory event per hour of sleep (RDI > 1) were at significantly greater risk of enuresis than were children with an RDI of less than 1. In other studies, more than one obstructive apnea per hour of sleep has been suggested to indicate OSA in children.[18]

The predisposition of boys to nocturnal enuresis, and the 3-to-1 ratio of primary to secondary enuresis are similar to descriptions of otherwise-normal children.[19] Wang and colleagues found nocturnal enuresis in 24 of 82 children (29%) referred for suspected OSA.[20] Eleven of those 24 had OSA confirmed with polysomnography, but no data were reported on the severity of the OSA. Brouillette and coworkers

Table 20–1. Patient Demographics

	Boys	Girls
N	90	70
With enuresis (%)	49	31*
Age (yr)	9.7 ± 3.6[†]	9.4 ± 3.6
BMI (kg/m^2)	22.2 ± 7.9	24.0 ± 9.8
RDI	11.3 ± 18.8	8.3 ± 13.4

*$P < .05$
†Mean ± SD
BMI, body mass index; RDI, respiratory disturbance
    index.

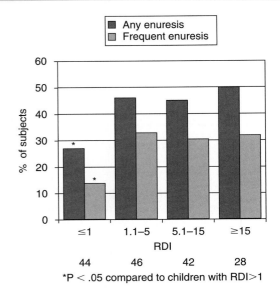

Figure 20–1. Prevalence of nocturnal enuresis in 160 children referred for suspected sleep-disordered breathing. Frequent enuresis was defined as wetting the bed 3 nights a week or more. (From Brooks LJ, Topol HI: Enuresis in children with sleep apnea. J Pediatr 2003; 142:515-518.)

found nocturnal enuresis in 8% of children with OSA compared to 4% of controls.[21] However, this was not a statistically significant difference, probably because of the small number of patients.

Finally, treatment of OSA with continuous positive airway pressure, dental devices, or adenotonsillectomy has been reported to ameliorate enuresis in adults[2-6] and children.[7-10,13,22]

Why might children with SDB be at risk for nocturnal enuresis? Proposed etiologies for nocturnal enuresis include insufficient arousal response, impaired urodynamics, and insufficient vasopressin production during sleep.

Children who wet the bed are reported by their parents to be more difficult to arouse from sleep than children without enuresis.[23] Weider and colleagues reported that "a number of patients [with upper airway obstruction] who could not be aroused before surgery were able to wake up and go to the bathroom by themselves after surgery."[13] SDB may therefore promote enuresis by decreasing the arousal response,[24] perhaps because of sleep fragmentation.[24-26]

Daytime urodynamics are similar in children with and those without enuresis.[27] However, the increased intra-abdominal pressure caused by respiratory efforts against an obstructed airway can be transmitted to the bladder. Cystometrography has demonstrated that bladder pressure during sleep may rise as high as 60 cm H_2O in conjunction with respiratory efforts against an obstructed upper airway, in contrast to pressures of about 5 cm H_2O during quiet wakefulness.[1] Thus, OSA may promote enuresis by increasing bladder pressure.

Finally, SDB can affect the secretion of urinary hormones such as atrial natriuretic peptide

(ANP) and antidiuretic hormone (ADH). Adults with OSA have elevated ANP and decreased ADH,[28-30] and the normal nocturnal decrease in urine output does not occur.[29-31] In patients with OSA, plasma ANP correlates negatively with cumulative apnea duration and lowest arterial oxygen saturation, and positively with the highest change in intrathoracic pressure.[28] This may result from the more negative intrathoracic pressures increasing atrial volume, thus stimulating ANP production. Acute hypoxemia may result from central or obstructive respiratory events, and it may stimulate ANP secretion.[32] Urine output, sodium excretion, and secretion of ANP all decrease, whereas renin and aldosterone increase, with successful treatment of OSA.[28,30,31,33,34]

Many of these studies describe patients referred for suspected SDB, and it is possible that nocturnal enuresis was a factor in the primary physician's decision to refer, thus inflating the reported prevalence of enuresis. Despite this, the evidence suggests that the association between nocturnal enuresis and OSA is real, with a reasonable physiologic basis.

Obstructive sleep apnea, which can usually be easily treated, should be considered in the differential diagnosis of nocturnal enuresis in children.

References

1. Yokoyama O, Amano T, Lee S, et al: Enuresis in an adult female with obstructive sleep apnea. Urology 1995;45:150-154.
2. Arai H, Furuta H, Kosaka K, et al: Polysomnographic and urodynamic changes in a case of obstructive sleep apnea with enuresis. Psychiatry Clin Neurosci 1999;55:319-320.
3. Everaert K, Pevernagie D, Oosterlinck W: Nocturnal enuresis provoked by an obstructive sleep apnea syndrome. J Urol 1995;153:1236.
4. Ulfberg J, Thuman R: A non-urologic cause of nocturia and enuresis: Obstructive sleep apnea syndrome. Scand J Urol Nephrol 1996; 30:135-137.
5. Steers WD, Suratt P: Sleep apnoea as a cause of daytime and nocturnal enuresis. Lancet 1997; 349:1604.
6. Kramer NR, Bonitati AE, Millman RF: Enuresis and obstructive sleep apnea in adults. Chest 1998; 114:634-637.
7. Wengraf C: Management of enuresis (letter). Lancet 1997;350:221-222.
8. Simmons FB, Guilleminault C, Dement WC, et al: Surgical management of airway obstructions during sleep. Laryngoscope 1977;87:326-338.
9. Timms DJ: Rapid maxillary expansion in the treatment of nocturnal enuresis. Angle Orthod 1990;60:229-233.
10. Sakai J, Herbert F: Secondary enuresis associated with obstructive sleep apnea (letter). J Am Acad Child Adolesc Psychiatry 2000;39:140-141.
11. Ersu R, Arman AR, Save D, et al: Prevalence of snoring and symptoms of sleep-disordered breathing in primary school children in Istanbul. Chest 2004;126:19-24.
12. Cinar U, Vural C, Cakir B, et al: Nocturnal enuresis and upper airway obstruction. Int J Pediatr Otorhinolaryngol 2001;59:115-118.
13. Weider DJ, Sateia MJ, West RP: Nocturnal enuresis in children with upper airway obstruction. Otolaryngol Head Neck Surg 1991;105:427-432.
14. Goodwin JL, Kaemingk KL, Fregosi RF, et al: Parasomnias and sleep disordered breathing in Caucasian and Hispanic children: The Tucson children's assessment of sleep apnea study. BMC Med 2004;2:14.
15. Brooks LJ, Topol HI: Enuresis in children with sleep apnea. J Pediatr 2003;142:515-518.
16. Oppel WC, Harper PA, Rider RV: The age of attaining bladder control. Pediatrics 1968;42:614-626.
17. Sheldon SH, Spire JP, Levy HB: Sleep-related enuresis. In Sheldon SH, Spire JP, Levy HB (eds): Pediatric Sleep Medicine. Philadelphia, WB Saunders, 1992, pp 151-166.
18. Marcus CL, Omlin KJ, Basinki DJ, et al: Normal polysomnographic values for children and adolescents. Am Rev Respir Dis 1992;146:1235-1239.
19. Rushton HG: Wetting and functional voiding disorders. Urol Clin North Am 1995;22:75-93.
20. Wang RC, Elkins TP, Keech D, et al: Accuracy of clinical evaluation in pediatric obstructive sleep apnea. Otolaryngol Head Neck Surg 1998; 118:69-73.
21. Brouillette R, Hanson D, David R, et al: A diagnostic approach to suspected obstructive sleep apnea in children. J Pediatr 1984;105:10-14.
22. Wang RC, Vordemark J: Effects of sleep apnea treatment upon enuresis in children. Surg Forum 1994;45:643-644.
23. Neveus T, Hetta J, Cnattingius S, et al: Depth of sleep and sleep habits among enuretic and incontinent children. Acta Paediatr 1999;88:748-752.
24. Berry RB, Kouchi KG, Der DE, et al: Sleep apnea impairs the arousal response to airway occlusion. Chest 1996;109:1490-1496.
25. Phillipson EA, Bowes G, Sullivan CE, Woolf, GM: The influence of sleep fragmentation on arousal and ventilatory responses to respiratory stimuli. Sleep 1980;3:281-288.
26. Downey B, Bonnet MH: Performance during frequent sleep disruption. Sleep 1987;10:354-363.
27. Norgaard JP, Rittig S, Djurhuus JC: Nocturnal enuresis: An approach to treatment based on pathogenesis. J Pediatr 1989;114:705-710.
28. Krieger J, Follenius M, Sforza E, et al: Effects of treatment with nasal continuous positive airway pressure on atrial natriuretic peptide and arginine vasopressin release during sleep in patients with obstructive sleep apnea. Clin Sci 1991;80:443-449.
29. Ichioka M, Hirata Y, Inase N, et al: Changes of circulating atrial natriuretic peptide and antidiuretic hormone in obstructive sleep apnea syndrome. Respiration 1992;59:164-168.
30. Lin C, Tsan K, Lin C: Plasma levels of atrial natriuretic factor in moderate to severe obstructive sleep apnea syndrome. Sleep 1993;16:37-39.
31. Rodenstein DO, D'Odemont JP, Pieters T, Aubert-Tulkens G: Diurnal and nocturnal diuresis and natriuresis in obstructive sleep apnea. Am Rev Respir Dis 1992;145:1367-1371.
32. Baertschi AJ, Adams JM, Sullivan MP: Acute hypoxemia stimulates atrial natriuretic factor secretion in vivo. Am J Physiol 1988;255:H295-H300.
33. Baruzzi A, Riva R, Cirignotta F, et al: Atrial natriuretic peptide and catecholamines in obstructive sleep apnea syndrome. Sleep 1991;14:83-86.
34. Follenius M, Krieger J, Krauth MO, et al: Obstructive sleep apnea treatment: Peripheral and central effects on plasma renin activity and aldosterone. Sleep 1991:14:211-217.

Treatment of Obstructive Sleep Apnea Syndrome in Children

21

Carole L. Marcus

Childhood obstructive sleep apnea syndrome (OSAS) is a common condition that can result in severe complications if not diagnosed and treated in a timely fashion. Nevertheless, most patients respond readily to treatment. The mainstay of treatment is tonsillectomy and adenoidectomy (T&A). Nasal continuous positive airway pressure (CPAP) is usually the second-line treatment for children who do not respond to T&A, or for those few children for whom T&A is not indicated. In selected cases, other treatment options may be useful.

WHEN TO TREAT

One of the biggest dilemmas in pediatric sleep medicine is the question of who warrants treatment. Very few outcome studies have been conducted in children. Some normative pediatric data are available.[1-4] However, these data tell us only what is statistically abnormal. We do not yet know which clinical or polysomnographic parameters predict a poor outcome—that is, which parameters are clinically important. It is generally accepted that children with severe OSAS should always be treated, as these children are at risk for serious complications such as cor pulmonale and failure to thrive. Many practitioners agree that children with primary snoring should not be subjected to surgery, although this group has not been rigorously studied. However, treatment of the child with mild abnormalities on polysomnography is controversial. In such cases, as with most medical conditions, treatment decisions should be based on the constellation of symptoms, physical examination, and laboratory results (polysomnography), rather than on polysomnography results alone. If the decision is made not to treat the child, then follow-up is important.

EMERGENCY TREATMENT

Most patients with diagnosed OSAS can await elective treatment. On a practical level, these children have often waited weeks or months before seeing a physician or undergoing a sleep study, and the decision is therefore made that they can wait for surgery. Although these patients do not seem to have acute problems, it should be realized that the short-term effects of untreated hypoxemia or obstructive apnea are unknown.

Occasionally, emergency treatment is warranted in children presenting with cardiorespiratory failure or severe hypoxemia. Many children can be successfully managed with nasopharyngeal tubes, pending definitive surgery,[5] or with CPAP.[6] Intubation is rarely needed. Sedation should be avoided, and supplemental oxygen should never be administered without careful monitoring for hypoventilation (see later).

TREATMENT MODALITIES

Tonsillectomy and Adenoidectomy

T&A is the first-line treatment for childhood OSAS. It is a relatively simple procedure with a low complication rate, and it usually results in a cure. Therefore, it is preferable to long-term use of CPAP, where compliance is often a problem. Nevertheless, T&A should not be undertaken lightly. As with any surgery, there is associated morbidity and even mortality. For these reasons, it is recommended that surgery be performed only after polysomnographic proof of OSAS has been obtained.[7,8]

Efficacy of T&A

OSAS results from the relative size and structure of the upper airway components, and the relationship between structural narrowing and neuromotor tone of the upper airway, rather than from the absolute size of the tonsils and adenoid. Thus, even in children with relatively small tonsils, or with additional risk factors for OSAS such as craniofacial syndromes, T&A is often successful in treating OSAS. This has been demonstrated in children with morbid obesity,[9,10] Down syndrome,[11] and cerebral palsy.[12] However, these patients should be reevaluated postoperatively to ensure that the OSAS has resolved and that further treatment is not necessary.

Several studies have evaluated the success rate for T&A in children with OSAS secondary to adenotonsillar hypertrophy. These studies are hard to compare directly, as they utilized different patient populations, recording techniques, definitions of respiratory events, time periods for postoperative evaluations, and types of surgery (e.g., some of the studies included patients who underwent adenoidectomy with monotonsillectomy). Nevertheless, the different studies all show that the overwhelming majority of patients have an improvement in both symptoms and polysomnographic findings postoperatively.[10,13-21] The most complete data are given by Suen and colleagues.[19] They studied 26 children with OSAS but without neurologic or craniofacial anomalies. Patients underwent follow-up polysomnography 6 to 50 weeks after T&A (personal communication from the authors), and showed a decrease in respiratory distress index (RDI) from 16 ± 10/hr to 2 ± 1/hr. Four patients continued to have an RDI of greater than 5 postoperatively, with one still having an RDI of 45 per hour. The preoperative RDI was a predictor of the response to surgery. Frank and coworkers[18] evaluated seven children 4 to 6 weeks after T&A and found that the average total number of apneas fell from 194 to 7. Bar and colleagues[22] studied 10 normal children an average of 3 months after T&A and found a decrease in the RDI from 8 ± 9 to 1 ± 2. Zucconi and coworkers[21] evaluated 14 patients with nap or overnight polysomnography 3 to 18 months postoperatively (surgery being adenoidectomy, adenoidectomy with monotonsillectomy, or T&A) and showed a decrease in the apnea-hypopnea index from 11 ± 10 to 3 ± 2/hr. Agren and colleagues[16] reported normalization of the oxygen desaturation index 1 year postoperatively.

Studies have shown that growth improves after T&A, even in children who were in the normal range beforehand.[20,22-25] In fact, even obese children gain weight postoperatively.[26] Enuresis has been reported to improve after surgery.[27] Studies of behavioral and cognitive function have, in general, shown an improvement after T&A. Ali and coworkers[28] found an improvement in the Conners Behaviour Scale, Matching Familiar Figures Test, and a continuous performance test postoperatively; children with snoring showed a lesser response after T&A, and controls (studied after a 6-month time period) did not change. Goldstein and colleagues[29] showed an improvement measured on the Child Behavior Checklist (controls were not evaluated). Gozal showed an improvement in academic scores after T&A in children with sleep-disordered breathing but no change in either normal controls or untreated children with sleep-disordered breathing.[30] In contrast to these studies, a study of behavioral symptoms after treatment, compared with an untreated control group, showed an improvement in daytime symptoms but no significant change in temperament or intelligence after surgery.[31]

Tonsillectomy or Adenoidectomy, or Both?

Many sleep specialists believe that both the tonsils and the adenoid should be removed, even if one or the other appears to be the more enlarged. This results from the belief that OSAS is caused by both structural and neuromotor abnormalities, and that therefore widening the airway as much as possible is desirable. There is also anecdotal evidence of a high persistence or recurrence rate in children treated with adenoidectomy or tonsillectomy alone. However, there are no randomized, controlled trials evaluating the different types of surgery. Nieminen and coworkers[17] noted that 73% of children with OSAS had a history of prior adenoidectomy; all improved after tonsillectomy. This suggests either that adenoidectomy alone was insufficient or that the adenoids grew back. Zucconi and colleagues[21] reported that three children who underwent adenoidectomy alone had only a transient improvement in OSAS, whereas 16 children who underwent T&A or adenoidectomy with monotonsillectomy did better. However, further details were not provided. In children with a submucous cleft palate, adenoidectomy may result in velopharyngeal incompetence; in this group, tonsillectomy alone is a consideration.

Adenoidal recurrence may occur, especially in very young children. One study evaluated adenoidal regrowth in a sample of children who had symptoms of nasal obstruction 2 to 5 years after adenoidectomy.[32] One patient had already undergone revision adenoidectomy. In the remaining patients, the authors reported lymphoid regrowth occupying 0% to 40% of the nasopharynx. Thus, if children develop a recurrence of OSAS after T&A, they should be evaluated to determine whether the adenoids have regrown and revision adenoidectomy is required.

Morbidity and Mortality

Acute general complications of T&A include hemorrhage (in approximately 3% of cases),[33] respiratory decompensation, anesthetic complications, pain, and poor oral intake. Death has been reported.[34] Preoperative sedation may precipitate acute upper airway obstruction.[35] Postoperative respiratory decompensation may result from transient worsening of OSAS secondary to postoperative edema and increased secretions; respiratory depression from anesthetic agents, narcotics, and the use of oxygen in children with a blunted hypoxic ventilatory drive; and the occurrence of postobstructive pulmonary edema.[36,37] The latter is a poorly understood phenomenon occurring with the relief of upper airway obstruction from any cause (such as croup, epiglottitis, or OSAS). Long-term complications of T&A, such as nasopharyngeal stenosis and velopharyngeal incompetence, occasionally occur.

A number of studies have evaluated the prevalence of postoperative respiratory complications. In patients with polysomnographically proven OSAS, prevalence rates of 16% to 27% have been reported.[6,38,39] Prevalence rates in those studies in which polysomnography was not performed are lower.[40,41] These studies probably included children with primary snoring as well as OSAS. Studies of postoperative complications have been remarkably consistent in their findings about which patients are at greatest risk for postoperative respiratory compromise. High-risk groups include children less than 3 years of age, children with underlying disease (craniofacial anomalies, obesity, cerebral palsy, or a history of prematurity), those with severe OSAS, and those with failure to thrive or cor pulmonale (both of which are associated with severe OSAS).[6,38,39,42-44] High-risk patients can nevertheless be treated safely if appropriate precautions are taken.[45] Recommendations include performing surgery in tertiary care centers where pediatric specialists and a pediatric intensive care unit are available, avoiding preoperative sedation, ensuring intravenous access prior to inducing anesthesia, and monitoring patients closely postoperatively, so that appropriate airway intervention can be performed as needed. Currently in the United States, T&A is usually performed as outpatient surgery. The American Academy of Pediatrics Clinical Practice Guideline[7] recommends that high-risk patients (Table 21–1) be hospitalized overnight after surgery and monitored continuously with pulse oximetry. CPAP can be used in the perioperative

---

Table 21–1.   Risk Factors for Postoperative Respiratory Complications in Children with OSAS Undergoing Adenotonsillectomy

Age younger than 3 years
Severe obstructive sleep apnea syndrome (OSAS) on polysomnography
Cardiac complications of OSAS (e.g., right ventricular hypertrophy)
Failure to thrive
Obesity
Prematurity
Recent respiratory infection
Craniofacial anomalies
Neuromuscular disorders

Reproduced with permission from American Academy of Pediatrics, Section on Pediatric Pulmonology, Subcommittee on Obstructive Sleep Apnea: Clinical practice guideline: Diagnosis and management of childhood obstructive sleep apnea syndrome. Pediatrics 2002;109:704-712.

period to stabilize patients prior to T&A and to treat postoperative complications.[6,46] It may reduce the need for postoperative intubation.

Follow-Up

All children should be reevaluated clinically after surgery. Those with severe OSAS preoperatively, continued risk factors for OSAS, or persistent symptoms should be considered for repeat polysomnography. Traditionally, it is stated that OSAS improves 6 to 8 weeks after T&A. However, this has not been studied systematically. Significant improvement may occur much earlier. Helfaer and colleagues performed repeat polysomnography the night after surgery on a group of children with OSAS.[47] This study was limited to children with mild to moderate disease and no underlying medical conditions. Postoperatively, patients showed an immediate reduction in the apnea-hypopnea index (from 5 ± 1 to 2 ± 1) and an improvement in arterial oxygen saturation during rapid eye movement sleep (from 78 ± 5% to 92 ± 1%).

Continuous Positive Airway Pressure

The vast majority of children with OSAS will be cured by T&A. However, a small number of patients will require further treatment. Typically, these patients have underlying medical conditions, such as obesity, craniofacial anomalies, or neuromuscular disease. However, occasional patients have idiopathic OSAS that persists after T&A despite the absence of any obvious risk factors.[48] In addition, some patients are not candidates for T&A, such as adolescents with minimal adenotonsillar tissue, or patients with severe bleeding disorders. In these patients, nasal CPAP can be a highly effective means of treatment.

Method of Action

During CPAP use, positive pressure is generated by a blower attached to a mask. For bilevel pressure, the inspiratory (IPAP) and expiratory (EPAP) pressures can be adjusted independently, so that the expiratory pressure is lower than the inspiratory pressure. Unlike conventional ventilators, the respiratory circuit has a single limb for both inspiration and expiration. A fixed leak near

the patient's mask prevents CO_2 rebreathing. CPAP increases the intraluminal upper airway pressure and elevates it above the upper airway critical closing pressure,[49] thereby stenting the airway open. It reduces upper airway[50] and diaphragmatic[51] inspiratory muscle activity. Because the upper airway is rich in sensory nerve endings, increased nasal airflow from CPAP can stimulate ventilation.[52] The use of nasal CPAP in adults with OSAS has been shown to result in improved cognitive and psychiatric function, decreased daytime somnolence, decreased waking hypercapnia, improved cardiovascular function, and possibly decreased mortality.[53]

Efficacy of CPAP in Children

In the United States, CPAP use is not approved for children weighing less than 30 kg. Nevertheless, there is widespread experience in the use of CPAP in children of all ages, including infants,[54,55] showing that it is safe and effective. Several large series have been published. One study reported CPAP use in 80 patients at the same institution,[46] and a multicenter study reported on CPAP use in 94 patients.[48] Both studies showed that CPAP was effective and tolerated in more than 80% of patients with OSAS, including children with craniofacial anomalies, obesity, or neurologic disorders. The required pressure varied from 4 to 20 cm H_2O, and this range was independent of age and underlying diagnosis. Presumably, the pressure level was proportional to the severity of OSAS, although different protocols at the varying institutions did not allow this to be evaluated systematically. Excluding patients in whom CPAP was only used perioperatively, or in whom additional treatment modalities were used, only 4% to 16% of patients improved sufficiently to discontinue CPAP over the several years of follow-up.[46,48] Long-term studies are needed.

Nasal CPAP has long been known to be effective in treating central apnea in infants; recent studies show that it is also effective in treating obstructive apnea in this age group.[54-56] Infants are more likely to be weaned off CPAP than older children.[54,55] Unfortunately, nasal masks are not commercially available in the United States for this age group, although an infant mask (ResMed, Sydney, Australia) is available in other countries.

Institution of CPAP Therapy

Although CPAP is effective in children, it requires time and patience on the part of both the family and the medical practitioner to get it to work. Several centers[46,57] begin CPAP at home on low pressures, to enable the child to gradually habituate to the system prior to bringing patients into the lab for a formal titration. It is important to make the CPAP use part of a child's bedtime routine. The alternative, placing the mask on a young child's face while the child is asleep, can result in frightened arousals during the night and leads to poor tolerance. Behavioral conditioning may be useful.[58,59] In children, pressure requirements change over time.[48,54] Therefore, it is necessary to frequently reevaluate pressure levels in response to growth. In addition, it is important to pay attention to mask and headgear fit as time passes.

Patients with OSAS whose CPAP was discontinued for 1 night may have a temporary improvement in breathing compared to their baseline, pre-CPAP treatment state. Polysomnography on the first night off CPAP demonstrates fewer and shorter obstructive apneas, decreased esophageal pressure swings, and less arterial oxygen desaturation.[60-62] This may result from a number of factors, including decreased sleep fragmentation, decreased upper airway edema, and resetting of the ventilatory drive. Because of this transient improvement, CPAP should be discontinued for at least several days prior to polysomnography in patients being evaluated for discontinuation of therapy.

Compliance

The major problem with CPAP use is poor compliance. A number of studies in adults have shown that approximately 15% to 20% of patients drop out immediately.[63,64] The remaining patients use CPAP for an average of 5 hours a night.[63-65] Comparable studies have not been performed in children, although a preliminary report suggests that their compliance may be similar.[66] It is recommended that compliance be assessed objectively by regular readings of the equipment hour meter. Compliance can be improved by increasing the comfort of the equipment and paying close attention to side effects. A ramp function that allows the machine to gradually increase pressure as the patient falls asleep may increase comfort. Bilevel pressure may be more comfortable than CPAP, although this requires further study in children. Only one study (in adults) has directly compared CPAP to bilevel ventilation for OSAS.[63] This study did not demonstrate a significant difference in effective use between the two methods. However, the CPAP group had a significantly larger dropout rate than the bilevel group. Furthermore, compliance in the bilevel group was affected by the difference between inspiratory and expiratory pressures, suggesting that different ventilation protocols may affect compliance. In practice, bilevel ventilation is often used for patients who find CPAP uncomfortable.

Side Effects

The most common side effects of CPAP use are nasal symptoms, including nasal congestion, rhinorrhea, dryness, and epistaxis (Table 21–2). These are caused by the cooling and drying effects of CPAP, which alters the nasal mucosa and impedes mucociliary clearance.[67] In one study, more than two thirds of adults using CPAP complained of nasal symptoms.[68] The most effective treatment is use of a heated humidifier; cool humidification is little better than placebo.[69] Attention to hygiene (cleaning the equipment and changing filters regularly) is important. Nasal steroids or saline drops may be efficacious in some patients. Other side effects include dry or irritated eyes resulting from mask leak. Dermatitis and pressure lesions from the mask may occur. This can be severe and can lead to decubitus ulcers, particularly in patients who are unable to adjust the mask themselves (e.g., those with cerebral palsy). Pressure lesions can be minimized by ensuring good mask fit, avoiding overtightening of the mask straps, using gel masks, placing spacers on the forehead rather than on the bridge of the nose, using skin hydrocolloid dressings, or alternating different types of masks. Gastric distension occurs occasionally but is usually self-limiting. More severe side effects, such as pneumothorax[70] or barotrauma affecting the eyes,[71] ears, and central nervous system,[72] have been reported very rarely.

Some considerations are specific to the use of CPAP in children. Central apneas can occur at

Table 21–2.   Treatment of Side Effects of Continuous Positive Airway Pressure (CPAP)

Side Effect	Treatment
Nasal symptoms (dryness, congestion, rhinorrhea, epistaxis)	Heated humidification Nasal steroids Saline nose drops
Skin ulceration	Correct mask fit. Avoid overtightening of head gear. Protect bridge of nose with hydrocolloid dressings. Gel masks Spacer on forehead instead of bridge of nose Alternate different interfaces (e.g., nasal cannula, nasal mask).
Eye irritation	Correct mask fit.
Inability to fall asleep while wearing CPAP	Pressure ramp
Central apnea	Bilevel ventilation with backup rate
Hypercapnia (rarely seen in children)	Nonrebreathing valve
Failure to trigger bilevel ventilation	Use ventilator with low triggering threshold or adjustable sensitivity levels. If suboptimal ventilation, consider increasing expiratory positive airway pressure and adding O_2.
Midfacial depression	Custom mask

higher pressure levels[46] because of an active Hering-Breuer reflex. This can be remedied by placing the patient on bilevel ventilation with a backup rate. Children may have problems triggering bilevel machines, as the triggering algorithms used are not suitable for the lower flow rate and faster respiratory rate seen in young or weak children. This must be taken into account when adjusting settings. Certain brands of equipment trigger better in young children than others. Mouth breathing during CPAP use is not a problem unless it interferes with ventilation, in which case a chin strap or full face mask can be used. However, there may be a risk of aspiration with the use of a full face mask, particularly in very young or developmentally impaired children. Occasionally, nasal damage (with nasal prongs)[73] or midfacial depression (with nasal masks)[74] occur in children who begin using CPAP at a young age.

Uvulopalatopharyngoplasty

Uvulopalatopharyngoplasty (UVPP) is a surgical procedure involving excision of the uvula and the posterior portion of the palate and tonsils, and trimming and reorientation of the tonsillar pillars. In adults, it has a success rate of approximately 50%.[75] The procedure is not commonly performed in children and has not been system-atically evaluated except in specific subpopulations. It is useful in patients in whom abnormal upper airway neuromuscular tone contributes to OSAS (e.g., patients with cerebral palsy and Down syndrome).[76-78]

Craniofacial and Other Surgeries

In complex patients with OSAS, particularly those with craniofacial anomalies, craniofacial surgery may be effective. This is especially indicated in patients who do not tolerate CPAP or who would also benefit from the cosmetic effect of surgery. Few large-scale studies have been published; most of them were by one group of surgeons.[79-82] This group has reported good success in treating patients with craniofacial anomalies, Down syndrome, or cerebral palsy using complex craniofacial surgery. They use an individualized surgical approach based on the site of obstruction. Patients are evaluated by physical examination, radiologic studies, and endoscopy. Those with abnormalities in the region of the nares to the velum are treated with combinations of adenoidectomy, septoplasty, and inferior turbinectomy. Those with obstruction in the region extending from the lips to the hypopharynx are treated with procedures such as tonsillectomy, UVPP, tongue reduction, mandibular osteotomy, and tongue–hyoid suspension. These procedures are best performed in experienced, multidisciplinary centers, as they are fraught with potential complications. Surgery may require prolonged intubation or temporary tracheostomy.

Select craniofacial procedures may be appropriate for patients with isolated anomalies. Mandibular distraction procedures can be performed in children with micrognathia, including infants with Pierre Robin syndrome or hemifacial microsomia[81] (Fig. 21–1). In this procedure, the mandible is divided and an external distraction device applied. Distraction is gradually applied via the device, typically by 1 mm/day. However, long-term complications, such as asymmetrical jaw growth, may occur. Midfacial advancement can improve both upper airway function and cosmetic appearance in children with craniofacial anomalies such as Crouzon syndrome. Tongue reduction has been used to treat patients with Down syndrome or other causes of macroglossia.[77,83] However, the effects of this surgery on swallowing and speech have not been formally investigated. Epiglottoplasty is useful in treating selected children with upper airway obstruction secondary to laryngomalacia,[84] although the overwhelming majority of children with laryngomalacia do not require treatment, as they improve with age.

Weight Loss

Weight loss is recommended for all obese patients. However, this is notoriously difficult to achieve. Even if weight loss does occur, it happens slowly. Therefore, interim treatment is required. T&A is often effective even in morbidly obese children,[9,85] and it is usually the first-line treatment unless there is minimal adenotonsillar tissue. CPAP can be used pending surgery. Patients with significant obesity should undergo postoperative polysomnography to determine whether further treatment, such as CPAP, is necessary.

Most of the data regarding weight loss and OSAS are from studies of adults. Major weight loss in adults, such as that seen with bariatric surgery, has been reported to result in resolution of apnea. Moderate weight loss (10% to 20% of body weight) is associated with a more modest improvement in OSAS.[86] One study evaluated the effects of bariatric surgery on OSAS in children.[87] Eleven children underwent surgery, with

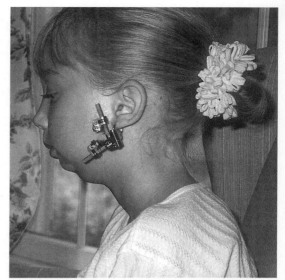
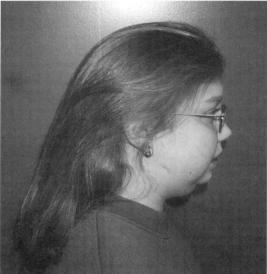

Figure 21–1. **Top,** An 8-year-old girl with obstructive sleep apnea syndrome secondary to micrognathia is shown immediately after a mandibular distraction procedure with the placement of external fixators. **Bottom,** The patient is shown several years after the procedure.

a resultant weight loss of 45% of body weight. Two children underwent simultaneous UVPP, and one child required a tracheostomy because of prolonged postoperative intubation. Nine patients received polysomnographic evaluation postoperatively and showed an improvement (from 73% to 93%) in mean arterial oxygen saturation. Additional details were not provided. Further study of bariatric surgery in morbidly obese children with severe apnea, who have failed other treatments, is warranted. Of concern, however, are several articles describing long-term recurrence of OSAS in obese patients who had lost weight, even though the weight loss had been maintained.[88,89] This may have resulted partly from the fact that the patients never attained a normal weight, even though they weighed less than they had originally.

Oral Appliances and Orthodontic Treatment

Oral appliances are recommended for adult patients with mild OSAS or those who are intolerant of CPAP,[90] but few studies have evaluated oral appliances in children. In one study,[91] children with mild to moderate OSAS and dysgnathia were fitted with an appliance. Twenty-six percent discontinued therapy. In the remainder, the apnea-hypopnea index decreased significantly but did not normalize. A second study showed a modest improvement in a group of children with mild obstructive apnea (apnea-hypopnea index decreased from 8 to 4 per hour).[92] Further study on oral and orthodontic appliances in children is warranted. At present, these devices should be used only by specialists with expertise in pediatric orthodontics, as they have the potential to alter the shape of the craniofacial skeleton in growing children. Conceivably, however, the early use of oral appliances could improve craniofacial characteristics that put children at risk for OSAS.

Rapid maxillary expansion using orthodontic appliances has been used successfully in one study of adults with obstructive apnea and maxillary constriction,[93] and in one study of children with obstructive apnea and maxillary constriction.[94] In the latter study, children with adenotonsillar hypertrophy were excluded (the criteria for diagnosing adenotonsillar hypertrophy were not stated). Thus, this appears to be a promising technique for a select population group.

Supplemental Oxygen

Two studies have evaluated the effect of supplemental oxygen on children with OSAS.[95,96] In both studies, supplemental oxygen resulted in improved arterial oxygen saturation, as expected. There were no clinically important differences in the number or duration of obstructive apneas when subjects breathed supplemental oxygen.[95,96] PCO_2 levels did not change for the group

as a whole. However, a few individuals showed a marked increase in PCO_2 when breathing supplemental oxygen; this could not be predicted by age, weight, or severity of OSAS (Fig. 21–2). Supplemental oxygen use will not alleviate the increased work of breathing or sleep fragmentation associated with OSAS, and this is therefore not an appropriate first-line treatment. However, these studies suggest that it may be useful as a temporizing measure, or when other treatments fail, in a few select individuals (e.g., in an infant with mild OSAS resulting from craniofacial anomalies, who is expected to improve with growth). Supplemental oxygen should never be administered to patients with OSAS without first measuring their change in PCO_2 in response to the oxygen.

Drugs

In general, pharmacologic agents are not useful in the management of OSAS. Systemic glucocorticosteroids have been used to shrink adenoidal tissue. However, only one study has evaluated this treatment. In an open-label, uncontrolled study, a 5-day course of prednisone did not

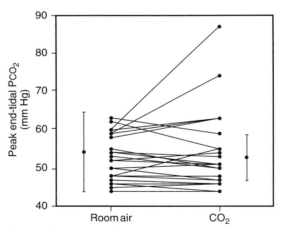

Figure 21–2. The peak end-tidal PCO_2 is shown for individual patients with obstructive sleep apnea syndrome while breathing room air compared with supplemental oxygen during sleep. Group means and standard deviations are shown in the side bars. Although there was no difference in the mean PCO_2 between the two conditions, several individuals had an increase in PCO_2 while breathing supplemental oxygen. (Adapted from Marcus CL, Carroll JL, Bamford O, et al: Supplemental oxygen during sleep in children with sleep-disordered breathing. Am J Respir Crit Care Med 1995;152(Pt 1):1297-1301.)

significantly improve OSAS.[97] Topical nasal steroids have been shown to have a modest effect in children with OSAS.[98] Following a 6-week course of treatment, patients had a modest improvement in apnea index from 11 ± 9 to 6 ± 8/hr. However, the individual response to treatment was varied, with a wide standard deviation, and many subjects went on to have T&A. The effect of withdrawing topical steroid treatment is not known. Thus, a trial of nasal steroids may be warranted in some patients with mild OSAS, but follow-up is essential. Further study is needed.

Environmental Conditions

There is a high prevalence of allergy in children with OSAS.[99] Theoretically, avoiding allergens may improve OSAS. Although passive smoking is associated with snoring,[100] one study failed to show a relationship between maternal smoking and OSAS.[101] Nevertheless, it seems prudent to minimize exposure to cigarette smoke.

Tracheostomy

Tracheostomy is the ultimate treatment for OSAS, as it bypasses the site of obstruction. However, it is associated with many complications, including speech problems, chronic tracheitis, and interference with the activities of daily life. Fortunately, with the increased use of CPAP and other treatment modalities, tracheostomy is now rarely required. It may be needed in children with upper airway obstruction during both wakefulness and sleep, particularly in children with cerebral palsy or severe craniofacial malformations.

CONCLUSION

A variety of effective treatment modalities are available for children with OSAS. However, many unanswered questions remain. What degree of OSAS warrants treatment? What is the correlation between polysomnographic abnormalities and clinical outcome? What is the long-term outcome of CPAP use in children? Which equipment is best suited for them? What are the success and complication rates of complex surgical procedures such as UVPP and tongue reduction in children? Are successfully treated patients at risk for recurrence of their disease as adults? Further long-term studies are desperately needed.

References

1. Marcus CL, Omlin KJ, Basinki DJ, et al: Normal polysomnographic values for children and adolescents. Am Rev Respir Dis 1992;146(Pt 1):1235-1239.
2. Acebo C, Millman RP, Rosenberg C, et al: Sleep, breathing, and cephalometrics in older children and young adults. Chest 1996;109:664-672.
3. Poets CF, Stebbens VA, Samuels MP, Southall DP: Oxygen saturation and breathing patterns in children. Pediatrics 1993;92:686-690.
4. Hunt CE, Corwin MJ, Lister G, et al: Longitudinal assessment of hemoglobin oxygen saturation in healthy infants during the first 6 months of age. Collaborative Home Infant Monitoring Evaluation (CHIME) Study Group [see comments]. J Pediatr 1999;135:580-586.
5. Kravath RE, Pollak CP, Borowiecki B: Hypoventilation during sleep in children who have lymphoid airway obstruction treated by nasopharyngeal tube and T and A. Pediatrics 1977;59:865-871.
6. Rosen GM, Muckle RP, Mahowald MW, et al: Postoperative respiratory compromise in children with obstructive sleep apnea syndrome: Can it be anticipated? Pediatrics 1994;93:784-788.
7. American Academy of Pediatrics, Section on Pediatric Pulmonology, Subcommittee on Obstructive Sleep Apnea: Clinical practice guideline: Diagnosis and management of childhood obstructive sleep apnea syndrome. Pediatrics 2002;109:704-712.
8. American Thoracic Society: Standards and indications for cardiopulmonary sleep studies in children. Am J Respir Crit Care Med 1996;153:866-878.
9. Kudoh F, Sanai A: Effect of tonsillectomy and adenoidectomy on obese children with sleep-associated breathing disorders. Acta Otolaryngol Suppl 1996;523:216-218.
10. Wiet GJ, Bower C, Seibert R, Griebel M: Surgical correction of obstructive sleep apnea in the complicated pediatric patient documented by polysomnography. Int J Pediatr Otorhinolaryngol 1997;41:133-143.
11. Marcus CL, Keens TG, Bautista DB, et al: Obstructive sleep apnea in children with Down syndrome. Pediatrics 1991;88:132-139.
12. Grundfast K, Berkowitz R, Fox L: Outcome and complications following surgery for obstructive adenotonsillar hypertrophy in children with neuromuscular disorders. Ear Nose Throat J 1990;69:756, 759-760.
13. Schechter MS: Technical report: Diagnosis and management of childhood obstructive sleep apnea syndrome. Pediatrics 2002;109:E69.

14. Shintani T, Asakura K, Kataura A: The effect of adenotonsillectomy in children with OSA. Int J Pediatr Otorhinolaryngol 1998;44:51-58.

15. Nishimura T, Morishima N, Hasegawa S, et al: Effect of surgery on obstructive sleep apnea. Acta Otolaryngol Suppl 1996;523:231-233.

16. Agren K, Nordlander B, Linder-Aronsson S, et al: Children with nocturnal upper airway obstruction: Postoperative orthodontic and respiratory improvement. Acta Otolaryngol 1998;118:581-587.

17. Nieminen P, Tolonen U, Lopponen H: Snoring and obstructive sleep apnea in children: A 6 month follow-up study. Arch Otolaryngol Head Neck Surg 2000;126:481-486.

18. Frank Y, Kravath RE, Pollak CP, Weitzman ED: Obstructive sleep apnea and its therapy: Clinical and polysomnographic manifestations. Pediatrics 1983;71:737-742.

19. Suen JS, Arnold JE, Brooks LJ: Adenotonsillectomy for treatment of obstructive sleep apnea in children. Arch Otolaryngol Head Neck Surg 1995;121:525-530.

20. Stradling JR, Thomas G, Warley AR, et al: Effect of adenotonsillectomy on nocturnal hypoxaemia, sleep disturbance, and symptoms in snoring children. Lancet 1990;335:249-253.

21. Zucconi M, Strambi LF, Pestalozza G, et al: Habitual snoring and obstructive sleep apnea syndrome in children: Effects of early tonsil surgery. Int J Pediatr Otorhinolaryngol 1993;26:235-243.

22. Bar A, Tarasiuk A, Segev Y, et al: The effect of adenotonsillectomy on serum insulin-like growth factor-I and growth in children with obstructive sleep apnea syndrome. J Pediatr 1999;135:76-80.

23. Marcus CL, Carroll JL, Koerner CB, et al: Determinants of growth in children with the obstructive sleep apnea syndrome. J Pediatr 1994;125:556-562.

24. Williams EF III, Woo P, Miller R, Kellman RM: The effects of adenotonsillectomy on growth in young children. Otolaryngol Head Neck Surg 1991;104:509-516.

25. Ahlqvist-Rastad J, Hultcrantz E, Melander H, Svanholm H: Body growth in relation to tonsillar enlargement and tonsillectomy. Int J Pediatr Otorhinolaryngol 1992;24:55-61.

26. Soultan Z, Wadowski S, Rao M, Kravath RE: Effect of treating obstructive sleep apnea by tonsillectomy and/or adenoidectomy on obesity in children. Arch Pediatr Adolesc Med 1999;153:33-37.

27. Weider DJ, Sateia MJ, West RP: Nocturnal enuresis in children with upper airway obstruction. Otolaryngol Head Neck Surg 1991;105:427-432.

28. Ali NJ, Pitson D, Stradling JR: Sleep disordered breathing: effects of adenotonsillectomy on behaviour and psychological functioning. Eur J Pediatr 1996;155:56-62.

29. Goldstein NA, Post C, Rosenfeld RM, Campbell TF: Impact of tonsillectomy and adenoidectomy on child behavior. Arch Otolaryngol Head Neck Surg 2000;126:494-498.

30. Gozal D: Sleep-disordered breathing and school performance in children. Pediatrics 1998;102:616-620.

31. Harvey JM, O'Callaghan MJ, Wales PD, et al: Six-month follow-up of children with obstructive sleep apnoea. J Paediatr Child Health 1999;35:136-139.

32. Buchinsky FJ, Lowry MA, Isaacson G: Do adenoids regrow after excision? Otolaryngol Head Neck Surg 2000;123:576-581.

33. Tami TA, Parker GS, Taylor RE: Post-tonsillectomy bleeding: An evaluation of risk factors. Laryngoscope 1987;97:1307-1311.

34. Wilkinson AR, McCormick MS, Freeland AP, Pickering D: Electrocardiographic signs of pulmonary hypertension in children who snore. BMJ 1981;282:1579-1581.

35. Yates DW: Adenotonsillar hypertrophy and cor pulmonale. Br J Anaesth 1988;61:355-359.

36. Galvis AJ: Pulmonary edema complicating relief of upper airway obstruction. Am J Emerg Med 1987;5:294-297.

37. Feinberg AN, Shabino CL: Acute pulmonary edema complicating tonsillectomy and adenoidectomy. Pediatrics 1985;75:112-114.

38. Ruboyianes JM, Cruz RM: Pediatric adenotonsillectomy for obstructive sleep apnea. Ear Nose Throat J 1996;75:430-433.

39. McColley SA, April MM, Carroll JL, Loughlin GM: Respiratory compromise after adenotonsillectomy in children with obstructive sleep apnea. Arch Otolaryngol Head Neck Surg 1992;118:940-943.

40. Rothschild MA, Catalano P, Biller HF: Ambulatory pediatric tonsillectomy and the identification of high-risk subgroups. Otolaryngol Head Neck Surg 1994;110:203-210.

41. Wiatrak BJ, Myer CM, Andrews TM: Complications of adenotonsillectomy in children under 3 years of age. Am J Otolaryngol 1991;12:170-172.

42. McGowan FX, Kenna MA, Fleming JA, O'Connor T: Adenotonsillectomy for upper airway obstruction carries increased risk in children with a history of prematurity. Pediatr Pulmonol 1992;13:222-226.

43. Biavati MJ, Manning SC, Phillips DC: Predictive factors for respiratory complications after tonsillectomy and adenoidectomy in children with

OSA. Arch Otolaryngol Head Neck Surg 1997;123:517-521.

44. Gerber ME, O'Connor DM, Adler E, Myer CM: Selected risk factors in pediatric adenotonsillectomy [see comments]. Arch Otolaryngol Head Neck Surg 1996;122:811-814.

45. Leiberman A, Tal A, Brama I, Sofer S: Obstructive sleep apnea in young infants. Int J Pediatr Otorhinolaryngol 1988;16:39-44.

46. Waters KA, Everett FM, Bruderer JW, Sullivan CE: Obstructive sleep apnea: The use of nasal CPAP in 80 children. Am J Respir Crit Care Med 1995;152:780-785.

47. Helfaer MA, McColley SA, Pyzik PL, et al: Polysomnography after adenotonsillectomy in mild pediatric obstructive sleep apnea. Crit Care Med 1996;24:1323-1327.

48. Marcus CL, Ward SL, Mallory GB, et al: Use of nasal continuous positive airway pressure as treatment of childhood obstructive sleep apnea. J Pediatr 1995;127:88-94.

49. Smith PL, Wise RA, Gold AR, et al: Upper airway pressure-flow relationships in obstructive sleep apnea. J Appl Physiol 1988;64:789-795.

50. Strohl KP, Redline S: Nasal CPAP therapy, upper airway muscle activation, and obstructive sleep apnea. Am Rev Respir Dis 1986;134:555-558.

51. Brochard L, Isabey D, Piquet J, et al: Reversal of acute exacerbations of chronic obstructive lung disease by inspiratory assistance with a face mask. New Engl J Med 1990;323:1523-1530.

52. McNicholas WT, Coffey M, Boyle T: Effects of nasal airflow on breathing during sleep in normal humans. Am Rev Respir Dis 1993;147:620-623.

53. American Thoracic Society: Indications and standards for use of nasal continuous positive airway pressure (CPAP) in sleep apnea syndromes. Am J Respir Crit Care Med 1994;150:1738-1745.

54. McNamara F, Sullivan CE: Obstructive sleep apnea in infants and its management with nasal continuous positive airway pressure. Chest 1999;116:10-16.

55. Guilleminault C, Pelayo R, Clerk A, et al: Home nasal continuous positive airway pressure in infants with sleep-disordered breathing. J Pediatr 1995;127:905-912.

56. Downey R III, Perkin RM, MacQuarrie J: Nasal continuous positive airway pressure use in children with obstructive sleep apnea younger than 2 years of age. Chest 2000;117:1608-1612.

57. Marcus CL: Ventilator management of abnormal breathing during sleep: Continuous positive airway pressure (CPAP) and nocturnal noninvasive intermittent positive pressure ventilation. In Loughlin GM, Carroll JL, Marcus CL (eds): Sleep and Breathing in Children: A Developmental Approach. New York, Marcel Dekker, 2000, pp 797-812.

58. Koontz KL, Slifer KJ, Cataldo MD, Marcus CL: Improving pediatric compliance with positive airway pressure therapy: The impact of behavioral intervention. Sleep 2003;26:1010-1015.

59. Rains JC: Treatment of obstructive sleep apnea in pediatric patients. Clin Pediatr 1995;34:535-541.

60. Sforza E, Lugaresi E: Daytime sleepiness and nasal continuous positive airway pressure therapy in obstructive sleep apnea syndrome patients: Effects of chronic treatment and 1-night therapy withdrawal. Sleep 1995;18:195-201.

61. Kribbs NB, Pack AI, Kline LR, et al: Effects of one night without nasal CPAP treatment on sleep and sleepiness in patients with obstructive sleep apnea. Am Rev Respir Dis 1993;147:1162-1168.

62. Boudewyns A, Sforza E, Zamagni M, Krieger J: Respiratory effort during sleep apneas after interruption of long-term CPAP treatment in patients with obstructive sleep apnea. Chest 1996;110:120-127.

63. Reeves-Hoche MK, Meck R, Zwillich CW: Nasal CPAP: An objective evaluation of patient compliance. Am J Respir Crit Care Med 1994;149:149-154.

64. Krieger J, Kurtz D, Petiau C, et al: Long-term compliance with CPAP therapy in obstructive sleep apnea patients and in snorers. Sleep 1996;19(Suppl):S136-S143.

65. Kribbs NB, Pack AI, Kline LR, et al: Objective measurement of patterns of nasal CPAP use by patients with obstructive sleep apnea [see comments]. Am Rev Respir Dis 1993;147:887-895.

66. Marcus CL, Davidson Ward SL, Lutz JM, et al: Compliance with CPAP vs bilevel pressure in children. Am J Respir Crit Care Med 2004;169:A732.

67. Constantinidis J, Knobber D, Steinhart H, et al: Fine-structural investigations of the effect of nCPAP-mask application on the nasal mucosa. Acta Otolaryngol 2000;120:432-437.

68. Pepin JL, Leger P, Veale D, et al: Side effects of nasal continuous positive airway pressure in sleep apnea syndrome: Study of 193 patients in two French sleep centers. Chest 1995;107:375-381.

69. Massie CA, Hart RW, Peralez C, Richards GN: Effects of humidification on nasal symptoms and compliance in sleep apnea patients using continuous positive airway pressure. Chest 1999;116:403-408.

70. Choo-Kang LR, Ogunlesi FO, McGrath-Morrow SA, Marcus CL: Recurrent pneumothoraces associated with nocturnal noninvasive ventilation in a patient with muscular dystrophy. Pediatr Pulmonol 2002;34:73-78.

71. Alvarez-Sala R, Garcia IT, Garcia F, et al: Nasal CPAP during wakefulness increases intraocular pressure in glaucoma. Monaldi Arch Chest Dis 1994;49:394-395.

72. Bamford CR, Quan SF: Bacterial meningitis: A possible complication of nasal continuous positive airway pressure therapy in a patient with obstructive sleep apnea syndrome and a mucocele. Sleep 1993;16:31-32.

73. Robertson NJ, McCarthy LS, Hamilton PA, Moss ALH: Nasal deformities resulting from flow driver continuous positive airway pressure. Arch Dis Child 1996;75:F209-F212.

74. Li KK, Riley RW, Guilleminault C: An unreported risk in the use of home nasal continuous positive airway pressure and home nasal ventilation in children: Mid-face hypoplasia. Chest 2000;117:916-918.

75. American Sleep Disorders Association: Practice parameters for the treatment of obstructive sleep apnea in adults: The efficacy of surgical modifications of the upper airway. Sleep 1995;19:152-155.

76. Kosko JR, Derkay CS: Uvulopalatopharyngoplasty: Treatment of obstructive sleep apnea in neurologically impaired pediatric patients. Int J Pediatr Otorhinolaryngol 1995;32:241-246.

77. Donaldson JD, Redmond WM: Surgical management of obstructive sleep apnea in children with Down syndrome. J Otolaryngol 1988;17:398-403.

78. Seid AB, Martin PJ, Pransky SM, Kearns DB: Surgical therapy of obstructive sleep apnea in children with severe mental insufficiency. Laryngoscope 1990;100:507-510.

79. Burstein FD, Cohen SR, Scott PH, et al: Surgical therapy for severe refractory sleep apnea in infants and children: Application of the airway zone concept. Plast Reconstr Surg 1995;96:34-41.

80. Cohen SR, Simms C, Burstein FD, Thomsen J: Alternatives to tracheostomy in infants and children with obstructive sleep apnea. J Pediatr Surg 1999;34:182-187.

81. Cohen SR, Lefaivre JF, Burstein FD, et al: Surgical treatment of obstructive sleep apnea in neurologically compromised patients. Plast Reconstr Surg 1997;99:638-646.

82. Lefaivre JF, Cohen SR, Burstein FD, et al: Down syndrome: Identification and surgical management of obstructive sleep apnea. Plast Reconstr Surg 1997;99:629-637.

83. Morgan WE, Friedman EM, Duncan NO, Sulek M: Surgical management of macroglossia in children. Arch Otolaryngol Head Neck Surg 1996;122:326-329.

84. Marcus CL, Crockett DM, Ward SL: Evaluation of epiglottoplasty as treatment for severe laryngomalacia [published erratum appears in J Pediatr 1991;118:168]. J Pediatr 1990;117:706-710.

85. Marcus CL, Curtis S, Koerner CB, et al: Evaluation of pulmonary function and polysomnography in obese children and adolescents. Pediatr Pulmonol 1996;21:176-183.

86. Strobel RJ, Rosen RC: Obesity and weight loss in obstructive sleep apnea: A critical review. Sleep 1996;19:104-115.

87. Breaux CW: Obesity surgery in children. Obes Surg 1995;5:279-284.

88. Sampol G, Munoz X, Sagales MT, et al: Long-term efficacy of dietary weight loss in sleep apnoea/hypopnea syndrome. Eur Respir J 1998;12:1156-1159.

89. Pillar G, Peled R, Lavie P: Recurrence of sleep apnea without concomitant weight increase 7.5 years after weight reduction surgery. Chest 1994;106:1702-1704.

90. American Sleep Disorders Association: Practice parameters for the treatment of snoring and obstructive sleep apnea with oral appliances. Sleep 1995;18:511-513.

91. Villa MP, Bernkopf E, Pagani J, et al: Randomized controlled study of an oral jaw-positioning appliance for the treatment of obstructive sleep apnea in children with malocclusion. Am J Respir Crit Care Med 2002;165:123-127.

92. Cozza P, Gatto R, Ballanti F, Prete L: Management of obstructive sleep apnoea in children with modified monobloc appliances. Eur J Paediatr Dent 2004;5:24-29.

93. Cistulli PA, Palmisano RG, Poole MD: Treatment of obstructive sleep apnea syndrome by rapid maxillary expansion. Sleep 1998;21:831-835.

94. Pirelli P, Saponara M, Guilleminault C: Rapid maxillary expansion in children with obstructive sleep apnea syndrome. Sleep 2004;27:761-766.

95. Marcus CL, Carroll JL, Bamford O, et al: Supplemental oxygen during sleep in children with sleep-disordered breathing. Am J Respir Crit Care Med 1995;152(Pt 1):1297-1301.

96. Aljadeff G, Gozal D, Bailey-Wahl SL: Effects of overnight supplemental oxygen in obstructive sleep apnea in children. Am J Respir Crit Care Med 1996;153:51-55.

97. Al-Ghamdi SA, Manoukian JJ, Morielli A, et al: Do systemic corticosteroids effectively treat obstructive sleep apnea secondary to adenotonsillar hypertrophy? Laryngoscope 1997;107:1382-1387.

98. Brouillette RT, Manoukian JJ, Ducharme FM, et al: Efficacy of fluticasone nasal spray for pediatric obstructive sleep apnea. J Pediatr 2001;138:838-844.

99. McColley SA, Carroll JL, Curtis S, et al: High prevalence of allergic sensitization in children with habitual snoring and obstructive sleep apnea. Chest 1997;111:170-173.

100. Corbo GM, Fuciarelli F, Foresi A, De Benedetto F. Snoring in children: Association with respiratory symptoms and passive smoking. BMJ 1989;299:1491-1494.

101. Redline S, Tishler PV, Schluchter M, et al: Risk factors for sleep-disordered breathing in children: Associations with obesity, race, and respiratory problems. Am J Respir Crit Care Med 1999;159:1527-1532.

Otolaryngologic Management of Sleep-Related Breathing Disorders

22

Julie L. Wei

Roberto L. Barretto

Mark E. Gerber

General and pediatric otolaryngologists are frequently asked to evaluate and consider surgical management in children with snoring, sleep-related breathing disorders, and possible obstructive sleep apnea (OSA). OSA and upper airway resistance syndrome (UARS) in the pediatric population are most often caused by adenoid and tonsillar (adenotonsillar) hypertrophy, which has a peak incidence from the ages of 2 to 5 years mirroring the incidence of pediatric OSA. However, other causes of upper airway obstruction must be ruled out and appropriately treated if present. Since the widespread availability and use of antibiotics, the morbidity and complications of tonsillitis have been reduced dramatically. Tonsillectomy and adenoidectomy are the most commonly performed curative procedures, and awareness of pediatric OSA syndrome (OSAS) and sleep apnea has resulted in a changing trend in the indication for pediatric adenotonsillectomy over the traditional infectious indication.[1] The definitions of OSA and UARS are described in detail in other chapters of this text; hence, this chapter will focus on the diagnosis, surgical indications, and outcome of adenotonsillectomy specifically relevant to OSA.

PATHOPHYSIOLOGY OF OSA

The pathophysiology of sleep-related breathing disorders, UARS, and OSA differs from patient to patient, depending on the presence of medical comorbidities, central versus obstructive apnea, and, if obstructive, the specific site of upper airway obstruction. The upper airway includes the nasal passages down to the glottic inlet, including potentially redundant soft tissue in the oropharynx and hypopharynx; therefore, evaluation must include areas other than the adenoid and tonsillar tissue.

Nasal obstruction secondary to allergic rhinitis or polyps may respond to conservative management. Stridor may signify laryngeal or tracheal pathology. Benign or malignant upper airway masses can present with snoring and sleep-disordered breathing. Comorbidities such as craniofacial abnormalities, neuromuscular deficiencies caused by cerebral palsy, and Down syndrome may play primary roles in the upper airway obstruction.[2] OSA specific to patients with craniofacial abnormalities and/or neurologically challenged children is carefully described in other chapters. Such patients require a more complex treatment plan through a multidisciplinary approach.

Nonsurgical management of pediatric OSA includes mechanical interventions such as continuous positive airway pressure (CPAP), bilevel positive airway pressure (BiPAP), and medical therapy. The indications and technical details related to CPAP and BiPAP are covered elsewhere. Medical therapy is specifically relevant in the treatment of obesity, allergy, sinonasal pathology, and adenotonsillar hypertrophy due to acute tonsillitis.

Obesity

Obesity is becoming more prevalent in the United States and is recognized as a significant health problem in children. However, in contrast to adults, most preadolescent children with OSA are of normal weight or even underweight. Nonetheless, obesity inducing or contributing to OSA is growing more prevalent in the pediatric population. Weight control alone has been shown to result in the partial cure of sleep-related breathing disorders.[3] For children with severe or morbid obesity, referral to a weight loss specialist or nutritionist and family education are critical in successfully reducing long-term sequelae of not only OSA but all obesity-related health problems.

Nasal Obstruction

The treatment of nasal pathology may improve obstructive symptoms. Many children present with a history of nasal congestion and nocturnal mouth breathing. This may be due to the nasal cycle, which is a natural phenomenon when breathing occurs via a single nasal passage such as in turbinate mucosa alternate engorgement or due to vasomotor rhinitis or allergies. In children who present with nasal airway obstruction, significant adenoid hypertrophy causing nasopharyngeal obstruction needs to be ruled out. Over-the-counter topical nasal decongestants and oral decongestants are not recommended for chronic use in the pediatric population. Nasal saline irrigation may be effective in relieving nasal congestion, especially during upper respiratory infections. Consistent daily use of topical nasal steroids may decrease the severity of snoring. Mometasone has been approved for children as young as 2 years of age, and fluticasone is approved for children 4 years of age or older. Intranasal steroid sprays may relieve nasal obstruction secondary to adenoid hypertrophy, providing symptomatic improvement in those without tonsillar hypertrophy. Aqueous intranasal beclomethasone (Beconase AQ) used twice daily for 16 weeks was shown to decrease the adenoid/choana ratio by 29% and reduce the nasal obstruction symptom score by 82%.[10]

Management of allergic rhinitis is essential if this is the cause of nasal congestion and the resulting upper airway obstruction. Avoidance, antihistamines, mast cell stabilizers, intranasal steroids, and immunotherapy, alone or in combinations are effective measures in controlling atopic disease.[4] Allergy testing may be helpful. Chronic sinusitis should also be considered in the patient with persistent rhinitis and nasal airway obstruction. In rare circumstances radiographic imaging studies such as coronal sinus computed tomographic screening may be helpful in the child with a history that is suggestive of but not conclusive enough to warrant medical management for sinusitis. Usually the clinical history and physical findings are sufficient to initiate a therapeutic trial regimen for sinusitis.

Appropriate sinusitis treatment should include broad-spectrum antimicrobial therapy. Ancillary measures such as topical nasal steroids and saline nasal washes may be beneficial. Adenoidectomy alone or with maxillary sinus irrigation has been shown to improve patients with purulent rhinorrhea and chronic nasal congestion secondary to chronic sinusitis and adenoiditis.

Before medical therapy for nasal obstruction, the presence of sinonasal and pharyngeal masses must be ruled out. The literature is replete with cases of benign and malignant neoplasms presenting clinically with snoring and symptoms suggestive of OSA. A thorough history and complete examination with heightened suspicions are necessary to identify these rare conditions and prevent a physician from simply attributing the symptoms of sleep-related breathing disorders to adenotonsillar hypertrophy.

Gastroesophageal Reflux/Gastrolaryngopharyngeal Reflux

Functional and pathologic gastroesophageal reflux (GER), and more specifically gastrolaryngopharyngeal reflux (GLPR), are widely recognized in the pediatric population and have been shown to be associated with both chronic sinusitis and upper airway edema in children. Direct visualization of the upper airway by flexible laryngoscopy in a child with GLPR may reveal edema of the pharyngeal and laryngeal mucosa as well as lingual tonsillar hypertrophy. These changes in turn may result in sleep-related breathing disorders and apnea in infants.[5,6] When the history and/or physical findings suggest that GLPR is involved, either a dual-channel, 24-hr pH probe study or a therapeutic trial of proton pump inhibitors or H_2 blockers is warranted.

DIAGNOSIS OF ADENOID AND TONSILLAR HYPERTROPHY

Adenoid hypertrophy is usually diagnosed by lateral neck x-ray, whereas tonsillar hypertrophy is clinically diagnosed by direct visualization. The history of mouth breathing may suggest nasal obstruction and adenotonsillar hypertrophy, but it is not specific to either adenotonsillar hypertrophy or OSA. Most children have prominent adenoid and tonsillar tissue relative to their small head size, but the majority of children do not have OSA. Children are susceptible to frequent viral infections involving the upper respiratory tract and will frequently have nasal congestion and rhinorrhea associated with the upper respiratory illnesses even without adenoid hypertrophy. The lateral neck x-ray will demonstrate nasopharyngeal airway narrowing secondary to prominent adenoid tissue, or alternatively, direct visualization using flexible fiber-optic nasopharyngoscopy will demonstrate adenoid hypertrophy if it is seen to occupy more than approximately 80% of the choana. Since both methods lack objectivity, the physician's observation, based on the clincal history and exam, should determine whether the patient undergoes polysomnography to assist in deciding if adenotonsillectomy is indicated.

When the oropharynx is inspected, the size, position, and characteristics of tonsils such as the presence of exudate, tonsilloliths, or crypts are noted. Tonsil size is determined clinically by the space both tonsils occupy in the oropharynx in view. Tonsils occupying less than 25% of the pharynx are routinely described by otolaryngologists as 1+, less than 50% 2+, less than 75% 3+, and finally, those occupying greater than 75% of the oropharyngeal space or tonsils making contact in the midline are 4+. This is a generalized classification for description. The decision to perform tonsillectomy should not be based on size alone. The tonsils may be endophytic and appear as 1+ or 2+ in the office exam, and the true size is often not appreciated until the time of surgery, when the patient is under anesthesia and the oropharynx is completely exposed using a mouth gag instrument. There is no strict correlation between the size of the tonsil and upper airway obstruction, and the oral exam may not represent the actual degree of obstruction compared with an exam of the posterior oropharynx with nasopharyngoscopy.

ACUTE TONSILLITIS

Patients with acute tonsillitis may have sudden or new-onset symptoms of snoring and OSA. Tonsillar hypertrophy secondary to acute bacterial or viral infection may be unilateral or bilateral, both of which may cause new or worsening symptoms of snoring and upper airway obstruc-

tion. Significant tonsillitis has been defined to include any of the following: temperature above 38.5° C, cervical adenopathy of greater than 2 cm, the presence of tonsillar exudate, or positive group A β-hemolytic streptococcus (GABHS). Patients evaluated for acute tonsillitis with concomitant symptoms of fever, odynophagia, dysphagia, and possible airway obstruction should be treated with a course of oral antibiotics if exudative tonsillitis is seen and/or a bacterial pathogen is confirmed by a rapid streptococcal swab test. Pain associated with acute tonsillitis can be safely and adequately treated with a single dose of oral or intramuscular dexamethasone in patients older than 15 years of age.[7] Acute mononucleosis may result in severe adenotonsillar hypertrophy with significant obstruction. A decision for adenotonsillectomy should take into consideration the patient's infection history and the frequency and severity of such airway obstruction as well as the likelihood of recurrence. Patients with acute tonsillar hypertrophy secondary to an infection should also be followed after infectious symptoms have resolved to ensure that there is resolution of adenoid and/or tonsillar hypertrophy and symptoms of upper airway obstruction.

CHRONIC ADENOTONSILLAR HYPERTROPHY

In one study of cases of chronic adenotonsillar hypertrophy, broad-spectrum antibiotics such as amoxicillin/clavulanate potassium given as a 30-day course have been shown to decrease adenotonsillar hypertrophy in the short term, but 83% of the patients had a return of their sleep-disordered breathing–related symptoms and went on to have surgical management for OSA at 24-month followup.[8] There may be a role for a prolonged course of antibiotics in providing short-term symptom relief or if the patient is not a surgical candidate due to medical comorbidities.

Dexamethasone 1 mg/kg/day over 3 to 5 days can result in a rapid reduction of tonsil and adenoid size, with an improvement in the symptoms of upper airway obstruction. However, short courses of oral prednisone have been shown to be ineffective in treating pediatric OSA caused by adenotonsillar hypertrophy.[9] Long-term use of corticosteroids is generally not recommended secondary to systemic side effects.

DIAGNOSIS OF OSA

While the clinical history and physical exam are important, they do not provide a reliable diagnosis of OSA. Several recent studies have demonstrated that OSAS diagnosed by history alone was confirmed in only 30% to 55.6% of patients when polysomnograms were perrformed.[10-14] These studies suggest that there is a poor correlation between history and OSA with polysomnography (PSG). However, they were conducted before high UARS was recognized and therefore most likely underestimated the incidence of sleep-disordered breathing. In general, it does appear that snoring as a symptom is not a reliable indicator of OSA. Primary snoring without associated abnormalities in sleep architecture, alveolar ventilation, or oxygenation is estimated to occur in up to 10% of the pediatric population.[15] PSG is considered the gold standard in diagnosing OSA. It is imperative to understand that OSAS is differentially defined in adults and children, and the criteria for an abnormal pediatric polysomnogram are different from those of adults.[16] An apnea index of 1 and an apnea-hypopnea index (AHI) of greater than or equal to 5 are considered abnormal; however, the clinical significance of these numbers is unknown. Due to the difficulties in confirming sleep-disordered breathing by history alone, PSG is a useful tool to assist in the confirmation of the diagnosis before considering surgical intervention.[17] The severity of the OSA based on the apnea index, respiratory disturbance index, lowest oxygen saturation, and maximum end-tidal CO_2 may direct the planning of postoperative care, such as observation in the intensive care unit and parental counseling of possible prolonged intubation during the immediate postoperative period. However, not every child with symptoms and an exam suggestive of upper airway obstruction secondary to adenotonsillar hypertrophy needs to have PSG-proven OSA before consideration of surgical intervention. First of all, there are simply not enough available sleep center resources to perform and interpret the number of pediatric polysomnograms necessary to evaluate every child with the symptoms of sleep-related breathing disorders. Second, clinically significant sleep-disordered breathing can be present even in the absence of an abnormal polysomnogram. UARS has recently been described in which negative intrathoracic pressure swings during inspiration lead to EEG arousals and sleep fragmentation and, more importantly, to subsequent daytime symptomatology similar to that of OSAS. In UARS the polysomnogram does not demonstrate significant apneas and hypopneas. It has been suggested to be more common than OSAS.[18] UARS may be formally diagnosed either by esophageal manometry, which measures respiratory effort and intrathoracic pressure, or end-tidal CO_2 capnography in conjunction with a suprasternal notch monitor, which detects increased intrathoracic pressure.

It is neither cost-effective nor possible to have every child who is a potential candidate for adenotonsillectomy obtain a polysomnogram, regardless of the severity of symptoms and the exam, or to undergo the aforementioned testing to diagnose UARS. The prevalence of UARS is underestimated in children, since it is not routinely assessed. However, since UARS leads to symptomatology similar to that of OSAS, clinical history alone that is suggestive of UARS can be an indication for surgical intervention. These patients demonstrate improvement in the elimination of snoring, sleep fragmentation, daytime somnolence or hyperactivity, and other symptoms associated with sleep-related breathing disorders after adenotonsillectomy. PSG should also be offered to families as an alternative approach to assist in providing additional objective data to help their decision making. For patients who are not surgical candidates due to medical comorbidity, PSG is necessary to determine the parameters for nonsurgical treatment options such as CPAP.

POLYSOMNOGRAPHY BEFORE SURGERY

There are currently no clear criteria according to which patients should undergo polysomnography before adenotonsillectomy. This decision is largely dependent on the physician bias and therefore should be based on the severity of the clinical history, the exam, and more specifically the presence of medical comorbidity, including obesity. For an otherwise healthy child without medical comorbidity, including obesity, and who does not have any history of intubation, hospitalization, or airway surgery, an oropharyngeal exam consistent with significant tonsillar hypertrophy may support the decision for adenotonsillectomy without first obtaining a polysomnogram. Complex patients who are at high risk for OSA may benefit from a baseline polysomnogram. In this population, additional postoperative PSG is useful to confirm the resolution of OSA, even in the absence of residual symptoms. Table 22–1 offers several predisposing factors for childhood OSA but is by no means a complete list. In addition, whenever the history does not match the examination, PSG is indicated.

INDICATIONS FOR ADENOTONSILLECTOMY

Successful surgical management of pediatric sleep-disordered breathing depends on identification and intervention at every level of obstruction, which may occur from the nasal vault down to the level of the glottis. A thorough history of symptoms, the physical exam, and at times flexible nasopharyngoscopy, laryngoscopy, and/or imaging studies will allow for the diagnosis of a site-specific obstruction and the formation of an appropriate surgical treatment plan. Most cases of sleep-disordered breathing in children are secondary to adenotonsillar hypertrophy, and symptoms are readily alleviated after adenotonsillectomy. Patients in whom the polysomnogram demonstrates both central and obstructive hypoventilation may require a multidisciplinary approach to achieve a satisfactory result. Decisions regarding when and how to intervene depend on several factors, among them the severity and site of obstruction; overall health of the child, including comorbid conditions; and family expectations. Treatment of pediatric sleep-disordered breathing varies depending on the severity. For very mild cases, observation alone with monitoring for worsening signs and symptoms may be sufficient. Surgical management has been shown to be beneficial not only to patients with mild cases secondary to adenotonsillar hypertrophy alone but also to patients with the aforementioned comorbid conditions. A combination of medical, surgical, and mechanical interventions may be necessary in treating moderate to severe cases.

Children who demonstrate mild or no evidence of OSA by polysomnography may still have UARS, causing sleep disturbances as well as

Table 22–1.	Factors Associated with High Risk for Obstructive Sleep Apnea
Neurologic Abnormalities	
Seizure disorder	Head injury
Cerebral palsy	Prematurity
Hydrocephalus	Central apnea
Arnold-Chiari	Meningomyelocele
malformation	Myotonic dystrophy
Craniofacial Abnormalities	
Micrognathia	Retrognathia
Macroglossia	Maxillary hypoplasia
Diseases	
Hypothyroidism	Crouzon's disease
Goiter	Gastroesophageal
Morbid obesity	reflux
Anatomic Obstructions	
Excessive soft tissue	Nasal stenosis
of the neck	Choanal atresia
Short neck	Septal deviation
Lingual tonsil	Laryngeal papillomas/
hypertrophy	tumors
Redundant	Subglottic stenosis
oropharyngeal	Subglottic
mucosa/long uvula	hemangioma
Adenoid hypertrophy	Nasal polyps
Tonsillar hypertrophy	Laryngeal web/
Pharyngeal flap	stenosis/mass
surgery	
Syndromes	
Achondroplasia	Beckwith-Wiedemann
Apert's	Treacher Collins
Down	Stickler's
Pierre Robin	Fetal alcohol
Prader-Willi	Marfan's
Klippel-Feil	Hemifacial microsomia

daytime chronic mouth breathing and behavior problems. A prospective study using parental questionnaires and sleep polysomnography demonstrated that adenotonsillectomy provides long-term benefits even in children in whom the obstruction did not meet the criteria for OSA (patients most likely have high upper airway resistance).[19] Many times the parents of children with sleep-disordered breathing have a high level of anxiety and disrupted sleep patterns secondary to their child's sleep dysfunction. Surgical intervention in these children can promptly improve the quality of the life for both the patient and the family.

TONSILLECTOMY AND ADENOIDECTOMY

Adenotonsillectomy is the most common major pediatric surgical procedure performed in the United States. Sleep-related breathing disorders secondary to adenotonsillar hypertrophy may have been more common than recurrent tonsillitis as an indication for surgery ever since the inception of the widespread use of antibiotic therapy. Daytime audible breathing and chronic mouth breathing are also common parental concerns leading to referral to an otolaryngologist. History taking should focus on night-time symptoms such as consistent nocturnal snoring, including observation of the degree of work of breathing; the presence of retractions or paradoxical abdominal respirations; obstructive pauses in airflow frequently followed by snorting or gasping for air; restless sleep; frequent arousals; and enuresis. Daytime symptoms include difficulty getting up in the morning, excessive irritability, hyperactivity, a poor attention span, somnolence, and even morning headaches. Children with more severe adenotonsillar hypertrophy may have audible breathing while awake, which is easily noted during an office visit.

PREOPERATIVE EVALUATION

Preoperative evaluation may vary depending on surgeon preference and hospital guidelines. Children who are otherwise healthy may obtain medical clearance for general anesthesia by a thorough history and physical exam from their primary physicians. Any patient with a complex medical history, including seizure, cardiac, endocrine, and pulmonary problems, should have an appropriate preoperative evaluation by the specialist treating the specific problem. Recommendations for perioperative, intraoperative, and/or postoperative management specific to each medical condition should be outlined and communicated to the surgeon before the procedure. Patients with complex medical comorbidities or who may be at an increased risk with general anesthesia should be evaluated by an anesthesiologist before the surgery. Many otolaryngologists rely on a detailed bleeding questionnaire to help screen for a possible bleeding disorder or the need for blood work and possible hematology consultation. When there are positive findings on the questionnaire, a screening set of coagulation studies is obtained, including a complete blood count, prothrombin time, partial thromboplastin time, and the recently available platelet function analysis, which is a replacement for bleeding time as a measure of platelet function. For African-American and other high-risk groups, a sickle cell screen should be considered if the patient has not been previously evaluated for sickle cell disease. There remains controversy regarding the need for routine, preoperative blood work before surgery, but due to the lack of cost-effectiveness as well as the inability to predict which patient is at risk for the reported 1% to 4% of postoperative hemorrhage, routine blood work before adenotonsillectomy is not usually performed.[20] Laboratory evaluations specific to coexisting medical conditions may be necessary to determine clearance for surgery and general anesthesia.

SURGICAL TECHNIQUES

Adenotonsillectomy is the most commonly performed procedure under general anesthesia by a variety of surgical techniques, including cold knife; electrosurgery, such as monopolar, bipolar, controlled radiofrequency, coablation, laser, and argon plasma coagulation; needlepoint or blade electrocautery; harmonic scalpel; and most recently the powered instrument microdébrider technique, described as subtotal or intracapsular tonsillectomy.[21-23] Electrosurgery and electrocautery differ in that electrosurgery uses a high-frequency electrical current that passes through tissue near the active electrode, causing the heating of the tissue and resulting in cutting, coagulation, and ablation of the tissue; in electrocautery the current passes through a heating element that conducts heat to the blade, creating a "hot blade" for cauterization or cutting of the tissue. Multiple studies have reviewed the differences among the various techniques. Except for reported differences in operating time and intraoperative bleeding, there are minimal statistically significant differences with respect to postoperative bleeding risk as well as outcome measures such as postoperative pain when a complete tonsillectomy is performed.[24-31]

A subtotal/partial tonsillectomy is also described as intracapsular. This technique preserves the tonsillar capsule and is believed to avoid direct surgical violation of the pharyngeal muscles, thus reducing postoperative pain and recovery time because there is less injury to and inflammation of the muscles and less disruption of nerve endings. A recent study concluded that when compared with the standard technique, intracapsular tonsillectomy is just as effective in relieving obstructive sleep-disordered breathing but produces statistically significantly less postoperative pain and fewer episodes of delayed hemorrhage and dehydration.[21] This study also reported that the numbers of days to return of normal activity and analgesic use were lower in the groups who underwent an intracapsular tonsillectomy. Future data from current, prospective, randomized studies may confirm that statistically significant differences exist between this and all previous techniques.

Adjunctive perioperative measures to improve postoperative results include the use of dexamethasone in a single perioperative dose. Meta-analysis of all blinded, randomized trials of perioperative dexamethasone use has demonstrated decreased postoperative emesis and an earlier return to a soft or regular diet in those that receive it. A single dose of 0.5 mg/kg of dexamethasone, up to 20 mg, given intraoperatively has been shown to be effective in reducing postoperative emesis and pain as well as improving oral intake.[32,33]

POSTOPERATIVE MANAGEMENT

Candidacy for Ambulatory Surgery

Several reviews of large series have demonstrated that adenoidectomy and tonsillectomy are safely performed as outpatient procedures on those children who meet the selection criteria.[34-40] One prospective study showed the safety of a six-hour postoperative recovery room observation period, and recommended a four-hour observation period based on their finding.[35]

Children with OSAS have been shown to have an increased risk of respiratory compromise immediately after surgery, with the most significant risk factors being age less than 3 years and an AHI of greater than 10.[41] Two other risk factors include having an abnormal electro-cardiogram and weight less than the 5th percentile for age.[41] An increased risk of respiratory compromise applies not only to children who have OSA secondary to adenotonsillar hypertrophy but also to those with OSA associated with craniofacial anomalies causing maxillary and/or mandibular hypoplasia and reduction in the pharyngeal airway. In addition to craniofacial anomalies, medical comorbidities involving neurologic problems such as seizure disorder, cerebral palsy, Down syndrome, and others cause such OSA to be more complex.[42]

One study identified postoperative respiratory compromise after adenotonsillectomy in 10 of 37 children with OSAS, and a review of patient characteristics resulted in a recommendation of overnight observation for patients who have any of the following high-risk clinical criteria: less than 2 years of age, craniofacial anomalies including midfacial hypoplasia or micrognathia/retrognathia, failure to thrive, hypotonia, cor pulmonale, morbid obesity, or a significant preoperative PSG abnormality.[43]

Several studies have demonstrated the increased incidence of postoperative airway complications in patients younger than 3 years of age; therefore, it is the common practice of most otolaryngologists to perform adenotonsillectomy as a 23-hour observation procedure in those younger than 3 years of age.[31,38,44,45] Other variables found to be statistically significant in predicting the risk of respiratory compromise after surgical intervention in pediatric patients include neuromuscular disorders, chromosome abnormalities, a history of restless sleep, difficulty in breathing while asleep, loud snoring with apnea, and an upper respiratory tract infection within 4 weeks of surgery.[31] All of the aforementioned risk factors warrant consideration for overnight observation after surgery.

Recovery Room and Postoperative Observation

Postoperatively, patients are typically observed in the recovery room for 30 to 45 minutes or until they are sufficiently stable for transfer to the ambulatory unit. Every ambulatory center has its own discharge criteria. The most common criteria include requiring demonstration of control of postoperative nausea and/or emesis and adequate pain control as well as an absence of obstructive snoring, oxygen requirements, and other signs of respiratory compromise. For patients under 3 years of age as well as those with an increased risk of respiratory compromise, the signs of respiratory compromise may occur at any time within the first 12 to 24 hours after the procedure but commonly occur in the recovery room. Young children and those with severe OSA are more likely to exhibit apneic episodes, stridor, an inability to maintain oxygen saturation over 90% despite supplemental oxygen, and upper airway obstruction requiring an artificial airway such as a nasopharyngeal trumpet or even endotracheal intubation. Inadequate air exchange can lead to CO_2 retention and narcosis, which further depress respiratory drive. This must be promptly recognized during the postoperative period and may be confirmed by using transcutaneous CO_2 monitoring. Such patients may require reintubation and respiratory support by means of a ventilator for 24 to 48 hours but are usually successfully extubated with an otherwise uneventful recovery period.

After fulfilling criteria in the recovery room, patients are typically transferred to an observation room for up to 4 hours. Attention to adequate analgesia, stable vital signs, the ability to void, and adequate oral intake determine whether a patient may be discharged home.

Patients are usually discharged home with a narcotic or non-narcotic analgesic and instructions for postoperative care. Those with severe OSA on preoperative PSG should be considered for postoperative PSG 6 weeks or later after surgical intervention to ensure that no further treatment is necessary. Postoperative PSG should also be considered in patients who have persistent or recurrent symptoms of upper airway obstruction and sleep-related breathing disorders after surgical intervention.

Postoperative use of antibiotics and analgesics, with or without narcotics, is based on the preferences of the surgeon. Narcotics (e.g., codeine and oxycodone) should be used judiciously postoperatively, especially in children younger than 3 years of age or those with neurologic disorders, medical comorbidities, or documented severe OSA. A recent study demonstrated equal efficacy between the administrations of ibuprofen and acetaminophen with codeine for pain control.[46] Another study demonstrated no difference in pain control and higher oral intake in the group that received acetaminophen alone, most likely due to the lack of potential nausea and vomiting and gastric irritation from the codeine.[47] In order to maximize the benefits of acetaminophen and minimize the potential side effects of a narcotic, the senior author uses a scheduled dose of acetaminophen every 4 hours (15 mg/kg) for the first few days after surgery. Hydrocodone is available without acetaminophen in many cough syrup formulations. A few of the formulations are liquid without an alcohol base. One of these is prescribed (dosing of hydrocodone at 0.15 mg/kg) to be given every 4 hours but only if needed for breakthrough pain that is not adequately relieved by the acetaminophen.

POTENTIAL COMPLICATIONS AFTER ADENOTONSILLECTOMY

Complications after adenotonsillectomy may be divided into immediate, short-term, and long term categories.[48] Primary and secondary hemorrhages after surgery are reported to be small but potentially significant risks in most series.[34,36,37,49] Primary hemorrhage occurs within 24 hours after surgery, while secondary hemorrhage usually occurs between postoperative days 5 and 10. There has been no identifiable, statistically significant risk factor for predicting post-tonsillectomy hemorrhage, with the exception of one study in which age greater than 21 was found to be associated with an increase in risk factor of 3%, almost twice that of those younger than 21 years of age.[49] Post-obstructive pulmonary edema results from a change in pulmonary hydrostatic pressure after an increase in intrathoracic pressure that develops after the removal of long-term upper airway obstruction. Other complications in the immediately postoperative period include dehydration secondary to pain and decreased oral intake, nausea and vomiting, atelectasis, aspiration, and temporary eustachian tube dysfunction or otalgia due to referred pain. Parents are typically instructed to aggressively encourage the oral intake of liquids, since it is speculated that hydration reduces hypertension as well as dry oropharyngeal mucosa and possibly traumatic eschar removal that may cause postoperative hemorrhage. Parents are also encouraged to keep the patients from being too physically active during the first few days after surgery as a measure to prevent hypertension, which may also cause postoperative hemorrhage.

Velopharyngeal insufficiency (VPI) may occur in the first few weeks to months after adenotonsillectomy and is more likely to occur in patients with a history of cleft palate, submucosal cleft palate, or a neuromuscular disorder with hypotonia. However, overaggressive resection of superior tonsillar pillars may cause shortening of the palate and may also produce the symptoms of VPI. Patients and/or parents may report hypernasality or fluid regurgitation into the nasopharynx. Most cases of post-adenotonsillectomy VPI are resolved with observation. For those with symptoms persisting for longer than 6 months, referral to speech therapy may be indicated. VPI as a complication after adenotonsillectomy could theoretically require surgical intervention but is rarely reported.

Nasopharyngeal stenosis is a rare but significant long-term complication secondary to scarring of raw mucosal surfaces during healing. Surgical repair may be necessary to re-establish an adequate nasal airway.[50]

OUTCOMES OF ADENOTONSILLECTOMY IN THE MANAGEMENT OF OSA AND UARS

Various parameters have been used in the evaluation and reporting of outcomes after adenotonsillectomy for the treatment of UARS and OSA. In one study, PSG performed before and after adenotonsillectomy demonstrated that surgery significantly decreased the number of obstructive apneas and the average number of total apneas during all sleep stages but did not have a significant effect on the duration and proportion of the various sleep stages.[51] One prospective study demonstrated that for mild OSA, defined as less than 15 OSA events per hour, 15 patients without underlying medical comorbidities demonstrated a reduction in the number of obstructive events and significant improvement in oxygen desaturation during rapid eye movement sleep on the operative night.[52] A retrospective case series evaluated 48 patients by comparing AHI, percent of sleep time with oxygen saturation below 90%, and percent of sleep time with end-tidal CO_2 of greater than 50 on the pre- and postoperative polysomnograms. This study included a diverse population of

patients such as those with cerebral palsy, Down syndrome, morbid obesity, and other syndromes who underwent adenotonsillectomy alone, adenotonsillectomy with uvulopalatopharyngoplasty (UPPP), or tonsillectomy as a part of UPPP only. Statistically significant differences were observed in all three parameters after surgical intervention.[53]

Before the availability and widespread use of PSG for the evaluation of OSA, adenotonsillectomy was shown to have far-ranging benefits, with a reduction in mouth breathing as well as improvement in behavioral problems even when the upper airway obstruction did not demonstrate severe OSA preoperatively.[19] This prospective study used pre- and postoperative sleep sonography (recorded respiratory sounds) during sleep as well as parental questionnaires to compare 100 children with a diagnosis of adenotonsillar hypertrophy with 50 age-matched control subjects. Other improvements reported include reduced dry mouth and halitosis, decreased mouth breathing, and decreased fussy morning behavior and daytime fatigue. All differences in parameters were shown to be statistically significant when comparing the outcomes of patients postoperatively with their symptoms preoperatively or with the control subjects.

In a review of 55 children with OSA treated with adenotonsillectomy, 86% of the patients markedly improved, defined as a 75% reduction in AHI; an 8% demonstrated improvement, defined as a 50% to 74% reduction in AHI; and a 3% demonstrated (slight) improvement, defined as a 25% to 49% reduction in AHI. Only one patient had less than a 25% reduction in AHI postoperatively.[54] In a different review of 134 children with OSA who underwent adenoidectomy and/or tonsillectomy, facial morphology was correlated with adenotonsillar hypertrophy. Significant improvement in AHI and the lowest oxygen saturation (LSAT) was found in 77.6% of patients. Those who did not demonstrate improvement tended to have smaller tonsils, narrower epipharyngeal spaces, and more poorly developed maxillary and mandibular protrusions.[55] This study also stratified the patients into age groups, and while the LSAT was improved in all age groups, significant improvements in AHI were noted in patients 1 to 3 years of age and 4 to 6 years of age but not in those 7 to 9 years of age. There were no statistically significant differences in improvement among members within an age group.

Adenotonsillectomy has been shown to effectively reverse cardiac changes in children with adenotonsillar hypertrophy by comparing the pre- and postoperative echocardiograms of patients with OSA as well as the postoperative echocardiography parameters with a control group.[56] They used echocardiography to compare children with adenotonsillar hypertrophy and sleep-related breathing disorders with a control group and found statistically significant differences in right and/or left ventricular enlargement as well as decreased left ventricular compliance.

In a review of 31 children with obesity and an expected body weight range of 130% to 260%, adenotonsillectomy was shown to decrease irregular breathing periods to almost zero and result in a mean of over 95% of the sleeping period during which oxygen saturation is greater than 90% in all patients.[3] Weight loss in these patients demonstrated a partial cure of sleep-related breathing disorders, while adenotonsillectomy was effective even when severe obesity remained.

While an adenotonsillectomy with or without additional surgery is expected to improve OSA in children with neuromuscular disorders, these patients are prone to increased postoperative airway complications and prolonged postoperative hospitalization and recovery. Such patients are likely to require insertion of a nasopharyngeal airway to maintain a patent upper airway, meticulous secretion management, and nasogastric feeding temporarily due to delayed and inadequate oral intake.[57] Avoidance of peri- and postoperative use of narcotics will decrease the depression of hypoxic respiratory drive. An awareness of increased potential for postoperative complications allows adequate discussion and preparation of the parents and family before surgery.

ADDITIONAL SURGICAL PROCEDURES

Patients with residual symptoms suggestive of upper airway obstruction after adenotonsillectomy, as well as those with a preoperative polysomnogram and an AHI of greater than 20, should be considered for a second polysomnogram typically 4 to 6 weeks after surgery. The

time period within which a second polysomnogram is performed depends on the availability of the study center and time to complete recovery from the adenotonsillectomy. Repeated PSG will again determine the severity of the airway obstruction and whether it is central or still obstructive, and the decision can then be made whether to pursue additional surgical intervention or medical therapy such as CPAP or BiPAP. Outcome studies have specifically focused on patients with medical comorbidities that increase the likelihood of having residual OSA despite standard adenotonsillectomy. Such conditions include Down syndrome, cerebral palsy, craniofacial syndromes, and neuromuscular disorders other than cerebral palsy. While it is beyond the scope of this chapter to discuss in detail the surgical techniques that are used more frequently in adults for the treatment of OSA, the outcomes of aggressive surgical intervention in these patients are reviewed.

In patients with Down syndrome, adenotonsillectomy as part of an aggressive management protocol including tongue reduction, tongue hyoid advancement, UPPP, and maxillary or mandibular advancement demonstrated improvement in the postoperative apnea index, respiratory disturbance index, and LSAT.[58] One prospective study evaluated the age-related outcomes of soft tissue and skeletal sleep apnea surgery for infants and children with severe OSA refractory to conservative medical and surgical measures.[59] The diagnoses among these patients included cerebral palsy, Down syndrome, Pierre Robin syndrome, and other craniofacial anomalies. This study demonstrated that children over 36 months of age demonstrated significant improvement in the respiratory disturbance index, apnea index, and LSAT postoperatively, whereas only the respiratory disturbance index improved significantly in those between 12 and 36 months of age. For children under 12 months of age, although there was a trend toward improvement in respiratory indexes, these patients experienced longer hospital stays, a greater mean number of extubation attempts, and a higher surgical failure rate than the older patients. The importance of a multidisciplinary approach and soft tissue/skeletal surgeries with adenotonsillectomy has been shown in several studies of various patient groups, specifically those who had residual OSA after medical management and adenotonsillectomy. For 15 of the 18 patients with cerebral palsy and OSA, aggressive surgical treatment allowed sparing of tracheostomy as the definitive procedure for OSA.[58] This study reported a postoperative reduction in the apnea index, respiratory disturbance index, and LSAT, which were all statistically significant compared with the same parameters on preoperative PSG.

Uvulopalatopharyngoplasty

UPPP may be necessary in children with long uvulae and redundant pharyngeal soft tissue with or without adenotonsillar hypertrophy. This surgical procedure has been shown to be effective in patients with OSA who also have neurologic disorders.[60,61] This is a much more prevalent treatment option in adults, since long-term or severe sequelae such as a speech abnormality or VPI from uvulectomy and/or UPPP have not been adequately studied in the pediatric population. In children whose anterior and posterior tonsillar pillars are prominent after tonsillectomy, the surgeon may consider suture approximation of the two pillars to tighten redundant pharyngeal mucosa, which may contribute to the upper airway obstruction, at the time of the tonsillectomy. Uvulectomy may rarely be performed independent of UPPP in conjunction with the adenotonsillectomy if it is found to be significantly elongated or edematous. As in adult patients, the main complication to avoid in this procedure is the overly aggressive resection of the soft palate, leading to VPI.

Septoplasty, Turbinate Reduction, and/or Sinus Surgery

The aforementioned procedures are all aimed at improving only the nasal airway and are performed when appropriate and necessary. The pediatric nasal septum is mostly cartilaginous, and injudicious surgical intervention may have a negative impact on long-term facial growth. Nasal septal dislocation secondary to traumatic birth may occur in the neonate, and closed reduction may be effectively done at the bedside after prompt diagnosis. Otherwise, septoplasty for a deviated nasal septum is rarely performed in the pediatric population, with the exception

of individual consideration given to those who have significant internal nasal deformities causing obstruction most commonly associated with nasal septal traumatic fractures. In summary, nasal surgery for the treatment of OSA in the pediatric population is uncommon.

Hypopharyngeal Airway Expansion–Related Procedures

Such procedures include geniohyoid advancement/expansion, tongue reduction, lingual tonsillectomy, lingual suspension, sliding genioplasty, and maxillary/mandibular distraction. For the pediatric population, with their relatively smaller craniofacial dimensions, the most common alternative surgical technique of relevance is maxillary/mandibular advancement for those with maxillary/mandibular hypoplasia causing significant pharyngeal airway compromise. With the improvement of external and internal distraction devices, such procedures may be critical in relieving or improving OSA and provide the opportunity for the patient to avoid a tracheostomy altogether or facilitate successful decannulation of patients who had previously required tracheostomy to relieve severe upper airway obstruction.[62] Again, with the exception of maxillary and mandibular distraction techniques, the aforementioned procedures are more relevant for treating adults with residual OSA after standard procedures such as septoplasty and UPPP.

Tracheostomy

Tracheostomy remains the most reliable and significant long-term surgical intervention for OSA refractory to all other interventions. Tracheostomy enables the complete bypass of all levels of upper airway obstruction and allows the use of night-time supplemental oxygen or ventilatory support for those patients requiring it. Tracheostomy is indicated if patients cannot tolerate consistent and successful CPAP/BiPAP use or if documented OSA persists on PSG despite more conservative surgical procedures such as adenotonsillectomy and UPPP. Children who have associated craniofacial anomalies, severe neurologic impairment such as cerebral palsy, and/or chronic pulmonary disease may meet multiple criteria for tracheostomy. This procedure may be necessary at the time of or before pharyngeal or craniofacial surgery for airway protection, with subsequent decannulation after resolution of OSA as evaluated by PSG. The decision to perform tracheostomy is not taken lightly. Despite the best of tracheostomy care, there are associated complications including accidental decannulation, central apnea due to loss of hypoxic respiratory drive, and mucous plugging resulting in ventilatory insufficiency.[62] Tracheostomy involves long-term equipment cost and significant levels of education for all those involved in the care of the patient.

FOLLOW-UP

For patients whose symptoms of OSA do not resolve, those with an AHI of greater than 20 preoperatively, and those with medical comorbidity including persistent or worsening obesity, follow-up PSG is imperative. While residual, severe OSA may be found even in asymptomatic children who are otherwise healthy, it is much more likely in those with pre-existing neurologic impairment. The decision to perform long-term monitoring with intermittent PSG should be made based on the clinical symptoms and history of OSA severity and may be necessary because the recurrence of OSA is possible and risk factors leading to recurrent OSA have not been well studied.

References

1. Rosenfeld R, Green R: Tonsillectomy and adenoidectomy: Changing trends. Ann Otol Rhinol Laryngol 1990;99:187-191.
2. Arnold J, Allphin A: Sleep apnea in the neurologically-impaired child. Ear Nose Throat J 1993;72:80-81.
3. Kudoh F, Sanai A: Effect of tonsillectomy and adenoidectomy on obese children with sleep-associated breathing disorders. Acta Otolaryngol Suppl (Stockh) 1996;523:216-218.
4. Demain JG, Goetz DW: Pediatric adenoidal hypertrophy and nasal airway obstruction: Reduction with aqueous nasal beclomethasone. Pediatrics 1995;95:355-364.
5. Phipps CD, Wood WE, Gibson WS, et al: Gastroesophageal reflux contributing to chronic sinus disease in children: A prospective analysis. Arch Otolaryngol Head Neck Surg 2000;126:831-836.
6. Plaxico DT, Loughlin GM: Nasopharyngeal reflux and neonatal apnea. Am J Dis Child 1981;135:793-794.
7. Wei JL, Kasperbauer JL, Weaver AL, et al: Efficacy of single-dose dexamethasone as adjuvant therapy for acute pharyngitis. Laryngoscope 2002;112:87-93.
8. Sclafani AP, Ginsburg J, Shah MK, et al: Treatment of symptomatic chronic adenotonsillar hypertrophy with amoxicillin/clavulanate potassium: Short- and long-term results. Pediatrics 1998;101:675-681.
9. Al-Ghamdi SA, Manoukian JJ, Morielli A, et al: Do systemic corticosteroids effectively treat obstructive sleep apnea secondary to adenotonsillar hypertrophy? Laryngoscope 1997;107:1382-1387.
10. Goldstein NA, Sculerati N, Walsleben JA, et al: Clinical diagnosis of pediatric obstructive sleep apnea validated by polysomnography. Otolaryngol Head Neck Surg 1994;111:611-617.
11. Leach J, Olson J, Hermann J, et al: Polysomnographic and clinical findings in children with obstructive sleep apnea. Arch Otolaryngol Head Neck Surg 1992;118:741-744.
12. Nieminen P, Tolonen U, Lopponen H, et al: Snoring children: Factors predicting sleep apnea. Arch Otolaryngol Suppl 1997;529:190-194.
13. Suen J, Arnold J, Brooks L: Adenotonsillectomy for treatment of obstructive sleep apnea in children. Arch Otolaryngol Head Neck Surg 1995;121:525-530.
14. Wang RC, Elkin TP, Keech D, et al: Accuracy of clinical evaluation in pediatric obstructive sleep apnea. Otolaryngol Head Neck Surg 1998;118:69-73.
15. Ali N, Pitson D, Stradling J: Natural history of snoring and related behaviour problems between the ages of 4 and 7 years. Arch Dis Child 1991;71:74-76.
16. Marcus CL, Omlin KJ, Basinki DJ, et al: Normal polysomnographic values for children and adolescents. Am Rev Respir Dis 1992;146:1235-1239.
17. Eliaschar I, Lavie P, Halperin E, et al: Sleep apneic episodes as indications for adenotonsillectomy. Arch Otolaryngol 1980;106:492-496.
18. Guilleminault C, Pelayo R, Leger D, et al: Recognition of sleep-disordered breathing in children. Pediatrics 1996;98:871-882.
19. Potsic WP, Pasquariello PS, Baranak CC, et al: Relief of upper airway obstruction by adenotonsillectomy. Otolaryngol Head Neck Surg 1986;94:476-480.
20. Manning SC: Coagulation profile as a predictor for post-tonsillectomy and adenoidectomy (T + A) hemorrhage. Int J Pediatr Otorhinolaryngol 1995;32:261-263.
21. Koltai PJ, Solares CA, Mascha EJ, et al: Intracapsular partial tonsillectomy for tonsillar

hypertrophy in children. Laryngoscope 2002;112 (8 pt 2):17-19.

22. Wiatrak BJ, Willging JP: Harmonic scalpel for tonsillectomy. Laryngoscope 2002;112(8 pt 2):14-16.

23. Plant RL: Radiofrequency treatment of tonsillar hypertrophy. Laryngoscope 2002;112(8 Pt 2): 20-22.

24. Hulcrantz E, Linder A, Markstrom A: Tonsillectomy or tonsillotomy? A randomized study comparing postoperative pain and long-term effects. Int J Pediatr Otorhinolaryngol 1999;51:171-176.

25. Lassaletta L, Martin G, Villafruela MA, et al: Pediatric tonsillectomy: Post-operative morbidity comparing microsurgical bipolar dissection versus cold sharp dissection. Int J Pediatr Otorhinolaryngol 1997;41:307-317.

26. Linder A, Markstrom A, Hulcrantz E: Using the carbon dioxide laser for tonsillectomy in children. Int J Pediatr Otorhinolaryngol 1999;50:31-36.

27. Pizzuto MP, Brodsky L, Duffy L, et al: A comparison of microbipolar cautery dissection to hot knife and cold knife cautery tonsillectomy. Int J Pediatr Otorhinolaryngol 2000;52:239-246.

28. Smith PS, Orchard PJ, Lekas MD: Predicting bleeding in common ear, nose, and throat procedures: A prospective study. R I Med J 1990; 73:103-106.

29. Weimert TA, Babyak JW, Richter HJ: Electrodissection tonsillectomy. Arch Otolaryngol Head Neck Surg 1990;116:186-188.

30. Wexler DB: Recovery after tonsillectomy: Electrodissection vs. sharp dissection techniques. Otolaryngol Head Neck Surg 1996;114:576-581.

31. Wiatrak BJ, Myer CM, Andrews T: Complications of adenotonsillectomy in children under 3 years of age. Am J Otolaryngol 1991;12:170-172.

32. Steward DL, Welge JA, Myer CM: Do steroids reduce morbidity of tonsillectomy? Meta-analysis of randomized trials. Laryngoscope 2001;111: 1712-1718.

33. Tom LW, Templeton JJ, Thompson ME, et al: Dexamethasone in adenotonsillectomy. Int J Pediatr Otorhinolaryngol 1996;37:115-120.

34. Colclasure JB, Graham SS: Complication of outpatient tonsillectomy and adenoidectomy: A review of 3,340 cases. Ear Nose Throat J 1990;69:155-60.

35. Gabalski EC, Mattucci KF, Setzen M, et al: Ambulatory tonsillectomy and adenoidectomy. Laryngoscope 1996;106(1 pt 1):77-80.

36. Lalakea ML, Marquez-Biggs I, Messner AH: Safety of pediatric short-stay tonsillectomy. Arch Otolaryngol Head Neck Surg 1999;125:749-752.

37. Nicklaus PJ, Herzon FS, Steinle EW IV: Short-stay outpatient tonsillectomy. Arch Otolaryngol Head Neck Surg 1995;121:521-524.

38. Postma DS, Folsom F: The case for an outpatient "approach" for all pediatric tonsillectomies and/or adenoidectomies: A 4-year review of 1419 cases at a community hospital. Otolaryngol Head Neck Surg. 2002;127:101-108.

39. Reiner SA, Sawyer WP, Clark KF, et al: Safety of outpatient tonsillectomy and adenoidectomy. Otolaryngol Head Neck Surg. 1990;102:161-168.

40. Rothschild MA, Catalano P, Biller HF: Ambulatory pediatric tonsillectomy and the identification of high-risk subgroups. Otolaryngol Head Neck Surg 1994;110:203-210.

41. McColley S, April M, Carroll J, et al: Respiratory compromise after adenotonsillectomy in children with obstructive sleep apnea. Arch Otolaryngol Head Neck Surg 1992;118:940-943.

42. Bower C, Richmond D: Tonsillectomy and adenoidectomy in patients with Down syndrome. Int J Pediatr Otorhinolaryngol 1995;33:141-148.

43. Rosen GM, Muckle RP, Mahowald MW, et al: Postoperative respiratory compromise in children with obstructive sleep apnea syndrome: Can it be anticipated? Pediatrics 1994;93:784-788.

44. Gerber ME, O'Connor DM, Adler E, et al: Selected risk factors in pediatric adenotonsillectomy. Arch Otolaryngol Head Neck Surg 1996;122:811-814.

45. Tom L, DeDio R, Cohen D, et al: Is outpatient tonsillectomy appropriate for young children? Laryngoscope 1992;102:277-280.

46. St. Charles CS, Matt BH, Hamilton MM, et al: A comparison of ibuprofen versus acetaminophen with codeine in the young tonsillectomy patient. Otolaryngol Head Neck Surg 1997;117:76-82.

47. Moir MS, Bair E, Shinnick P, et al: Acetaminophen versus acetaminophen with codeine after pediatric tonsillectomy. Laryngoscope 2000;110: 1824-1827.

48. Johnson LB, Elluru RG, Myer CM: Complications of adenotonsillectomy. Laryngoscope 2002;112 (8 pt 2):35-36.

49. Wei JL, Beatty CW, Gustafson RO: Evaluation of posttonsillectomy hemorrhage and risk factors. Otolaryngol Head Neck Surg 2000;123:229-235.

50. McDonald TJ, Devine KD, Hayles AB: Nasopharyngeal stenosis following tonsillectomy and adenoidectomy: Report of six cases and their repair. Arch Otolaryngol 1973;98:39-41.

51. Frank Y, Kravath RE, Pollak CP, et al: Obstructive sleep apnea and its therapy: Clinical and polysomnographic manifestations. Pediatrics 1983;71:737-742.

52. Helfaer MA, McColley SA, Pyzik PL, et al: Polysomnography after adenotonsillectomy in mild pediatric obstructive sleep apnea. Crit Care Med 1996;24:1323-1327.

53. Wiet GJ, Bower C, Seibert R, et al: Surgical correction of obstructive sleep apnea in the complicated pediatric patient documented by polysomnography. Int J Pediatr Otorhinolaryngol 1997;41:133-143.

54. Nishimura T, Morishima N, Hasegawa S, et al: Effect of surgery on obstructive sleep apnea. Acta Otolaryngol Suppl (Stockh) 1996;523:231-233.

55. Shintani T, Asakura K, Kataura A: The effect of adenotonsillectomy in children with OSA. Int J Pediatr Otorhinolaryngol 1998;44:51-58.

56. Gorur K, Doven O, Unal M, et al: Preoperative and postoperative cardiac and clinical findings of patients with adenotonsillar hypertrophy. Int J Pediatr Otorhinolaryngol. 2001;59:41-46.

57. Grundfast K, Berkowitz R, Fox L: Outcome and complications following surgery for obstructive adenotonsillar hypertrophy in children with neuromuscular disorders. Ear Nose Throat J 1990; 69:756, 759-760.

58. Cohen SR, Lefaivre JF, Burstein FD, et al: Surgical treatment of obstructive sleep apnea in neurologically compromised patients. Plast Reconstr Surg 1997;99:638-646.

59. Januszkiewicz JS, Cohen SR, Burstein FD, et al: Age-related outcomes of sleep apnea surgery in infants and children. Ann Plast Surg 1997;38: 465-477.

60. Derkay CS, Maddern BR: Innovative techniques for adenotonsillar surgery in children: Introduction and commentary. Laryngoscope 2002;112(8 pt 2):2.

61. Kosko J, Derkay C: Uvulopalatopharyngoplasty: Treatment of obstructive sleep apnea in neurologically impaired pediatric patients. Int J Pediatr Otorhinolaryngol 1995;32:241-246.

62. Cohen SR, Suzman K, Simms C, et al: Sleep apnea surgery versus tracheostomy in children: An exploratory study of the comparative effects on quality of life. Plast Reconstr Surg 1998;102: 1855-1864.

Primary Snoring in Children

Susanna A. McColley

23

PRIMARY SNORING

Primary snoring (PS) describes nightly or frequent snoring that is not associated with apnea, hypoventilation, or sleep fragmentation.[1] By definition, the diagnosis is made by polysomnography, with objective measurement of sleep and respiratory function. These criteria differentiate PS from obstructive sleep apnea syndrome (OSAS), which is associated with various degrees of hypoxemia, hypercapnia, and sleep fragmentation related to complete or partial upper airway obstructive events.

Clinical history alone cannot differentiate PS from OSAS.[2] In a study of 83 snoring children referred to a tertiary pediatric sleep clinic, parents completed a standardized, nurse-administered questionnaire that asked questions regarding snoring frequency, observed apnea, struggling to breathe, and other daytime and nighttime symptoms. Children then underwent nocturnal polysomnography to assess for sleep-disordered breathing. Although there were several differences in symptom frequencies between the children with PS and those with OSAS, both single and multiple questions showed poor sensitivity and specificity in discriminating between PS and OSAS.

UPPER AIRWAY RESISTANCE SYNDROME

Although PS is a polysomnographic diagnosis, a diagnosis of PS suggests that no adverse sleep-related or daytime sequelae are associated with snoring in the absence of gas exchange abnormalities or abnormal sleep architecture. In other words, some children with snoring have no interruption of normal sleep patterns, no cardiorespiratory compromise, and no neuropsychological morbidity. It follows that no treatment is required. Because snoring is common, affecting approximately 10% of children and up to 40% of adults, the presence of snoring without adverse consequences is likely to occur. However, discussion of PS as a distinct diagnosis is complicated by the emergence of the upper airway resistance syndrome (UARS) as a distinct clinical entity.

UARS is defined as partial upper airway obstruction that is not associated with gas exchange abnormalities but is accompanied by increased respiratory effort (conventionally measured by changes in intrathoracic pressure via esophageal manometry) terminated by electroencephalographic arousal; the primary symptom in adults is daytime somnolence.[3] Snoring occurs in most affected individuals, but physiologic findings of UARS have been noted in patients without snoring, especially in those who have had palatal surgery for upper airway obstruction. UARS is associated with increased upper airway collapsibility during sleep.[4] Guilleminault and colleagues initially reported the clinical and polysomnographic characteristics of UARS in 25 children who were referred for evaluation of snoring, excessive daytime somnolence, and behavioral problems.[5] They demonstrated marked differences in the referred group compared to 25 healthy control children. Subsequently, numerous studies have demonstrated these polysomnographic findings in adults with daytime somnolence. Daytime somnolence is significantly improved with nasal continuous positive airway pressure therapy, as objectively measured by the multiple sleep latency test.[3]

In adults, excessive daytime somnolence has a number of significant sequelae, including an increased risk of motor vehicle and work-related accidents and impaired mood. Hypertension is also frequently seen in adults with UARS. Children identified as having UARS have a variety of daytime symptoms, including symptoms of attention deficit hyperactivity disorder and academic problems. Most studies of snoring children have not defined or described UARS as a clinical entity separate from OSAS or PS, and many have not performed detailed physiologic recording. However, many studies have suggested significant neurocognitive abnormalities in habitually snoring children,[6-8] including attention deficit hyperactivity disorder, academic problems, and behavioral problems. Available data do not allow clear separation between patients with UARS and those with OSAS.

Although sleep physiologists often view sleep-disordered breathing as a spectrum, with primary snoring being the mildest and OSAS the most severe form,[1] no studies demonstrate a clear relationship between the degree of sleep-disordered breathing and symptoms or physiologic sequelae. Furthermore, although the diagnosis of primary snoring has traditionally been made on the basis of polysomnographic findings alone, the available evidence suggests that absence of daytime symptoms should be an additional diagnostic criterion.

EPIDEMIOLOGY

A number of epidemiologic studies from diverse geographic locations have been published describing the prevalence of snoring in children. Most of these have utilized parental report via either questionnaire or interview format. Most have not included objective measurements of respiration during sleep, or they have included such measures only in a subset of children felt to be at high risk for OSAS.

A summary of epidemiologic studies of snoring in children is presented in Table 23–1. The prevalence of habitual snoring ranges from a minimum of 3.2% in Iceland to a maximum of 12.1% in England. This contrasts with the 40% frequency of regular snoring in adults. Studies that have attempted to identify a subgroup of children with OSAS show a prevalence of this disorder of between 0.7% and 2.9%. None of these epidemiologic studies have attempted to distinguish UARS from PS. Rosen[19] studied 326 otherwise healthy children with snoring. Fifty-nine percent of children had OSAS, 25% had PS, 6% had UARS, and 10% had no snoring. It is notable that 28% of the children in the study were obese.

NATURAL HISTORY

Limited data are available regarding the natural history of primary snoring in children. Marcus and coworkers[20] repeated polysomnography in 20 children 1 to 3 years after the initial diagnosis of PS; none had undergone airway surgery. All of these children had persistent snoring; in 20%, snoring had increased, and in 70% there was no change. Overall, there was no change in apnea index, oxyhemoglobin saturation, or peak end-tidal P_{CO_2}. However, two children had mild OSAS on repeat testing. The authors concluded that most children with PS do not progress to having OSAS, and those who do progress have only mild OSAS. Daytime symptoms in persistently snoring children were not reported.

Topol and Brooks[21] studied nine children with primary snoring 3 years after initial polysomnographic diagnosis of PS; a control group of nine age-matched, nonsnoring subjects were also studied for comparison. As in the study by Marcus and colleagues, there was no overall change in respiratory parameters between the first and second polysomnograms; one snoring subject had significant worsening of the respiratory disturbance index. Interestingly, the control group had significantly better sleep efficiency and fewer brief arousals than the snoring group, which suggests that some of the children with PS may actually have been affected by UARS.

DIAGNOSIS

History and Physical Examination

A sleep history that includes a question regarding nocturnal snoring should be included in health maintenance or well child care visits.[22] The hallmark of primary snoring is nightly or near-nightly snoring without physiologic or neurocognitive consequences. Once a history of habitual snoring is elicited, further history taking and a physical examination serve to assess sleep-related or daytime symptoms that may be associated with significant upper airway obstruction during sleep. Children who have numerous episodes of observed obstructive apnea, daytime somnolence, and problems with behavior, attention, or school performance require prompt referral for diagnostic testing and treatment for OSAS or UARS.

Table 23–1. Epidemiology of Snoring in Children

First Author (Year)	Number (Age Range)	Country	Methods*	Habitual Snoring† Prevalence	OSAS Prevalence
Ali (1993)[9]	782 (4-5 yr)	England	Postal questionnaire; home overnight video and oximetry in a subset of "high risk" and control	12.1%	0.7%
Ali (1994)[10]	504 (6-7 yr)	England	Follow-up study of children in preceding study; repeat postal questionnaire only	11.4%	Not examined
Gislason (1995)[11]	454 (6 mo-6 yr)	Iceland	Postal questionnaire; overnight respiratory monitoring in children suspected of having sleep apnea	3.2%	2.9%
Teculescu (1992)[12]	190 (5-6.4 yr)	France	Interview questionnaire	10%	Not examined
Corbo (1989)[13]	1615 (6-13 yr)	Italy	Self-administered questionnaire	7.3%	Not examined
Corbo (2001)[14]	2209 (10-15 yr)	Italy	Self-administered questionnaire	5.6%	Not examined
Hultcrantz (1995)[15]	500 (4 yr)	Sweden	Interview; PSG in children with habitual snoring	6.2%	Data incomplete
Smedje (1999)[16]	1844 (5-7 yr)	Sweden	Self-administered questionnaire	7.7%	Not examined
Anuntaseree (2001)[17]	1008 (6-13 yr)	Thailand	Self-administered questionnaire; PSG in patients snoring "most nights"	8.5%	0.7%
Ferreira (2000)[18]	976 (6-11 yr)	Portugal	Self-administered questionnaire	8.6%	Not examined

*All questionnaire and interview data were obtained from parents.
†Habitual snoring is defined as frequent or nightly snoring, or snoring at least 3 nights per week, in the absence of upper respiratory infection.
OSAS, obstructive sleep apnea syndrome; PSG, polysomnography.

The physical examination may be normal, or it may reveal signs of upper airway obstruction such as mouth breathing and tonsillar hypertrophy. Dolichocephaly and midface hypoplasia are associated with snoring and OSAS. Obesity appears to be a predisposing factor in both snoring and OSAS, whereas growth failure may signify severe sleep-disordered breathing.

Nocturnal Polysomnography

Primary snoring is defined by polysomnographic criteria. To differentiate PS from OSAS or UARS, it is important to carefully evaluate sleep staging and the frequency of electroencephalographic arousals. Normal polysomnographic findings, including the absence of increased arousal frequency or abnormal tachypnea during sleep, suggest PS. Although the gold standard for diagnosis of UARS is measurement of esophageal pressure, this technique is invasive. Other techniques have been evaluated but are not in widespread clinical use. Therefore, an otherwise asymptomatic child with snoring and a normal polysomnogram can be assumed to have PS. On the other hand, a child with normal polysomnographic findings and abnormal symptoms may have UARS, and treatment should be considered.

TREATMENT

By definition, primary snoring requires no specific treatment. Because of the rare progression from primary snoring to OSAS, children should be monitored clinically and reevaluated if symptoms increase over time. Because pediatric sleep-disordered breathing is a spectrum, individual treatment decisions must be based on individual symptoms and physical findings, not on polysomnographic findings alone.

FUTURE DIRECTIONS

Further studies of snoring in children are needed. The wide variability in published prevalence may be secondary to the influence of ethnicity and environment in different populations; further definition of prevalence differences would be useful in identifying patients at risk and in public health policy decisions. Better definition of the clinical consequences of snoring, and specific comparisons between patients with PS and those with UARS, are needed. Longer-term natural history studies are essential, including health and functional outcomes in adolescents and adults who had childhood snoring.

References

1. Greene MG, Carroll JL: Consequences of sleep-disordered breathing in childhood. Curr Opin Pulm Med 1997;3:456-463.
2. Carroll JL, McColley SA, Marcus CL, et al: Inability of clinical history to distinguish primary snoring from obstructive sleep apnea syndrome. Chest 1995;108:610-618.
3. Exar EN, Collop NA: The upper airway resistance syndrome. Chest 1999;115:1127-1139.
4. Gold AR, Marcus CL, Dipalo F, Gold MS: Upper airway collapsibility during sleep in upper airway resistance syndrome. Chest 2002;121:1531-1540.
5. Guilleminault C, Winkle R, Korobkin R, Simmons B: Children and nocturnal snoring: Evaluation of the effects of sleep related respiratory resistive load and daytime functioning. Eur J Pediatr 1982;139:165-171.
6. Chervin R, Dillon J, Bassetti C, et al: Symptoms of sleep disorders, inattention, and hyperactivity in children. Sleep 1997;20:1185-1192.
7. Gozal D: Sleep-disordered breathing and school performance in children. Pediatrics 1998;102:616-620.
8. Gozal D, Pope DW: Snoring during early childhood and academic performance at ages thirteen to fourteen years. Pediatrics 2001;107:1394-1399.
9. Ali NJ, Pitson DJ, Stradling JR: Snoring, sleep disturbance, and behaviour in 4-5 year olds. Arch Dis Child 1993;68:360-366.
10. Ali NJ, Pitson D, Stradling JR: Natural history of snoring and related behaviour problems between the ages of 4 and 7 years. Arch Dis Child 1994;71:74-76.
11. Gislason T, Benediktsdottir B: Snoring, apneic episodes and nocturnal hypoxemia among children 6 months to 6 years old. Chest 1995;107:963-966.
12. Teculescu D, Caillier I, Perrin P, et al: Snoring in French preschool children. Pediatr Pulmonol 1992;13:239-244.
13. Corbo GM, Fuciarelli F, Foresi A, De Benedetto F: Snoring in children: association with respiratory symptoms and passive smoke. BMJ 1989;299:1491-1494.
14. Corbo G, Forastiere F, Agabiti N, et al: Snoring in 9- to 15-year-old children: Risk factors and clinical relevance. Pediatrics 2001;108:1149-1154.
15. Hultcrantz E, Lofstrand-Tidestrom B, Ahlquist-Rastad J: The epidemiology of sleep related breathing disorder in children. Int J Pediatr Otorhinolaryngol 1995;32(Suppl):S63-S66.

16. Smedje H, Broman J-E, Hetta J: Parents' reports of disturbed sleep in 5-7-year-old Swedish children. Acta Paediatr 1999;88:858-865.

17. Anuntaseree W, Rookkapan K, Kuasirikul S, Thongsuksai P: Snoring and obstructive sleep apnea in Thai school-age children: Prevalence and predisposing factors. Pediatr Pulmonol 2001;32:222-227.

18. Ferreira AM, Clemente V, Gozal D, et al: Snoring in Portuguese primary school children. Pediatrics 2000;106(5). Available at http://www.pediatrics.org/cgi/content/full/106/5/e64.

19. Rosen CL: Clinical features of obstructive sleep apnea in otherwise healthy children. Pediatr Pulmonol 1999;27:403-409.

20. Marcus CL, Hamer A, Loughlin GM: Natural history of primary snoring in children. Pediatr Pulmonol 1998;26:6-11.

21. Topol HI, Brooks LJ: Follow-up of primary snoring in children. J Pediatr 2001;138:291-293.

22. Section on Pediatric Pulmonology, Subcommittee on Obstructive Sleep Apnea Syndrome: Clinical practice guideline: Diagnosis and management of childhood obstructive sleep apnea syndrome. Pediatrics 2002;109:704-712.

Sleep in Neurologic Disorders

Stephen H. Sheldon
Daniel G. Glaze

24

Disorders of the brain are often associated with severe sleep disturbances. Frequently, children with neurologic disabilities experience chronic sleep–wake problems related to circadian timing of sleep, sleep-related seizure disorders, sleep-related movement disorders, and sleep-related breathing disorders. Many respond poorly to traditional therapeutic intervention. Established treatments include behavioral management, chronotherapy, phototherapy, faded response-cost programs, sedatives, hypnotics, and antidepressants. These are often unsuccessful in the youngster with a chronic disabling condition of the central nervous system (CNS). Some therapeutic approaches may even exacerbate symptoms or result in respite for only a few days.

Patients present with symptoms that may include profound sleep onset difficulties at desired bedtimes, inability to consolidate sleep, inability to maintain sleep, irregular sleep–wake schedules, rapidly changing sleep–wake schedules, obstructive sleep apnea syndrome, problems with central control of breathing, seizures, movement disorders, and arousal disorders. Presence of multiple symptoms is the rule rather than exception. Sleep deprivation and fragmentation of sleep continuity occur, and considerable performance problems, as well as delay in the response to rehabilitative efforts, can result. Interestingly, these disorders of sleep and the sleep–wake cycle not only deeply affect the patient and his/her quality of life but commonly result in sleep disturbances and decreased quality of life for the entire family.

CORRELATES OF CENTRAL NERVOUS SYSTEM DEVELOPMENT

The CNS is the principal organ system governing sleep, sleep's components, and the sleep–wake cycle. Major CNS alterations occur throughout fetal life, neonatal life, infancy, and childhood. Understanding these changes is essential in assessing the patient with CNS dysfunction during wakefulness and during sleep. Indeed, a comprehensive awareness of maturational changes during sleep may provide insight into management.

Genetic and environmental factors are important in determining morphologic and electrophysiologic development of the CNS. Differentiation begins very early in the evolution of the embryo, with a thickening of the dorsal ectoderm into the neural plate. The cells in this single layer rapidly increase in number and stratify, and two folds and a neural groove develop. This central groove fuses to become the neural tube, giving rise to the substance of all neural elements whose cell bodies and supporting elements lie within the brain and spinal cord.[1]

During regional differentiation of the CNS, structural flexure begins. Three regions can be identified: cephalic flexure (region of the midbrain), cervical flexure (junction of the brain and spinal cord), and pontine flexure (junction of the metencephalon and myelencephalon). The lumen of the neural tube undergoes dramatic changes during this period of development that correspond to regional specialization. The lumen in the area of the telencephalon will ultimately become the lateral ventricles. The lumen within the telencephalon and diencephalon will become the third ventricle. The cerebral aqueduct develops from the lumen in the mesencephalon. The lumen of the metencephalon and myelencephalon becomes the fourth ventricle.

Neuronal activity appears to be important in the migration of neurons to appropriate positions within the CNS, the degree of dendritic branching, and the strength of synaptic interconnections.[2] Mitosis and migration continue throughout development, and completion of the

269

location of individual neurons occurs about 1 year after postconception term. Two internal processes result in a high degree of neuronal activity: the waking state and active (rapid eye movement [REM]) sleep. It is possible that these two states are important during prenatal and early postnatal life for appropriate ultrastructural development of the CNS.

Centers responsible for control of sleep and the sleep–wake cycles are contained in areas that develop from the diencephalon. Appropriate diencephalic maturation is essential for normal sleep to occur. All neuronal activity that eventually reaches the cortex passes through the diencephalon, with the sole exception of those originating from olfaction. The third ventricle is contained within the diencephalon. During the seventh week of development, a small evagination appears from the caudal wall of the third ventricle. This eventually becomes glandular and forms the pineal body that is responsible for secretion of melatonin.

Melatonin plays an important role in regulating the sleep–wake cycle, presumably through entrainment to light–dark cycling. Secretion is highly responsive to afferent neural activity via the retinohypothalamic tract. Secretion increases in a dark environment and decreases when the retinas are exposed to light. Although data regarding the function of melatonin are conflicting, evidence exists that it affects the timing of sleep through its effect on circadian organization.[3] Exogenous melatonin has been noted to be useful in regulating sleep in children with some sleep disorders[4] and in improving sleep in some neurologically handicapped children.[5] It seems likely, therefore, that disorders of development of the diencephalon, as well as acquired disorders that affect development or function of cells in the caudal wall of the third ventricle, can result in significant sleep–wake disorders.

After the seventh postconception week, thalamic regions undergo differentiation, and neuronal fibers separate the massive gray matter of the walls of the thalamus into numerous thalamic nuclei. Similarly, the wall of the hypothalamus contains hypothalamic nuclei, the optic chiasm, the suprachiasmatic nucleus, and the neural lobe of the stalk of the body of the pituitary gland. The hypothalamus eventually becomes the executive region for regulation of all autonomic activity including core body temperature, temperature regulation, and sleep. Because the suprachiasmatic nucleus becomes the governing region for the circadian timing of many major physiologic functions (the biological clock), it seems clear that dysfunctional development of, or injury to, the ventral region of the diencephalon can result in profound symptoms related to the sleep–wake cycle.

The cerebral hemispheres become prominent during the sixth postconception week. They expand rapidly until they cover the diencephalon and mesencephalon. The telencephalon becomes the most specialized and complex portion of the brain and can be quite sensitive to changes in intrauterine environment. In the presence of decreased neuronal electrical activity secondary to hypoxemia from any cause, abnormal concentrations of cellular elements, decreased dendritic branching, and a lack of the synaptic strength needed to develop essential and mature neural networks may result.

DISORDERS OF MATURATIONAL DEVELOPMENT

Culebras[6] has comprehensively described neuroanatomic and neurologic correlates of a wide variety of sleep abnormalities. Lesions of the medial mesencephalon almost invariably cause a reduction in the level of alertness. Symptomatic cataplexy, characterized by active inhibition of skeletal muscle tone, has been described in patients with rostral brainstem tumors that invade the floor of the third ventricle.[7] Disorders of the lower mesencephalon and upper pons tegmentum involving the region around the locus ceruleus are responsible for symptoms of REM sleep without atonia.[8] Extensive pontine tegmental lesions cause a reduction in total sleep time, alterations in or abolition of non-REM (NREM) sleep states and REM sleep, and paralysis of lateral gaze.[9]

Disorders involving the medullary regions of the CNS commonly affect respiratory centers. A wide variety of sleep-related breathing problems are seen in youngsters with Arnold-Chiari malformation.[10,11] Central apnea, increased periodic breathing during REM and NREM sleep, central hypoventilation syndrome, and prolonged expiratory apneas can occur. If motor centers controlling pharyngeal musculature are involved, obstructive sleep apnea may also be present.

Many other correlations can be identified. Hypothalamic lesions have been associated with hypersomnia. Diffuse lesions of the thalamus lead to either ipsilateral decrease or complete abolition of sleep spindles and represent a useful electrographic sign of thalamic abnormalities.[12] The cerebral hemispheres, although not primordial in the generation or maintenance of NREM and REM sleep, do have a modulating influence. Patients with extensive cortical laminar necrosis fail to exhibit slow waves or spindles during NREM sleep but can express cortical desynchronization during REM sleep.[13] Finally, space-occupying lesions of the CNS may cause sleep–wake disturbances or specific sleep disorders by virtue of their location. They may also cause symptoms indirectly through the development of increased intracranial pressure, hydrocephalus, or both.

POLYSOMNOGRAPHIC CORRELATES

The clinical discipline of pediatric sleep medicine and the study of sleep disorders in infants and children are becoming increasingly focused on brain dysfunction. Study of the sleeping brain has been termed by Culebras as "neurosomnology."[14] The physiologic functions of most other organ systems differ significantly from the waking state, and there are clear ontogenetic changes that occur in sleep and its structure. Studying longitudinal changes of multiple physiologic variables during sleep in the laboratory might be termed developmental polysomnography.[15] Evaluation of maturation of sleep within the context of normal and abnormal human development might provide a sensitive method of analysis.

It has been shown that electroencephalography (EEG) is an excellent tool for measuring brain maturation.[16] Each conceptional age reveals a characteristic pattern. The important features of normal EEG ontogeny, therefore, tend to reflect normal development. An apparent delay of the appearance of these EEG patterns might reflect an arrest or a delay in maturation of the CNS. It has been proposed that close attention to stages of brain maturation in normal and abnormal EEGs, as well as the normal progression of state development during sleep, might allow more accurate timing of brain insult in infants with neurologic sequelae.

Comprehensive polysomnography utilizing an EEG array that provides greater detail than the standard montage recommended for adult polysomnography is recommended for the neonatal and pediatric patient. However, diagnosing ontogenetic EEG variations must be performed with caution, as abnormalities in the EEG reflect general pathophysiologic processes but show little specificity for any particular disease.[17]

Other polysomnographic variables can be important in the assessment of developmental maturation. Adding eye movement recordings and electromyography to the EEG might improve specificity. Recording of eye movements during sleep helps to identify the sleep state. Eye movement density and bursts of saccades may hold special significance in prediction of mental development and morbidity secondary to neonatal illness. Becker and Thoman[18] evaluated the occurrence of REM storms in newborn infants and again at 3, 6, and 12 months of chronologic age. The number of rapid eye movements within each 10-second interval of active sleep was rated on a scale based on the frequency and intensity of the eye movements. Bayley scales of mental development were administered to the cohort of infants at 12 months of age. Interestingly, a significant negative correlation was found between the frequency of REM storms and Bayley scores. By 6 months of age, REM storms seemed to express dysfunction or delay in the development of central inhibitory feedback control for sleep organization and phasic sleep-related activities.

The degree of phasic electromyographic activity during sleep may also reflect maturity of the developing brainstem. Gross movements, localized body movements, and phasic muscle activity are controlled by the CNS at different organizational levels. Phasic motor activity is ontogenetically simpler and decreases early during development. Gross movements are quite complex and require a greater degree of central integration. The type and frequency of muscle activity during sleep might, therefore, add to information about the integrity of the CNS. Hakamada and coworkers[19] studied various types of motor activity in term newborns with significant illnesses. Generalized body movements, localized tonic movements, and generalized phasic movements were evaluated. Patients with minimally depressed EEG background activity showed an increase in generalized movements and localized tonic movements during quiet sleep. In contrast, patients with markedly severe EEG abnormalities showed an increase in phasic movements. It was concluded that a significant decrease in generalized body movements, or an increase in generalized phasic muscle activity, might indicate a poor prognosis for particular infants. However, the presence of even small amounts of localized tonic movements suggest preservation of cortical function. Nonetheless, diagnostic use of polysomnography and its components becomes most cost effective when applied to specific problems.

SLEEP DISORDERS IN INFANTS AND CHILDREN

Sleep disorders that occur in adults also occur in children. Disorders of sleep and the sleep–wake cycle differ from adult disorders in etiology, pathophysiology, morbidity, and treatment. Indeed, symptomatology can be dramatically different, and childhood sleep disorders are frequently overlooked or overshadowed by clinical problems that appear and are evaluated during the day. It must be remembered that disordered sleep can underlie meaningful daytime symptoms and can exacerbate other medical disorders.

There is often considerable delay in diagnosing disordered sleep in the neonate, infant, or child. Brouillette and colleagues[20] described significant delays in the diagnosis of sleep disordered breathing and demonstrated profound morbidity. In 22 patients with documented obstructive sleep apnea, mean delay in referral for 20 patients first evaluated after the neonatal period was 23 ± 15 months. Almost three quarters of the patients studied developed serious sequelae including cor pulmonale, failure to thrive, permanent neurologic deficits, behavioral disturbances, hypersomnolence, and developmental abnormalities.

The following paragraphs discuss common primary sleep-related disorders in children. These include obstructive sleep apnea, central sleep apnea, and other breathing disorders that occur during sleep, sleep-related seizures, partial arousal disorders, movement disorders associated with sleep, and sleep–wake schedule disorders. Focus is placed on clinical presentation, laboratory diagnosis, and management considerations.

Sleep-Disordered Breathing in Infants and Children

Eight types of respiratory pauses or respiratory dysfunction during sleep can be described. The clinical significance of each varies according to the conceptional age of the youngster, the developmental status, and the presence of other medical or congenital abnormalities. Respiratory pauses include obstructive apnea, central apnea, mixed apnea, expiratory apnea, post-sigh apnea, and periodic breathing. Central hypoventilation and obstructive hypoventilation may not be associated with pauses in breathing but may significantly affect ventilatory function.

An obstructive apnea is defined as an absence of nasal and oral airflow from the nose and mouth despite continuing chest and/or abdominal effort (Fig. 24–1). Lack of airflow may be brief, lasting 6 seconds or less, depending on the rate of respiration. If there are at least two obstructed respiratory efforts, the apnea may be clinically significant. Obstructive apnea can be prolonged and associated with cardiac deceleration (generally occurring during the last third of the apnea), oxygen desaturation, and elevation of end-tidal CO_2 ($E_T co_2$) after airflow resumes.

Definition of central apnea varies according to the age of the patient. In premature and very young infants, central apnea is defined as absence of nasal and oral airflow *and* respiratory efforts lasting 20 seconds or longer. It may also be clinically significant if shorter than 20 seconds but associated with heart rate changes or oxygen desaturation (Fig. 24–2). Prolonged central apnea, related to an absence of both inspiratory and expiratory neuronal activity, appears to be quite unusual in otherwise normal infants and children during NREM/quiet sleep. Brief central apnea is normal during REM/active sleep. When prolonged central apneas occur during quiet sleep, central hypoventilation syndrome or a primary underlying central nervous system or brainstem abnormality may be present.

Mixed apnea contains polysomnographic components of both central and obstructive respiratory pauses (Fig. 24–3). There is some evidence, however, that the "central" component of a mixed apnea is either prolonged expiration or an expiratory apnea.[21] It may also represent a combination of both.

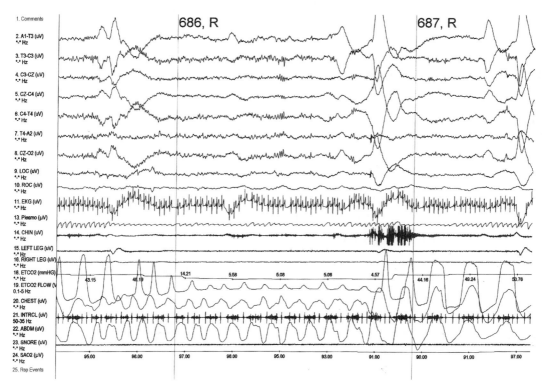

Figure 24–1. This 60-second epoch demonstrates a prolonged obstructive apnea during REM sleep. Note the significant decrease in airflow (>50% reduction) in the end-tidal carbon dioxide ($E_T co_2$) flow channel (19). There is continued and increasing respiratory effort in the chest and abdominal channels (20 and 22) and continued intercostal electromyographic activity (21). After the event, there is an arousal and a return to normal respiration. Note the shift in the phase angle of chest and abdomen prior to the apnea, during the apnea, and after the apnea. During the apnea, effort shifts 180 degrees, and paradoxical breathing can be noted. There is mild oxygen desaturation with spontaneous and rapid return to oxygen saturation baseline. There is also a mild elevation of the $E_T co_2$ during recovery breathing after the event. Numbers in parentheses indicate channels in the figure.

Expiratory apnea has received little attention in the medical literature. It is defined as an absence of polysomnographically recorded nasal and oral airflow in the presence of continued expiratory effort against an occluded or partially obstructed upper airway. A prolonged expiratory phase of breathing can be demonstrated (Fig. 24–4). Almost all expiratory apneas are preceded by an augmented breath, or a sigh.[22] Upper airway occlusion may occur at any level, from the nasopharynx to the larynx. Preliminary evidence in some children indicates that a reflex glottic adduction may occur in the presence of continued diaphragmatic contraction. Increased parasympathetic tone may be present, affecting the diaphragm via the vagus nerve and increas-

ing vocal cord adduction via the recurrent laryngeal nerve. A significant fall in the heart rate seems to occur during the first third of the respiratory pause in a manner similar to that seen during the Valsalva maneuver. There is little change in the arterial oxygen saturation (Sao_2) regardless of the length of the apnea. This might be explained by a temporary increase in lung volume and positive expiratory pressure. The potential importance of recognizing expiratory apnea is evident when assessing apnea or bradycardia during home monitoring of the infant, as well as in some patients with underlying CNS and autonomic nervous system abnormalities.

Although expiratory apneas are typically preceded by a sigh, post-sigh apneas seem to be

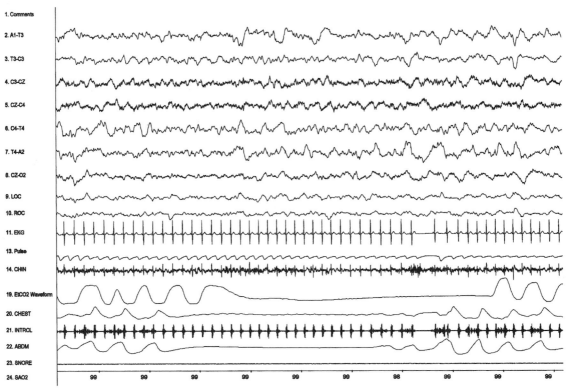

Figure 24–2. Central apnea with a sinus pause noted in the electrocardiogram (EKG). In this 30-second epoch recorded during non-REM slow-wave sleep, a somewhat prolonged central apnea is noted. Air ceases, and there is also cessation of effort demonstrated in the chest, intercostal electromyography, and abdominal effort channels. Note that airflow on this tracing was measured using an end-tidal carbon dioxide ($E_T CO_2$) waveform. Because a side-stream method of analysis is required (with the sampling chamber in the instrument rather than directly in the air stream as seen in main-stream analysis), there is about a 3-second sampling delay. Effort seems to stop before flow stops, and effort begins before flow begins. This is artifact secondary to this sampling delay in $E_T CO_2$ waveform, and the apnea is central rather than mixed. Note the 1.5-second sinus pause in the EKG at the end of the event. Oxygen desaturation did not occur during this respiratory pause.

associated with little or no upper airway obstruction (Fig. 24–5). An augmented breath is followed by an apnea that appears to be central. There is little change in heart rate, almost no oxygen desaturation, and an absence of hypercarbia during and after the event. In certain cases, continued rise in $E_T CO_2$ can be demonstrated. Identification of these respiratory pauses is also important in evaluating infants with apnea and in follow-up of infants being monitored at home.

Periodic breathing is a pattern of respiration characterized by three or more respiratory pauses of 3 seconds or longer, separated by normal breathing for less than 20 seconds.[23] Periodic breathing is a normal pattern of respiration in premature infants during active/REM and quiet/NREM sleep (Fig. 24–6). The proportion of the total sleep time occupied by periodic breathing decreases as the youngster matures. Periodic breathing is most often confined to active/REM sleep in the term newborn. Persistence later in infancy and childhood may be abnormal and reflect immaturity or an abnormality of brainstem respiratory control. Unfortunately, clear norms regarding appropriate percentages of periodic breathing across age groups are not yet available.

Obstructive Sleep Apnea Syndrome

The hallmark of obstructive sleep apnea in children is snoring. Snoring, however, can be absent even in the presence of severe obstructive sleep

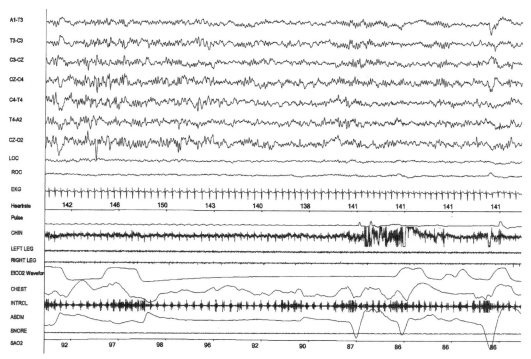

Figure 24–3. This 30-second epoch demonstrates a mixed apnea. It reveals a pause in respiratory effort accompanied by a pause in airflow. However, at least two respiratory efforts (resumption of chest effort, abdominal effort, and intercostal muscle electromyographic activity) occur prior to resumption of airflow. The return of effort is significantly greater than the 3-second sampling delay of end-tidal carbon dioxide (E_Tco_2). The event is followed by an arousal, but no electrocardiographic (EKG) changes occurred. This event, however, was associated with a fall in oxygen saturation (Sao_2) greater than 4% from the baseline, and the nadir Sao_2 reached 86%.

apnea. Breathing is often punctuated with pauses and snorts. Difficulty breathing during sleep, restless sleep, diaphoresis, morning headaches, excessive morning thirst, nightmares, sleep terrors, and enuresis may be associated symptoms. Daytime abnormalities include sleepiness, hyperactivity, poor school performance, abnormal behavior, aggressiveness, pathologic shyness, and social withdrawal. Learning problems, frequent upper airway infections, failure to thrive, or obesity may occur. In severe cases, pulmonary hypertension and cor pulmonale can develop.

Obstructive sleep apnea during childhood is often associated with an anatomic abnormality of the upper airway. The most common cause of upper airway obstruction in children is hypertrophy of the tonsils and adenoids.[24] Malformations of the mandible and maxillae can also cause upper airway obstruction during sleep. Central and peripheral neurologic abnormalities can also result in obstructive sleep apnea as a result of dysfunction of pharyngeal muscular movements.

The upper airway serves a variety of functions during the respiratory cycle, including protection of the lower airway and phonation. Little is known about the physiologic function and reflex activity of the upper airway and larynx in breathing during sleep in neonates, and there is a paucity of studies regarding normal and abnormal pharyngeal and laryngeal respiratory function in prepubertal children. During the normal respiratory cycle, the laryngeal airway is widely patent during inspiration, and it narrows during expiration.[25] Changes in the glottic aperture during the respiratory cycle result from phasic activity of the posterior cricoarytenoid muscles and the pharyngeal constrictor muscles.[26] The posterior cricoarytenoid muscles function to widen the glottis and are the principal abductor of the vocal cords. Along with the pharyngeal

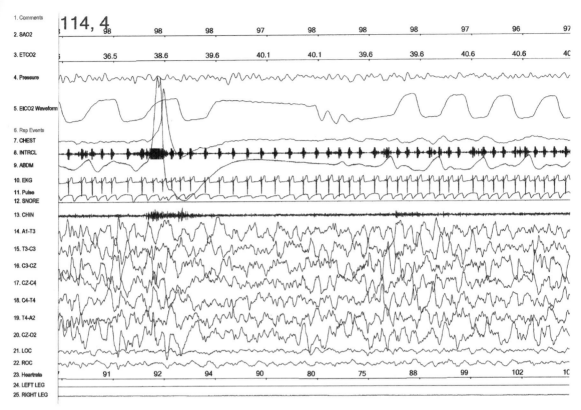

Figure 24–4. Although they are not frequently discussed, expiratory apneas do occur. There is apparent resumption of expiratory neuronal activity and effort despite the occlusion of the upper airway. This is often preceded by an augmented breath (sigh) or an arousal, or both. The event shown illustrates several characteristic features. There is an augmented breath during arousal (electromyography shows chin muscle increases, and there is a brief increase in the heart rate). During the immediate postinspiratory period, there is persistence of expiratory flow as demonstrated by the prolonged alveolar plateau on the end-tidal carbon dioxide ($E_T$co$_2$) waveform. There is also an initial fall in the R-R interval, with return to the baseline as the event continues and then resolves. This is quite different from a postsigh respiratory pause and a true central apnea, because during these events there is a progressive deceleration in the heart rate, followed by an increase in the heart rate during the arousal after the event has ceased.

constrictor muscles, the lateral cricoarytenoid, oblique and transverse arytenoid, and thyroarytenoid muscles function to close the glottis by adduction of the vocal cords. Controlled decline in the activity of the posterior cricoarytenoid muscles acts in consort with a decrease in activity of thoracic inspiratory muscles to cause expiratory braking, a reflex-controlled regulation of expiratory airflow and end expiratory volume.[27] Appropriate function of the upper airway in regulating the respiratory cycle is critical. There is increasing evidence that the upper airway has to dilate before the diaphragm initiates inspiration. Children with neurologic deficits or an auto-nomic nervous system abnormality may be at high risk for abnormalities of respiration. Obstructive apnea predominates in children with neurologic abnormalities, but other types of apnea often occur.

Apnea of Prematurity

Apnea of prematurity (AOP) is defined as excessive periodic breathing with pathologic apnea in a premature infant. Almost half of all premature infants manifest periodic breathing during the neonatal period. Periodic breathing occurs with greater frequency as gestational age decreases

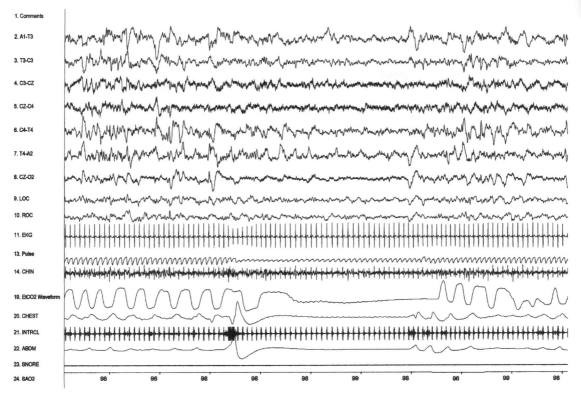

Figure 24–5. This 30-second epoch demonstrates a postsigh respiratory pause. There is an augmented breath (sigh), with rapid return of the flow to the zero baseline. There is little change in the electrocardiogram, and there are no other physiologic effects of this event.

and is present in almost all newborns less than 28 weeks gestation.[28] AOP occurs in about half of all infants with periodic breathing. It is thought to be related to immaturity of the brainstem respiratory centers, central and peripheral chemoreceptors, and pulmonary reflexes.

Even though many respiratory pauses in the premature infant are central, there is evidence suggesting that half of all apneas in premature infants may be obstructive or mixed in origin.[29] In these immature and often ill newborns, complex neuromuscular events required to maintain pharyngeal patency during respiration are easily overwhelmed.[30]

AOP is often responsive to medical treatment. Treatment of recurrent, clinically significant apnea in a premature infant should ensure adequate oxygenation and ventilation. Physical stimulation may be all that is necessary. Continuous positive airway pressure (CPAP), supplemental oxygen, or mechanical ventilation may also be required.

Methylxanthines are currently the most widely used medications in the treatment of AOP.[31] Theophylline has been shown to reduce the number of apneic episodes and lessen development of respiratory failure.[32] Theophylline, however, does not shorten the clinical course of AOP. Caffeine has also been shown to produce a significant increase in ventilation, tidal volume, and mean inspiratory flow. Caffeine appears to increase ventilation mainly by increasing central inspiratory drive. Both caffeine and theophylline have similar effects on episodes of apnea; however, caffeine seems to have an earlier effect on respiratory rate. Side effects of tachycardia, arousal, and gastrointestinal intolerance are more frequently observed with theophylline when compared to caffeine.[33] Theophylline has also been shown to be associated with a decrease in cerebral blood flow.[34] Caffeine provides stable plasma levels and has a significantly longer plasma half-life, allowing the prescription of only one daily maintenance dose.

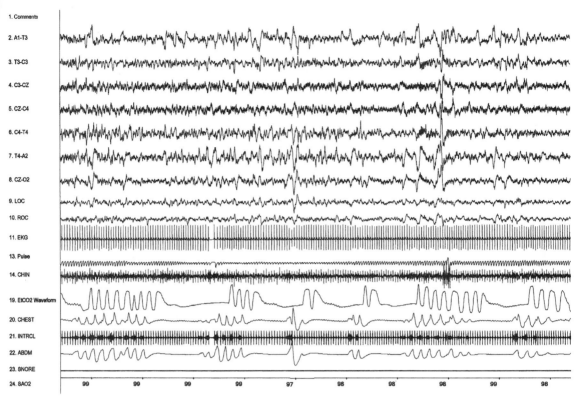

Figure 24–6. This 120-second epoch demonstrates periodic breathing, defined as three or more respiratory pauses that are at least 3 seconds long and that are separated by less than 20 seconds of normal breathing. This is normal in the premature infant in both quiet sleep and active sleep. As the babies are born closer to full term, periodic breathing tends to decrease in prevalence throughout the sleep period and is typically specific to active sleep. Prolonged periods of periodic breathing during quiet sleep in the term or near-term infant might suggest the presence of a central control of breathing problem, and further clinical investigation may be indicated. Care must be taken that the baby was actually asleep at the time the spells of periodic breathing were noted in the respiratory channels. Crying can appear very much like periodic breathing; technologist notes and video evaluation are extremely helpful in differentiating between the two.

Nasal CPAP is quite effective in resolving obstructive apneas in premature and very young infants. Central apneas, on the other hand, are unaffected by nasal CPAP, although oxygenation has been shown to increase, whether or not apnea is present.[35] For central apneas in the premature infant, methylxanthine treatment appears to be significantly superior to CPAP.[36]

Doxapram, a potent respiratory stimulant, has been used experimentally to treat AOP. It appears to affect both peripheral chemoreceptors and central respiratory centers.[37] Doxapram infusions have been used in preterm infants when therapeutic concentrations of theophylline had failed to control episodes of central apnea.[38]

Obstructive Hypoventilation and High Upper Airway Resistance

Obstructive hypoventilation occurs when there is chronic upper airway obstruction associated with high upper airway resistance. Overt apnea may not be present (Fig. 24–7). If obstructive apneas and hypopneas occur, they tend to be most significant during REM sleep. Often, however, the number of apneas and or hypopneas per hour of sleep is within age-appropriate normal limits. Respiratory rate during sleep is often increased and oxygen saturation may be normal. E_TCO_2 is, however, significantly elevated and remains high because of upper airway occlusion.

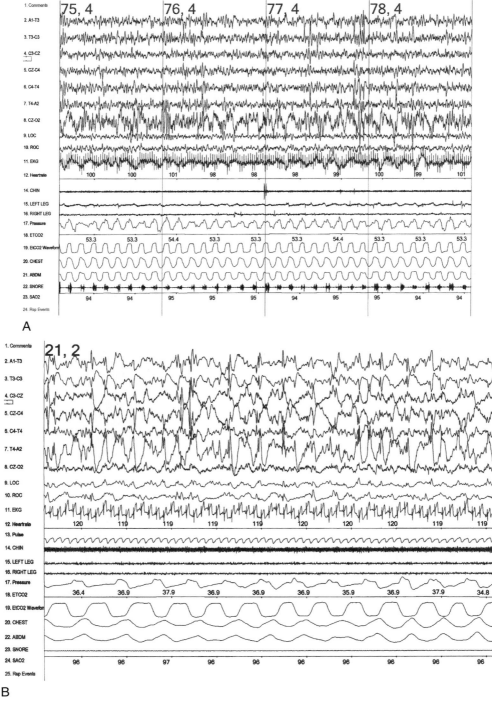

Figure 24–7. **A,** This 120-second epoch recorded during slow-wave sleep demonstrates obstructive hypoventilation. Airflow appears normal, but the end-tidal carbon dioxide (E_TCO_2) is elevated to greater than 50 mm Hg. This represents alveolar hypoventilation. However, considerable snoring is noted in this patient, and considerable apneas and hypopneas were noted during REM sleep. Therefore, the elevation of the E_TCO_2 is most likely caused by obstructive hypoventilation. **B,** This 30-second epoch, recorded from a patient who had suffered from hypoxic-ischemic encephalopathy, demonstrates continuous epileptiform activity of sleep. The record could not be adequately scored for NREM sleep state because persistent and consistent spike and wave activity was noted in NREM sleep.

It has been recommended that obstructive hypoventilation be considered when E_TCO_2 measurements remain above 46 mm Hg for more than 60% of the total sleep time or when the E_TCO_2 rises above 53 mm Hg.[39]

Central Hypoventilation

Central hypoventilation is an uncommon disorder manifested by insufficient ventilatory effort due to inadequate output from the brainstem centers that control breathing—that is, there is a failure of the automatic control of breathing. Hypoventilation in the absence of lung disease or dysfunction of respiratory muscles exacerbates during sleep. Respiratory rate may appear normal, but tidal volume during sleep is extremely low. On the other hand, some children with central hypoventilation have normal or increased tidal volumes but a significantly reduced respiratory rate. Hypoventilation may also occur during wakefulness.

Infants with central hypoventilation syndrome may appear otherwise normal. Spontaneous breathing occurs, especially during sleep, or the infant may breathe erratically. When mechanical ventilation is instituted, weaning is difficult. Blunted response to hypercapnia and hypoxemia is often demonstrable.

Clinically, infants may present early in life with apparent apneic episodes. However, symptoms may be manifested later in infancy and include cyanosis and pulmonary hypertension. The clinical course is chronic, and life-long ventilatory support is often required, particularly during sleep. Some infants improve with time and may be able to support ventilation during wakefulness. Others deteriorate over time and require 24-hour mechanical ventilatory support.

Diagnosis of Sleep-Disordered Breathing

Accurate diagnosis of respiratory pauses during sleep is based on continuous monitoring of respiratory, cardiovascular, and electroencephalographic parameters across the child's habitual sleep period. Severity of breathing disorders during sleep often varies in a circadian manner. The highest incidence of pathologic apnea, even in very young infants, occurs during the early morning hours.[40] Polysomnographic monitoring is most reliable when performed during the major sleep period at night and attended by a technician. Premature newborns and term neonates may be evaluated adequately during daytime hours if several continuous sleep–wake cycles are monitored.

The parameters that should be monitored continuously during polysomnography include nasal and oral airflow by capnography, chest and abdominal respiratory effort, oxygen saturation, and measurement of E_TCO_2. Oxygen saturation is monitored using pulse oximetry. Continuous electrocardiography (lead II) is also recorded. This provides continuous feedback of the cardiovascular effects of respiratory pauses. Continuous monitoring of the EEG, with an expanded electrode array, chin muscle and anterior tibialis electromyography, electro-oculogram, and objective recording of patient behavior during the sleep study is essential. When indicated, esophageal pH may also be continuously monitored. Recording multiple physiologic variables provides an accurate identification of sleep state–related respiratory changes as well as identification of apneas associated with other significant sleep-related disorders (e.g., sleep-related seizure activity, gastroesophageal reflux).

Pneumography (respiratory effort monitoring by thoracic impedance, and heart rate monitoring) should be avoided as a diagnostic method.[23] Pneumograms have been widely used for screening in asymptomatic premature and term infants. Unfortunately, integrity of respiration during sleep can be significantly underestimated by this type of recording. Sensitivity and specificity of pneumography is poor. False-positive and false-negative results are common. Partial airway obstruction may cause false breath detection, and breaths immediately after a sigh, or biphasic augmented breaths are often missed.[41] In addition, unless nasal and oral airflows are recorded, only central apneas can be detected. Monitoring only thoracic impedance may result in failure to detect obstructive apnea, can confuse cardiac pulse artifact with respiratory effort, and cannot detect abdominal respiratory efforts.

Impedance pneumography done in the home is almost as costly as comprehensive technician-attended polysomnography conducted in the laboratory. Pneumograms should be reserved for evaluation of infants who trigger frequent home monitor alarms, in which circumstances it may help by differentiating true from false activation of the monitor. *Technician-attended polysomnography is still considered the most reliable and effective method available for describing respiration during sleep* and for identification of normal versus abnormal upper airway function during sleep.

Paroxysmal Disorders

Sleep-related paroxysmal disorders may be differentiated into epileptiform and nonepileptiform abnormalities. Interictal EEG evaluations may not be helpful in diagnosis. Often, spells do not occur in the laboratory and comprehensive assessments and management must be based on clinical grounds. Continuous monitoring of EEG and other physiologic functions during polysomnography in the sleep laboratory may be quite helpful in differentiating seizure disorders from nonepileptic paroxysmal disturbances.

Seizures

An abundant variety of paroxysmal motor disorders may occur during sleep. These recurring spells must be differentiated from sleep-related nonepileptic motor activity. The sleep of patients with true seizures is typically fragmented.[42] Abnormal sleep patterns may, however, indicate a toxic effect of medication or CNS injury.

Interictal epileptiform activity tends to increase during light stages of NREM sleep and is inclined to be suppressed during REM sleep. This is particularly true in patients suffering from partial complex seizures.[43] Sleep deprivation increases the rate of focal interictal epileptiform discharges most markedly in stage 2 NREM sleep. Some epileptic seizures appear almost exclusively during sleep. For example, a syndrome of continuous spike and wave activity during sleep occurs in young children and is associated with hyperkinesias, neuropsychological disturbances, and progressive aphasia—the Landau-Kleffner syndrome.[44]

Much literature confirms the observation that epileptic seizures occur in relation to specific sleep stages and the sleep–wake cycle.[45] Sleep deprivation has been commonly used to promote seizures in the laboratory, especially in patients with temporal lobe seizure disorders.[46] Although seizures are recognized clinically only during the day, fluttering of the eyelids can be observed during sleep in conjunction with paroxysmal bursts of 3 cycles per second spike-and-wave activity.[47] Partial complex seizures originating in the frontal lobe occur most characteristically during NREM sleep. Among patients with sleep-related complex seizures studied by Cadilhac,[48] almost two thirds occurred during NREM sleep. Approximately 16% of seizures studied were isolated to REM sleep, and 20% occurred in both NREM and REM sleep states. There is also a strong correlation between seizures and sleep in patients with benign partial epilepsy with centrotemporal spikes (Rolandic epilepsy).[45]

In addition to the facilitatory effect of sleep on seizure activity, seizure frequency may be affected by the presence of other sleep-related disorders. For example, in a group of patients with obstructive sleep apnea syndrome and partial epilepsy, six of seven patients studied by Devinsky and colleagues[49] revealed a significant reduction in the frequency of seizure activity and seizure severity after successful treatment of the sleep-related breathing abnormality.

Clinical differentiation between epileptic and nonepileptic spells that occur during sleep can often be difficult. Stores[50] reviewed this issue and was able to divide patients fitting this diagnostic dilemma into three categories. A first group consisted of patients with nonepileptic primary sleep disorders that are often associated with motor phenomena and similar presentations, including some nightmares and sleep terrors, NREM sleep partial arousal disorders, and REM-sleep motor disorders. The second group consisted of patients with primary sleep disorders with motor components that can be incorrectly diagnosed as epilepsy, including the partial arousal disorders, REM-sleep motor disorder, sleep-related rhythmic movement disorders (such as jactatio capitis nocturnes), some symptoms associated with obstructive sleep apnea, automatic behaviors, idiopathic CNS hypersomnia, and sleep-related enuresis. Finally, the third group of patients have some epileptic disorders that occur during sleep and may be mistaken for sleep disorders. These consist of nocturnal complex partial seizures of the temporal lobe and, particularly of frontal lobe origin, nocturnal hypnogenic dystonia, episodic nocturnal wanderings, and nonconvulsive status epilepticus.

Paroxysmal Hypnogenic Dystonia

Paroxysmal hypnogenic dystonia was first described by Lugaresi and Cirignotta in 1981.[51] It is a rare disorder characterized by stereotypic, choreoathetotic movements and dystonic posturing during NREM sleep. Symptoms may begin in childhood and be mistaken for normal (or abnormal) behavior patterns or other stereotypic movement disorders. Episodes may be brief, lasting less than a minute, or may be prolonged, persisting for hours. Eyes are often open and vocalizations may occur. If episodes occur frequently or are recurrent during a single sleep period, significant sleep disruption may occur. There are rhythmic, sometimes violent, stereotypic movements (e.g., kicking, thrashing) of the limbs and/or trunk, associated with dystonic posturing of the hands, feet, arms, legs, and/or face. At the termination of an episode, patients may be coherent, but they rapidly return to sleep.

Polysomnography usually reveals episodes arising out of stage 2 NREM sleep (although it has been reported to occur in slow-wave sleep as well). An EEG pattern of arousal may occur a few seconds before an episode. Significant movement artifact is seen on the EEG. Whether clear epileptiform activity occurs during a spell is somewhat controversial. Radiographic studies and magnetic resonance imaging are notably normal. It is unknown whether hypnogenic paroxysmal dystonia is associated with CNS (or other) pathology.

Symptoms generally run a chronic course and may persist for many years. Carbamazepine, in small doses, has ameliorated symptoms in some patients.

Parasomnias

Parasomnias are classified as dysfunctions associated with sleep, sleep stages, or partial arousals from sleep. They are a group of disorders with strikingly dissimilar presentations, but they share many clinical and physiologic characteristics. Often, parasomnias present clear symptomatology (e.g., sleepwalking, head-banging, bruxism). Manifestations appear early in childhood and might be considered by parents and health care practitioners as normal, benign, or behavioral in origin. As the child ages, benign characteristics can become exaggerated and dramatic. However, few pathophysiologic abnormalities can be identified, despite occasionally severe paroxysmal features.[52]

As with all other disorders of sleep and wakefulness, evaluation begins with a comprehensive history and physical examination. Special attention must be placed on a detailed description of the events. Neurodevelopmental landmarks must be carefully assessed. Sleep–wake schedules, habits, and patterns require delineation. Morning wake time, evening bedtime, bedtime rituals, and nap time rituals should be described. The presence of excessive daytime sleepiness, snoring, or restlessness during sleep should be ascertained. Whether there are or are not concurrent medical illnesses and whether the patient is taking any medications or drugs should be obtained in the clinical interview.

In the complete physical examination, emphasis should be placed on a comprehensive neurologic and developmental assessment. The existence of developmental delays or symptoms suggestive of neurologic disorders might indicate an organic basis for the patient's presenting symptoms. Evidence of other medical disorders should be assessed as possible contributing or coexistent factors.

Laboratory evaluations should be guided by the presenting signs and symptoms. A urine drug screen may be helpful if the symptoms might be a side effect of medication. Polysomnography is often indicated. An expanded EEG electrode array is recommended. A more extensive EEG montage than typically recorded during polysomnography is often helpful in differentiating a nonepileptic parasomnia from sleep-related seizures. Concomitant video recording of the patient while sleeping is indispensable and can clearly demonstrate motor manifestations and chronicle stereotypic movements. Attempts should be made to obtain at least 400 minutes of natural *nocturnal* sleep. It is often helpful to have the patient drink fluids and avoid urination prior to settling, as bladder distention may precipitate some parasomnias. The need for all-night EEG recordings, routine EEG, and radiographic studies depends on the presenting situation, nighttime manifestations, and clinical symptoms.

Nonepileptic Stereotypic Parasomnias

Although the phenomenon of stereotypic movements during sleep has been recognized for many years, little is known of the etiology. Stereotypic nonepileptic parasomnias are characterized by repetitive, meaningless movements or behaviors. Large muscle groups are involved and manifestations include rhythmic, repetitive movements such as body rocking, head-banging, head-rolling, and body-shuttling. They are typically associated with transition from wakefulness to sleep, may be sustained into light sleep, and/or occur after arousal from sleep. Children are usually developmentally, behaviorally, and medically normal. Movements may be alarming in appearance, and parents often become concerned for the child's physical and mental well-being. Injury sometimes occurs.

Stereotypic movements occur in normal infants and children. Lack of rhythmic activity during infancy has occasionally been associated with developmental delays. When stereotypic movements during wakefulness persist into older childhood and adolescence, a coexisting psychogenic component may be present. Stereotypic movements may be a form of attention getting, or a mechanism of self-stimulation or self-soothing, in developmentally disabled children.

Rhythmic movements can be observed in two thirds of normal children by 9 months of age. The incidence of head-banging occurs in 3% to 6.5% of the normal population; body rocking, in 19.1% to 21%; and head-rolling, in 6.3%. By 18 months of age, the prevalence of rhythmic movements decreases to less than 50%, and by 4 years of age to approximately 8%. This consistent decrease and spontaneous resolution of symptoms as the child grows and develops is consistent with a maturational origin of the disorder.

At times, motor activity and head-banging can be violent, and physical injury can occur, although it is uncommon. Cutaneous ecchymosis and callus formation can result. However, more serious injuries, including subdural hematoma and retinal petechiae, have been reported. Rhythmic movements usually decrease in intensity and often resolve spontaneously between 2 and 4 years of age. Rarely, symptoms persist into adolescence and adulthood.

Diagnosis is based on identification of characteristic symptoms in the absence of other medical or psychiatric disorders. Polysomnography demonstrates typical rhythmic movements during the immediate presleep period and may persist into stage 1 NREM sleep. Occasionally,

activity is noted after spontaneous arousal. It can occur during slow-wave sleep, but it is rare during REM sleep. Focal, paroxysmal, and epileptiform EEG activity associated with the stereotypic activity are absent; however, a full-montage EEG may be necessary to rule out epilepsy. Sleep architecture, stage progression, and stage volumes are typically normal.

Partial Arousal Disorders

Arousal disorders are thought to be caused by impaired or "partial" arousal from slow-wave sleep. A hierarchical model may exist, as it appears that a continuum of manifestations of each of these disorders of sleep is present. Symptoms most often begin in childhood and resolve spontaneously, although occasionally they persist into adolescence and adulthood. Manifestations are quite alarming and injury often occurs.

Arousal disorders present with bizarre, dramatic symptoms and share a number of common features. All seem to occur during stage 3/4 sleep. Confusion, disorientation, and amnesia for the events are present, and at times the episodes are precipitated by external stimuli. In contrast, forced arousal from REM sleep is more often followed by rapid awakening, clear thought processes, and vivid dream recall.

Partial arousal disorders occur more frequently during periods of stress, in the presence of fever, after sleep deprivation, and in patients with hypersomnolence syndromes. Partial arousals normally occur at the end of slow-wave sleep periods during ascent to lighter sleep stages. Because of the depth of slow-wave sleep and the high arousal threshold in children, these arousal disorders may represent conflicting interaction between the mechanisms generating slow-wave sleep and arousal. Chronobiologic triggers that control sleep stage cycling may be more likely to result in a partial arousal if the sleep schedule is chaotic. There may be internal desynchronization, and the internal arousal stimulus may come at the "wrong" time, resulting in incomplete arousal and manifest characteristics of both states. As the child develops, these CNS mechanisms mature, synchronization occurs, and symptoms resolve spontaneously.

Confusional arousals consist of partial arousals from slow-wave sleep during the first half of the sleep period. Episodes are sudden, startling, and may be precipitated by forced awakenings. Children may appear to be awake during the episode, but they do not respond appropriately to commands and resist being consoled. Confusion and disorientation are prominent. Attempts to abort the "attack" may, in fact, make the symptoms more severe and violent.

Factors that result in increased slow-wave sleep or those that impair arousal may precipitate or exacerbate confusional arousals. Hypersomnia secondary to rebound from sleep deprivation, narcolepsy syndrome, idiopathic hypersomnia, or obstructive sleep apnea may exacerbate symptoms. Confusional arousals/sleep drunkenness is frequently seen in patients with narcolepsy syndrome after prolonged daytime naps (those that are longer than 60 minutes and that contain slow-wave sleep). Stress, anxiety, fever, and excessive exercise may precipitate attacks. Organic pathology is rarely noted, although CNS lesions of the periventricular gray matter, reticular activating system, and posterior hypothalamus have been reported in some patients. Injuries during confusional arousals are common if there is displacement of the patient from the bed.

The onset of symptoms is usually prior to 5 years of age. Children gradually arouse from slow-wave sleep, and they may moan or mumble unintelligibly. Symptoms then crescendo significantly. Patients may thrash about in bed or fall from the bed to the floor. During the episode, the child appears profoundly confused and disoriented. Combativeness and aggressiveness may occur and consolation or restraint may result in exacerbation of symptoms. Episodes may be brief, lasting for only a few minutes, or they may be prolonged and last for several hours. There is usually retrograde and/or anterograde amnesia for the event. There may be associated night terrors or somnambulism. Enuresis may occur during or following the episode, resulting in difficulties in differentiating these spells from partial complex seizures.

Diagnosis is based on identification of confusion, disorientation, agitation, or combativeness on arousal, most often during the first one third to one half of the night. Associated amnesia for the event is present. There is rarely a clearly identifiable medical or psychiatric disorder present on clinical evaluation. Partial complex seizure disorders with confusional automatisms

need to be ruled out. Polysomnography reveals sudden arousal from slow-wave sleep, brief periods of delta activity, stage 1 theta patterns, recurrent microsleeps, or a poorly reactive alpha activity, or any combination of these. Focal, paroxysmal, and epileptiform activity are absent from the EEG. Symptoms may peak during middle childhood and then undergo spontaneous remission. The clinical course is usually benign (although frightening). Physical injury can occur and the child must be protected from trauma during the episode.

Somnambulism: Sleepwalking

Somnambulism may vary in presentation from simple sitting up in bed to agitated running and aggressive, violent behavior during sleep. The complex series of automatic behaviors manifested may appear, on the surface, purposeful. As with other partial arousal disorders, somnambulistic episodes occur out of slow-wave sleep, during the first third of the sleep period. Episodes may be quite alarming. Patients are uncoordinated and clumsy during the walking episode, and injuries are common. Because of the high incidence of trauma during events, agitated somnambulism should be considered a potentially fatal disorder and the major goal of management is to protect the child from harm.

Somnambulism has been reported to occur in 1% to 15% of the population. It occurs with greatest frequency during childhood, decreasing significantly during adolescence, and it is uncommon in adults. Episodes vary in frequency, intensity, and length, making parental reports quite inaccurate; the true incidence is therefore unknown. There appears to be an equal sex distribution. There also appears to be a significant familial pattern, although clear genetic transmission has not been identified.

Somnambulism usually begins in middle childhood, between 4 and 8 years of age, although onset may occur at any time after the child develops the ability to walk. Symptoms range from simple sitting up in bed to extremely agitated, semi-purposeful automatisms and frantic running. Most often the child will wander around the house and can perform complex tasks, such as unlocking doors, taking food from the refrigerator, and eating. At times, children leave the house. Often, the behaviors are meaningless and unusual. Verbalizations may occur but are usually garbled, confused, and meaningless. Eyes are often open and the child may appear awake, but behaviors are only semi-purposeful. Choreiform movements of the arms and head may occur. Often, enuretic episodes occur and the child may urinate (or attempt to urinate) at unusual places around the house. During a somnambulistic spell, the child is extremely difficult to wake, although complete arousal is possible. If awakened, confusion and disorientation are usually present. Motor activity can cease spontaneously, and the child may lie down and return to sleep at unusual places around the home, or the child may return to bed without ever becoming alert.

A number of factors may precipitate somnambulistic events. Fever and sleep deprivation are notable. Any disorder that can produce significant disruption of slow-wave sleep, such as obstructive sleep apnea, may precipitate events. In addition, sleep walking can often be precipitated by urinary bladder distention in the susceptible patient. External noise may also trigger an event. A number of medications can exacerbate the disorder, including thioridazine, Prolixin, perphenazine, desipramine, and chloral hydrate.

Polysomnography typically reveals an arousal from stage 3 or stage 4 sleep during the first half of the sleep period. Most of the background EEG activity is obscured by muscle artifact. Seizure activity is notably absent.

Although it is clinically difficult, somnambulism should be differentiated from other disorders of arousal, such as confusional arousals and night terrors. Displacement from the bed and calm nocturnal wanderings are less common with confusional arousals. Night terrors are more typically associated with the appearance of intense fear and panic and are less likely to be associated with displacement from bed (although displacement from bed is more common with night terrors than nightmares). Intense autonomic discharges and an initial scream herald a sleep terror and are not present in somnambulism. Nocturnal seizure disorders typically reveal epileptiform discharges during the events; however, the interictal EEG may be normal. REM sleep behavior disorder has been described in children, characteristically occurs during REM sleep, and is associated with clear verbalizations and seemingly purposeful movements.

Sleep Terrors

Sleep terrors are third in a continuum of partial arousals from slow-wave sleep. The onset of a sleep terror (in contrast to the gradual onset of confusional arousals) is sudden, abrupt, striking, and frightening. These arousals are associated with profound autonomic discharges and behavioral manifestations of intense fear. The exact prevalence of sleep terrors, like that of other partial arousals, is unknown.

Onset of symptoms is usually between 2 and 4 years of age. Although most frequent during childhood, sleep terrors can occur at any age. As with other nonepileptic parasomnias, precipitating factors include fever, bladder distention, sleep deprivation, and CNS depressant medication. Symptoms tend to significantly decrease during puberty and rarely persist into adolescence and adulthood. Psychopathology is rare in children.

A sleep terror begins suddenly. The child typically sits upright in bed and emits a piercing scream. Severe autonomic discharge occurs. Eyes are usually widely open and pupils may appear dilated. Tachycardia, tachypnea, diaphoresis, and increased muscle tone are present. During the episode, the child is unresponsive to efforts to console, and parental efforts often exacerbate autonomic and motor activity. During a spell, the youngster may run hysterically around the house. The child may run wildly into walls, furniture, or windows. Episodes of extreme agitation are commonly associated with injury. Unintelligible vocalizations and enuresis can occur. As with other partial arousal disorders, the child awakened from a spell may be confused and disoriented, and there is amnesia for the event. In contrast to confusional arousals, episodes of sleep terrors are usually brief, lasting only a few minutes, and they subside spontaneously.

Diagnosis is based on identification of these symptoms and exclusion of organic pathology. Polysomnography reveals sudden arousal from slow-wave sleep during the first third of the major sleep period. Sleep terrors, however, can occur out of slow-wave sleep at any time during the night. Partial arousals without motor manifestation occur more frequently in children with sleep terrors than in unaffected children. Autonomic discharges during these partial arousals are identified by the presence of tachycardia without full-blown symptoms.

Sleep terrors require differentiation from sleep-related epilepsy with automatisms. In these patients, EEG may show abnormal discharges from the temporal lobe, although nasopharyngeal leads may be required to identify the focus of abnormal activity. Epileptic events may also be distinguished from disorders of partial arousal by the presence of a combination of clinical features, stereotypic behaviors, and the fact that they may occur during any part of the sleep period as well as during wakefulness. Identification of epileptiform activity, however, does not completely rule out the presence of a partial arousal, as they may occur concomitantly in the same patient.

Management of Parasomnias

There is no clear consensus regarding when a partial arousal parasomnia requires treatment. Symptoms are most often mild, occur less than once per month, and result in injury to neither the child nor the parents. In mild cases, explanation of partial arousal disorders and parental reassurance may be all that is necessary. Sleep hygiene also should be discussed. Parents should be encouraged to let the event run its course and to intervene minimally. Interventions should focus on preventing injury and simply guiding the child back to bed. Too vigorous intervention may prolong the episode.

Parents can be alerted of a quiet somnambulistic episode by the use of an alarm system (e.g., a bell placed on the doorknob of the child's room). Appropriate sleep hygiene is essential. Sleep deprivation should be avoided and regular sleep–wake schedules maintained. Brief daytime naps might be attempted and a period of quiet activity or relaxation techniques instituted prior to bedtime. Fluids after the night-time meal should be limited and the child encouraged to empty the bladder immediately prior to bedtime. Fevers, if present, should be appropriately treated.

Severity of partial arousals is considered *moderate* when symptoms occur less than once per week and do not result in harm to the patient or to others. In these cases, reassurance and a behavioral approach (including behavior training, sleep hygiene, psychotherapy, and/or hypnosis) have been successful.

In *severe* cases, when episodes occur almost nightly or are associated with injury, nondrug approaches are considered first. Drug treatment, when used, should be prescribed for a short period of time and should be used in conjunction with sleep hygiene and behavioral management. The patient can be weaned from medication when symptoms have been under good control for approximately 3 to 6 months.

The most commonly prescribed medication is diazepam. However, lorazepam and clonazepam in small doses are also quite effective. Dosage should be adjusted to the needs of the child. Prolonged use of medication increases the potential for side effects and complications. The young child generally responds well to both behavioral and medicinal approaches.

Parasomnias Associated with REM Sleep

Parasomnias previously discussed have been related to dysfunctions associated with sleep state transitions and partial arousal from NREM stage 3 and stage 4 sleep. Parasomnias have also been reported to occur out of stage REM sleep. In many cases, manifestations are dissimilar and can be differentiated on clinical grounds alone. Certain REM sleep parasomnias, however, share the symptoms of partial arousal disorders. Some frequently occur in children (e.g., nightmares), whereas others are extremely rare and have only recently been described in children (e.g., REM sleep behavior disorder). Disorders rarely encountered during childhood are included (e.g., REM sleep behavior disorder) because their importance to the practitioner may become clear when they are more completely understood and dysfunction associated with the sleeping state is further delineated in children.

Nightmares

A nightmare is a frightening dream that may awaken the youngster from REM sleep. There is usually vivid, clear recall of disturbing dream content. Anxiety and mild autonomic manifestations occur. Often, an anxiety dream contains elements of danger to the individual; a sudden arousal from REM sleep occurs; and after awakening, the youngster is oriented to the environment with clear sensorium. Dream content usually involves an experience of immediate and credible threat to survival, security, or self-esteem.

Dream anxiety attacks occur in REM sleep and are often associated with the longest, most intense REM period, during the last third of the night. Major body movements are rare (because of REM hypotonia), but REM sleep fragmentation, increased phasic activity, and frequent movement arousals and awakening from sleep with clear mentation are typical. Manifestations are generally mild and vocalizations are rare. Although autonomic activity increases during nightmares, it is generally mild, differentiating it from a sleep terror. There is good recall for the disturbing dream, and the child functions well on waking. In contrast to sleep terrors, nightmares are brief. A prolonged waking episode with difficulty returning to sleep is common after a nightmare. In addition, nightmares are generally unassociated with violent outbursts, there is no displacement from the bed (until the child awakens), and injuries are quite rare. Return to sleep is generally delayed, and the child often responds well to parental intervention.

Diagnosis of anxiety dreams is based on the identification of the mild manifestations of disturbing dreams occurring during the early morning hours, absence of intense autonomic activation, clear recall of the dream, appropriate functioning and alertness on awakening, and a good response to parental interventions. Polysomnography may reveal an abrupt arousal from REM sleep. The REM period from which the child awakens is usually the longest and most intense period of the night. It occurs later in the sleep period, during early morning hours, and is associated with mild tachycardia and tachypnea. Increased rapid eye movement density may be noted. Focal, paroxysmal, and epileptiform EEG activities are absent.

Nightmares must be differentiated from sleep terrors, REM sleep behavior disorder, and epilepsy. Sleep terrors are usually more vivid, they are frightening to the observer, they occur during the first third of the sleep period, and they are associated with severe autonomic discharges. There is fragmented recall, the child is confused on waking, somnambulism and agitated sleepwalking are common, and many children suffer injuries.

REM sleep behavior disorder has been recently described in childhood. Symptoms are similar to those seen in the adult patient. In the adult, the sudden arousal from REM sleep is associated with significant purposeful motor activity. Similar symptoms may be seen in patients with post-traumatic stress disorder, where there is state dissociation including, but not limited to, increased chin muscle tone, increased phasic activity, increased major body movements during REM sleep, and increased periodic limb movements. Partial complex seizure disorders may occur during any stage of sleep and wake, and automatisms and stereotypy are common. Seizure episodes are associated with abnormal EEG activity.

Sleep Paralysis

Sleep paralysis is characterized by absence of voluntary motor activity occurring at the beginning of a sleep period (hypnagogic) or immediately after awakening from sleep (hypnopompic). The patient is conscious and aware of the environment but feels paralyzed. All muscle groups are involved, but the diaphragm and extraocular muscles are spared. Active inhibition of alpha and gamma motor neurons is present and is similar to that seen during REM sleep and cataplexy. Sleep paralysis typically lasts only several minutes and subsides spontaneously. Occasionally, attacks can be aborted by rapid movements of the eyes or by being touched. Hypnagogic or hypnopompic hallucinations are unusual but can occur and add to anxiety.

Isolated episodes of sleep paralysis can occur in unaffected individuals. Frequent spells are reported in patients with narcolepsy and in familial sleep paralysis. Onset is usually during adolescence, but symptoms may begin during childhood. Children have difficulty describing the events and may appear asleep during the episode. Parents are unaware of the sleep paralysis spell, because the atonia can be aborted by touching or shaking.

The clinical course varies significantly. Most cases are isolated and may be exacerbated by sleep deprivation, excessive sleepiness, stress, irregular sleep–wake schedules, or acute changes in sleep phase. Sleep paralysis runs a more chronic course in patients with narcolepsy and in the familial form of the disorder.

Diagnosis of sleep paralysis is based on identification of presenting symptoms. These may be quite difficult to interpret in children. Complaints of an inability to "get up" or inability to "wake up" may be more common in children. The youngster complaining to the parent of an inability to move after sleep offset is rarely encountered. Sleep paralysis associated with narcolepsy can be differentiated from the isolated form by the absence of chronic excessive daytime sleepiness, sleep attacks, hypnagogic hallucinations, and cataplexy. Atonic generalized seizures occur during wakefulness and may or may not be associated with changes in level of consciousness. Syncope occurs during wakefulness as well and is most commonly associated with altered levels of consciousness.

Polysomnography usually reveals significant decrease in skeletal muscle tone in the presence of a normal waking EEG pattern and conjugate eye movements. Occasionally, patients enter sleep during an episode of sleep paralysis and reveal an EEG pattern consistent with stage 1 sleep. True sleep-onset REM periods may occur.

REM Sleep Behavior Disorder

REM sleep behavior disorder (RBD) or REM sleep motor anomaly (RMA) has been described in adults.[53] There is evidence that a similar syndrome also occurs during childhood.[54] Nonetheless, RBD is an unusual disorder characterized by the appearance of elaborate, sometimes purposeful movement during REM sleep. There is a paradoxical increase in muscle tone, and patients seem to be acting out their dreams. Violent behavior such as punching, kicking, leaping out of bed, and running are reported and often correspond with dream mentation. Injuries to the patient and to bed partners are common.

Cases of RBD/RMA have been reported in pediatric patients,[54] and further understanding of this disorder may reveal the incidence and prevalence to be higher than current descriptions suggest. The majority of cases are idiopathic, but neurologic disorders have been identified in approximately 40% of affected adults.

Polysomnography reveals increased muscle tone that persists throughout sleep. There is often a paradoxical increase in muscle tone during REM sleep, increased phasic activity, and excessive limb or body jerking. Complex behaviors occur out of REM sleep, but no epileptiform activity is noted on EEG during the complex movements. Interestingly, REM sleep behavior disorder in adults responds well to benzodiazepines, especially clonazepam.

Imperative in management of youngsters with nonepileptic partial arousal disorders is a stepwise approach. Education of parents and reassurance may be the only requirement. It is essential the child be protected from injury, especially if spells are frequent, there is displacement from the bed, or the child is significantly agitated and violent. Behavioral management includes close attention to sleep hygiene, adequate total sleep time, and limited nocturnal fluids. Fever should be evaluated and treated appropriately. Sleep deprivation should be avoided. Sources of stress and anxiety should be identified and appropriately addressed. If motor manifestations are present, an alarm system should be established so that the parents/caretakers can be forewarned of episodes. A bell on a doorknob may be all that is needed. If medications are indicated, benzodiazepines are typically the drugs of first choice. Clonazepam in small doses (e.g., 0.25 mg orally at bedtime) is quite effective for both NREM and REM disorders. Unfortunately, because of the long half-life of clonazepam, a hangover effect can occur and the youngster may do poorly and exhibit excessive sleepiness the following day. Lorazepam in similarly small doses has been quite successful. Small doses of diazepam at bedtime may be most appropriate for partial arousal parasomnia, which occurs only during the first third of the sleep period time. If RBD/RMA is suspected, appropriate psychological, neurologic, and psychiatric evaluations should be considered. As previously stated, RBD/RMA has been associated with post-traumatic stress disorder in adults, and preliminary data may support a similar phenomenon in children.

Cerebral Palsy

Sleep problems commonly occur in patients with cerebral palsy (CP). Alterations of the sleep–wake cycle and specific primary sleep disorders may increase morbidity. Often, the quality of life of the youngster and the family is profoundly affected.

Physiologic changes occurring during sleep affect specific reflexes in children with CP. Alterations in the H-reflex during sleep were studied in 13 children with cerebral palsy (eight with spastic tetraplegia, two with a mixed form of cerebral palsy without spasticity, three with hypotonic diplegia or tetraplegia).[55] In unaffected children, the maximum H-reflex progressively decreases in amplitude from wakefulness to REM sleep. In hypertonic patients, there is only a slight decrease in the H-reflex in NREM sleep and no significant change in REM sleep; the amplitude of the H-reflex is always greater than that in the control group. In dystonic and hypotonic patients, the results obtained are similar to those of the control group. In spastic patients (as opposed to the control and the dystonic and hypotonic groups), normal balance between the function of supraspinal systems regulating the amplitude of the spinal reflexes during wake and sleep is altered, probably through the scarce functionality of the supraspinal inhibitory structures.

Activity in youngsters with CP is often less than physical activity in healthy peers. Children with spastic diplegia were compared with normal controls in an analysis of their physical activity during the day versus in sleep.[56] It was determined that children with spastic diplegia are considerably less active than their healthy peers. *This is often significant in stabilization of the sleep–wake cycle, as there is a correlation of regularly scheduled physical activity during the day and improvement of sleep at night.* Regular exercise as part of a comprehensive sleep hygiene program is important in stabilization of the sleep–wake cycle and can improve sleep in some youngsters.

Disturbances in the sleep–wake cycle have also been evaluated electroencephalographically in children with CP. Classification of the background EEG was well correlated with disturbances in the sleep cycle, which was also related to the interval after the hypoxic insult.[57] The relationship between sleep states and EEG patterns also had a close correlation with the classification and became progressively disturbed with increasing severity of the background EEG. Each grade of the background EEG abnormality had a different prognostic significance according to the time of the recording. The one in the first week offered the best prognostic value. A disturbance of sleep—if it exists—always runs parallel with the course of the disease.[58]

Sleep EEG patterns were compared in 23 mentally retarded children (from 4 months to 5 years old) with CP, and 39 reference mentally retarded children with no abnormality except psychomotor retardation.[59] The children with CP (unlike those without CP) exhibited absence of EEG patterns characteristic of wakefulness, NREM sleep states that could not be differentiated, absence of NREM characteristics and NREM sleep without spindles, and absence of REM sleep. In addition, short sleep times and long waking times during the night were often noted.

Melatonin concentration in blood, urine, or saliva may become a useful marker of the circadian rhythm in disorders of biologic rhythms.[60] Of particular interest to pediatric clinicians is the potential application of melatonin treatment in establishing or reestablishing circadian rhythms in infants and children maintained for long periods under artificial light conditions, as encountered in intensive care units, and in the treatment of sleep and other rhythm disorders associated with developmental delay or blindness. Care must be taken when using melatonin in youngsters with neurologic deficits, especially those with intractable seizure disorders. There may be a proconvulsant effect of exogenous melatonin in some children with cerebral palsy and seizure disorder.[61] Until there is a clear understanding of the efficacy and side effects of melatonin, it should be reserved for those youngsters with chronic neurologic disabilities not associated with epilepsy, and for sightless youngsters who are unresponsive to light–dark cycling.

Infants and children with myelomeningocele, hydrocephalus, and Arnold-Chiari malformation often exhibit symptomatic apnea or hypoventilation. In a study of 18 asymptomatic infants, Ward and colleagues[11] showed that asymptomatic infants with myelomeningocele had longer total sleep time, longer episodes of longest apnea, greater duration of apnea greater than or equal to 6 seconds as percent of total sleep time, and lower mean heart rate than did control infants. This suggested that asymptomatic infants with myelomeningocele have a high incidence of ventilatory pattern abnormalities during sleep. This is currently being studied in a multicenter retrospective analysis of respiratory patterns in children with this CNS abnormality.

To assess hypoxic and hypercapnic arousal response in children with myelomeningocele and apnea, Ward and colleagues[62] evaluated 11 infants in the presence of controlled hypoxemia and 6 infants with controlled hypercarbia challenges. During hypoxemia, only two infants with myelomeningocele aroused in comparison to eight of nine control infants. Similarly, during hypercarbia, arousal occurred in only three infants with myelomeningocele compared to all seven control infants. Three infants with myelomeningocele subsequently died. It was concluded that infants with myelomeningocele, Arnold-Chiari malformation, and apnea or hypoventilation have arousal deficits to normal respiratory stimuli.

Circadian Rhythm Disorders

Children suffering from chronic debilitating neurologic disabilities frequently experience disorders of the sleep–wake cycle related to intrinsic biologic (circadian) rhythms. In addition to disordered sleep architecture and composition, many youngsters (and their families) endure significant disorganization of the timing of sleep. Disorders of timing of sleep may result in a significant lifestyle disarray, affect daytime functioning and performance, and contribute to resistance to therapeutic interventions during daytime hours.

Delayed Sleep Phase Syndrome

Sleep phase delay is common during childhood and is seen in many youngsters with and without abnormalities of neurologic status. Bedtime struggles are common, and sleep onset difficulties can be profound. Once asleep, continuity and architecture may be normal, unless early morning waking is required or sleep maintenance difficulties are also present. The child who has early morning responsibilities may experience extreme difficulty arousing. Excessive daytime sleepiness most likely occurs, especially during early morning hours. This may be manifested by actual sleep attacks (unintentional sleep episodes), attention problems, behavioral abnormalities, or hyperactivity. Youngsters with delayed sleep phase syndrome function best in the afternoon or early evening hours. Spontaneous sleep offset (when no responsibilities are present) tends to be quite late in the morning, often extending into the afternoon. On weekends, recovery may occur because of the ability to sleep later in the day, only to have the problem recur during weekdays. Treatment principally focuses on sleep hygiene. Firm, stable time of morning sleep offset is essential. Advancing bed-

time will follow. Faded bedtimes with response cost is an appropriate behavioral intervention. If youngsters are not asleep within a reasonable period of time (e.g., 20 to 30 minutes after lights out), they may be removed from bed to perform quiet tasks until drowsiness is identified. They should then be placed back into bed. Slowly advancing bedtime after sleep onset occurs relatively rapidly will assist in changing and ultimately fixing the timing of the major sleep period. Although there is typically a rapid response to this type of intervention, it may take somewhat longer in the youngster with developmental or neurologic disability. Medication is sometimes required in children with significant neurologic abnormalities, and it may delay sleep onset. Chloral hydrate and benzodiazepines are most commonly prescribed. If chloral hydrate is used, the dosage should be adequate to assist in sleep onset.

References

1. Martin JH, Jessell TM: Development as a guide to the regional anatomy of the brain. In: Kandel ER, Schwartz JH, Jessell TM: Principles of Neural Science (3rd ed). New York, Elsevier, 1991, pp 296-308.
2. Oksenberg A, Marks G, Farber J, et al: Effect of REM sleep deprivation during the critical period of neuroanatomical development of the cat visual system. Sleep Res 1986;15:53.
3. Armstrong SM, Cassone VN, Chesworth MJ, et al: Synchronization of mammalian circadian rhythms by melatonin. J Neural Trans Suppl 1986;21:375-394.
4. Dahlitz M, Alvarez B, Vignau J, et al: Delayed sleep phase syndrome response to melatonin. Lancet 1991;333:1121-1124.
5. Jan JE, Espezel H, Appleton RE: The treatment of sleep disorders with melatonin. Dev Med Child Neurol 1994;36:97-107.
6. Culebras A: Neuroanatomic and neurologic correlates of sleep disturbances. Neurology 1992;42 (Suppl 6):19-27.
7. Stahl SM, Layzer RB, Aminoff MJ, et al: Continuous cataplexy in a patient with a midbrain tumor: The limp-man syndrome. Neurology 1980;30:1115-1118.
8. Hendricks JC, Morrison AR, Mann GL: Different behaviors during paradoxical sleep without atonia depend on pontine lesion site. Brain Res 1982;239:81-105.
9. Autret A, Laffont F, de Toffol B, et al: A syndrome of REM and non-REM sleep reduction and lateral

gaze paresis after medial tegmental pontine stroke: CT scans and anatomical correlation in four patients. Arch Neurol 1988;45:1236-1242.

10. Balk RA, Hiller FC, Lucas EA, et al: Sleep apnea and the Arnold-Chiari malformation. Am Rev Respir Dis 1985;132:929-930.

11. Ward SL, Jacobs RA, Gates EP, et al: Abnormal ventilatory patterns during sleep in infants with meningomyelocele. J Pediatr 1986;109:631-634.

12. Jurko MF, Andy OJ, Webster CL: Disordered sleep patterns following thalamotomy. Clin Electroencephalogr 1971;2:213-217.

13. Autret A, Carrier H, Thommasi M, et al: Etude physiopathologique et neuro-pathologique d'un syndrome decortication cerebrale. Rev Neurol (Paris) 1975;131:491-504.

14. Culebras A: The neurology of sleep. Neurology 1992;42(Suppl 6):6-8.

15. Sheldon SH: Evaluating sleep in infants and children. New York, Lippincott-Raven, 1996, p 276.

16. Tharp BR: Electrophysiological brain maturation in premature infants: An historical perspective. J Clin Neurophysiol 1990;7:302-314.

17. Binnie CD, Prior PF: Electroencephalography. J Neurol Neurosurg Psychiatry 1994;57:1308-1319.

18. Becker PT, Thoman EB: Rapid eye movement storms in infants: Rate of occurrence at 6 months predicts mental development at 1 year. Science 1981;212:1415-1416.

19. Hakamada S, Watanabe K, Hara K, et al: Body movements during sleep in full-term newborn infants. Brain Dev 1982;4:51-55.

20. Brouillette RT, Fernbach SK, Hunt CE: Obstructive sleep apnea in infants and children. J Pediatr 1982;100:31-40.

21. Sanders MH, Rogers RM, Pennock BE: Prolonged expiratory phase in sleep apnea: A unifying hypothesis. Am Rev Respir Dis 1985;131:401-408.

22. Sheldon SH, Onal E, Lilie J, Spire JP: Sleep-related post-inspiratory upper airway obstruction in children. Sleep Res 1993;22:270.

23. National Institutes of Health Consensus Development Conference: Infantile apnea and home monitoring. Bethesda, Md, US Department of Health and Human Services, October 1, 1987, NIH Publication No 87-2950.

24. Sheldon SH, Spire JP, Levy HB: Pediatric Sleep Medicine. Philadelphia, WB Saunders, 1992, p 142.

25. Mathew OP, Remmers JE: Respiratory function of the upper airway. In Saunders NA, Sullivan CE (eds): Sleep and Breathing. New York, Marcel Dekker, 1984, pp 163-200.

26. Bartlett D Jr: Effects of hypercapnia and hypoxia on laryngeal resistance to airflow. Respir Physiol 1979;37:293-302.

27. Remmers JE, Bartlett D Jr: Reflex control of expiratory airflow and duration. J Appl Physiol 1977;42:80-87.

28. Bouterline-Young HJ, Smith CA: Respiration of full-term and premature infants. Am J Dis Child 1953;80:753.

29. Dransfield DA, Spitzer AR, Fox WW: Episodic airway obstruction in premature infants. Am J Dis Child 1983;137:441-443.

30. Milner AD, Boon AW, Saunders RA, Hopkin IE: Upper airway obstruction and apnoea in preterm babies. Arch Dis Child 1980;55:22-25.

31. Kelly DH, Shannon DC: Treatment of apnea and excessive periodic breathing in the full-term infant. Pediatrics 1981;68:183-186.

32. Bairam A, Boutroy MJ, Badonnel Y, Vert P: Theophylline versus caffeine: Comparative effects in treatment of idiopathic apnea in the preterm infant. J Pediatr 1987;110:636-639.

33. Sims ME, Yau G, Rambhatla S, et al: Limitations of theophylline in the treatment of apnea of prematurity. Am J Dis Child 1985;139:567-570.

34. Rosenkrantz TS, Oh W: Aminophylline reduces cerebral blood flow velocity in low birth weight infants. Am J Dis Child 1984;138:489-491.

35. Miller MJ, Carlo WA, Martin RJ: Continuous positive airway pressure selectively reduces obstructive apnea in preterm infants. J Pediatr 1985;106:91-94.

36. Jones RAK: Apnoea of immaturity: I. A controlled trial of theophylline and face mask continuous positive airway pressure. Arch Dis Child 1982;57:761-765.

37. Hirsch K, Wang SC: Selective respiratory stimulating action of doxapram compared to phenylenetetrazol. J Pharmacol Exp Ther 1974;189:1-11.

38. Barrington KJ, Finer NN, Peters KL, Barton J: Physiologic effects of doxapram in idiopathic apnea of prematurity. J Pediatr 1986;108:124-129.

39. Marcus CL, Omlin KJ, Basinki DJ, et al: Normal polysomnographic values for children and adolescents. Am Rev Respir Dis 1992;146:1235-1239.

40. Guilleminault C: Sleep apnea in infancy. In Guilleminault C (ed): Sleep and Its Disorders in Children. New York, Raven Press, 1987, pp 213-224.

41. Brouillette RT, Morrow AS, Weese-Mayer DE, Hunt CF: Comparison of respiratory inductive plethysmography and thoracic impedance for apnea monitoring. J Pediatr 1987;111:377-383.

42. Baldy-Moulinier M, Touchon J, Besset A, et al: Sleep architecture and epileptic seizures. In Degen R, Neidermeyer E (eds): Epilepsy, Sleep and Sleep Deprivation. Amsterdam, Elsevier, 1984, pp 109-118.

43. Rossi GF, Colicchio G, Pola P: Interictal epileptic activity during sleep: A stereo-EEG study in

patients with partial epilepsy. Electroencephalogr Clin Neurophysiol 1984;58:97-106.

44. Hirsch E, Marescaux C, Maquet P, et al: Landau-Kleffner syndrome: A clinical and EEG study of five cases. Epilepsia 1990;31:756-767.

45. Bourgeois B: The relationship between sleep and epilepsy in children. Semin Pediatr Neurol 1996;3:29-35.

46. Rajna P, Veres J: Correlation between night sleep duration and seizure frequency in temporal lobe epilepsy. Epilepsia 34;1993;574-579.

47. Niedermeyer E: Sleep electroencephalogram in petit mal. Arch Neurol 1965;12:625-630.

48. Cadilhac J: Complex partial seizures and REM sleep. In Sterman MB, Shouse MN, Passouant P (eds): Sleep and Epilepsy. New York, Academic Press, 1982, pp 315-324.

49. Devinsky O, Ehrenberg B, Barthlen GM, et al: Epilepsy and sleep apnea syndrome. Neurology 1994;44:2062-2064.

50. Stores G: Confusions concerning sleep disorders and epilepsies in children and adolescents. Br J Psychiatry 1991;158:1-7.

51. Lugaresi E, Cirignotta F: Hypnogenic paroxysmal dystonia: Epileptic seizure or a new syndrome? Sleep 1981;4:129-138.

52. Sheldon SH: Pediatric Sleep Medicine. Philadelphia, WB Saunders, 1992, pp 119-135.

53. Schenck CH, Hurwitz TD, Mahowald MW: REM sleep behavior disorder. Am J Psychiatry 1988; 145:652.

54. Sheldon SH, Jacobsen JJ: REM sleep motor disorder in children. J Child Neurol 1998;13:257-260.

55. Cherubini E, Frascarelli M, Riccardi B, et al: [Changes in the monosynaptic reflex during wakefulness and sleep of children with cerebral paralysis.] Riv Neurol 1978;48:228-241.

56. van den Berg-Emons HJ, Saris WH, de Barbanson DC, et al: Daily physical activity of school children with spastic diplegia and of healthy control subjects. J Pediatr 1995;127:578-584.

57. Watanabe K, Miyazaki S, Hara K, Hakamada S: Behavioral state cycles, background EEGs and prognosis of newborns with perinatal hypoxia. Electroencephalogr Clin Neurophysiol 1980;49: 618-625.

58. Laffont F, Autret A, Minz M, et al: Polygraphic study of nocturnal sleep in three degenerative diseases: ALS, oligo-ponto-cerebellar atrophy, and progressive supranuclear palsy. Waking Sleeping 1979;3:17-30.

59. Shibagaki M, Kiyono S, Takeuchi T: Nocturnal sleep in mentally retarded infants with cerebral palsy. Electroencephalogr Clin Neurophysiol 1985;61:465-471.

60. Cavallo A: The pineal gland in human beings: Relevance to pediatrics. J Pediatr 1993;123:843-851.

61. Sheldon SH: Proconvulsant effects of melatonin in children with chronic neurological handicapping conditions. The Lancet 1998;351:1254.

62. Ward SL, Nickerson BG, van der Hal A, et al: Absent hypoxic and hypercapneic arousal responses in children with myelomeningocele and apnea. Pediatrics 1986;78:44-50.

Disorders of Arousal in Children

Gerald M. Rosen
Mark W. Mahowald

25

PARASOMNIAS

Parasomnias represent a broad group of sleep disorders that are defined as undesirable phenomena occurring predominantly during sleep. These sleep disorders are of great interest to sleep specialists, primary care providers, and patients (and their parents) because this group comprises some of the most common and bizarre sleep problems seen in children. The International Classification of Sleep Disorders (ICSD),[1] published in 1990, includes the following four subcategories of parasomnia: arousal disorders, sleep–wake transition disorders, parasomnias usually associated with rapid eye movement (REM) sleep, and other parasomnias. The ICSD is currently under revision, and in the revised nosology the sleep–wake transition disorders, which include rhythmic movement disorders, will be reclassified in the sleep-related movement disorder category. This topic is covered in Chapter 26. Parasomnias associated with REM sleep, which include REM sleep behavior disorder and recurrent nightmares, is covered in Chapter 26 and other parasomnias, which include enuresis, in Chapter 27. This chapter addresses arousal disorders.

DISORDERS OF AROUSAL IN CHILDREN

Disorders of arousal constitute a common group of sleep disorders seen in children[2] that was first described as a distinct clinical entity by Broughton in 1968.[3] Disorders of arousal constitute a clinical spectrum that varies from a child who quietly sits up in bed, mumbles briefly, and then lies back down and returns to sleep to the adolescent who has a sudden arousal that begins with a bloodcurdling scream followed by headlong flight. All of the disorders of arousal share a common pathophysiology and have many similarities in family history, genetic predisposition, timing during the sleep cycle, and clinical features.

CLINICAL DESCRIPTION

The clinical features common to most children experiencing any of the disorders of arousal include the timing during the night-time sleep cycle, misperception of and unresponsiveness to the environment, automatic behavior, a high arousal threshold, varying levels of autonomic arousal, and variable retrograde amnesia. The disorders of arousal typically begin abruptly at the transition from the first period of slow-wave sleep (non-REM [NREM] stage 4) (Figs. 25–1 and 25–2) of the night, which accounts for the typical timing 60 to 90 minutes after sleep onset at the end of the first ultradian sleep cycle. The duration of each event can vary from less than 1 minute to over 90 minutes. In most cases, the arousal will terminate when the child returns to sleep without ever fully awakening. Although only a single event usually occurs on a given night, some children may have multiple ones. When there are multiple events, they will typically recur at 60- to 90-minute intervals during the first half of the night that correspond to subsequent transitions out of slow-wave sleep at the end of each subsequent ultradian sleep cycle. Successive events on the same night tend to be progressively milder.

Although the clinical manifestations of the disorders of arousal occur along a spectrum, for ease of description and to establish a common nomenclature, the ICSD has divided the spectrum of arousal disorders into three distinct entities: sleepwalking, confusional arousals, and sleep terrors. This nomenclature will be used throughout the present chapter. At the mildest

293

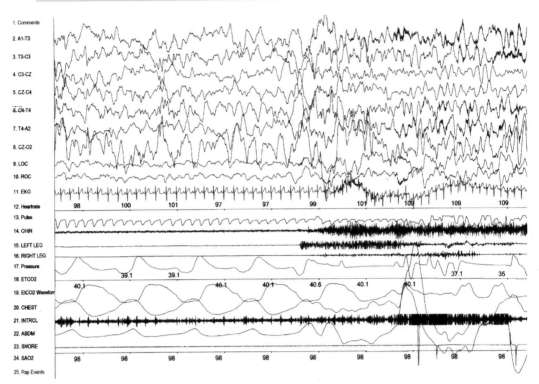

Figure 25–1. Polysomnogram of a disorder of arousal that occurred precipitously out of slow-wave sleep.

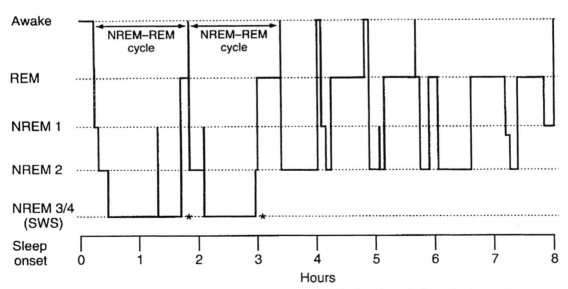

Figure 25–2. Idealized sleep hypnogram showing ultradian rhythm through the night. NREM–REM cycles are approximately 90 minutes; the majority of SWS occurs early in the sleep period, and the majority of REM sleep occurs late in the sleep period. Disorders of arousal generally occur during the transition out of SWS (asterisks). NREM, non-REM; REM, rapid eye movement; SWS, short-wave sleep. (Rosen GM, Ferber R, Mahowald MW: Evaluation of parasomnias in children. Child Adolesc Psychiatr Clin North Am 1996;5:601-616.)

end of the spectrum, a child will simply awaken from sleep, sit up in bed, look around briefly, lie back down, and return to sleep. These arousals are rarely noticed unless the child sleeps with a parent. This type of arousal is usually not characterized as a problem by parents and is seldom brought to the attention of the child's physician. These arousals may be noted as an incidental finding in children who are studied by overnight polysomnography for other reasons.

Sleepwalking

The presentation of sleepwalking is similar at all ages and includes, at a minimum, a partial arousal from sleep with some ambulation. The young child may simply awaken and crawl about in the crib before returning to sleep. These events generally go unnoticed unless the child sleeps with another family member. An older child may get up and walk to the parents' room or may simply be found asleep at a location different from where s/he went to bed, with no recollection of having left his/her bed. Some unusual behavior, such as urinating in an inappropriate place such as the closet or next to the toilet, is common. Such a child may be easily led back to bed, with little evidence of a complete awakening and no recall of the event the next day. Sleepwalking can be triggered in most children by simply waking and then standing them up within the first few hours of sleep onset. Sleepwalking is not dangerous in and of itself, but children may put themselves in danger during a sleepwalking episode by climbing out a window or leaving their homes. During presumed sleepwalking, children have drowned while camping near water and have frozen to death after leaving their homes in the winter.

Sleepwalking is common in children, as documented in two large-scale, population-based studies by Klackenberg[4] in Sweden and Laberge and colleagues[2] in Quebec. Klackenberg longitudinally studied a group of 212 randomly selected children in Stockholm from ages 6 to 16 years. The prevalence of quiet sleepwalking occurring at least once during the 10-year data collection period in this group was 40%. The yearly incidence varied from 6% to 17%, although only 3% had more than one episode per month. In Klackenberg's study, the sleepwalking persisted for 5 years in 33% of children and for over 10 years in 12%.

Laberge and associates studied 1353 randomly selected children in Quebec whose parents completed sleep questionnaires regarding the presence of parasomnias in their children yearly from the time they were 10 to 13 years of age and retrospectively from when their children were ages 3 to 10 years. In this group, occasional or frequent sleepwalking was present in 14% of all children at some time between the ages of 3 and 13 years. The yearly incidence of sleepwalking from Laberge's study, as shown in Table 25–1, varied from 3% to 9%. In the majority of these children, the sleepwalking began and ended between the ages of 3 and 10 years. At 13 years of age 3% of the children were still sleepwalking. The sleepwalking persisted beyond the age of 13 years in 24% of these children. There was no gender difference in sleepwalking prevalence. In the studies of both Laberge and coworkers and Klackenberg, sleepwalking was frequently seen in those children who had confusional arousals at a younger age.

Table 25–1.   **Prevalence of Parasomnias at Various Ages in the Same Children**

Age	Sleepwalking (%)	CA&NT (%)	Sleeptalking (%)
3-10	9.2	14.7	37.1
11	7	3.8	32.5
12	6.8	2.3	30.1
13	3.3	1.2	29.2
Overall	13.8	17.3	55.5

CA&NT, confusional arousals and night terrors.
Modified with permission from Laberge L, Tremblay RE, Vitaro F, Montplasir J: Development of parasomnias from childhood to early adolescence. Pediatrics 2000;106:67-74.

Confusional Arousals

Confusional arousals may seem quite bizarre and frightening to parents. The arousal usually starts with some movements and moaning, progressing to crying and often in association with intense thrashing about in the bed or crib. An infant may be described simply as crying inconsolably. These arousals are common in infants and toddlers. The child is typically described as appearing confused, with the eyes open or closed. These events can last anywhere from a few minutes to over 1 hour, with 5 to 15 minutes being typical. Even if the child calls for the parents, s/he often does not recognize them. Even vigorous attempts to wake the child are often unsuccessful. Holding and cuddling usually do not provide reassurance; instead, the child often resists, twists, and pushes away and may become more agitated. It is the parents' inability to comfort their child, who appears to be in great distress, that is often of the greatest concern to them.

In the study of Laberge and colleagues,[2] the prevalence of occasional or frequent confusional arousals between the ages of 3 and 13 years was 17%. The yearly incidence varied from 1% to 14%. In 85% of the children in their study, the confusional arousals first appeared between the ages of 3 and 10 years, and in the majority of these children, the confusional arousals disappeared before the age of 10 years. The confusional arousals persisted beyond 13 years of age in 6.7% of the children who had confusional arousals at a younger age. Sleepwalking and confusional arousals were often seen in the same child at different ages in the studies of both Laberge[2] and Klackenberg.[4] Thirty-six percent of the children with sleepwalking in the study of Laberge and coworkers had confusional arousals as preschoolers, and all of the children with confusional arousals in Klackenburg's study had at least one episode of sleepwalking. Laberge and colleagues used the term "night terrors" to describe the events that are called "confusional arousals" in the present chapter. Confusional arousals is used here to conform to the definitions described in the ICSD Classification of Sleep Disorders.[1]

Sleep Terrors

Sleep terrors are the most dramatic and least common of the disorders of arousal. They are seen more often in older children and young adults. The events usually begin precipitously with the child bolting upright with a scream. There is generally a high level of autonomic arousal. The eyes are usually open, the heart is racing, and often there is diaphoresis and mydriasis. The facial expression is one of intense fear. A youngster may jump out of bed and run blindly as if to frantically avoid some unseen threat. These events are usually shorter than confusional arousals, generally terminating within a few minutes. The child may awaken at the conclusion of the sleep terror or may simply return to sleep without ever having completely awakened. The child may report some recollection, but it is most often fragmented and not characteristic of the imagery reported from dreams and nightmares. As measured by the Social Behavior Questionnaire,[5] anxiety was associated with confusional arousals and sleep terrors in the study of Laberge and associates[2] and has been noted by other authors in case reports of children and adolescents.[6,7]

PATHOPHYSIOLOGY OF DISORDERS OF AROUSAL

Disorders of arousal can best be understood within the context of the basic neurophysiology of sleep. This is described in detail in Chapter 4. However, those aspects of sleep–wake regulation that are particularly relevant to the understanding of disorders of arousal will be discussed here. Sleep is an active, complex, highly regulated neurologic process that is generated by and primarily for the benefit of the brain. Sleep is composed of two fundamentally different sleep states: REM and NREM sleep. REM sleep, NREM sleep, and wakefulness each have very different patterns of cerebral blood flow, glucose utilization, predominant neurotransmitter systems, neuronal activation, and thalamic functioning. From the perspective of brain function, REM and NREM sleep are as different from each other as each is from wakefulness. From this perspective, there are three different "states of being" in which humans can exist: REM sleep, NREM sleep, and wakefulness.[8-12] The determination of the state of being may be made using a variety of criteria. For clinical evaluations, electrographic criteria are generally used—the electroencephalogram, electro-oculogram, and chin electromyogram—

as described in the sleep stage–scoring manual of Rechtschaffen and Kales.[13] However, behavioral criteria may also be used to differentiate wakefulness, NREM sleep, and REM sleep[14] in humans, and single-cell neuronal discharge patterns can be used to characterize states of being in experimental animals.[8]

Each state has its own unique neuroanatomic, neurophysiologic, neurochemical, and neuropharmacologic correlates. There are a number of physiologic markers for each state that tend to occur in concert and cycle in a predictable and uniform manner, resulting in the behavioral appearance of a single prevailing state. Because sleep is a fundamental property of numerous neuronal groups rather than a phenomenon that requires the whole brain, it is possible for different parts of the brain to be in the different states of wakefulness, REM sleep, and NREM sleep at the same time. This concept is fundamental to the understanding of a number of sleep disorders, including the disorders of arousal. If different parts of the brain can be in different states simultaneously, then the physical, clinical, and polysomnographic manifestations of these states can also occur simultaneously. When this occurs, the event can be described as a mixed or dissociated state.[14]

Sleep is a dynamic state. There are continuous currents driving and defining the propensity toward NREM sleep, REM sleep, and wakefulness. The rhythmic alternation among these three states defines two important biologic rhythms, the circadian and ultradian rhythms. The alternation of wakefulness, REM sleep, and NREM sleep over the 24-hour light–dark cycle defines the circadian rhythm, whereas the interweaving of these states over the sleep period defines the ultradian rhythm (Fig. 25–2). Circadian cycling is controlled by a hypothalamic pacemaker located in the suprachiasmatic nucleus.[15] Sleep–wake cycling is the most obvious manifestation of the circadian rhythm, but equally important are diurnal variations in body temperature, hormone secretion, drug metabolism, pulmonary function, immune response/reactivity, blood pressure, intestinal motility, gastric acid secretion, and the propensity to enter REM sleep. As the brain cycles among NREM sleep, REM sleep, and wakefulness, a dynamic reorganization occurs among multiple neuronal networks and neurotransmitters at many levels

of the neuraxis. A complex switch orchestrated in the midbrain and thalamus takes place.[9,10] The transition among states usually occurs smoothly and completely and is not behaviorally apparent, but this is not always the case. The transition may be gradual and incomplete, resulting in the behavioral appearance of a mixed state. This is the neurophysiologic correlate of the clinical situation that is referred to as *state dissociation*. Narcolepsy, REM sleep behavior disorder,[14] and disorders of arousal can all be best understood as clinical examples of mixed or dissociated states of being.

During the disorders of arousal, some facets of wakefulness appear during the transition out of slow-wave sleep. This usually occurs at the end of the first ultradian sleep cycle. As a consequence, the transition out of slow-wave sleep, which is usually quiet, becomes dramatic and perhaps violent. The child appears caught between deep slow wave sleep and wakefulness. His/her behavior at this time has elements that we associate with wakefulness (walking, talking, complex motor behaviors) and sleeping (misperception of and unresponsiveness to the environment, high arousal threshold, amnesia, automatic behavior) occurring simultaneously. The EEG during a partial arousal from sleep is typically characterized by waking and sleeping rhythms with the simultaneous occurrence of alpha, theta, and delta frequencies and likely shows that different areas of the brain are in different states simultaneously. This dissociated state is inherently unstable, and eventually one state is fully declared. In most cases, the child appears to simply return to quiet sleep. Alternatively, the child may awaken but will have no recall of the arousal and will usually rapidly return to sleep. The causes of the disorders of arousal are multifactorial. The genetic predisposition, homeostatic drive, sleep–wake cycling/synchronization, and behavioral/emotional state all seem to play some role in the clinical appearance of the disorders of arousal. Of these factors, genetic predisposition is probably the most important. A positive family history in a first-degree relative is present in 60% of the children with these disorders[16] compared with 30% in the general population. Sleep–wake cycling and synchronization are affected by age, homeostatic factors, circadian factors, hormones, and drugs. Affective disorders, anxiety, and environmental stress have all been identified as important factors in the appearance of the disorders of arousal in clinical studies,[2-4,6,7] although the mechanisms by which these factors lead to the arousal is not known.

GENETICS OF DISORDERS OF AROUSAL

A familial predisposition toward the disorders of arousal has been recognized since these disorders were first described. The genetics of the disorders of arousal has been explored by Hublin and coworkers[17,18] in population-based twin studies and by Lecendreux and colleagues[19] in the human leukocyte antigen testing of patients who sleepwalk and normal control subjects. Hublin and colleagues calculated the phenotypic variance of sleepwalking attributable to genetic factors at 65%, which he believed was the result of many genes, each with minor effects. This is consistent with the results of human leukocyte antigen testing for sleepwalking by Lecendreux and associates.

The neurophysiologic mechanisms by which genetics influences the appearance of the disorders of arousal is not known. One possible explanation, for which there is good theoretical support and some experimental evidence, is that the familial predisposition toward the disorders of arousal is mediated by the genetic control of the kinetics of the sleep homeostatic process. This process has been shown to be under strong genetic control in animal studies.[20] Studies in mice have demonstrated that sleep loss leads to an increase in homeostatic drive, with a change in slow-wave sleep activity as measured by delta power, in a dose–response fashion that varies with the duration of prior wakefulness and is different in different genotypes. A quantitative trait-loci analysis revealed that this trait is the product of multiple genes. Human EEG studies have also shown that slow-wave sleep and EEG slow-wave activity are markers for measuring homeostatic drive.[21-23] Increases in slow-wave sleep and slow-wave activity occur after sleep deprivation and decline after sleep. In laboratory animals, the increase in the homeostatic drive caused by sleep deprivation is not obliterated after the suprachiasmatic nucleus has been destroyed; suggesting that the site of control for the homeostatic system is different from that for the circadian system. Although the suprachi-asmatic nucleus does not control the homeostatic process, the circadian system interacts with the homeostatic system to regulate the timing of sleep and wakefulness and hence the duration of each. The synchronization of the homeostatic and circadian systems has been shown to be essential for the attainment of optimum sleep and wakefulness. This interaction is described in a comprehensive article by Dijk and Lockley.[22] Adequate sleep duration occurs only when the circadian and homeostatic systems are fully synchronized. The clinical implication of this observation is that a child with an irregular and/or chaotic sleep–wake schedule will simply not be able to have optimum synchronization of the homeostatic and circadian systems; this inevitably leads to sleep disruption and sleep deprivation, which leads to a clinical event in the child predisposed to the disorders of arousal.

POLYSOMNOGRAPHY IN DISORDERS OF AROUSAL

Polysomnographic studies have shown that individuals with the disorders of arousal, when compared with normal control subjects, have no consistent differences in sleep macroarchitecture[23,24]—that is, sleep efficiency, sleep stage percentages, and sleep latencies, among its other characteristics. However, there are differences in the sleep microarchitecture, including cyclic alternating patterns in arousal rates,[25,26] arousals from slow-wave sleep,[23,26] and slow-wave sleep activity delta counts between the sleep of patients with the disorders of arousal and that of control subjects. These differences are the most prominent during the first ultradian sleep cycle, which is when the disorders of arousal usually occur. There were (1) an increased number of brief EEG arousals from slow-wave sleep, (2) a decrease in slow-wave sleep activity delta counts at the end of the first ultradian cycle, and (3) an increase in arousals from the cyclic alternating patterns compared with control subjects. The subjects for these research studies were carefully screened for the presence of other sleep disorders, specifically sleep-disordered breathing, sleep deprivation, and restless legs syndrome.

In one large case series of children referred to a sleep clinic for an evaluation of the disorders of arousal, there was an association between sleep-disordered breathing and the disorders of arousal or restless legs syndrome with periodic leg movements and these same disorders.[27] The disorders of arousal disappeared after adenotonsillectomy in the children with sleep-disordered breathing and after drug treatment in the children with restless legs syndrome, suggesting that these clinical causes of sleep disruption can unmask a disorder of arousal.[27]

All of these lines of evidence suggest that the fundamental abnormality that underpins the disorders of arousal is the instability of slow-wave sleep. This conclusion is supported by the clinical observation and experimental evidence that in individuals predisposed to the disorders of arousal, an event is much more likely to occur after a night of sleep deprivation[28] that increases the homeostatic drive and would be expected to make an unstable homeostatic system more unstable or after sleep fragmentation from sleep apnea or the periodic movements of sleep.

CLINICAL EVALUATION OF CHILDREN WITH DISORDERS OF AROUSAL

Children do not present to a clinician with a diagnosis but rather with a clinical problem. It is the responsibility of the clinician to arrive at the diagnosis through a careful history and the appropriate use of diagnostic studies. The children described in this chapter will generally present with the complaint of unusual nocturnal awakenings. It is important to recognize that there are many causes of this disorder in children. The most important tool for evaluating children with unusual nocturnal awakenings is a complete sleep and medical history. The sleep history will usually allow the clinician to distinguish between the different causes of unusual nocturnal arousals and to formulate an appropriate evaluation and treatment plan. The pediatric sleep history is covered in Chapters 2 and 5. Those facets of the sleep history that are the most important in the evaluation of the disorders of arousal are listed in Table 25–2. Any problem that causes sleep disruption, which results in awakenings, or affects sleep duration or synchronization can lead to the appearance of the disorders of arousal in a child who is thus predisposed.

There are a number of distinguishing clinical characteristics in the histories of children with

the disorders of arousal. The salient features are listed and discussed below.

Timing: Events generally though not always occur about 90 minutes after sleep onset. If a second event occurs during the night, it typically occurs 90 minutes after the first, at the time of the transition out of slow-wave sleep. Arousals occurring on or soon after awakening are more likely to represent unusual sleep-related seizures.[29]

Description of the event: The onset can be gradual, with sleepwalking and confusional arousals, or sudden, with sleep terrors. The behavior during an event is often bizarre and may be complex but is not stereotypical. The child is not normally responsive to the environment, although s/he may be partially responsive. A child will not typically recognize parents and often cannot be comforted by them. The events generally terminate with a return to sleep and without a complete awakening.

Frequency: The frequency of occurrence is highly variable, from several times a night to once in a lifetime; multiple episodes in a single night may occur but are uncommon.

Level of consciousness: This child is generally not arousable.

Memory of event: Most children will have no recall the day after the event.

Daytime sleepiness: Most children have no evidence of daytime sleepiness the next day.

Family history: The family history is often positive in parents and siblings for any of the disorders of arousal.

Table 25–3 lists those conditions that mimic the disorders of arousal and those that may trigger them. The conditions that may mimic the disorders of arousal include seizures; cluster headaches; psychiatric disorders such as nocturnal panic attacks, post-traumatic stress disorder, and nocturnal dissociative disorder; nightmares; REM sleep behavior disorder; and the rhythmic movements of sleep. The conditions that may trigger these disorders in a child who may be predisposed include obstructive sleep apnea, the periodic movements of sleep, gastroesophageal reflux, and behavioral/psychiatric disorders. Sleep deprivation and an irregular sleep–wake schedule are the most common, easily corrected, nonspecific triggers for the disorders of arousal.

Table 25–2.   Sleep History

Circadian

Sleep log for 2 weeks (time in bed, sleep onset, awakening time) (weekdays/weekends)
Vacation sleep schedule
24-hour daily schedule of activities (school, work, meals, play)
Amount of light in room
Seasonal variations
Preferred sleep time and duration

Sleep Environment

Describe bedroom (What is in it? Who is there? How much natural light is there? Is there a television or radio?)

Sleep Onset

How does the child fall asleep?
Who is present at sleep onset and what do they do?
Are there curtain calls, fears, hypnagogic hallucinations, sleep-onset paralysis, restless legs, head banging, body rocking?

Arousals

Time of night	Frequency
Triggers	Association with injury
Description of arousal	Way in which it terminates
Level of agitation/ ambulation	Manner in which the child returns to sleep?
Association with eating/drinking	Recall the next day
Level of consciousness	Age of onset
Duration	

Other Sleep Behavior

Seizures, enuresis, diaphoresis, restlessness, snoring, cough, choking, apnea, periodic movements of sleep, vomiting, nightmares, bruxism

Waking Behavior

Hypnopompic hallucinations, paralysis, headaches

Daytime Sleep

Naps, cataplexy, excessive daytime sleepiness, settings where sleep occurs

Medical

Neurologic: Migraine headaches, attention-deficit disorder, seizures, tics, mental retardation, narcolepsy, neuromuscular disease
Psychiatric: Depression, anxiety, dissociative disorders, conduct disorder, panic disorder, physical/sexual abuse, post-traumatic stress disorder
Ear, Nose, Throat: Ear infections, ear effusions, nasal airway obstruction, sinusitis, streptococci infections, swallowing problems
Cardiorespiratory: Asthma, cough, heart disease, pneumonia
Gastrointestinal: Vomiting, diarrhea, constipation, swallowing problems
Growth: Failure to thrive
Allergies: Milk, seasonal, asthma, eczema
Drug: Legal/illegal
School/behavior: School/developmental problems, behavioral problems
Acute medical illness

Family History

Sleep apnea/snoring
Arousals (sleepwalking, confusional arousals, night terrors, restless legs/periodic movements)
Psychiatric condition (depression)
Social issues (stress at home, divorce, family violence, drug/ethyl alcohol use)
Narcolepsy, hypersomnolence
Restless legs syndrome
Delayed/advanced sleep phase

POLYSOMNOGRAPHY

The role of polysomnography in the evaluation of the disorders of arousal is limited because the sleep macroarchitecture in children with these disorders is generally normal. However, some differences in polysomnographic recorded sleep have been reported in children with these disorders, such as hypersynchronous delta,[30] preced-ing the arousal. This is a nonspecific finding that is also seen in children undergoing polysomnog-raphy for other reasons. The primary role of polysomnography in the evaluation of children with the disorders of arousal is to rule out other sleep disorders, such as obstructive sleep apnea, the periodic movements of sleep, gastroe-sophageal reflux, nocturnal psychogenic disso-ciative states, REM sleep behavior disorder, and

Table 25–3.   Conditions That Mimic* or Trigger† Disorders of Arousal

Neurologic	Sleep
*Seizures	*Nightmares
*Cluster headaches	*Rhythmic movements of sleep
Medical	*Rapid eye movement sleep behavior disorders
†Obstructive sleep apnea	†Periodic movements of sleep
†Gastroesophageal reflux	†Sleep deprivation
Behavioral/Psychiatric	†Irregular sleep–wake schedule
*Conditioned arousals	
*Post-traumatic stress disorder	*Conditions that mimic disorders of arousal.
*Nocturnal dissociative state	†Conditions that trigger disorders of arousal.
*Nocturnal panic	

nocturnal seizures, which may either trigger or mimic the disorders of arousal.

If nocturnal seizures are suspected as the cause of the awakenings as a result of the history of the stereotypical nature or the timing of the arousals throughout the sleep period or if there is an increased likelihood of seizures because of a concomitant neurologic problem, further diagnostic studies should be obtained. In most clinical settings, sleep-related seizures can be best evaluated with sleep-deprived EEG or an overnight study in an EEG telemetry unit. These children should be evaluated in a sleep lab only if the lab staff are experienced in the diagnosis and treatment of sleep-related seizures. This complex topic of sleep-related epilepsy is discussed in Chapter 24 and has recently been reviewed by Mallow.[29]

TREATMENT OF CHILDREN WITH DISORDERS OF AROUSAL

The most appropriate treatment for the child with an unusual nocturnal arousal will depend on the diagnosis. It goes without saying that before considering a treatment strategy, one must have completed a comprehensive medical, neurologic, and sleep evaluation such as the one described in this chapter. If the disorders of arousal are thought to be the most likely cause of the awakenings, the treatment should begin with the education of the child and the parents, reassurance, and safety. The following recommendations represent essential components in any effective treatment plan for children with the disorders of arousal.

The **education** of the parents and their children about the benign, self-limiting nature of the disorders of arousal is always the starting point of treatment. It is often helpful to discuss the pathophysiology of these disorders in a manner that is comprehensible to both the child and parents.

The **demystification** of the symptoms is an important part of the education of the parents and child about the disorders of arousal. The parents often misconstrue the problem and fear that the intensity of the arousal reflects severe, unresolved conflicts and are symptoms of psychological distress. Although it is true that psychological stressors contribute to the appearance of these disorders, they are rarely the only cause.

The child's **safety** is of paramount concern in managing children with the disorders of arousal. These disorders are not dangerous in and of themselves, but during such an event children can put themselves in danger by walking out of the house during winter or by running through a plate glass door. In most cases these concerns can be addressed using a simple, commonsense approach. The child should not sleep on the upper level of a bunk bed, obstructions should be removed from the room, double-cylinder locks may need to be installed on the doors of the house, or a security system alerting the parents that a door or window has been opened may need to be installed.

Sleep extension and regularizing the child's sleep schedule should always be considered as part of the treatment of the disorders of arousal. Sleep deprivation and an irregular sleep-wake schedule are very common problems for children and are often causally related to the appearance of these disorders. Correcting these problems often leads to the resolution of the arousal.

A history of **caffeine use** should be determined, and if found, its elimination is recommended.

The child's **bedtime routine** should be pleasant for both the parent and the child and ideally ends with his/her transition to sleep within 15 minutes of bedtime. If there is conflict at bedtime, sleep onset latency is prolonged, or if the child is fearful or requires close contact with a parent, these issues will need to be addressed.

Medication has also been described as an effective treatment for the disorders of arousal in several series of case reports, although it has not been the subject of well controlled studies. Clonazepam[31,32] has been the most widely used medication for the treatment of these disorders. However, there is a general hesitancy by many clinicians to begin pharmacotherapy for these disorders in children because in most cases the events are benign and self-limiting and have no direct, adverse impact on the child. In a child with frequent, disruptive, or potentially dangerous arousals, medication may be a good short-term strategy while other nonpharmacologic modalities are initiated. If medication is used, it should be given 1 to 1½ hours before the anticipated sleep onset to ensure that there are adequate drug levels in the brain at the beginning of the night, when these disorders are most likely to occur. The beginning dose of clonazepam is generally 0.25 mg. Tricyclic antidepressants have also been anecdotally reported to be effective in the case reports of children with the disorders of arousal.[33,34]

Two behavioral treatments for confusional arousals have been described anecdotally in the literature. **Scheduled awakening** was first suggested by Lask[35] as a treatment for the disorders of arousal; although it is not clear why this intervention is helpful, several case reports have described its efficacy.[36,37] The recommended treatment is simple enough: The child is awakened 15 to 30 minutes before the time of the usual arousal and needs to open his/her eyes and at least mumble a response before being allowed to return to sleep. The parents continue this intervention nightly for 1 month. In some cases this simple intervention has been effective. However, it should be noted that in some cases these scheduled awakenings actually trigger an arousal. **Relaxation and/or mental imagery** and biofeedback have both been described in several series of case reports as being useful treatments for the disorders of arousal.[38]

Psychotherapy and **counseling** are important interventions for the child who has evidence of significant psychological distress. This is true for any child in whom these problems are discovered when these psychological factors are considered to have an adverse impact on the child's or family's life. However, children are rarely able to compartmentalize their emotional lives as well as adults, so it is uncommon for the only manifestation of significant psychological difficulties to be the nocturnal awakenings.

SUMMARY

To the casual observer, the disorders of arousal represent a paradox during which an individual appears to engage in waking behavior while still asleep. With the understanding that sleep and wakefulness are not always mutually exclusive states of being, the paradox disappears. The concept of a mixed state or state dissociation provides an explanation for these events that is founded in the current understanding of the neurophysiology of sleep. The disorders of arousal are common problems, especially in young children, and can usually be fully evaluated and treated by a knowledgeable sleep clinician without the use of high technology.

References

1. Thorpy MJ, Chairman, Diagnostic Classification Steering Committee of the American Sleep Disorder Association: The International Classification of Sleep Disorders: Diagnostic and Coding Manual, 1990.
2. Laberge L, Tremblay RE, Vitaro F, Montplasir J: Development of parasomnias from childhood to early adolescence. Pediatrics 2000;106:67-74.
3. Broughton RJ: Sleep disorders: Disorders of arousal? Science 1968;159:1070-1078.

4. Klackenberg G: Somnambulism in childhood—prevalence, course and behavioral correlates: A prospective longitudinal study (6-16 years). Acta Paediatr Scand 1982;71:495-499.

5. Tremblay RE, Loeber R, Gagnon C, et al: Disruptive sleep with stable and unstable high fighting behavior patterns during junior elementary school. J Ab Child Psychol 1991;19:285-300.

6. Simonds JF, Parago H: Sleep behavior and disorders in children and adolescents evaluated at psychiatry clinics. Dev Behav Pediatr 1984;6:6-10.

7. Dahl RE, Puig-Antich J: Sleep disturbance in children and adolescent psychiatric disorders. Pediatrician 1990;167:32-37.

8. Jones B: Basic mechanisms of sleep-wake states. In Kryger MH, Roth T, Dement W (eds): Principles and Practice of Sleep Medicine. Philadelphia, WB Saunders, 1994, pp 145-162.

9. Basics of sleep behavior. In Chase M, McCarley R, Rechtschaffen A, Roth T (eds): Los Angeles, UCLA Sleep Research Society, 1993, pp 17-78.

10. Hobson J, Schiebel A: The brainstem care: Sensorimotor integration and behavioral state control. Neurosci Res Prog Bull 1980;18.

11. Hobson J, Steriade M: Neuronal basis of behavioral state control. In Bloom F (ed): Handbook of Physiology, vol 4. Bethesda, Md, American Physiological Society, 1986, pp 701-823.

12. Hobson J, Lydic R, Baghdoyan H: Evolving concepts of sleep cycle generation: From brain centers to neuronal populations. Behav Brain Sci 1986;9:371-448.

13. Rechtschaffen A, Kales A: A Manual of Standardized Terminology: Techniques and Scoring System for Sleep States of Human Subjects. Los Angeles, UCLA Brain Information Service/Brain Research Institute, 1968.

14. Mahowald MW, Schenck CH: Dissociated states of wakefulness and sleep. Neurology 1992;42:44-52.

15. Harrington M, Rusak B, Mistlberger R: Anatomy and physiology of the mammalian circadian system. In Kryger M, Roth T, Dement W (eds): Principles and Practice of Sleep Medicine, 3rd ed. Philadelphia, WB Saunders, 2000.

16. Richman N: Surveys of sleep disorders in children in a general population. In Guilleminault C (ed): Sleep and Its Disorders in Children. New York, Raven Press, 1987, pp 115-127.

17. Hublin C, Kaprio J, Partinen M, et al: Prevalence and genetics of sleepwalking: A population-based twin study. Neurology 1997;48:177-181.

18. Hublin C, Kaprio J, Partinen M, et al: Parasomnias: Co-occurrence and genetics. Psychiatr Gen 2001; 11:65-70.

19. Lecendreux M, Bassetti C, Dauvilliers Y, et al: HLA and genetic susceptibility to sleepwalking. Mol Psychiatry 2003;8:114-117.

20. Franken P, Chollet D, Tafti M: The homeostatic regulation of sleep need is under genetic control. J Neurosci 2001;21:2610-2621.

21. Dijk DJ, Czeisler CA: Contribution of the circadian pacemaker and the sleep homeostat to sleep propensity, sleep structure, electroencephalographic slow waves, and sleep spindle activity in humans. J Neurosci 1995;15:3526-3538.

22. Dijk DJ, Lockley SW: Functional genomics of sleep and circadian rhythm: Integration of human sleep-wake regulation and circadian rhythmicity (invited lecture). J Appl Physiol 2002;92:852-862.

23. Gaudreau H, Joncas S, Zadra A, Montplaisir J: Dynamics of slow-wave activity during the NREM sleep of sleepwalkers and control subjects. Sleep 2000;23:755-760.

24. Guilleminault C, Poyares D, Aftab FA, et al: Sleep and wakefulness in somnambulism: A spectral analysis study. J Psychosom Res 2001;51: 411-416.

25. Zuconi M, Oldani A: Arousal fluctuation in non-rapid eye movement parasomnias: The role of cyclic alternating pattern as a measure of sleep instability. J Clin Neurophysiol 1995;12: 147-154.

26. Smirne S, Ferini-Strambi L: Clinical applications of cyclic alternating pattern. In Comi G, Lucking C, Kimura J, Rossini PM (eds): Clinical Neurophysiology: From Receptors to Perception. Philadelphia, Elsevier Science, 1999, pp 109-112.

27. Guilleminault C, Palombini L, Pelayo R, Chervin R: Sleepwalking and sleep terrors in prepubertal children: What triggers them? Pediatrics 2003; 111:e17-e25.

28. Joncas S, Zadra A, Paquet J, Montplaisir J: The value of sleep deprivation as a diagnostic tool in adult sleepwalkers. Neurology 2002;58:936-940.

29. Mallow BA: Paroxysmal events in sleep. J Clin Neurophysiol 2002;19:522-534.

30. Espa F, Ondze B: Sleep architecture, slow wave activity and sleep spindles in adult patients with sleepwalking and sleep terrors. Clin Neurophysiol 1999;111:929-939.

31. Mahowald M, Schenck C: NREM parasomnias. Neurol Clin North Am 1996;14:675-696.

32. Schenk C, Boyd J, Mahowald M: A parasomnia overlap disorder involving sleepwalking, sleep terrors, and REM sleep behavior disorder in 33 polysomnographically confirmed cases. Sleep 1997;20:972-981.

33. Dahl R: The pharmacologic treatment of sleep disorders. Psych Clin North Am 1992;15:161-178.

34. Balon R: Sleep terror disorder and insomnia treated with trazadone: A case report. Ann Clin Psychiatry 1994;6:161-163.

35. Lask B: Novel and non-toxic treatment for night terrors. Br Med J 1988;297:592.

36. Tobin J: Treatment of somnambulism with anticipatory awakening. J Pediatr 1993;122:426-427.

37. Frank C, Spirito A: The use of scheduled awakenings to eliminate childhood sleepwalking. J Pediatr Psychol 1997;22:345-353.

38. Kohen DP, Mahowald MW, Rosen GM: Sleep-terror disorder in children: The role of self hypnosis in management. Am J Clin Hypnosis 1991;4:233-244.

The Parasomnias

26

Stephen H. Sheldon

Parasomnias are classified as dysfunctions associated with sleep, sleep stages, and partial arousal from sleep. The International Classification of Sleep Disorders (ICSD),[1] published in 1990, includes the following four subcategories of parasomnias: arousal disorders, sleep–wake transition disorders, parasomnias usually associated with rapid eye movement (REM) sleep, and other parasomnias. The ICSD is currently under revision, and in the revised nosology the sleep–wake transition disorders, which include rhythmic movement disorders, will be reclassified in the category of sleep-related movement disorders.

These disorders of sleep are strikingly dissimilar in presentation but share many clinical and biologic characteristics. The symptoms appear early in childhood. The steady, gradual transformation and resolution of symptoms suggest that the etiology of parasomnias may be maturational. Few pathophysiologic abnormalities can be identified despite the severe and often intense symptoms. Spontaneous remission as the child ages is common.

Longitudinal observations have shown that many parasomnias may appear gradually or have a sudden onset. The frequency of parasomnia spells can vary and can range from single rare episodes to nightly events persisting for a protracted period of time. During wakefulness, no obvious clinical abnormalities are present and the patients appear medically and developmentally normal, only to express bizarre and sometimes violent behaviors during sleep.

ETIOLOGY

The etiology of parasomnias is unknown. A maturational etiology has been hypothesized. However, any theoretical basis for the underlying cause of parasomnias must address the common features. The additional characteristics affecting classification in the pediatric patient include those parasomnias typically associated with non-REM (NREM) slow-wave sleep (SWS), those typically associated with REM sleep, those typically associated with the transition from wakefulness to sleep, and other parasomnias. Classification is typically made with the emphasis on observable behaviors.[2]

CLINICAL AND LABORATORY EVALUATION OF A CHILD WITH A PARASOMNIA

Evaluation begins with a comprehensive history and physical exam. Special emphasis must be placed on a detailed description of the nocturnal events, including but not limited to the following variables.

1. Usual time of occurrence of the spell
2. Description of behaviors, movements, or symptoms manifested
3. Whether intervention efforts by the caretaker improve or exacerbate symptoms
4. Whether the child leaves the bed
5. Recall or amnesia of the event(s)
6. Occurrence of symptoms during daytime naps
7. Presence or absence of symptoms during wakefulness
8. Presence of stereotypical movements or rhythmic behaviors during the spell

Basic neurodevelopmental landmarks must be carefully assessed for the presence of daytime waking behavioral or developmental abnormalities. Typical sleep–wake schedules, habits, and patterns require delineation. Habitual morning waking time, evening bedtime, and bedtime and nap time rituals should be described. The presence of excessive daytime sleepiness, snoring, or other respiratory symptoms[3] may assist in determining exacerbating factors. The presence of concurrent medical illnesses and medication history should be obtained in the clinical interview.

A complete physical exam must be performed. Emphasis should be placed on a comprehensive neurologic and developmental evaluation. The existence of developmental delays or symptoms suggestive of neurologic disorders might indicate an organic basis for the presenting symptoms. Other sleep disorders are common in children with parasomnias, and resolution of the primary underlying sleep disorder often results in resolution of the parasomnia spells.[3] A urine drug screen might be helpful if the symptoms are considered to be due to a side effect of medication.

Video recording of the spell by the parents can provide significant information. Video polysomnography is often indicated.[4,5] An expanded EEG electrode array assists in differentiating a parasomnia from sleep-related seizures and might provide information localizing focal pathology (Fig. 26–1). Concomitant video recording of the patient while s/he is asleep may demonstrate clinical manifestations and chronicle movements.[6] The study should begin no later than 10:00 PM to avoid artificially short sleep onset latency and end no earlier than 6:00 AM to avoid missing the last REM episode. The patient should be allowed to awaken spontaneously so that a realistic natural recording may be obtained. It is often helpful to have the patient drink fluids and avoid urination before settling, since bladder distention may precipitate some parasomnias.[7] In analyzing the polysomnogram, special emphasis is placed on the identification of other sleep-related pathologies that might precipitate the parasomnia. Attention should also be devoted to analyzing the amplitude of slow waves, synchronization of slow-wave activity,[8] arousal rhythms occurring during

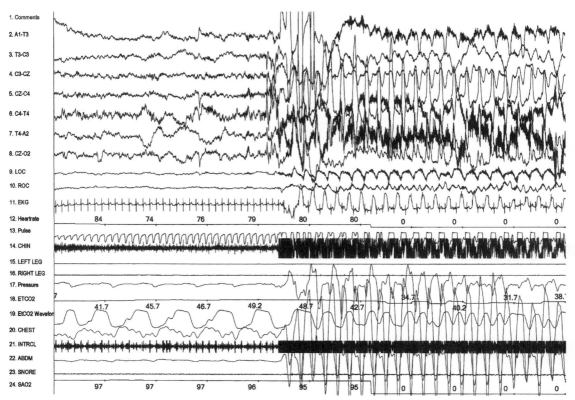

Figure 26–1. Recording of centrotemporal spikes characteristic of benign epilepsy of childhood (benign rolandic epilepsy). In this 120-second epoch, spike activity can be seen in the left temporal region; the series of spikes were followed by an arousal (not a seizure).

SWS (Fig. 26–2), and intrusion of 4 to 7 Hz EEG activity into SWS. Partial arousals, frequent arousal rhythms without a state change, and hypersynchronous theta intrusion into SWS (theta–delta pattern) (Figs. 26–3 and 26–4) have been associated with but not diagnostic of arousal disorders.[9] The need for all-night EEG recordings, routine sleep-deprived EEG, and radiographic studies depends on the presenting situation, night-time manifestations, and clinical symptomatology.

SLEEP–WAKE TRANSITION DISORDERS

Sleep–wake transition disorders (SWTDs) represent a group of sleep disorders that are manifested by falling asleep, the transition between sleep states, or the transition from sleep to wakefulness. At times they may be thought of as state dissociations or overlapping states. The presentation varies considerably from rare and mild movements during state transitions to frequent and sometimes injurious movements having the potential to result in discomfort, pain, anxiety, embarrassment, and disturbance of the youngster's sleep as well as that of the entire family. Included in this classification of disorders are rhythmic movement disorders (head banging and body rocking), sleep starts, sleep talking, and isolated sleep paralysis.

Rhythmic Movement Disorders

Rhythmic movement disorders involve stereotypical body rocking or head banging that occurs during the transition from wakefulness to sleep.[10-17] These movements may also occur during arousals from sleep and may persist into NREM sleep. The movements vary in intensity and can sometimes be quite violent. The etiology is unknown. Rhythmic movements surrounding the sleep period are common and have been reported in approximately two thirds of normal children. There appears to be a male-to-female ratio of 4:1. They are typically self-limiting and are resolved spontaneously in the vast majority of youngsters by 4 years of age.[18]

The diagnosis of rhythmic movement disorders is based on the identification of characteristic symptoms in the absence of other medical and/or psychiatric disorders. Polysomnography is rarely required for diagnosis, but when used it demonstrates the typical rhythmic movements during the immediate presleep period that may extend into early stage 1 sleep. They may also be seen during arousals from sleep and sleep cycle transitions. Occasional movements may be seen during SWS, but it is rare during REM sleep.[19] Focal, paroxysmal, and/or other epileptiform activity associated with the stereotypical activity are absent. Video recordings can be quite helpful in characterizing these rhythmic movements.

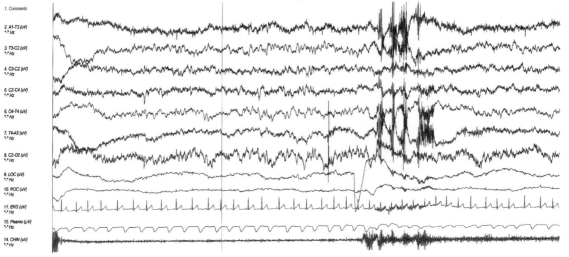

Figure 26–2. Recording of frequent arousal rhythms seen during short-wave sleep in children with non–rapid eye movement parasomnia. In this epoch the rhythm is depicted as a significant theta burst.

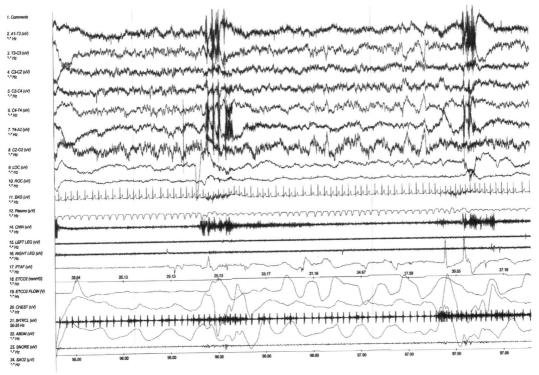

Figure 26–3. Recording of a 30-second epoch demonstrating a theta-delta pattern during slow-wave sleep in a 13-year-old child. Note the intrusion of theta band activity during delta sleep. This theta-delta pattern has been observed in some patients with non–rapid eye movement (NREM) motor parasomnias. It may be consistent with but not diagnostic of NREM motor disorders.

Home video recordings can also be very helpful in classification. An occasional sleep-deprived or prolonged EEG recording may be required to rule out seizure disorders. Once asleep, sleep architecture, state progression, and stage volumes are typically normal (Fig. 26–5).

Although vigorous head banging may seem quite aggressive, injury is rare. Occasional bruising and/or abrasions might occur. The spontaneous degradation of symptoms and spontaneous resolution occur. A variety of treatments have been suggested; however, most reports are anecdotal, and there have been few treatment regimens that have been replicable. Treatment has included such varied modalities as intentional rhythmic movements before bedtime, rhythmic sounds in the sleeping environment, antihistamines, benzodiazepines, and carbamazepine. The degree of success varies with each treatment regimen. Children should be protected from injury, and other disorders must be ruled out, such as autism, pervasive developmental disorder, and hypnogenic dystonia.

Sleep Starts

Sleep starts (hypnic myoclonia) has also been termed *hypnagogic jerks*.[1] This transition problem from wakefulness to sleep is characterized by a sudden, single, brief muscular contraction of the legs and occasionally the arms, head, and postural muscles.[20] Sensory hallucinations (hypnagogic hallucinations) often occur before the sleep start, and the subjective perception of falling may occur, ending with the myoclonic jerk. Sleep starts are common, occur in most individuals, and are not pathologic unless they are frequent and result in sleep onset insomnia.[21] They also must be differentiated from seizures, especially if they occur in patients with known epilepsy.[22]

Hypnic myoclonia may occur at any age and may be frightening when observed by a parent, especially if it is associated with a vocalization or cry. Injury from the massive movement is rare, but foot injuries secondary to kicking a bedpost or crib rail may occur.

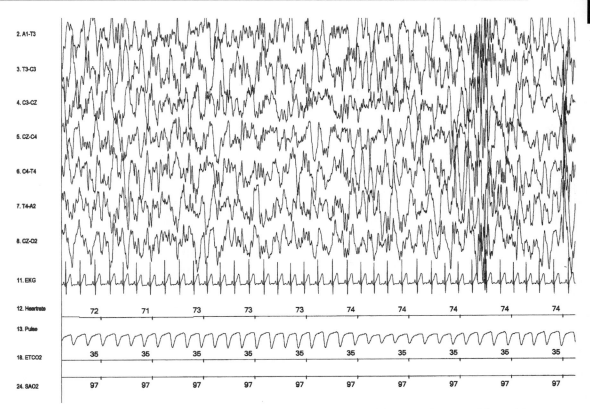

Figure 26–4. Recording of arousal rhythms appearing as bursts of hypersynchronous delta activity during short-wave sleep, which can be seen during the final one third of the 30-second epoch. This activity has also been reported in some children before an episode of enuresis.

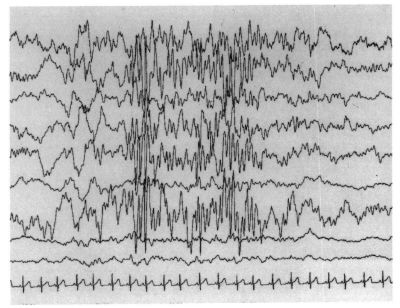

Figure 26–5. Rhythmic movement disorder demonstrated by a 60-second epoch on a recording of a youngster who had been evaluated for sleep-related head-banging. This event typically occurs during the transition from wakefulness to sleep but may also be seen during sleep. In this epoch the patient suddenly became aroused, with a rhythmic movement artifact noted in all channels. Video recording of this patient revealed the rhythmic shuttling of his whole body against the headboard of the bed.

Sleep Talking

Sleep talking (somniloquy) is very common during childhood. It is typically of little concern to parents and caretakers. Significant outbursts and loud talking or utterances are rare but occasionally may be significant enough to disturb the sleep of parents or other family members.[23-25] Somniloquy is not associated with pathologic states but may be related to other parasomnias, such as sleep terrors, confusional arousals, and sleepwalking.

The diagnosis is based on identification of the typical manifestations of coherent speech, incoherent mumbling, or utterances during the sleep period. Amnesia of the event is typical. The clinical course is usually self-limiting, but symptoms may persist. Polysomnography reveals that somniloquy can occur in any stage of sleep.

PARASOMNIAS USUALLY ASSOCIATED WITH REM SLEEP

Parasomnias also occur during REM sleep. In most cases, the manifestations are markedly dissimilar to those of the NREM sleep parasomnias and sleep–wake transition disorders. Most can be differentiated on clinical evaluation alone. Certain REM sleep parasomnias may occasionally share symptoms similar to partial arousal disorders. The frequency varies considerably from commonly seen REM sleep parasomnias (e.g., nightmares) to others that are rarely described in childhood (e.g., REM sleep behavior disorders). Disorders rarely encountered during childhood are included because their importance to the practitioner might become clear when they are more completely understood and the dysfunctions associated with the sleeping state are further delineated in children.

Nightmares

A nightmare (anxiety dream) occurs during REM sleep and is characterized by a frightening dream that often results in a prolonged period of wakefulness.[26,27] There is typically clear recall of the dream, manifestations of anxiety may be present, and there may be some mild autonomic nervous system discharge. There is sudden arousal from REM sleep, arousal to a full waking state, full orientation to the environment, and a clear sensorium.

Nightmares most commonly occur during the last one half to one third of the sleep period, during the longest and most intense REM episode. The "dream story" is often complex and may involve a credible threat to survival, security, or self-esteem. The dreams are usually vivid, with a clear, action-packed story line. The dream recall is appropriate to the child's developmental and maturational level. The child is most often fully awake and alert after the nightmare, and the reaction is emotional rather than associated with the intense autonomic nervous system discharges seen in association with sleep terrors. Children are often easily comforted after an arousal from a nightmare, and the return to sleep is delayed.

Nearly all children experience nightmares. Prevalence data are not clear. The age of onset appears to parallel the development of dreams in childhood. There seems to be equal sex distribution and no clear familial pattern.

Movements are rare during nightmares due to normal REM sleep hypotonia; however, arousal from sleep with clear mentation is typical. Manifestations are generally mild and vocalizations rare.

The diagnosis of anxiety dreams is based on the identification of the mild and characteristic manifestations of disturbing dreams occurring during the early morning hours, absence of intense autonomic activation, clear recall of the dream, a story-like quality to the dream report, appropriate functioning and alertness on awakening, and a good response to parental interventions. Other diagnostic techniques are rarely required, and nightmares are typically easily differentiated from sleep terrors on solely clinical grounds (Table 26–1).

If polysomnography is conducted, an abrupt awakening from REM sleep is seen, followed by a prolonged period of wakefulness after sleep onset. There may be mild tachycardia. Increased eye movement density during REM sleep may accompany the nightmare. Muscle tone is low, and there may be increased frequency of phasic muscle twitches. Focal, paroxysmal, and epileptiform activities are absent.

Occasional nightmares are common during childhood. However, if they become frequent, persist for prolonged periods of time, or are associated with daytime behavioral or performance dysfunction, underlying medical or psychological causes should be considered.

Table 26–1.   Comparison of Sleep Terrors and Nightmares

Characteristic	Sleep Terror	Nightmare
Time of night	First third to first half of the sleep period	Last half to last third of the sleep period
Sleep stage	Slow-wave sleep	REM sleep
Associated activity	Movement and significant motor activity is common.	Movements during nightmares are rare.
Severity	Severe outbursts	Mild to moderate crying
Vocalizations	Common	Mild and rare
Autonomic nervous system	Intense autonomic discharges including but not limited to tachycardia, tachypnea, diaphoresis, and pupillary dilation	Mild autonomic activity
Recall for the event	None/amnesia for the event	There is good recall for the nightmare. There is a story quality to the dream report (typically a good dream that turned bad).
State on awakening	Confused/disoriented	Fully awake and functioning
Injuries/violence	Common	Rare
Associated sleepwalking	About 18% are associated with agitated sleepwalking.	None

REM, rapid eye movement

Treatment is based on reassurance and education. The maintenance of appropriate sleep hygiene is essential. Identifying and minimizing underlying causes, especially those that are anxiety or stress related, are essential to appropriate management. Additional medical and/or psychological evaluation and management may be required.

Isolated Sleep Paralysis

Isolated sleep paralysis is characterized by a period of inability to voluntarily move occurring at the beginning of the sleep period (hypnagogic) or immediately on awakening from sleep (hypnopompic).[28,29] The child is conscious and awake and vigilant toward the environment. All muscle groups except the diaphragm and extraocular muscles are typically involved. Active inhibition of alpha motor neurons is present, and this inhibition is similar (if not identical) to that which is associated with normal REM sleep. Patients often have a sensation of difficulty breathing due to inhibition of the accessory muscles of respiration, and the episodes are characteristically frightening.

Sleep paralysis spells are most often brief, last only a few minutes, and subside spontaneously. At times spells can be aborted by contact from another person or by volitional rapid movements of the eyes. Hypnagogic or hypnopompic hallucinations are unusual during spells of sleep paralysis but can occur and increase the anxiety related to the episode.

Normal individuals experience isolated occurrences of sleep paralysis . More frequent events are seen in patients with narcolepsy syndrome (as part of the tetrad of excessive daytime sleepiness/sleep attacks, cataplexy, hypnagogic hallucinations, and sleep paralysis) and in *familial* sleep paralysis. There is equal sex distribution in this isolated form and a female preponderance in the familial form.

The onset usually occurs during adolescence, but the symptoms may begin during childhood. Children have difficulty describing the event and may appear asleep throughout its duration. The parents may be unaware of its occurrence, since touching or shaking might abort the hypotonia. The symptoms may be mistaken for resistance to awakening. Children who resist awakening arouse cranky and obstinate. On the other hand, children awakening from an episode of sleep paralysis might be frightened and cry.

The clinical course varies significantly among individuals. Most cases are isolated and are provoked by sleep deprivation, excessive sleepiness, stress, and an irregular sleep–wake schedule or after acute changes in the sleep phase. Sleep paralysis runs a more chronic course in patients with narcolepsy syndrome and in the familial form of the disorder.

The diagnosis is based on the identification of presenting symptoms, which may not be obvious. Sleep paralysis associated with narcolepsy syndrome can be differentiated from the isolated form by the presence of other symptoms related to the clinical tetrad. Atonic generalized seizures occur during wakefulness and may or may not be associated with changes in the level of consciousness. Syncope occurs during wakefulness as well and is commonly associated with altered levels of consciousness.

Polysomnography might reveal a significant decrease in chin muscle tone in the presence of normal waking EEG rhythm. Conjugate eye movements may be present as well. Patients may occasionally enter sleep during an episode of sleep paralysis and reveal an EEG pattern consistent with stage 1 sleep. True sleep-onset REM periods may occur at night, and a multiple sleep latency test may be required to differentiate these episodes from narcolepsy syndrome.

REM Sleep Motor Disorder

REM sleep motor disorder (RMD), originally described in adults as REM sleep behavior disorder, has also been described in childhood.[30] RMD is an unusual abnormality seen in REM sleep that is characterized by elaborate, sometimes purposeful movements accompanied by vocalizations. There is a paradoxical increase in muscle tone that might be considered the absence of REM sleep atonia, resulting in patients "acting out their dreams." Violent behaviors occasionally occur, with patients punching, kicking, and/or leaping out of bed. These behaviors are associated with vivid dream recall. Injuries to the patient or to bed partners are common. Episodes usually occur

during the first REM period of the night, approximately 90 minutes after sleep onset.

RMD usually begins during late adulthood and progresses over a variable period of time. Children may also be affected, and a greater understanding of this disorder may reveal the incidence and prevalence to be higher than current descriptions suggest. A majority of cases are idiopathic; however, neurologic disorders have been reported in approximately 40% of affected adults. The signs and symptoms have also been reported in post-traumatic stress disorder.

Polysomnography reveals increased muscle tone that persists throughout sleep, especially REM sleep. There are increased phasic muscle activity, excessive limb movements and body jerking, and periodic limb movements. Complex behaviors occur during REM sleep. No epileptiform activity is noted on EEG. Interestingly, RMD in both children and adults responds well to benzodiazepines, especially clonazepam.

Sleep Bruxism

Sleep bruxism is the forceful grinding or rhythmic clenching of the teeth or rhythmic movements of the mandible during sleep.[31]

These rhythmic movements are the result of involuntary, repetitive contractions of the masseter, temporalis, and pterygoid muscles. When teeth grinding occurs, there is loud, unmistakable noise produced. Predisposing factors for the development of bruxism have been reported to include minor abnormalities of the teeth, malocclusion, stress, and anxiety. Some anecdotal data have shown that rhythmic movement and protrusion of the mandible also occur during arousals associated with occlusive sleep-disordered breathing.

The prevalence of bruxism is unclear, but it has been estimated that 5% to 20% of children have manifested symptoms. Bruxism has been reported in over 50% of children, with a mean age of onset of 10.5 years. Dental evidence of bruxism can be identified in 10% to 20% of the general population There appears to be an equal sex distribution, and the condition is most commonly seen in children and young adults. Similar to many parasomnias, a familial pattern without clear genetic transmission can be shown. There are no longitudinal studies demonstrating the natural course of bruxism.

Episodes of rhythmic jaw movements occur either periodically or paroxysmally in bursts of 5 to 15 seconds or longer and are often repeated many times during the sleep period. The daytime symptoms are common and include jaw pain, craniofacial pain, painful teeth, morning headaches, chronic wear to the crowns of the teeth, periodontal tissue damage, and bleeding from the gums. Resorption of alveolar bone, hypertrophy of the masseter and temporalis muscles, and temporomandibular joint dysfunction can occur. Sleep bruxism can also be mistaken for atypical migraine cephalgia, especially when the response to traditional treatment has been poor.

The diagnosis is made by the identification of the loud, unmistakable sound of bruxism in the absence of other medical or psychiatric disorders that may produce abnormal movements during sleep. Obstructive sleep-disordered breathing should also be assessed, especially in the presence of morning headaches, frequent nocturnal awakenings (with or without headaches), snoring, restless sleep, daytime sleepiness, hyperactivity, attention span problems, and performance difficulties.

Polysomnography reveals paroxysmal, rhythmic muscle activity manifested by about 1 Hz muscle artifact over the temporalis muscle (Fig. 26–6). This rhythmic activity may also be seen in the chin muscle electromyogram or masseter muscle groups. If it is associated with occlusive sleep-disordered breathing, the muscle activity occurs during the arousal immediately after the obstructive respiratory event (Fig. 26–7).

A number of therapeutic approaches have been recommended, yet a most important factor

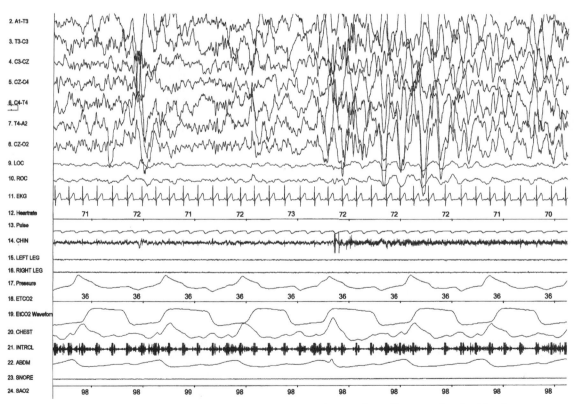

Figure 26–6. Recording showing a rhythmic temporalis muscle artifact associated with airway obstruction. In this 60-second epoch the artifact is noted during an arousal after an episode of apnea, and this brief activity can again be seen during an arousal after hypopnea. The exact cause of this activity is not known, but in patients with obstructive sleep-disordered breathing, it may be mandibular movement in an attempt to assist in opening the airway.

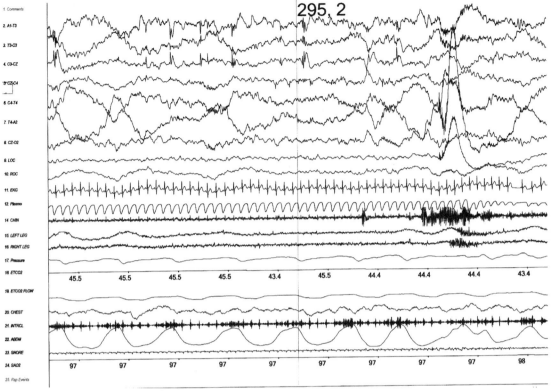

Figure 26–7. Transcoronal electrode array showing bruxism activity involving the rhythmic movement of the temporalis and masseter muscles. Bruxism is often associated with an obnoxious teeth-grinding noise. This disorder may occur during the day and/or during sleep and may be associated with significant wearing of the crowns and enamel of the teeth. There may or may not be similar activity seen in an electromyographic recording of the chin muscle. In this epoch the muscle movement is seen over the temporal leads.

is appropriate dental management. A mouth guard may be worn to prevent damage to the teeth. However, the mouth guard does not seem to prevent episodes of bruxism and is used primarily as a preventive dental intervention. If stress or anxiety is prominent, efforts to minimize the precipitating causes may be helpful. Treatment of dental and/or other anatomic abnormalities, if present, may not alter its course. If bruxism is associated with occlusive sleep-disordered breathing, this should be appropriately managed.

References

1. American Sleep Disorders Association: International Classification of Sleep Disorders: Diagnostic and Coding Manual (rev). Rochester, Minn, American Sleep Disorders Association, 1997.

2. Brooks S, Kushida CA: Behavioral parasomnia. Curr Psychiatr Reports 2002;4:363.

3. Guilleminault C, Palombini L, Pelayo R, Chervin RD: Sleepwalking and sleep terrors in prepubertal children: What triggers them? Pediatrics 2003; 11:e17.

4. Zucconi M, Oldani A, Ferini-Strambi L, et al: Nocturnal paroxysmal arousals with motor behaviors during sleep: Frontal lobe epilepsy or parasomnia? J Clin Neurophysiol 1997;14:513.

5. Dyken ME, Yamada T, Lin-Dyken DC: Polysomnographic assessment of spells in sleep: Nocturnal versus parasomnias. Semin Neurol 2001;21:377.

6. Zucconi M, Ferini-Strambi L: NREM parasomnias: Arousal disorders and differentiation from nocturnal frontal lobe epilepsy. Clin Neurophysiol 2000;41:1221.

7. Broughton R: Childhood sleep walking, sleep terrors and enuresis nocturna: Their pathophysiology

and differentiation from nocturnal epileptic seizures. Sleep 1978. Basel, S Karger, 1980, p 103.

8. Parrino L, Smerieri A, Terzano MG: Combined influence of cyclic arousability and EEG synchrony on generalized interictal discharges within the sleep cycle. Epilepsy Res 2001;44:7.

9. Sheldon SH, Riter S, Detrojan M: Atlas of Sleep Medicine in Infants and Children. Armonk, NY, Futura, p 208.

10. deLissovoy V: Head banging in early childhood: A study of incidence. J Pediatr 1961;58:803.

11. Kravitz H, Rosenthal V, Teplitz Z, et al: A study of head-banging in infants and children. Dis Nerv Sys 1960;21:203.

12. Lewis MH, Baumeister AA, Mailman RB: A neurobiological alternative to the perceptual reinforcement hypothesis of stereotyped behavior: A commentary on "self-stimulatory behavior and perceptual reinforcement." J Appl Behav Anal 1987;20:253.

13. Lourie RS: The role of rhythmic patterns in childhood. Am J Psychiatry 1949;105:653.

14. Lovaas I, Newsom C, Hickman C: Self-stimulatory behavior and perceptual reinforcement. J Appl Behav Anal 1987;20:45.

15. Sallustro MA, Atwell CW: Body rocking, head banging, and head rolling in normal children. J Pediatr 1978;93:704.

16. Schwartz SS, Gallagher RJ, Berkson G: Normal repetitive and abnormal stereotyped behavior of nonretarded infants and young mentally retarded children. Am J Ment Def 1986;90:625.

17. Klackenburg G: Rhythmic movements in infancy and early childhood. Acta Paediatr Scand 1971;224(Suppl):74.

18. Kaneda R, Furuta H, Kazuto K, et al: An unusual case of rhythmic movement disorder. Psychiatr Clin Neurosci 2000;54:348.

19. Kohyama J, Matsukura F, Kimura K, Tachibana N: Rhythmic movement disorder: Polysomnographic study and summary of reported cases. Brain Dev 2002;24:33.

20. Oswald I: Sudden bodily jerks on falling asleep. Brain 1959;82:92.

21. Broughton R: Pathological fragmentary myoclonus, intensified sleep starts and hypnagogic foot tremor: Three unusual sleep-related disorders. In Koella WP (ed): Sleep 1986. New York, Fischer-Verlag, 1988, p 240.

22. Fusco L, Pachatz C, Cusmai R, Vigevano F: Repetitive sleep starts in neurologically impaired children: An unusual non-epileptic manifestation in otherwise epileptic subjects. Epileptic Dis 1999;1:63.

23. Rechtschaffen A, Goodenough D, Shapiro A: Patterns of sleep talking. Arch Gen Psychiatry 1962;7:418.

24. Saskin P, Whelton C, Moldofsky H, Akin F: Sleep and nocturnal leg cramps. Sleep 1988;11:307.

25. Laberge L, Tremblay RE, Vitaro F, Montplaisir J: Development of parasomnias from childhood to early adolescence. Pediatrics 2000;106:67.

26. Fisher CJ, Byrne J, Edwards R, Kahn E: A psychophysiological study of nightmares. JAMA 1970;18:747.

27. Ferber R: Sleeplessness in children. In Ferber R, Kryger M (eds): Principles and Practice of Sleep Medicine in the Child. Philadelphia, WB Saunders, 1995, p 79.

28. Guilleminault C: Narcolepsy and its differential diagnosis. In Guilleminault C (ed): Sleep and Its Disorders in Children. New York, Raven Press, 1987, p 182.

29. Penn NE, Kripke DF, Scharff J: Sleep paralysis among medical students. J Psychol 1981;107:247.

30. Sheldon SH, Jacobsen J: REM-sleep motor disorder in children. J Child Neurol 1998;13:257.

31. Monaco A, Ciammella NM, Marci MC, et al: The anxiety in bruxer child: A case-control study. Minerva Stomatol 2002;51:247.

Sleep-Related Enuresis   27

Stephen H. Sheldon

Sleep-related enuresis (SRE) is characterized by the involuntary and recurrent voiding of urine during sleep. Biologic sequelae are uncommon, but psychological and emotional comorbidity are substantial. To minimize the consequences, an understanding of the etiology, diagnostic procedures, and treatment is required.

Between 3 million and 7 million school-aged children suffer from SRE.[1] Prevalence data are similar in all industrialized societies.[2] Symptoms of SRE are often secreted, and generalizations to large populations should be accepted as approximations rather than as reflections of actual incidence and prevalence.

SRE may be *primary* or *secondary* depending on the pattern of symptom presentation. Primary SRE is the involuntary discharge of urine during sleep, typically at night, that has been present since birth and has not been interrupted by significant asymptomatic periods. Secondary enuresis refers to symptoms of involuntary voiding, typically at night, when there has been an intervening period of at least 3 asymptomatic months followed by recurrence.[3,4] Secondary SRE is more commonly associated with organic or psychological factors than is primary SRE. Approximately 80% of enuretic children wet only at night, 5% wet only during wake during the day, and about 15% are enuretic both during wake and sleep.[5] Again, organic and psychological causes are more common when there is also a pattern of incontinence during wakefulness.

The age at which SRE becomes abnormal is controversial. The child's coping ability and commitment to solving the problem are important. The family's overall cohesion and frustration with the child who wets the bed at night can influence parental perceptions about the consequences of enuresis on the child and the family.[6] Most agree that 5 years of age is the lower limit where concern over bedwetting should begin

and intervention should be considered.[7] SRE is present in approximately 30% of 4 year olds but in only 10% of 6 year olds, 3% of 12 year olds, and 1% of 15-year-old adolescents. Spontaneous remission rates of about 14% to 19% per year have been reported.[8] Boys tend to be affected about twice as frequently as girls when less than 11 years of age. After age 11 years, the sex distribution appears to be equal.[9] Additionally, there appears to be a familial predisposition. The highest frequency of SRE occurs in children when both mother and father were enuretic as children.[10]

ETIOLOGY

The exact cause of primary SRE is unknown. It is most likely that a variety of factors exist and contribute to persistence of SRE after the age at which daytime continence occurs. Because spontaneous resolution of SRE occurs at a relatively regular and steady rate thorough middle childhood, the underlying cause is thought to relate to delayed maturation of bladder mechanisms, and perhaps to a delay in the development of portions of the central nervous system required or maintenance of continence.

Although there is no conscious control over the smooth muscle of the bladder, voluntary control over voiding involves the maintenance of control over skeletal musculature that may directly influence smooth muscle. During wakefulness, recognition of bladder distension most likely involves autonomic afferent stimuli originating in the bladder wall.

Sleep-related continence appears to be related to several factors. First, functional bladder capacity (i.e., the volume at which perception of the need for micturition occurs) must increase to a level that can adequately maintain volume throughout the entire sleep period without

317

spontaneous contractions. An adequate functional volume is about 300 to 360 cc, and it is generally reached by 2 to 7 years of age.[11] Children with primary SRE tend to have delayed functional bladder capacity when compared to nonenuretic children. These children's smaller functional bladder capacity is insufficient to maintain sleep-related continence even though they are 4½ years of age or older.[12]

Spontaneous detrusor muscle contractions tend to be more frequent in enuretic children.[13] These spontaneous bladder contractions are inhibited through complex interactions of voluntary muscle groups. When contractions are uninhibited, involuntary detrusor muscle contraction might occur during sleep.

Antidiuretic hormone secretion peaks during nocturnal hours. This circadian variation results in decreased free-water clearance, a decrease in the volume of urine production at night, and an increase in urine osmolality during the sleep period. Night-time increase in antidiuretic hormone secretion has been shown to be significantly diminished in some enuretic children with primary enuresis.[14-16] Investigations involving children with SRE compared with unaffected controls pointed to a central action of desmopressin, a defect at the central arginine vasopressin receptor, or abnormality in the pathway of sensory signals.[17]

Nonenuretic children and adults arouse when the bladder reaches its functional capacity. Although the mechanism of this arousal is not clear, it is most likely viscerally mediated via impulses originating in the bladder muscle.[18] This arousal response results in waking and conscious perception of the need to void. This results in activation of voluntary muscle groups that are involved in maintenance of urinary continence.

None of these postulated mechanisms function alone. The underlying cause of SRE most likely involves an interaction of factors related to ongoing development of the urinary tract, endocrine system, autonomic nervous system, and areas of the central nervous system responsible for arousal and waking.

Underlying psychological factors are uncommon causes for primary SRE and seem to occur in less than 1% of prepubertal children.[19,20] Symptoms related to emotional problems, however, appear in about 10% to 15% of children and appear in enuretic children more commonly than in nonenuretic youngsters. Emotional symptoms might include, but are not limited to, thumb sucking, nail biting, tantrums, stuttering, eating disorders, and poor self-esteem.[21,22] With primary SRE, these symptoms tend to resolve with resolution of the SRE.[23] On the other hand, psychological etiologies are more common in children with secondary SRE. Situational stress, separation from parents, abuse or neglect, anxiety, and birth of a new sibling have all been associated with secondary SRE.[1,21,24-26]

Achieving continence during sleep is part of the constitutional development of the child. Despite the lack of clear documentation for the concept of maturational delay as an underlying cause, it is based on longitudinal clinical observations. First, in the absence of clinical intervention, complete sleep-related continence will occur at about 15% per year prior to puberty. Functional bladder capacity increases as maturation progresses, despite a normal anatomic bladder capacity.[27] Uninhibited bladder contractions that occur in enuretic children improve as the youngster grows and matures.[13,28] Coordinated contractions of multiple skeletal muscles is necessary to initiate the urinary stream, as well as to maintain continence.[29] Control over these muscle groups follows a clear developmental pattern similar to the development of other motor skills. Arousal from sleep is required when bladder distension occurs. This arousal response is quite high in smaller children, and the threshold for arousal from internal and external stimuli decreases as maturation occurs.

Although straightforward genetic factors have not been identified, a familial pattern of primary SRE has been demonstrated.[23,30-32] Many parents of children with primary SRE were also enuretic as children. When both parents suffered from SRE, almost three fourths of their children were also enuretic. This is dramatically different from children of parents who were not enuretic as children. When neither parent was enuretic as a child, only 15% of their offspring suffer from SRE. Twin studies have also shown that when one twin sibling suffers from SRE, there is a greater predisposition for younger siblings to also suffer from similar symptoms.

Genetic factors may be pertinent in some cases. The pattern of involvement seems to be consistent with an autosomal dominant characteristic with incomplete penetrance. Genetic studies suggest linkage of primary SRE to specific markers on chromosomes 12, 13, and 22.[33-36] An association between genotype and phenotype, and identification of intermediary phenotypes or traits of children with SRE need to be documented.[37] Nonetheless, the expectations of enuretic parents for their children may contribute to some degree of familial clustering of symptoms.

There has been some suggestion that early introduction of toilet training is unsuccessful, as are rigid or punitive training practices. Development of diurnal and sleep-related urinary continence cannot be taught. Waking and sleep-related continence is acquired by a complex interaction between maturation of physiologic systems and learning by trial and error (or success). Too-rigid toilet training and introduction of toilet training too early may be associated with SRE.[38,39] However, other studies have shown no correlation between the success or failure of toilet training efforts and the development of SRE.[40-42]

Arousal from sleep seems to be difficult in children with SRE. Although the arousal threshold from slow-wave sleep may seem to underlie SRE in some children, youngsters with SRE tend to sleep no more deeply than nonenuretic children, and the structure of their sleep is not substantially different.[7] Enuresis occurs in all sleep stages, and spells appear to be random or related to time of night rather than sleep state.[43,44] Although sleep of enuretic children does not seem to differ significantly from that of nonenuretic youngsters, those who suffer from primary SRE spend a slightly longer time in bed and have an increased number of sleep cycles. Children who have enuretic spells during rapid eye movement (REM) sleep are found to have more REM sleep than comparison children. Tachycardia is often seen to precede the enuretic spell. Although the sleep of children with SRE seems to be polysomnographically normal, these children can exhibit signs of autonomic arousal prior to voiding.[45]

ORGANIC FACTORS ASSOCIATED WITH SLEEP-RELATED ENURESIS

Urinary tract infection (UTI) is 10 times more common in prepubertal girls suffering from habitual SRE than in age-matched girls without SRE.[20] Boys are much less likely to be prone to UTI than girls, even in the presence of uninhibited bladder contractions. Although most UTIs are symptomatic, occult infection can occur and typical symptoms such as fever, dysuria, and diurnal urinary frequency may not be present. It is still unclear whether SRE in patients with a UTI is a symptom of a chronic underlying infection or a result of the pathophysiologic mechanism responsible for SRE. After adequate treatment of the UTI, SRE often remains present and continues long after the infection has resolved.[8]

Anatomic abnormalities of the urinary tract have been associated with SRE. Any distal obstruction may be associated with the development of bedwetting.[1,2,28] The presence of urinary tract abnormalities is very low in primary SRE, and expensive invasive urologic procedures are most often not needed in the evaluation of children with SRE. However, consideration must be given to the possibility of the presence of an organic abnormality when diurnal symptoms suggest difficulty initiating or stopping the urine stream, dysuria, daytime enuresis, or excessive urinary frequency.

Extrinsic pressure on the bladder from a variety of causes may result in enuresis. Extrinsic pressure on the bladder decreases its functional and anatomic volume, and a large fecal mass or extrinsic space-occupying lesion can result in a long-term disorder of bladder control.[1] In a patient with chronic constipation, the resolution of the fecal mass pressing on the bladder often results in resolution of the enuresis.

Patients with medical conditions that result in polyuria often present with SRE as an initial problem. Indeed, any condition that results in polyuria can cause SRE. Enuresis as a primary complaint occurs commonly in patients with diabetes mellitis or diabetes insipidus. There is a higher than normal frequency of SRE in children with sickle cell anemia, sickle cell trait, and other hemoglobinopathies.[3,46] Enuresis is commonly present in children with sleep-disordered breathing (see Chapter 20). In addition, enuresis commonly occurs in children who suffer from non-REM sleep parasomnias, such as sleep terrors, sleepwalking, and confusional arousals.

Some neurologic disorders may result in enuresis. Enuresis may be associated with spinal cord lesions, including but not limited to meningomyelocele, tumors, and agenesis. Enuresis may also occur as a manifestation of a seizure disorder.

Medications that result in a higher urine volume, such as diuretics, may also result in SRE. Medications may be prescribed as short-term or long-term medical regimens for other medical conditions. Nonetheless, unintentional ingestion of diuretics should also be considered in the initial evaluation.

DIAGNOSIS OF SLEEP-RELATED ENURESIS

Successful treatment of SRE is based on an accurate diagnosis. The diagnostic workup begins with a comprehensive history and physical examination. Secondary SRE (specifically if associated with symptoms suggesting a urinary tract abnormality), UTI, polyuria, polyphagia, polydipsia, seizure disorder, obstructive sleep apnea syndrome, history of prior surgery related to the genitourinary tract, allergies, or diurnal enuresis, should raise the suspicion of organic disease. Initial workup should also include an assessment of possible psychopathology or abnormalities in family dynamics. The family history should be evaluated for evidence of enuresis in the patient's mother or father. Sleep habits and patterns also require assessment. Maintenance of sleep logs or a sleep diary for about 2 to 4 weeks may provide insight into the accuracy of the sleep–wake history and will provide a graphic longitudinal description of the child's sleep and wake behaviors as well as a graphic depiction of the pattern of bedwetting.

Measurement of the bladder's functional urine volume during the period of graphic measurement of the youngster's sleep provides information regarding functional capacity. If the functional bladder capacity is normal, primary SRE is unlikely, and a search for other etiologies might be considered.

Laboratory evaluations begin with a urinalysis and urine culture. These tests may be all that is required in the initial evaluation. The urine specific gravity; the presence of glucose in the urine, pyuria, or proteinuria; and the presence of casts in the urinary sediment should be assessed. A urine culture as part of the initial workup to rule out occult UTI is important. Other expen-

sive or invasive procedures are not typically required in the initial evaluation. Additional testing should be guided by the differential diagnosis after the initial assessment.

Ultrasonography, vesicle sphincter electromyography, and cystoscopy might be considered in some children who continue to be enuretic after 3 months of treatment. If radiographic or cystoscopic examinations are normal, continued enuresis may be associated with detrusor or sphincter muscle problems.

If loud snoring, restless sleep, and sleep-related diaphoresis are present, comprehensive nocturnal polysomnography might be considered as part of the patient's comprehensive evaluation. However, polysomnographic evaluation is rarely required in the diagnosis of primary SRE and should be reserved for those situations in which an underlying sleep-related disorder is strongly suspected. Indeed, diagnosis is most often based on assessment of the history and physical examination alone.

TREATMENT

Treatment of SRE is based on a rational approach to diagnosis and management of any underlying organic or pathologic condition. Treatment of underlying sleep-disordered breathing often results in resolution of the enuresis. Any psychiatric or psychological cause must be addressed prior to or in conjunction with the institution of any developmental, maturational, or behavioral management program. Successful enuresis management programs utilize combined methods of intervention. Regardless of the treatment program of choice, behavior management and bladder training are typically included and are important aspects of any intervention.

Treatment must begin with an assessment of whether the child has primary or secondary enuresis. The majority of patients presenting with this complaint suffer from primary SRE and require parental support, empathy, and patience. As the spontaneous cure rate for children between the ages of 5 and 16 years is about 15% per year, it is commonly recommended that no treatment be provided. Nonetheless, when the child or parent desires a more rapid resolution or when secondary, emotional problems occur, treatment may also involve behavior modification, enuresis alarms, and retention control exercises. Fluid restriction, pharmacotherapy, psychotherapy, hypnosis, or biofeedback, or a combination of these interventions, may be entertained.[47] Behavioral intervention is more likely to be successful in children over the age of 6. Between the ages of 3 and 5 years, reassurance, motivational counseling, and simple bladder training exercises may manage the problem. Continued input from the health care professional and support during treatment contribute to compliance.

Persistence and consistency must be encouraged and supported in any motivational and behavioral counseling program. In the absence of support and close followup, poor compliance is likely and persistence of the problem can be expected to occur.

When a program involving any form of behavioral management begins, sufficient time must be spent to reassure the youngster and the parents that the symptom of primary enuresis is not their fault. Expectation of results of the management program must be realistic, and there must be clear communication regarding the time required for problem resolution. Support and positive reinforcement by the health care professional is essential. When expectations are clear and well understood, the likelihood of success increases. The tone of the counseling should remain positive. Resolution may take months. Persistently working toward an agreed-on goal should be the primary focus of management rather than an instantaneous cure of the SRE. Parents and caretakers should avoid punishment or exhibiting disappointment when the occasional wet night occurs, as is common during management. Interventions such as randomly waking the child from sleep to void should be discouraged; this generally results in prolongation of the problem. Management must focus on treatment of the child's problem and not "treatment of the bed."[5]

Respondent conditioning is very helpful. Parents and children should agree on a reward system that is readily attainable at the beginning of management. Rewarding the child for a dry bed in the morning can be more discouraging than supportive because this is often beyond the youngster's capability at the outset of the program. The reward need not be large or expensive. Most importantly, the goal must be attainable by the child, and the reward must be provided consistently and immediately after the desired behavior is performed.

Initial management includes bladder-training exercises during the day. Exercises consist of asking the child to terminate the urine stream about halfway through the void, counting to 5, and then finishing the void. This final completion is important because residual urine in the bladder may result in the development of a UTI. Rewards should be given for accomplishing each of these behaviors.

Dry-bed exercises using guided imagery techniques also have been suggested. At bedtime, the child is instructed to lie in bed for a few moments, visualizing being asleep and feeling bladder fullness. Assistance from the parents is required. Visualization of arousal and awakening is then suggested and the child gets out of bed, goes to the toilet, and voids. This technique should continue for several months, depending on the child's response. Counseling the youngster and family that setbacks should be expected, at the beginning of treatment and throughout its course, improves compliance. Resolution of symptoms occurs at a rate of approximately 35% per year with the use of this regimen alone.[7] Nevertheless, if there is no progress or change in symptoms after about 3 months, other interventions might be considered.

Enuresis alarms are also commonly used in behavioral interventions. Although medications were once a common approach, health care professionals now appear to be more likely to recommend behavioral techniques in managing SRE.[7,48]

A variety of instruments are available, some more successful than others. Much of the success involves motivation of the child and family. Enuresis alarms involve a system that produces a loud sound when the sensor becomes wet. All alarm systems function using the same principle of *operant conditioning*, with the physiologic function of bladder distension, detrusor muscle contraction, and voiding coupled to an external stimulus. The sound (i.e., the stimulus) is intended to awaken (i.e., the response) the child, who will then stop voiding and will finish the void in the toilet. Eventually, by coupling the stimulus to the response of arousal, children awaken at the sensation of bladder distention.[5]

At first, the child may have difficult waking to the sound of the buzzer or bell. Indeed, confusional arousals might result. Parents should help the child awaken and guide the child to the bathroom to attempt to void in the toilet. If parents are consistent and persistent in their response to the sound of the alarm, soon the youngster will begin to spontaneously wake with the alarm.

When treatment with an enuresis alarm begins, the child typically completely empties the bladder. Gradually, there will be a perceptible decrease in the volume of urine voided prior to arousal and an increase in the volume voided in the toilet. This progressive decrease in the amount of urine voided into the bed continues until only a small spot of urine is voided, just enough to trigger the alarm. Then only the underclothing may be wet but not the bed. Dry nights will then begin to occur and increase in frequency until nocturnal continence is achieved. After about 1 month of consecutive dry nights, the alarm may be discontinued.

Behavioral modification, motivational counseling, and bladder training exercises may be used along with the enuresis alarm. Initial change in the pattern of bedwetting typically begins after about 3 to 6 weeks of treatment. Youngsters' responses can vary considerably, depending on the presence or absence of comorbid conditions, motivation of the youngster, and consistency of parental assistance. Some youngsters become dry quickly and others require much longer time. In children where longer treatment regimens have been required, it is unclear whether the resolution was a result of the treatment or because of timing of maturation of nocturnal bladder continence.

As with all treatment regimens, exacerbations may occur. It is important for the child and the parents to understand that these are possible and can be expected in many children, and they should not become discouraged. Reinstitution of the treatment protocol typically results in a very rapid response.

Few contraindications exist. The child must be able to hear the alarm, and its volume must be greater than the arousal threshold. Hearing-impaired children or children of hearing-impaired parents may not be responsive to this method of management. Children and parents must be considerably motivated. Children who are fearful or resistant to the alarm are less likely to respond favorably. Children must be developmentally

capable of responding appropriately to the alarm. The younger the child, the less likely it is that the results will be positive. Finally, the enuresis alarm should not be used as a means of toilet training. Diurnal continence results from a complicated interaction of multiple reflexes, cognitive ability to inhibit bladder contraction, and conditioning. Nocturnal continence requires time and patience. Parents' expectations should be appropriate to the intervention.

Resolution of SRE using enuresis alarms has been reported at approximately 65% to 80%, with relapse rates of approximately 10% to 15%.[49] Comparative trials reveal that the enuresis alarm may be superior to pharmacotherapy and may be more effective in treatment of primary SRE when utilized with a behavior modification program. This technique may increase functional bladder capacity and result in sustained confidence.[50,51]

Most often, the enuresis alarm is combined with a positive reinforcement program, retention control training, and positive practice using guided imagery. A combined approach to the management of enuresis is superior to the use of an alarm alone.

Medications used in the treatment of SRE have included antidepressants, antidiuretics, antispasmodics, and prostaglandin synthesis inhibitors. Desmopressin, 10 to 40 micrograms intranasally or 200 to 600 micrograms orally, has been successful in the treatment of primary SRE. Although desmopressin usually reduces the frequency of wetting, only a small minority of patients obtains complete dryness using this medication.[15,52,53] Treatment effects usually last only as long as the drug is taken. Recurrences are common. Side effects are uncommon. Significant hyponatremia associated with seizures has been reported.[54,55] There does not appear to be a relationship between a family history of SRE and response to desmopressin.[32] Utilization of desmopressin with an enuresis alarm or other behavioral intervention may be the best overall therapy, and this combined approach appears to be superior to either given alone.[56,57]

Oxybutynin chloride has a direct spasmolytic effect on the bladder and is helpful in controlling some children with SRE that is caused by uninhibited bladder contractions. Oxybutynin has a direct effect on bladder smooth muscle, and contractions are directly inhibited. Traditionally, it has been utilized in children with incontinence secondary to neurogenic bladder. It has been shown to be effective in controlling diurnal enuresis and uninhibited detrusor muscle contractions, and it has been used in some centers in combination with desmopressin and behavioral interventions in comprehensive SRE management programs.

Tricyclic antidepressants, particularly imipramine, have been the most commonly prescribed medication for the treatment of SRE. Their effectiveness appears to be derived from increased alpha-adrenergic stimulation of proximal tubules of the kidneys.[58,59] Unfortunately, the response rate is quite variable and the long-term cure rate is only about 25%. Relapses are common. Tricyclic antidepressants significantly affect the sleep cycle and result in REM sleep suppression. There is a narrow therapeutic window, and fatal overdose is a significant possibility.[60]

In one randomized, double-blind, placebo-controlled trial, carbamazepine was shown to be useful in the treatment of primary SRE.[61] However, comprehensive polysomnography or EEG was not done prior to randomization, making the results questionable.

Other forms of interventions using alternative techniques have been reported. Electroacupuncture has been reported to result in 65% more dry nights than in control children.[62] However, only 5 of 23 youngsters were considered responders to treatment (responders defined as having a greater than 90% reduction in the number of wet nights at a 6-month evaluation). Interestingly, according to the youngsters' parents, the sleep arousal threshold had decreased in about 50% of these children.

The success rate of any management program may be attributed in part to the spontaneous cure rate or to the patient's response to increased attention to the problem. Emotional support of the child is probably one of the most critical elements of any treatment program.

References

1. Schaefer CE: Childhood Encopresis and Enuresis. New York, Van Nostrand Reinhold, 1979, p 89.
2. Schmidtt ED: Nocturnal enuresis: An update on treatment. Pediatr Clin North Am 1982;29:21.
3. Nino-Murcia G, Keenan SA: Enuresis and sleep. In Guilliminault C (ed): Sleep and Its Disorders in Children. New York, Raven Press, p 253.
4. Wyker AW: Standard diagnostic considerations. In Gillenwater JY, Grayhack JT, Howard SS, et al (eds): Adult and Pediatric Urology. Chicago, Year Book Medical, 1987, p 62.
5. Sheldon SH: Sleep-related enuresis. Child Adolesc Psychiatr Clin North Am 1996;5:661-672.
6. Landgraf JN, Abidari J, Cilento BG, et al: Coping, commitment, and attitude: Quantifying the everyday burden of enuresis on children and their families. Pediatrics 2004;113:334.
7. Sheldon SH, Spire JP, Levy HB: Pediatric Sleep Medicine. Philadelphia, WB Saunders, 1992, pp 151-166.
8. Forsythe WI, Redmond A: Enuresis and spontaneous cure rate: Study of 1129 enuretics. Arch Dis Child 1974;49:259.
9. Meadow SR: Enuresis. In Edelman CH (ed): Pediatric Kidney Disease. Boston, Little, Brown, 1978, p 1176.
10. Cohen MW: Symposium on behavioral pediatrics. Pediatr Clin North Am 1975;22:3.
11. Esperanca N, Gerrard JW: Nocturnal enuresis: Studies in bladder function in normal children and enuretics. Can Med Assoc J 1969;101:721.
12. Muellner SR: Development of urinary control in children: Some aspects of the cause and treatment of primary enuresis. JAMA 1960;172:1256.
13. Koff SA, Murtagh DS. The uninhibited bladder in children: Effect of treatment on recurrence of urinary tract infection and on vesicoureteral reflux resolution. J Urol 1983;130:1138-1141.
14. Norgaard JP, Rittig S, Djurhuus JC: Nocturnal enuresis: An approach to treatment based on pathogenesis. J Pediatr 1989;114(Pt 2):705.
15. Folwell AJ, Macdiarmid SA, Crowder HJ, et al: Desmopressin for nocturnal enuresis: Urinary osmolality and response. Br J Urol 1997;80:480.
16. Aikawa T, Kasahara T, Uchiyama M: The arginine vasopressin secretion profile of children with primary nocturnal enuresis. Eur Urol 1998;33(Suppl 3):41.
17. Eggert P: What's new in enuresis? Acta Paediatr Taiwan 2002;43:6-9.
18. Sheldon SH, Spire JP, Levy HB: Pediatric Sleep Medicine. Philadelphia, WB Saunders, 1992, pp 151-166.
19. Rutter M, Yule W, Grahm P: Enuresis and behavioral deviance. In Kolvin I, MacKeith RC, Meadow SR (eds): Bladder Control and Enuresis. London, Heinemann Medical Books, 1973, pp 137-147.
20. Taylor PD, Turner RK: A clinical trial of continuous, intermittent and overlearning "bell and

pad" treatment for nocturnal enuresis. Behav Res Ther 1975;13:281-293.

21. Benjamin LS, Stover DO, Geppert TV, et al: The relative importance of psychopathology, training procedure and urological pathology in nocturnal enuresis. Child Psychiatry Hum Dev 1971;1:215.

22. Faschingbauer TR: Enuresis: Its nature, etiology, and treatment—A review of the literature. JSAS Catalog of Selected Documents for Psychology 1975;5:194.

23. Hallgren B: Enuresis: A clinical and genetic study. Acta Psychiatr Scand Suppl 1957;114:1.

24. Douglas JWS: Early disturbing events and later enuresis. In Klovin I, MacKeith RC, Meadows SR (eds): Bladder Control and Enuresis. London, Heinemann Medical Books, 1973.

25. Werry JS: Enuresis: A psychosomatic entity? Can Med Assoc J 1967;97:319.

26. Sheldon SH, Levy HB, Ahart S: Sleep disorders in abused and neglected children (Unpublished data.) 1990.

27. Troup CW, Hodgson NB: Nocturnal functional bladder capacity in enuretic children. J Urol 1971;129:132.

28. Lapides J, Diokno AC: Persistence of the infant bladder as a cause of urinary infection in girls. J Urol 1970;103:243.

29. Muellner SR: Physiology of micturition. J Urol 1951;65:805.

30. White N: A thousand consecutive cases of enuresis: Results of treatment. Child Fam 1971;10:198.

31. Young GC: The family history of enuresis. J R Inst Public Health 1963;26:197.

32. Schaumberg HL, Rittig S, Djurhuus JC: No relationship between family history of enuresis and response to desmopressin. J Urol 2001;166:2435-2437.

33. Eiberg H: Total genome scan analysis in a single extended family for primary nocturnal enuresis: Evidence for a new locus (ENUR3) for primary nocturnal enuresis on chromosome 22q11. Fur Urol 1998;33(Suppl 3):34.

34. Arnell H, Hjalmas K, Jagervall N, et al: The genetics of primary nocturnal enuresis: Inheritance and suggestion of a second major gene on chromosome 12q. J Med Genet 1997;34:360.

35. von Gontard A, Hollmann F, Eiberg H, et al: Clinical enuresis phenotypes in familial nocturnal enuresis. Scand J Urol Nephrol 1997;183(Suppl):11.

36. Eiberg H: Total genome scan analysis in a single extended family for primary nocturnal enuresis: Evidence for a new locus (ENUR3) for primary nocturnal enuresis on chromosome 22q11. Eur Urol 1998;33(Suppl 3):34.

37. von Gontard A, Schaumburg H, Hollmann E, et al: The genetics of enuresis: A review. J Urology 2001;166:2438.

38. Benajmin LS, Serdahely W, Geppert TV: Night training through parents' implicit use of operant conditioning. Child Dev 1971;42:963.

39. Bindelgltas PM, Dee GH, Enos FA: Medical and psychosocial factors in enuretic children treated with imipramine hydrochloride. Am J Psychiatry 1968;124:125.

40. Broughton RJ: Sleep disorders: Disorders of arousal? Science 1968;159:1070.

41. Despert J: Urinary control and enuresis. Psychosom Med 1944;6:294.

42. Klackenberg G: Primary enuresis: When is a child dry at night? Acta Paediatr Scand 1955;44:513-518.

43. Kales A, Kales JD, Jacobson A, et al: Effect of imipramine on enuretic frequency and sleep stages. Pediatrics 1977;60:431.

44. Mikkelsen EJ, Rapoport JL, Nee L, et al: Childhood enuresis: I. Sleep patterns and psychopathology. Arch Gen Psychiatry 1980;37:1139-1144.

45. Bader G, Neveus T, Kruse S, Sillen U: Sleep of primary enuretic children and controls. Sleep 2002;25:579.

46. Readett DR, Morris JS, Serjeant GR: Nocturnal enuresis in sickle cell haemoglobinopathies. Arch Dis Child 1990;65:290.

47. Mattelaer P, Mersdorf A, Rohrmann D, et al: Biofeedback in the treatment of voiding disorders in childhood. Acta Urol Belg 1995;63:5-7.

48. Vogel W, Young M, Primack W: A survey of physician use of treatment methods for functional enuresis. J Dev Behav Pediatr 1996;17:90-93.

49. Moffatt ME: Nocturnal enuresis: A review of the efficacy of treatments and practical advice for clinicians. J Dev Behav Pediatr 1997;18:49-56.

50. Monda JM, Husmann DA: Primary nocturnal enuresis: A comparison among observation, imipramine, desmopressin acetate and bedwetting alarm systems. J Urol 1995;154:745-748.

51. Oredsson AF, Jorgensen TM: Changes in nocturnal bladder capacity during treatment with the bell and pad for monosymptomatic nocturnal enuresis. J Urol 1998;160:166-169.

52. Moffatt ME, Harios S, Kirshen AJ, Burd L: Desmopressin acetate and nocturnal enuresis: How much do we know? Pediatrics 1993;92:420-425.

53. Skoog SJ, Stokes A, Turner KL: Oral desmopressin: A randomized double-blind placebo controlled study of effectiveness in children with primary nocturnal enuresis. J Urol 1997;158:1035-1040.

54. Thompson S, Rey JM: Functional enuresis: Is desmopressin the answer? J Am Acad Child Adolesc Psychiatry 1995;34:266-271.

55. Robson WL, Jackson HP, Blackhurst D, Leung AK: Enuresis in children with attention-deficit hyperactivity disorder. South Med J 1997;90:503-505.

56. Bradbury MG, Meadow SR: Combined treatment with enuresis alarm and desmopressin for nocturnal enuresis. Acta Paediatr 1995;84:1014-1018.

57. Bradbury M: Combination therapy for nocturnal enuresis with desmopressin and an alarm device. Scand J Urol Nephrol 1997;183(Suppl):61-63.

58. Fritz GK, Rockney RM, Yeung AS: Plasma levels and efficacy of imipramine treatment for enuresis. J Am Acad Child Adolesc Psychiatry 1994;33:60-64.

59. Hunsballe JM, Rittig S, Pedersen ES, et al: Single dose imipramine reduces nocturnal urine output in patients with nocturnal enuresis and nocturnal polyuria. J Urol 1997;158:830-836.

60. Harari MD, Moulden A: Nocturnal enuresis: What is happening? J Paediatr Child Health 2000;36:78-81.

61. Al-Waili NS: Carbamazepine to treat primary nocturnal enuresis: A double-blind study. Eur J Med Res 2000;5:40-44.

62. Bjorkstrom G, Hellstrom AL, Andersson S: Electro acupuncture in the treatment of children with monosymptomatic nocturnal enuresis. Scand J Urol Nephrol 2000;34:21-26.

Pharmacology of Sleep Disorders in Children

28

John H. Herman
Stephen H. Sheldon

This chapter reviews the differential diagnosis of sleep disorders in children and describes under what circumstances sedative/hypnotic medications are useful for their treatment. It reviews classes of medications that affect sleep, with the implications of their use in a pediatric population highlighted. It also reviews the mechanism of the sleep-promoting or -disrupting effects of various classes of psychoactive compounds.

CRITICAL ASPECTS OF PEDIATRIC SLEEP PHARMACOLOGY

Insomnia and hypersomnolence in children are related to the neurotransmitters γ-aminobutyric acid (GABA), serotonin, dopamine, norepinephrine, histamine, and acetylcholine. The compounds that affect sleep share the common property of being excitatory or inhibitory in the brain in one or more of the above neurotransmitter systems.

The receptor mechanisms for the actions of the sleep-promoting medications include the ligands of the benzodiazepine receptor site, which allosterically modulates the GABA receptor and its chloride ion channel; serotonin 5-hydroxytryptamine $(5\text{-HT})_{2A}$ antagonists; anticholinergics/antimuscarinics; antihistamines; and α-adrenergic antagonists.

Examples of the classes of medication active at these sites include benzodiazepines and benzodiazepine-like substances that bind to the benzodiazepine recognition site; GABA agonists such as mood stabilizers; GABA reuptake inhibitors, which are also mood stabilizers; and benzodiazepine-mimicking compounds, including zaleplon and zopiclone. Serotonin 5-HT_{2A} antagonists include antidepressants such as trazodone and nefazodone. Anticholinergic medications include tricyclic antidepressants such as amitriptyline and clomipramine. Antihista-

mines are present in a wide variety of compounds, including tricyclic antidepressants. Sedating antihistamines include hydroxyzine and diphenhydramine. α-Adrenergic antagonists are present in antidepressants and blood pressure medications.

The classes of medication that disrupt sleep include dopamine agonists, adenosine antagonists, cholinergic agents, and serotonin reuptake inhibitors. Norepinephrine and dopamine reuptake blockade also results in sleep disruption. Adenosine antagonists such as caffeine disrupt sleep.

The selection of a sedating or stimulating psychopharmacologic agent for a child is always *diagnosis based.*

In children, pharmacologic agents are typically used only when behavioral interventions are not effective.

The selection of a pharmacologic agent requires a sleep diagnosis to be firmly established for which the agent is suitable. A thorough interview with the patient and parents or others involved in managing the child's sleep is required. A differential evaluation must include a complete sleep history, establishing the severity of the sleep difficulty, its frequency, and its duration. The times of the night that the sleep difficulty and undisturbed sleep occur should be established. The extent to which the child is sleepy or is sleeping during the day should be reviewed. The impact of the sleepiness or tiredness on school performance is important. Differences between the number of hours of sleep on school day and non–school day nights is also important because many children are partially sleep deprived on school days and obtain rebound sleep on weekends.

Circadian rhythm disorders must be ruled out before considering difficulty initiating and maintaining sleep (DIMS). Sleep hygiene problems, such as inappropriate noise or light in the sleeping environment, should be reviewed.

Listed below are some of the diagnoses that may lead to DIMS in a child, and subsequent sections will review the treatment approaches focusing on pharmacologic interventions.

Sleep onset association disorder
Settling disorder of infancy/childhood
DIMS secondary to sleep phobia
Sleep-related panic attacks
Childhood-onset psychophysiologic insomnia
Phase delay syndrome
Phase advance syndrome
DIMS secondary to anxiety disorder
DIMS secondary to mood disorder
DIMS secondary to psychosis/schizophrenia
Night terrors
Nightmares
Sleepwalking
Head banging, jactatio capitis nocturna
Confusional arousal
DIMS in association with attention deficit hyperactivity disorder (ADHD)

A comprehensive understanding of the child's emotional state at the time of the sleep difficulty, whether it is sleep onset insomnia or nocturnal awakening, is important. Chronic sleep-related anxiety, fear, a depressed mood, worrying thoughts, and apprehension each may be indicative of a psychiatric diagnosis. The behavioral repertoire of the child on awakening should be established. Does the child remain in his or her own bed or enter the parent's bedroom? The manner in which the parents respond to the child's sleep difficulties is also important. Do they capitulate to the child's wish to remain in their bed, or do they take the child to his or her bed?

The extension of any night-time symptoms into daytime behavior should also be explored. If the symptoms of an anxiety or mood disorder appear to be related to the sleep difficulty, are there comparable symptoms present during the day and in different situations? Many children express profound anxiety as bedtime approaches, have disturbed sleep for the first portion of the sleep period, and then settle into undisturbed sleep until morning awakening. Some of these children may show no apprehensiveness with separation or in other circumstances.

It is important to determine whether either biologic parent or any first-degree relatives have or have had sleep difficulties similar to those of the child. Detailed questioning will frequently reveal a first-degree relative with a similar sleep problem. Inquiry into its course and treatment is helpful. Anxiety, depressive, and bipolar disorders each have a demonstrable family linkage. Adoption studies suggest a strong genetic component in the risk for these disorders.

If it is established that the patient (child) has comorbid psychiatric symptoms and a family member or members have similar symptoms, the sleep specialist is not diagnosing a psychiatric disorder in the child but deducing the etiology of the sleep disorder and fashioning an approach that considers psychiatric symptoms.

When both the psychiatric symptoms and DIMS are present, establishing the time course of the two is important in diagnosing the sleep disorder. If the sleep disorder emerges concurrent with the emotional symptoms and subsides when they subside, then treating the emotional disorder will most likely result in amelioration of the sleep symptoms. If the sleep disorder precedes the emotional disorder, then it may be an initial emerging symptom or an independent disorder.

Before administering a sleeping agent to a child, the child's family should complete a sleep log for at least 2 weeks to provide a baseline measurement of the chief complaint. A target symptom for which the drug is prescribed, such as sleep onset latency, sleep duration, or sleep fragmentation, should be selected. A realistic level of improvement, such as reducing sleep onset latency from greater than 1 hour to less than 30 minutes, should be discussed with the family. The family should maintain the sleep log after the drug trial begins to enable the assessment of the effectiveness of the drug with regard to the specific selected complaint.

Caution in Children When Using Psychoactive Compounds

All medications used in the treatment of insomnia or parasomnia require close monitoring. Sleep-inducing medications may precipitate night terrors, sleepwalking, confusional arousal, and daytime somnolence, which has the potential to exacerbate psychiatric and behavioral problems and disrupt attention and learning.[1]

The recurrence of parasomnias on withdrawal of sedating medications is common, especially if withdrawal is rapid.[1] Gradual withdrawal over several weeks may be required.

Sleep-Inducing Agents

The term *sedative-hypnotic* refers to the ability of a medication to sedate (or tranquilize) and induce sleep (hypno-). When sedative medications are used to decrease anxiety, they are referred to as anxiolytics. A number of agents are approved as anxiolytics, among them various antidepressants such as doxepin and paroxetine, benzodiazepines such as alprazolam and diazepam, and buspirone, a $5-HT_{1A}$ augmenting agent. Virtually every hypnotic approved by the Food and Drug Administration is a benzodiazepine or a compound that binds to the benzodiazepine receptor site. Many agents approved as anxiolytics, antidepressants, and antipsychotics have drowsiness as a side effect, and some physicians prefer these agents over benzodiazepines despite the absence of demonstrated efficacy.

Effects of GABA Allosteric Modulators on Sleep

Barbiturates, which are first-generation hypnotics, increase stage 1 sleep and decrease paradoxical (rapid eye movement [REM]) sleep. Virtually all benzodiazepines, including triazolam, midazolam, and diazepam, also decrease sleep onset latency, increase non-REM (NREM) stages 1 and 2 sleep, and decrease REM sleep except for midazolam, which increases both stage 1 and REM sleep at low doses. Zolpidem and zopiclone decrease REM sleep but do not increase stage 1 sleep.[2] Nearly all of these compounds have been shown to reduce the proportion of slow-wave activity. The activation of $GABA_A$ receptors is involved in the initiation and maintenance of NREM sleep and the generation of sleep spindles but disrupts the processes underlying slow-wave sleep (SWS).

BENZODIAZEPINES AND SLEEP

All benzodiazepines share certain effects in common—hypnotic, anxiolytic, muscle relaxant, and anticonvulsive—but some have greater emphasis on one or the other of these common effects. Therefore, certain benzodiazepines are more effective as anxiolytics and others as hypnotics. The speed at onset determines whether a benzodiazepine will be effective in treating sleep onset insomnia, and the medication half-life determines whether it is effective in treating disorders of maintaining sleep or early morning awakening. Benzodiazepines with a short half-life tend to exert more amnestic effects, and those with a long half-life result in more daytime sleepiness.

ZALEPLON

Zaleplon (Sonata), a nonbenzodiazepine that binds to the benzodiazepine receptor, has an ultrashort half-life, making it useful in the treatment of sleep onset insomnia. Recent publications support its greater safety in children than zolpidem and benzodiazepines.[3] Zaleplon is 14.3 times more potent in binding to membrane preparations of the cerebellum than to those of the spinal cord. It produces significant increases in muscimol binding similar to those of diazepam, and it is antagonized by flumazenil. Zaleplon shows little affinity for other receptors, and it produces large increases in EEG power of the delta frequency band without affecting the alpha or beta frequency band. In contrast, intravenous administration of triazolam and zopiclone increases the energy of the beta frequency band. The zaleplon-induced increase in the delta frequency band is antagonized by pretreatment with flumazenil, which does not affect the spontaneous EEG alone. These results suggest that zaleplon is a selective, full agonist of the ω_1-receptor subtype; thus, zaleplon may induce SWS.[4]

ZOLPIDEM

Zolpidem (Ambien) has a relatively short half-life and no demonstrable morning hangover and may be preferable to benzodiazepines with longer half-lives, especially in children. It has powerful hypnotic properties but little anxiolytic effect. Zolpidem is a widely used hypnotic agent acting at the $GABA_A$ receptor benzodiazepine site. It is especially useful in the treatment of middle-of-the-night insomnia or early morning awakening because of its half-life of 2 to 3 hours. On recombinant receptors, zolpidem displays a high affinity for only the α_1-$GABA_A$ receptors and an intermediate affinity for α_2- and α_3-$GABA_A$ receptors. It does not bind to α_5-$GABA_A$

receptors. The sedative action of zolpidem is exclusively mediated by α_1-GABA receptors. Similarly, the activity of zolpidem against GABA antagonist–induced tonic convulsions is also completely mediated by α_1-GABA$_A$ receptors. The sedative/hypnotic and anticonvulsant activities of zolpidem are due to its action on α_1-GABA$_A$ receptors and not on α_2- and α_3-GABA$_{2A}$ receptors.[5]

Triazolam

Triazolam (Halcion) is useful for the treatment of insomnia in children because of its short half-life but is to be avoided because of its amnestic effects.

Tricyclic Antidepressants and Sleep

Tricyclic antidepressants should be selected with sedative properties taken into consideration. The sedating or activating properties of antidepressants are side effects of the medication. Sedation with certain compounds will occur on the first night of administration, which is beneficial in many instances and in contrast to the therapeutic effect of the medication, which may require 2 to 6 weeks to emerge.

Pediatric patients presenting with hypersomnolence or insomnia whose onset coincided with that of an affective disorder should be administered an antidepressant that addresses both their sleep complaint and mood disorder. If sleep was normal until the advent of the mood disorder, then treating the mood disorder typically restores sleep to its levels before the mood disorder episode. That is, all antidepressants, whether they affect sleep or not, will probably result in improvement in the patient's sleep as the mood disorder is treated. If a sleep complaint emerges or continues independent of a mood complaint in the past, it will be most efficacious to select an antidepressant with an appropriate sleep- or wake-up–enhancing profile.

Some antidepressants powerfully promote or interfere with sleep. Tricyclic antidepressants have been used to treat children for many years. There is little evidence that they are effective antidepressants in children. However, those with sedating properties may be preferred in cases in which insomnia is present.

Most sedation
Amitriptyline

Lomipramine
Doxepin
Trimipramine

Moderate sedation
Imipramine
Nortriptyline

Least sedation
Amoxapine
Desipramine
Protriptyline

For the hypersomnolent, anergic, depressed child with psychomotor slowing, protriptyline is the most activating tricyclic antidepressant. Agitation and anxiety are its two most prevalent side effects. Doxepin, which is approved for both depression and anxiety, is effective in depressed individuals with insomnia, especially with mixed anxiety/depression symptoms.

Selection of Serotonin-Specific Reuptake Inhibitors (Not So Specific)

Selective serotonin reuptake inhibitors (SSRIs) cause insomnia by stimulating 5-HT$_{2A}$ receptors in brainstem and forebrain sleep-promoting centers. 5-HT$_{2A}$ receptor stimulation results in increased wakefulness and disruption of SWS.

More stimulation
Fluoxetine
Sertraline

Less stimulation
Fluvoxamine
Paroxetine

No stimulation
Citalopram

Several members of this class of medication have demonstrated efficacy in children in controlled trials. Various studies have shown that SSRIs disrupt sleep. Their administration generally results in reduced SWS, greatly reduced REM sleep, and increased stage 1 sleep. The mechanism of action is believed to be the activation of 5-HT$_{2A}$ receptors.

Bupropion and Sleep

Bupropion's mechanism of action is as a norepinephrine and dopamine reuptake inhibitor. It inhibits sleep by increasing dopamine and norepinephrine at the synaptic cleft and is the least preferred for insomniac patients. It is the most preferred for retarded depression, which presents with cognitive slowing and hypersomnia. It is also frequently prescribed for patients who do not respond to serotonergic agents, including SSRIs and tricyclic antidepressants. Bupropion can be added to SSRIs to increase their clinical efficacy.

Serotonin and Norepinephrine Reuptake Inhibitors

Venlafaxine (Effexor), a dual reuptake inhibitor, and serotonergic and noradrenergic reuptake inhibitors may be more rapid in onset and more effective in severe depression. It is the most preferred in depressed patients who present with hypersomnia, cognitive slowing, and anergia. Venlafaxine causes insomnia at medium doses and severe insomnia at high doses due to blockade at the NE, 5-HT and DA receptors.

Noradrenergic and Specific Serotonergic Antidepressants

The mechanism of action of mirtazapine (Remeron) is as a noradrenergic and specific serotonergic 5-HT$_{2A}$ antagonist. It is sleep enhancing due to its 5-HT$_{2A}$ antagonism, antihistaminergic actions, and alpha$_2$ antagonist property, which disinhibits both the NE and 5-HT receptors. It is specifically indicated in depressed patients with insomnia.

Serotonin Antagonists/Reuptake Inhibitors

Serotonin 5-HT$_{2A}$ antagonists/reuptake inhibitors are sleep enhancing. Nefazodone, a member of this class, causes norepinephrine reuptake blockade and acts as an antagonist at the serotonin 5-HT$_{2A}$ receptor. A major side effect is sedation. Perhaps the most sedating of all antidepressants is trazodone, which both acts as an antagonist at the 5-HT$_{2A}$ receptor and blocks histamine receptors, leading to two sedating mechanisms.

Antiseizure Medications and Sleep

Valproic acid (Depakene) is used as an antiseizure medication and in the treatment of bipolar disorder. It has sedating effects and may be used effectively in the treatment of insomnia associated with behavioral agitation. Carbamazepine (Tegretol) is also used principally as an anti-seizure medication and in the treatment of bipolar disorder. It also has sedating effects. Gabapentin (Neurontin) is sedating and appears to increase SWS.

Atypical Antipsychotics and Sleep

Atypical antipsychotics that are sedating include ziprasidone, quetiapine, and olanzapine. Risperidone, another atypical antipsychotic, has insomnia as a side effect. Clozapine (Clozaril) is not discussed because of the risk of agranulocytosis. Atypical antipsychotics at low doses are extremely useful in treating severe agitation in combination with insomnia. Because they lack many of the side effects of typical neuroleptics, they are more frequently administered to individuals who do not meet the criteria of the Diagnostic and Statistical Manual–IV for psychosis or schizophrenia but are agitated due to disrupted sleep.

Combination Medications for Depression and Insomnia

Sedating agents such as trazodone, nefazodone, a sedating atypical antipsychotic, or a benzodiazepine may be added to an SSRI at bedtime for the treatment of insomnia with depression. The dose of the SSRI should be considered, as the addition of a second agent may result in increased side effects.

Most benzodiazepines have half-lives that are too long to be effective in children.

Pharmacologic Treatment of Specific Sleep Disorders in Children and Adolescents

Sleep Onset Insomnia, Settling Disorders, and Sleep-Related Anxiety

Before prescribing medication, a differential diagnosis should be performed differentiating a true insomnia from a variety of other sleep and psychiatric disorders that result in difficulty in initiating sleep. Sleep onset insomnia in a child consists of minimum bedtime resistance and an elongated period of wakefulness without attempts at interaction with caretakers. In contrast, settling disorders are characterized by bedtime struggles and/or repeated attempts at interaction with caretakers. Settling disorders may be conceptualized as normal, early developmental variations of oppositional defiant disorder. Sleep-related anxiety is characterized by an increase in autonomic and central nervous system symptoms of anxiety and fear related to bedtime and sleep. Sleep-related anxiety may be a normal variation of the anxiety disorders as the child struggles to deal with the early developmental task of individuation/separation.

It is important to differentiate among sleep onset insomnia, settling disorders, and sleep-related anxiety, as each is treated differently. Sleep onset insomnia is treated with behavioral therapy approaches such as stimulus control therapy, sleep restriction therapy, relaxation therapy, and sleep hygiene. It may also be treated with sedating medications in certain circumstances. If sleep maintenance is not an issue, a medication with a rapid onset and short half-life, such as zaleplon, is preferred.

Settling disorders are treated with a variety of techniques. These behavioral techniques require close cooperation among all caretakers involved in the child's sleep initiation. Medications are not indicated and have not been found to be efficacious in treating settling disorders. Prolonged settling disorders may indicate other psychiatric diagnoses.

Sleep-related anxiety is treated with approaches virtually the opposite of settling disorders. A caretaker in the child's presence, typically on a palate next to the child's bed, is required to minimize anxiety. Antianxiety benzodiazepines with a rapid onset, such as diazepam, may be helpful for brief periods. The dose should be low enough so as not to induce daytime somnolence.

Most children with sleep onset insomnia, in contrast to those with a settling disorder, will not be brought to the attention of a physician because they tend to remain in their own beds and not disturb caretakers. Adults with childhood-onset insomnia come to the attention of physicians only after they reach their twenties or older, when poor sleep quality results in daytime fatigue. In contrast to sleep onset insomnia, much more frequently observed is psychophysiologic insomnia, which consists of DIMS.

Children with sleep difficulties had significantly increased odds of anxiety/depression based on the mother's but not the teacher's reports. The association increased with age and was independent of the mother's history of major depressive disorder. The association between sleep difficulties and anxiety/depression was greater than that for other psychiatric problems.[6]

Circadian phase disorders and psychiatric disorders often have sleep onset insomnia as a presenting complaint, as do anxiety disorders and depression. Although delayed sleep phase syndrome may be treated with melatonin administered in the early evening, behavioral techniques, namely exposure to early morning bright light, are usually a first-line treatment in children (see Table 9–2 in Chapter 9).

A 5-mg dose of melatonin at 6:00 PM is safe for short-term use in uncomplicated sleep onset insomnia and significantly more effective than placebo in advancing sleep onset and dim-light melatonin onset and increasing sleep duration in elementary school children. These results were confirmed in children with chronic sleep onset insomnia in a placebo-controlled trial. Sustained attention was not affected.[7] Other pharmacologic choices are described below.

Benzodiazepines are indicated mainly for transient or short-term insomnia, for which prescriptions should be limited to a few days, occasional or intermittent use, or courses not to exceed 2 weeks, if possible. Temazepam, loprazolam, and lormetazepam, which have a medium duration of action, are suitable. Diazepam is also effective in single or intermittent doses. Potent, short-acting benzodiazepines such as triazolam appear to carry a greater risk of adverse effects.[8]

Sleep Phobia

Children sometimes develop a specific phobic reaction to sleeping alone, with all the characteristics of a specific phobia, such as fear of flying or fear of blood for adults. The phobia includes a panicky reaction, with autonomic activation and apparent terror, as if the child's life is in danger. This reaction is distinct from settling disorders, in which an overwhelming sense of palpable terror is not present, and anxiety disorders, in which the symptoms are present in many situations throughout the day.

Specific phobias in adults are treated with behavioral therapy, typically a deconditioning model. The same approach is the most effective in children, which consists of introducing the child to sleeping in his or her own room in a gradual and nonthreatening manner. Medications are a second-line treatment, most typically a benzodiazepine with anxiolytic properties.

The sleep specialist must carefully devise a plan, the first step of which is to achieve separation that is tolerated without overwhelming anxiety by the parents as well as the child. This outcome may be realized with a parent on a cot in the child's room. Considerable skill is required to develop a stepwise program that is neither too draconian nor overcapitulates to the child's demands.

Settling Disorders

Sleep difficulties characterized by the need for interaction with caretakers, namely having a parent in the child's bed or the child wishing to be in the parents' bed, are best treated behaviorally. These difficulties are settling disorders, in which the child repeatedly seeks the parents' presence. A settling disorder should be differentiated from a sleep phobia, as the latter is marked by overwhelming panic that would be exacerbated by a technique such as allowing a child to cry for a set period of time. Ferber describes techniques for dealing with settling disorders, which are variations of behavioral therapy techniques. Flexibility of approach is the hallmark of these interventions, the object of which is to find one that is tolerable for both the parents and the child.

Children aged 6 to 12 months with severe, chronic sleep disorders such as DIMS were compared to peers without sleep problems. At the age of 5.5 years, 7 of the 12 children in the sleep disorder group met the criteria for the diagnosis of ADHD. None of the control children met these criteria.[9] Sleep problems at 4 years of age predict behavioral/emotional problems in midadolescence after controlling for sex, adoption status, and behavioral/emotional status. The correlation between sleep problems and depression/anxiety increased significantly from age 4 years to midadolescence.[10]

Medications appear to be effective in treating night-time awakening in the short term, but long-term efficacy has not been demonstrated. In contrast, specific behavioral interventions have consistently shown both short-term efficacy and the possible long-term effects of dealing with settling problems and night-time awakening.[11]

Hyperactivity is associated with both increased body movement during sleep and sleepwalking; behavioral problems are related to bedtime struggles. The symptoms of depression and anxiety are associated with night terrors, difficulty falling asleep, and daytime somnolence.[12]

Behavioral extinction techniques as well as parent education are effective in preventing sleep problems. They are now considered to be well established treatments. Graduated extinction and scheduled awakenings appear to be effective behavioral treatments.[13]

Less sleep at night is associated with a psychiatric diagnosis in children, and less night-time sleep *and* less sleep in a 24-hour period are associated with increased behavior problems and more externalization of problems.[14] Others have focused on the relationship between the regulation of sleep and the control of attention, emotion, and behavior.[15]

Confusional Arousal

No controlled studies of the effects of medication have been performed. In severe cases, clinical reviews indicate that benzodiazepines and tricyclics are effective.[16] Because antihistamines are sedating and do not consistently have anxiolytic effects, they may increase the likelihood of parasomnia.

Night Terrors

Night terrors should be distinguished from nightmares (i.e., anxiety dreams) and sleep-related panic attacks. Night terrors occur early in the night with no morning recollection and are characterized by intense autonomic arousal and disoriented behavior. Nightmares typically occur later in the sleep period but are more variable in their time of occurrence, and typically a vivid dream with a narrative plot is reported. Night terrors emerge from stages 3 and 4 sleep, and nightmares emerge from REM sleep. Sleep-related panic attacks are similar to night terrors in the severity of perceived dread but are characterized by morning recall and the concurrent development of fear of the bedroom and sleep, which are associated in the child's mind with the possibility of recurrence.

A sleep and behavioral/psychiatric disorder questionnaire showed that adolescents with sleep terrors and sleepwalking have an increased prevalence of neurotic traits, psychiatric disorders, and behavioral problems. Sleep terrors and sleepwalking in childhood are probably principally related to genetic and developmental factors and their continuation; in particular, their onset in adolescence may be related to psychological factors.[17]

It is not clear whether the hypnotic or anxiolytic properties of benzodiazepines constitute the mechanism of action of these drugs in treating night terrors. There are no controlled studies of the effects of these medications. Diazepam at bedtime is the standard treatment, but midazolam, oxazepam, lorazepam, or clonazepam, is sometimes preferred.[16]

One study of night terror episodes[18] featured confused behaviors, motor activity, and absent or fragmented recall. Polysomnography documented arousal from SWS in 9 of 10 patients. All of the original patients reported psychiatric symptoms. All 6 patients who received the subsequent structured evaluation met the lifetime criteria for Axis I conditions (most commonly affective and substance abuse disorders) and had elevated scores on the personality scale of the Millon Clinical Multiaxial Inventory–II. Night terrors were not limited to psychiatric episodes. The episodes that occur in adults are similar to those that are described in children. While they are distinct from sleep-related panic attacks, night terrors appear to occur in adults with histories of psychopathology.[18]

Sleep-Related Panic Attacks

In this placebo-controlled trial, clonazepam was an efficacious and safe short-term treatment for panic disorder. Discontinuation during and after slow tapering was well tolerated.[19]

Panic attacks may be induced during stages 3 and 4 sleep by the administration of high doses of caffeine to sleeping subjects.[20]

Fluoxetine has been found to be effective in the treatment of a variety of anxiety disorders in children who were not responsive to psychotherapy, including separation anxiety, social phobia, generalized anxiety disorder, and panic disorder. Improvement occurs over a 5-week period. Doses vary and should be individualized for each clinical situation.[21]

Children with panic disorder show greater changes in heart and respiratory rates when lactate is infused during sleep.[22] Patients with a history of sleep panic have higher rates of generalized anxiety disorder, social phobia, and major depression. The presence of sleep-related panic attacks may delineate a subgroup of panic disorder patients who have early difficulties with anxiety and comorbid mood and anxiety disorders as adults.[23]

Panic disorder frequently appears first during adolescence and may occur concurrent with sleep-related panic attacks or night terrors. Besides panic attacks and avoidance behavior, adolescents often have sleep initiation and continuation disturbances. They suffer from insomnia, nocturnal panic attacks, and fear of going to bed or falling asleep.[24,25]

Concurrent acute onset of night terrors, somnambulism, and spontaneous daytime panic attacks meeting the criteria for panic disorder is reported in a 10-year-old-boy with a family history of panic disorder (unpublished anecdote). Both the parasomnias and the panic disorder were fully responsive to therapeutic doses of imipramine. A second case of night terrors and infrequent full-symptom panic attacks is noted in another 10-year-old boy whose mother has panic disorder with agoraphobia. The clinical resemblance and reported difference between night terrors and panic attacks are described. The absence of previous reports of this comorbidity is notable. It is hypothesized that night terrors and panic disorder involve a similar constitutional vulnerability to dysregulation of brainstem-altering systems.

Sleepwalking

There are no controlled studies of the effects of medication. Clinical reviews indicate triazolam, lorazepam, diazepam, and clonazepam or imipramine, desipramine, and clomipramine may be used at bedtime. Another medication that has some demonstrated efficacy is carbamazepine.[16]

Nocturnal Enuresis

In this disorder, only the results of long-term followup are meaningful. Most studies of desmopressin (DDAVP) show it to be statistically more effective than placebo after 2 to 4 weeks of use. This finding is not clinically useful, as symptom resumption frequently follows withdrawal. Both DDAVP and imipramine are effective in short-term studies.[26] Those most likely to be permanently dry with DDAVP are older children who respond to 20 µg and do not wet the bed frequently.[27] Oxybutynin (Ditropan) for bladder spasms is the most effective when nocturnal enuresis is combined with daytime incontinence.[28]

Treatment with tricyclic antidepressant drugs (imipramine, amitriptyline, lomipramine and desipramine) reduces bedwetting by about one night per week. DDAVP and tricyclic antidepressants appear to be equally effective while on treatment, but this effect is not sustained after treatment is stopped. Alarms appear to be more effective in the long term.[29]

Treatment with DDAVP is more effective than retention control training in decreasing the number of wet nights but not effective in children with a low functional bladder capacity. Daytime functional bladder capacity predicts a response to DDAVP but not to retention control training.[30]

In a 9-week study, there is a greater effect of DDAVP combined with alarm therapy than either alone. However, combined treatment and either DDAVP or alarm therapy for 9 weeks have a 6 month follow-up success rate of about 37%.[31]

Treatment of Insomnia with Moderate to Severe Developmental Disabilities

Eighteen of 20 children with developmental disabilities had shorter sleep latencies when receiving melatonin than placebo in a double-blind, 6-week trial. The greater the sleep latency at baseline, the more it decreased with melatonin. However, melatonin does not increase sleep duration, nor does it decrease the number of awakenings. No side effects have been reported when melatonin is used in this manner.[32]

Sleeplessness after Pineal Tumor Extraction

Melatonin replacement therapy is beneficial for those patients who have deficient melatonin synthesis from both DIMS and circadian rhythm disorders.[33]

Sleepless Children Who Do Not Tolerate Oral Medication

Eight children who were inpatients at Children's Hospital in Boston or at Children's Hospital at Stanford (aged 5 to 16.6 years) and were unable to tolerate oral medications received intravenous amitriptyline for neuropathic pain, depression, and sleep disturbance and as an adjuvant agent for opioid analgesia. One patient experienced an extrapyramidal reaction that was successfully managed with diphenhydramine.[34]

Insomnia in Children Secondary to Anxiety Disorders

Listed above are settling disorders, sleep onset insomnia, and sleep phobia. In contrast to each of these sleep problems, insomnia secondary to an anxiety disorder entails generalized anxiety in a wide variety of circumstances, chronic worrying, and frequently oversensitivity to the feelings of others. These children may have a variety of the symptoms of anxiety and a family history of anxiety disorders.

Currently favored medications for anxiety disorders, including generalized anxiety disorder, panic disorder, phobias, and phobic disorders, are antidepressants, especially SSRIs, and buspirone. The heterocyclic doxepin and the SSRI paroxetine are both approved for anxiety disorders and have sedating side effects. In addition, anxiety disorders frequently overlap with depressive disorders, varying from major depressive disorder with subsyndromal anxiety in generalized anxiety disorder with dysthymia. Both depressive symptoms and anxiety level may vary independent of each other.

If the onset of insomnia is coincident with an exacerbation of anxiety symptoms, then it should first be addressed with antianxiety medications, frequently SSRIs such as paroxetine, which is sedating, and the heterocyclic doxepin. For generalized anxiety disorder, the serotonergic 5-HT$_{1A}$ agonist buspirone is a first-line treatment. Clonidine is helpful in blocking the noradrenergic aspects of anxiety, such as tachycardia, sweating, and tremor.

Benzodiazepines are useful in the treatment of the subjective aspects of anxiety, especially when a rapid response is required. They are helpful in treating residual insomnia after symptom relief from the underlying anxiety disorder has been addressed. The risk–benefit ratio must be considered carefully before prescribing an agent from this class to a child because of the possibility of daytime sedation, abuse, and addiction. Short–half-life benzodiazepine receptor agonists such as zaleplon are preferred because of less daytime sedation. Long–half-life medications in this class, such as clonazepam, are preferred when their daytime anxiolytic effects are sought.

Long-term Medication for Difficulties Initiating and Maintaining Sleep in Children

In the treatment of long-standing DIMS in children, antidepressants are the most frequently used class of medication. Brief treatment most frequently uses antihistamines. The most sedating antidepressants are amitriptyline, doxepin, nefazodone, and trazodone.

In laboratory studies in adults, SSRIs (fluoxetine, paroxetine, fluvoxamine, and sertraline) significantly disrupt sleep, with the exception of citalopram (Celexa).

Zolpidem (Ambien) and zaleplon (Sonata) are nonbenzodiazepines that are active at the benzodiazepine receptor site. They have less morning sedation and result in fewer withdrawal symptoms than classic benzodiazepines. Zolpidem at bedtime is indicated for late-night sleep maintenance and early morning awakening; both start at 5-mg doses for adults. Zaleplon, with its ultrashort half-life, is indicated for sleep onset insomnia. The use of these medications in children has not been studied extensively, but their favorable side effect profiles, including less daytime sedation, suggest that they might be well tolerated.

All of the antidepressants that increase the sleep tendency suppress REM sleep, with the exception of nefazodone and trazodone. The behavioral, developmental, and physiologic effects of long-term benzodiazepine administration in children have not been studied.

Treatment of Resistant, Severe DIMS

Medications with different mechanisms of action, including antihistaminergic, anticholinergic, serotonergic, benzodiazepine, and antiseizure agents, should be rotated. A combination of medications, each at low doses, from two or three classes may be preferred over increasing the dose.

It is becoming more common to prescribe atypical antipsychotics with sedating profiles to children and adolescents who have agitation and DIMS that do not respond to other treatments. Unlike the classic neuroleptics, these medications have fewer extrapyramidal side effects, especially at low doses. These agents include ziprasidone (Geodon), quetiapine (Seroquel), and olanzapine (Zyprexa) but not risperidone (Risperdal), which has insomnia as a side effect.

Disrupted Sleep in Children with Attention Deficit Hyperactivity Disorder

The parents of children with ADHD state that their children show a high rate of sleep problems, more than those described by the parents of normal control subjects. Sleep differences in ADHD are not verified by actigraphy or sleep diary data, with the exception of longer sleep duration and increased bedtime resistance. Interactions during bedtime routines are more challenging in ADHD, which may be the basis of the perceived sleep problems.[35]

Most sleep disturbances in ADHD are secondary to stimulant treatment and comorbid anxiety and behavior disorders. ADHD cannot be explained as a consequence of sleep disruption.[36] Children with ADHD are not different from control subjects on polysomnographic sleep variables, but video analysis shows more upper and lower limb movements.[37]

Although no polysomnographic differences are found, boys with ADHD fall asleep more rapidly on the multiple sleep latency test than children without symptoms of ADHD. Its results correlate with hyperactivity, impulsivity, and inattentiveness. Children with ADHD are more sleepy during the day due to a deficit in alertness and not poorer sleep quality.[38]

Children with bipolar disorder differ from those with ADHD in the presence of mania-specific symptoms, including grandiosity, and they typically show ultrarapid or ultradian cycling. The sleep disorders of bipolar children are best treated with mood stabilizers.[39]

Sleep disturbances in children with ADHD should be addressed behaviorally and/or by modifying stimulant schedules and doses and not by sedatives/hypnotics unless an independent sleep diagnosis is verified.

References

1. Broughton RJ: NREM arousal parasomnias. In Kryger MH, Roth T, Dement WC (eds): Principles and Practice of Sleep Medicine, 3rd ed. Philadelphia, WB Saunders, 2000.

2. Gottesmann C, Gandolfo G, Arnaud C, Gauthier P:The intermediate stage and paradoxical sleep in the rat: Influence of three generations of hypnotics. Eur J Neurosci 1998;10:409-414.

3. Israel A, Kramer J: Safety of zaleplon in the treatment of insomnia. Ann Pharmacother 2002;36: 852-859.

4. Noguchi H, Kitazumi K, Mori M, Shiba T: Binding and neuropharmacological profile of zaleplon, a novel nonbenzodiazepine sedative/hypnotic. Eur J Pharmacol 2002;434:21-28.

5. Crestani F, Martin JR, Mohler H, Rudolph U: Mechanism of action of the hypnotic zolpidem in vivo. Br J Pharmacol 2000;131:1251-1254.

6. Johnson EO, Chilcoat HD, Breslau N: Trouble sleeping and anxiety/depression in childhood. Psychiatry Res 2000;94:93-102.

7. Smits MG, Nagtegaal EE, van der Heijden J, et al: J Child Neurol 2001;16:86-92.

8. Ashton H: Guidelines for the rational use of benzodiazepines: When and what to use. Drugs 1994;48:25-40.

9. Thunstrom M: Severe sleep problems in infancy associated with subsequent development of attention-deficit/hyperactivity disorder at 5.5 years of age. Acta Paediatr 2002;91:584-592.

10. Gregory AM, O'Connor TG: Sleep problems in childhood: A longitudinal study of developmental change and association with behavioral problems. J Am Acad Child Adolesc Psychiatry 2002;41:964-971.

11. Ramchandani P, Webb VV, Stores G: A systematic review of treatment of settling problems and night waking in young children. West J Med 2000;173: 33-38.

12. Smedje H, Broman JE, Hetta J: Associations between disturbed sleep and behavioral difficulties in 635 children aged six to eight years: A study based on parent's perceptions. Eur Child Adolesc Psychiatry 2001;10:1-9.

13. Mindell JA: Empirically supported treatments in pediatric psychology: Bedtime refusal and night wakings in young children. J Pediatr Psychol 1999;24:465-481.

14. Lavigne JV, Arend R, Rosenbaum D, Smith A, et al: Sleep and behavior problems among preschoolers. J Dev Behav Pediatr 1999;20:164-169.

15. Dahl RE: The development and disorders of sleep. Adv Pediatr 1998;45:73-90.

16. Broughton R: Principles and Practice of Sleep Medicine. 2000.

17. Gau SF, Soong WT: Psychiatric comorbidity of adolescents with sleep terrors or sleepwalking: A case-control study. Aust NZ J Psychiatry 1999; 33:734-739.

18. Llorente MD, Currier MB, Norman SE, et al: Night terrors in adults: Phenomenology and relationship to psychopathology. J Clin Psychiatry 1992;53:392-394.

19. Moroz G, Rosenbaum JF: Efficacy, safety, and gradual discontinuation of clonazepam in panic disorder: A placebo-controlled, multicenter study using optimized dosages. J Clin Psychiatry 1998;60:604-612.

20. Koenigsberg HW, Pollak CP, Ferro D: Can panic be induced in deep sleep? Examining the necessity of cognitive processing for panic. Depress Anxiety 1998;8:126-130.

21. Fairbanks JM, Pine DS, Tancer NK, et al: Open fluoxetine treatment of mixed anxiety disorders in children and adolescents. J Child Adolesc Psychopharmacol 1997;7:17-29.

22. Koenigsberg HW, Pollak CP, Fine J, et al: Cardiac and respiratory activity in panic disorder: Effects of sleep and sleep lactate infusions. Am J Psychiatry 1994;151:1148-1152.

23. Labbate LA, Pollack MH, Otto MW, et al: Sleep panic attacks: An association with childhood anxiety and adult psychopathology. Biol Psychiatry 1994;36:57-60.

24. Lepola U, Koponen H, Leinonen E: Sleep in panic disorders. J Psychosom Res 1994;38(Suppl 1): 105-111.

25. Garland EJ, Smith DH: Simultaneous prepubertal onset of panic disorder, night terrors, and somnambulism. J Am Acad Child Adolesc Psychiatry 1991;30:553-555.

26. Yang S, Chiou YH, Lin CY, et al: Treatment guidelines of enuresis in Taiwan. Acta Paediatr Taiwan 2001;42:271-277.

27. Kruse S, Hellstrom AL, Hanson E, et al: Treatment of primary symptomatic nocturnal enuresis with desmopressin: Predictive factors. BJU Int 2001; 88:572-576.

28. Neveus T: Oxybutynin, desmopressin and enuresis. J Urol 2001;166:2459-2462.

29. Glazener CM, Evans JH, Peto RE: Tricyclic and related drugs for nocturnal enuresis in children. Cochrane Database Syst Rev 2000;CD002117.

30. Hamano S, Yamanishi T, Igarashi T, et al: Functional bladder capacity as predictor of response to desmopressin and retention control training in monosymptomatic nocturnal enuresis. Eur Urol 2000;37:718-722.

31. Leebeek-Groenewegen A, Blom J, Sukhai R, van der Heijden B: Efficacy of desmopressin combined with alarm therapy for monosymptomatic nocturnal enuresis. J Urol 2001;166:2456-2458.

32. Dodge NN, Wilson GA: Melatonin for treatment of sleep disorders in children with developmental disabilities. J Child Neurol 2001;16:581-584.

33. Jan J, Tai J, Hahn G, Rothstein RR: Melatonin replacement therapy in a child with a pineal tumor. J Child Neurol 2001;16:139-140.

34. Collins JJ, Kerner J, Sentivany S, Berde CB: Intravenous amitriptyline in pediatrics. J Pain Symptom Manage 1995;10:471-475.

35. Corkum P, Tannock R, Moldofsky H, et al: Actigraphy and parental ratings of sleep in children with attention-deficit/hyperactivity disorder (ADHD). Sleep 2001;24:303-312.

36. Mick E, Biederman J, Jetton J, Faraone SV: Sleep disturbances associated with attention deficit hyperactivity disorder: The impact of psychiatric comorbidity and pharmacotherapy. J Child Adolesc Psychopharmacol 2000;10:223-231.

37. Konofal E, Lecendreux M, Bouvard MP, Mouren-Simeoni MC: High levels of nocturnal activity in children with attention-deficit hyperactivity disorder: A video analysis. Psychiatry Clin Neurosci 2001;55:97-103.

38. Lecendreux M, Konofal E, Bouvard M, et al: Sleep and alertness in children with ADHD. J Child Psychol Psychiatry 2000;41:803-812.

39. Geller B, Williams M, Zimerman B, et al: Prepubertal and early adolescent bipolarity differentiate from ADHD by manic symptoms, grandiose delusions, ultra-rapid or ultradian cycling. J Affect Disord 1998;51:81-91.

Index

Note: Page numbers followed by f and t refer to figures and tables, respectively.